T0355278

Oxford Textbook of
Violence Prevention

Epidemiology, Evidence, and Policy

Edited by

Peter D. Donnelly
Professor of Public Health Medicine
School of Medicine
University of St Andrews
Scotland, UK
and
President/CEO designate
Public Health Ontario
Toronto, Canada

Catherine L. Ward
Associate Professor of Psychology
Department of Psychology
University of Cape Town
Cape Town, South Africa

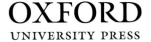

OXFORD
UNIVERSITY PRESS

OXFORD
UNIVERSITY PRESS

Great Clarendon Street, Oxford, OX2 6DP,
United Kingdom

Oxford University Press is a department of the University of Oxford.
It furthers the University's objective of excellence in research, scholarship,
and education by publishing worldwide. Oxford is a registered trade mark of
Oxford University Press in the UK and in certain other countries

Published in the United States of America by Oxford University Press
198 Madison Avenue, New York, NY 10016, United States of America

British Library Cataloguing in Publication Data
Data available

Library of Congress Control Number: 2014937975

ISBN 978–0–19–967872–3

Printed in China by
C&C Offset Printing Co. Ltd

This book is dedicated to the memory of the more than 500,000 people murdered this year, their family and friends; and to the 500,000 more who will die next year and every year until we make global violence reduction a scientific and political priority.

Foreword

The *Oxford Textbook on Violence Prevention* describes how public health can help to prevent violence, and is an important new resource for policymakers, practitioners, and researchers interested in violence and health. Published 12 years after the World Health Organization's landmark *World Report on Violence and Health*, it updates the scientific literature on understanding and preventing violence, and readers will be rewarded by having in hand an overview of the latest developments in the field. The timing of its publication also gives it the potential to shape the global violence prevention agenda in important ways.

Violence prevention is still new to many countries and remains sensitive to economic forces and political dynamics. Over the last decade, while violence prevention activities have expanded, the role of the health sector has not followed suit. Recession-related budget cuts have forced public health to shrink back from novel challenges like violence prevention into the comfort zone of more conventional disease prevention and health promotion.

Recognizing the need to counter that trend, Member States of the World Health Organization have for the first time since 2003 requested the Organization and themselves to scale up the health sector's involvement in violence prevention activities. In May 2014, the 67th World Health Assembly—the annual gathering of ministers of health—adopted a resolution that committed governments to strengthening their health sector efforts to prevent violence. The resolution also requested the World Health Organization to produce a global plan of action to better articulate the role of the health system in a multi-sectoral response. By providing the latest scientific information, this publication will assist in carrying out these requests.

While most violence prevention efforts go towards addressing violence against women and against children, other forms of violence such as youth violence and elder abuse have received less attention—despite their large impact on public health. Hence this volume also calls for due attention to all forms of violence, and for ensuring that resources allocated for their prevention are commensurate with the size of the problem and the potential for intervention. It is therefore a welcome reminder to beware of ignoring the epidemiologically important in favour of the politically salient.

The year 2014 marks the first year after the death of Nelson Mandela, who wrote in his foreword to the 2002 *Word Report on Violence and Health* that "We must address the roots of violence. Only then will we transform the past century's legacy from a crushing burden into a cautionary lesson." Please join me in honoring Nelson Mandela's legacy by using this volume to ensure that before the next century is upon us, we have addressed the roots of violence.

Etienne Krug
Director
Department of Violence and Injury
Prevention and Disability
World Health Organization

Acknowledgements

We are indebted to two peer-reviewers, who kindly undertook to read all the chapters and provide feedback that has been immensely valuable in shaping the content of this book. They are Harriet MacMillan, Professor in the Departments of Psychiatry and Behavioural Neurosciences, and Pediatrics, at McMaster University, Canada; and Elizabeth Ward, Director, Disease Prevention and Control in the Ministry of Health, Jamaica.

We are also grateful to Karen Ross (University of St Andrews) and Jane Kelly (University of Cape Town) for extraordinary editorial assistance.

We are grateful to OUP commissioning editor Nicola Wilson, OUP assistant commissioning editor Caroline Smith and Prakash Balasubramanian, Project Manager, Newgen for their professional support throughout this complicated project.

Editing this book was supported in part by a grant from the University of Cape Town's Research Committee (URC) to Catherine L. Ward.

Contents

List of Contributors

Naeemah Abrahams
Deputy Unit Director
Gender and Health Research Unit
Medical Research Council
Cape Town, South Africa

Peter Anderson
Professor of Substance Use, Policy and Practice
Institute of Health and Society
Newcastle University
Newcastle, UK and
Professor of Alcohol and Health
Faculty of Health, Medicine and Life Sciences
Maastricht University
Maastricht, Netherlands

Lillian Artz
Associate Professor and Director
Gender, Health and Justice Research Unit
Faculty of Health Sciences
University of Cape Town
Cape Town, South Africa

Jane Barlow
Professor of Public Health in the Early Years
Warwick Infant and Family Wellbeing Unit
Warwick Medical School
Coventry, UK

Astrid Berg
Associate Professor of Psychiatry
Department of Psychiatry and Mental Health
University of Cape Town, Cape Town and
Associate Professor Extraordinary
Department of Psychiatry
University of Stellenbosch
Stellenbosch, South Africa

Kavi Bhalla
Assistant Professor
International Injury Research Unit
Johns Hopkins Bloomberg School of Public Health
Baltimore, Maryland, USA

Debbie Bradshaw
Unit Director
Burden of Disease Research Unit
Medical Research Council
Cape Town, South Africa

Alexander Butchart
Coordinator, Prevention of Violence
Department of Violence and Injury Prevention and Disabilities
World Health Organization
Geneva, Switzerland

Richard F. Catalano
Bartley Dobb Professor for the Study and Prevention of
    Violence and
Director of Social Development Research Group
School of Social Work
University of Washington
Seattle, Washington, USA

Jonathan P. Caulkins
H. Guyford Stever Professor of Operations Research and
    Public Policy
Heinz College
Carnegie Mellon University
Pittsburgh, Pennsylvania, USA

Vania Ceccato
Associate Professor in Urban Safety
School of Architecture and the Built Environment
Royal Institute of Technology
Stockholm, Sweden

Jeffrey E. Clutter
Research Associate
Institute of Crime Science
University of Cincinnati
Cincinnati, Ohio, USA

Heléne Combrinck
Associate Professor
Centre for Disability Law and Policy
University of the Western Cape
Cape Town, South Africa

Theodore J. Corbin
Associate Professor of Emergency Medicine
Drexel University College of Medicine/School of Public Health
Center for Nonviolence and Social Justice
Philadelphia, Pennsylvania, USA

Phaedra Corso
UGA Foundation Professor of Human Health
College of Public Health
University of Georgia
Athens, Georgia, USA

Andrew Dawes
Associate Professor Emeritus
Department of Psychology
University of Cape Town
Cape Town, South Africa

Liesbeth De Donder
Professor in Adult Educational Sciences
Faculty of Psychology and Educational Sciences
Vrije Universiteit Brussels
Brussels, Belgium

Ross Deuchar
Professor of Criminology and Criminal Justice
School of Social Sciences
University of the West of Scotland
Scotland, UK

Karen Devries
Lecturer in Social Epidemiology
Department of Global Health and Development
London School of Hygiene and Tropical Medicine
London, UK

Peter D. Donnelly
Professor of Public Health Medicine
School of Medicine
University of St Andrews
Scotland, UK and
President/CEO designate
Public Health Ontario
Toronto, Canada

Robin S. Engel
Professor and Director
Institute of Crime Science
University of Cincinnati
Cincinnati, Ohio, USA

Dorothy L. Espelage
Professor of Educational Psychology
College of Education
University of Illinois at Urbana-Champaign
Champaign, Illinois, USA

Abigail A. Fagan
Associate Professor
Sociology and Criminology and Law
University of Florida
Gainesville, Florida, USA

Gene Feder
Professor of Primary Care
School of Social and Community Medicine
University of Bristol
Bristol, UK

Michael Flood
Senior Lecturer in Sociology
School of Social Sciences, Media and Communication
University of Wollongong
New South Wales, Australia

Ellen E. Foley
Associate Professor of International Development and
    Social Change
Department of International Development, Community,
    and Environment
Clark University
Worcester, Massachusetts, USA

Beverly L. Fortson
Behavioral Scientist
Research and Evaluation Branch
Division of Violence Prevention
Centers for Disease Control and Prevention
Atlanta, Georgia, USA

Claudia García-Moreno
Lead Specialist, Gender and Gender-based violence
Department of Reproductive Health and Research
World Health Organization
Geneva, Switzerland

Anna J. Gavine
Research Fellow
School of Medicine
University of St Andrews
Scotland, UK

Erika Gebo
Associate Professor of Sociology
Department of Sociology
Suffolk University
Boston, Massachusetts, USA

Christine Goodall
Senior Clinical Lecturer
Honorary Consultant in Oral Surgery
Dental School, School of Medicine
College of Medical, Veterinary, and Life Sciences
University of Glasgow
Scotland, UK

John M. Hagedorn
Professor
Department of Criminology, Law, and Justice
University of Illinois-Chicago
Chicago, Illinois, USA

James E. Harrison
Professor and Director of the Research Centre for Injury Studies
School of Medicine
Flinders University
Adelaide, South Australia

Susan Hawkridge
Senior Lecturer in Child and Adolescent Psychiatry
Department of Psychiatry
Stellenbosch University
Stellenbosch, South Africa

Lori Heise
Senior Lecturer in Social Epidemiology
Department of Global Health and Development
London School of Hygiene and Tropical Medicine
London, UK

Scott W. Henggeler
Professor of Psychiatry and Behavioral Sciences
Family Services Research Center
Medical University of South Carolina
Charleston, South Carolina, USA

Isabel Iborra
Professor of Psychology
Department of Psychology
Universidad Católica de Valencia
Valencia, Spain

Thomas Jacobson
MPP Student/Research Assistant
Luskin School of Public Affairs
University of California Los Angeles
Los Angeles, California, USA

Robin J. Kimbrough-Melton
Research Professor
Colorado School of Public Health
University of Colorado
Aurora, Colorado, USA

Mark A. R. Kleiman
Professor of Public Policy
Luskin School of Public Affairs
University of California Los Angeles
Los Angeles, California, USA

Guy Lamb
Director of Safety and Violence Initiative
University of Cape Town
Cape Town, South Africa

Jorja Leap
Adjunct Professor of Social Welfare
Luskin School of Public Affairs
University of California, Los Angeles
Los Angeles, California, USA

Denise Martin
Senior Lecturer in Criminology and Criminal Justice
School of Social Sciences
University of the West of Scotland
Scotland, UK

Richard Matzopoulos
Specialist Scientist
Burden of Disease Research Unit
Medical Research Council and
Honorary Research Associate
School of Public Health and Family Medicine
University of Cape Town
Cape Town, South Africa

Nadine McKillop
Research Fellow
School of Criminology and Criminal Justice
Griffith University
Mt Gravatt, Queensland, Australia

Gary B. Melton
Professor of Paediatrics
University of Colorado School of Medicine and
Professor of Community and Behavioral Health
Colorado School of Public Health
Aurora, Colorado, USA

James A. Mercy
Special Advisor for Global Activities
Division of Violence Prevention
Centers for Disease Control and Prevention
Atlanta, Georgia, USA

Melissa T. Merrick
Behavioral Scientist
Surveillance Branch
Division of Violence Prevention
Centers for Disease Control and Prevention
Atlanta, Georgia, USA

Christopher Mikton
Technical Officer, Prevention of Violence
Department of Violence and Injury Prevention and Disability
World Health Organization
Geneva, Switzerland

Francesco Mitis
Technical Officer
Division of Noncommunicable Diseases and Life-Course
World Health Organization Regional Office for Europe
Copenhagen, Denmark

Alison Morris-Gehring
Research Fellow
Department of Global Health and Development
London School of Hygiene and Tropical Medicine
London, UK

xviii LIST OF CONTRIBUTORS

Ian Neethling
Senior Scientist
Burden of Disease Research Unit
Medical Research Council
Cape Town, South Africa

Fergus G. Neville
Research Fellow in Public Health Sciences
School of Medicine
University of St Andrews
Scotland, UK

Christina Pallitto
Scientist
Department of Reproductive Health and Research
World Health Organization
Geneva, Switzerland

Bridget Penhale
Reader in Mental Health of Older People
School of Health Sciences
Faculty of Medicine and Health Sciences
University of East Anglia
Norwich, UK

Max Petzold
Professor in Biostatistics
Centre for Applied Biostatistics
Sahlgrenska Academy
University of Gothenburg
Gothenburg, Sweden

Megan Prinsloo
Senior Scientist
Burden of Disease Research Unit
Medical Research Council
Cape Town, South Africa

Jonathan Purtle
Assistant Professor
Drexel University School of Public Health
Center for Nonviolence and Social Justice
Philadelphia, Pennsylvania, USA

John A. Rich
Professor
Drexel University School of Public Health
Center for Nonviolence and Social Justice
Philadelphia, Pennsylvania, USA

Linda J. Rich
Director of Education and Consultation
Drexel University College of Medicine
Center for Nonviolence and Social Justice
Philadelphia, Pennsylvania, USA

Laurie Ross
Associate Professor of Community Development and Planning
Department of International Development, Community, and Environment
Clark University
Worcester, Massachusetts, USA

Brad Rowe
Research Analyst
Luskin School of Public Affairs
University of California Los Angeles
Los Angeles, California, USA

Lynnmarie Sardinha
Research Associate in Domestic Violence and Health
School of Social and Community Medicine
University of Bristol
Bristol, UK

Mohamed Seedat
Professor of Psychology and Head
Institute for Social and Health Sciences University of South Africa
Johannesburg, South Africa and
Director of Medical Research Council-University of South Africa
Violence, Injury and Peace Research Unit
Cape Town, South Africa

Soraya Seedat
Professor of Psychiatry
Department of Psychiatry
Stellenbosch University
Stellenbosch, South Africa

Dinesh Sethi
Programme Manager
Division of Noncommunicable Diseases and Life-Course
World Health Organization Regional Office for Europe
Copenhagen, Denmark

Simukai Shamu
Senior Scientist
Gender and Health Research Unit
Medical Research Council and
Honorary Lecturer
School of Public Health
University of the Western Cape
Cape Town, South Africa

Margaret Shaw
Consultant
Crime and Social Policy and
Former Director of Analysis and Exchange
International Centre for the Prevention of Crime
Montreal, Canada

Stephen Smallbone
Professor of Criminology and Criminal Justice
School of Criminology and Criminal Justice
Griffith University
Mt Gravatt, Queensland, Australia

Heidi Stöckl
Lecturer in Social Epidemiology
Department of Global Health and Development
London School of Hygiene and Tropical Medicine
London, UK

Shahnaaz Suffla
Senior Scientist
Medical Research Council-University of South Africa
Violence, Injury and Peace Research Unit
Cape Town, South Africa

Nathaniel H. Taylor
Research Professional
College of Public Health
University of Georgia
Athens, Georgia, USA

Richard E. Tremblay
Professor of Early Childhood Development
School of Public Health
Physiotherapy and Population Science University College Dublin
Dublin, Ireland and
Emeritus Professor
Departments of Pediatrics and Psychology
University of Montreal
Montreal, Canada

Catherine L. Ward
Associate Professor of Psychology
Department of Psychology
University of Cape Town
Cape Town, South Africa

Charlotte Watts
Professor of Social and Mathematical Epidemiology
Department of Global Health and Development
London School of Hygiene and Tropical Medicine
London, UK

Damien J. Williams
Lecturer in Public Health Sciences
School of Medicine
University of St Andrews
Scotland, UK

SECTION 1

An introduction to the study of violence as a public health issue

CHAPTER 1

Interpersonal violence: a global health priority

Peter D. Donnelly and Catherine L. Ward

Violence in Pre-History

The perpetration of violence is the stuff of human history.
(Moreno 2011)

From our earliest days as a species, humankind has had to fight: for survival, against predatory animals, against rival bands and clans, and even perhaps against competing sub-species of hominid. Competition for food and resources could be so extreme in some circumstances that the losers literally became the food (Saladié et al. 2012). But more generally, competition for resources whether territory, materials, access to strategic or sacred places or reproductive partners, or the work of enslaved labourers placed an early evolutionary premium on an ability to fight and when required to kill.

As we move forward into the recorded period, history books are replete with tales of vicious battles, genocide, and global wars—but also tell of individual acts of barbarism driven by ambition, self-interest, and greed. Our catalogue of literature over the ages frequently depicts vengeful, resolute, and unforgiving leaders whose success is often judged by their ability to subjugate and conquer through violent means.

And yet, it is humankind's ability to form cooperative communities rather than the ability to fight that has provided our species with a distinctive and definitive evolutionary advantage. Such social altruism may itself be the product of genetically conserved traits advantageous in primitive environmental conditions (Baschetti 2007). Without it, a move from small hunter-gatherer bands to settled agricultural communities would not have been possible. In its absence the division and specialization of labour central to economic and intellectual progress would have been inconceivable and the first faltering steps in the creation of civic society and rational governance could not have been taken.

The Development of Law and Justice Systems

It is in that development of civic society and structural forms of government that one can detect the earliest attempts at regulating, if not overtly attempting to reduce, violence. As the capricious 'justice' of the warlord or absolute monarch is gradually replaced by state-sanctioned systems, the cultural requirement to exact revenge and engage in vendettas is reduced and the temptation to use violence in pursuit of personal gain has to be balanced against the possibility of apprehension, trial, and, often severe, sanction.

As systems of government and criminal justice progressed so a focus on deterrence and punishment became balanced with a concern for rehabilitation. The extreme nature of the legal sanctions (e.g. crucifixion, hanging, drawing, and quartering or being stoned to death) is gradually replaced by lengthy imprisonment or at least less gruesome (but still objectionable) means of administering judicial execution. A general international acceptance emerges that prisoners do not forfeit all of their human rights upon conviction and international standards have come to require that judicial decisions should be politically independent. However, in many parts of the world these precepts do not apply and injustice and cruel and arbitrary punishment remain common (http://www.amnesty.org).

More philosophically the debate on the purpose of sentencing for crimes of violence remains contested. The correct balance between deterrence, punishment, and the exercise of natural justice (with its implied beneficial effect in reducing private revenge) on the one hand and rehabilitation on the other is a live political issue in many countries around the world. So too is the issue as to whether violent perpetrators are 'mad', i.e. mentally ill in some way, or 'bad', i.e. morally reprehensible. Even in cases where mental illness is excluded there will be debate about whether we are dealing with bad behaviour or a bad person and whether the origins of either or both are to be found in nature or nurture. The judicial treatment of juveniles is particularly contentious in that regard (*New York Times* 2012).

It is against such a complicated historical, legal, moral, and sociological backdrop that those who set out to reduce violence in the twenty-first century must operate. And even if one accepts Stephen Pinker's assertion that when considered over a 10,000-year period 'The decline in violence may be the most significant and least appreciated development in the history of our species' (Pinker 2011, p. 692) and that today 'we may be living in the most peaceable era in our species existence' (Pinker 2011, p. xxi), with over half a million homicides a year (Krug et al. 2002) there is clearly still much work to be done. Nor can we assume that societies will automatically continue to progress towards reduced levels of violence; for as we will see later in this book some of the inherent drivers of violence: poverty, inequality, injustice, and discrimination, remain firmly in place, and in some instances are increasing.

Why Violence should no Longer be Needed

At its simplest the argument for seeking to further reduce violence is that we no longer need violence. Where there are systems in place to ensure that people have at their disposal the means for survival then the immediate recourse to violence to achieve survival is unnecessary. The means for survival however are more than just shelter, warmth, food, and security. It must involve the right to fully participate in society including, but not limited to, the right to vote in a functioning democracy and to have access to impartial, fair, and affordable justice. Many would also argue that meaningful citizenship requires fair access to education, healthcare, and essential social services, and that in most societies that dictates realistic opportunity for paid employment for those who are able and access to appropriate benefits for those who are not. The absence of these factors can logically be considered a form of structural violence against individuals or communities. Corruption and prejudice may focus that structural violence upon certain disadvantaged groups identified by race, age, or gender. Many diseases and health-related conditions, not simply violence, cannot be fully understood without recourse to the concept of structural violence and the historical context within which it operates (Farmer 2004).

So how should 'violence' be defined? Behavioural definitions tend to concern themselves with the difference between aggression and violence, with aggression being a broader category. Both concepts have three essential features: the intent to cause harm, the belief that the behaviour will cause harm, and the belief that the victim would wish to avoid the aggressive behaviour. Violence is at the more serious end of this—while all violent behaviour is aggressive, the reverse is not true: an adult beating up another is violence, while a toddler's hitting her mother is aggressive but not violent (Anderson and Bushman 2002). Aggressive young people can of course grow up to become perpetrators of violence, as Tremblay argues in Chapter 5 of this volume, and this is an important argument developmentally—but it remains that not all aggressive acts are violent.

The World Health Organization (WHO) approaches this from a public health perspective, and provides the definition that is central to how we have framed this book: 'The intentional use of physical force or power, threatened or actual, against oneself, another person, or against a group or community, that either results in or has a high likelihood of resulting in injury, death, psychological harm, maldevelopment or deprivation' (Dahlberg and Krug 2002, p. 5). These definitions all rule out accidentally causing harm: the central concept is the intention to cause harm (Anderson and Bushman 2002; Dahlberg and Krug 2002). The WHO definition of course leaves the door open for three types of violence: self-directed, interpersonal, and collective violence (Dahlberg and Krug 2002). Here, we focus only on interpersonal violence: while there is some overlap in the risk and protective factors that influence self-directed and interpersonal violence (Krug et al. 2002), it is worth a book on its own; and while we acknowledge that collective violence is an important problem, we only address it in the form of gang violence, where it too shares risk and protective factors with interpersonal violence (see Gebo, Chapter 29, this volume).

It is no coincidence that if one wishes to find the highest rates of homicide in the world one only has to look at areas where such structural violence is in place; for murder is in practice largely a disease of poverty and inequality. So to find the world's epicentres of untimely and unnecessary death it is only necessary to seek poverty, inequality, social exclusion, and injustice. In truth the early deaths from homicide of over 500,000, mostly impoverished young men, each year constitutes the world's most inexcusable health inequality.

But what is the role for health in reducing violence in such circumstances? Traditionally health has held a somewhat marginal role. It has concerned itself with the process of picking up the pieces; that is, caring for the wounded. The specialist field of forensic psychiatry would be brought in to adjudicate sanity, particularly in relation to an accused's ability to plead or in an attempt to assess culpability. However, increasingly clinicians began to ask questions about whether medical conditions caused by violence could be prevented in the same way as the prevalence of medical conditions caused by other factors could be reduced.

'Medical' metaphors for understanding violence prevention are implicit in many violence prevention activities (Dodge 2008): if the spread of measles can be prevented by quarantining the ill, can we prevent violence by quarantining deviant youth from prosocial young people? If preventive surgery can straighten a leg and so prevent a child from limping, can corrective interventions 'straighten young people out', so that they are no longer aggressive? If a polio vaccine can prevent children from contracting the disease at all, are there early interventions that prevent children from becoming aggressive? Or is aggression a chronic disease (like asthma), and interventions should be targeted towards ameliorating symptoms and helping children and parents cope?

A Public Health Approach to Violence

They were aided and abetted in this endeavour by specialists in public health. Public health as a specialty is variously defined and sub-classified (Griffiths et al. 2005) but in general can be seen as the art and science of delaying death and preventing ill health through the organized efforts of society. It has its origins in the control of outbreaks of communicable disease but now works across all diseases and underlying causes of ill health as well as playing a significant role in planning, organizing, and evaluating health service provision and outcome. Although grounded in the science of epidemiology and originally medically dominated, public health has greatly benefitted in recent decades from an approach that embraces a variety of disciplines and methodological approaches. And so taking a modern public health approach to a problem as complicated as violence reduction may for example involve blending qualitative and quantitative methods and calling on the skills of an anthropologist to work alongside an epidemiologist. This inter- (or even trans-) disciplinary approach is gaining popularity in many disciplines, but particularly those that address complex problems (Kessel and Rosenfield 2008) such as violence, where (for instance) brain structure and genetics (with the roots of scientific understanding in the 'hard science' end of biological sciences), early child rearing (typically studied by behavioural scientists), and social norms (the domain of social scientists) all come together to influence the likelihood of aggression.

But what exactly is a public health approach to the prevention of violence? And how does that differ from a health perspective?

Public health is collectivist by nature and draws on the organized efforts of society. Unlike a standard health approach with its focus on therapy and cure, public health has a leaning towards prevention and the minimization of harm. Great store is placed on avoiding the blaming of victims. Individual autonomy is respected but those who choose to expose themselves to risk are not condemned as stupid or feckless. Rather the working assumption is always that the situation in which they find themselves makes healthy choices hard to make.

In terms of violence there are striking overlaps between risk factors for perpetration and victimization. Poor childhoods scarred by physical, emotional, and sometimes sexual abuse are often compounded by parental substance abuse, desertion, or incarceration. Poor educational provision and low educational attainment limits further education and employment opportunities. Communities where violence is tolerated drive young men and sometimes women into gangs in search of protection and a sense of belonging. The interpersonal resources to avoid peer pressure are often lacking and the perpetration of violence can become a way of earning respect.

It is all to easy to see the downward spiral of exposure to poor parenting and domestic abuse, early oppositional disobedience, school truancy, early drug and alcohol use, and escalating involvement in violence when one looks at individual case studies. And yet as societies somehow we miss, or perhaps choose to ignore, the structural violence imposed on the communities from which these young people come.

Programmes Focused on Violence Reduction

The inspirational work of Homeboy industries in Los Angeles (http://www.homeboyindustries.org) is at least in part captured by one of their slogans: 'Nothing stops a bullet like a job'. In Glasgow, UK, (http://www.actiononviolence.com) they may worry more about knives and machetes, but the sentiment rings true. Young people want meaningful work. Having a job is shorthand for so many things. It is a reason to get up in the morning, a reason not to be stoned or drunk the night before, a source of self-respect, a way to have money and thus autonomy, and a stake in society. The only mystery is why this surprises us, for this is what we all sought as graduates or school leavers. The truth is that young men and women involved in gangs are much more like those of us who write and read books like this than most would imagine. They want many of the same things we do but whilst we organize society in a way that fails to protect them in their earliest years and allows them to be damaged as young children and then compounds matters by excluding them from their legitimate needs, then it is perhaps not surprising that they sometimes feel they need to resort to violence. To seek to understand is certainly not to condone, but it is a necessary first step in developing a Public Health-driven approach to prevention.

A number of chapter authors in this book refer to the ecological model, a model which originated in developmental psychology (Bronfenbrenner 1979; Figure 1.1). Its power lies in placing the violent behaviour exhibited by an individual within a series of widening contexts, thus allowing us to understand that multiple influences may operate on an individual at once:

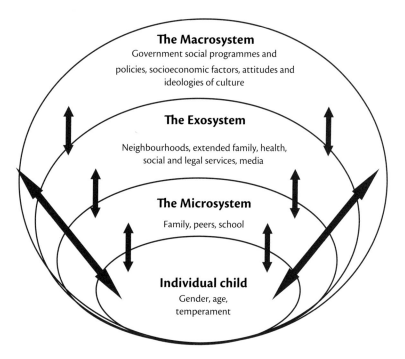

Fig. 1.1 The ecological model.

- First the individual concerned who like all of us is a complicated mixture of nature and nurture, who may have been exposed to alcohol and drugs even before birth, whose earliest experiences may be damaging, and whose epigenetic inheritance is still poorly understood.

- Secondly the 'everyday' contexts that are most influential—family, school, peer groups—the contexts in which we have our daily interactions. For instance, many young men grow up without satisfactory male role models. The feminization of the caring workforce in troubled areas (probably partly because of poor pay) compounds the absence of males in lives typified by absent fathers.

- Thirdly, we need to consider the community in which the individual lives, often typified by poverty, social exclusion, and low educational attainment.

- Finally, the society in which that community exists, which all too often exhibits disastrous flaws such as corruption, administrative incompetence, and institutional racism thus compounding the structural violence imposed on individuals.

In interacting with each other, influences from these various contexts may increase the effects of others (for instance, child-rearing environments—father's criminality—may interact with genes to multiply the likelihood of the child's obtaining a criminal record; a stable family living situation can reduce the effects of family socioeconomic status on the likelihood of a poor outcome for children; Bronfenbrenner 1986).

But a public health approach does not need to fully understand the complex bio/psycho/social basis of the problem; no more than did John Snow—in many ways the Father of public health—need to understand the details of the causation of cholera to stem the 1854 London epidemic by removing the pump handle from the contaminated source so that it could no longer be accessed. It was enough for him to know that it was something to do with that particular source of water. If we are inspired by his example we can make progress now even whilst we fill in the details of what precise insult causes which deficit—a tactic typical of a public health approach that does not regard pragmatic as a dirty word.

But what then in practical terms does a public health approach involve?

Firstly, there is a need for a formal assessment of the problem. This usually involves defining and counting cases, whether those be deaths or incidents of assault. But it may equally well involve listening carefully to typical young people living their lives in these troubled communities, or observing and carefully mapping spirals of violent action and reaction in the endless and pointless dance of retaliation driven by (usually) young men's perceived need to maintain status in the eyes of others. This is not just about counting instances, but also about understanding those factors that cause the problem (or cause good outcomes). Traditionally, the terms 'risk' and 'protective' factors have been used to indicate those that increase (risk factors) or decrease (protective factors) the likelihood of a poor outcome (risk factors). Often risk and protective factors are the opposite poles of a continuum—for instance, aggressive peers increase the likelihood of violence while prosocial peers decrease its likelihood. More recently, however, there has been a move to differentiate between factors that decrease the likelihood of a poor outcome in a context of risk (protective factors) and those that increase the likelihood of a good outcome in any context (promotive factors), although considerable definitional confusion remains (Stouthamer-Loeber et al. 2004).

Next one needs to learn what works. Fundamentally prevention science assumes that this means targeting risk factors (to decrease them) and protective/promotive factors (to increase them; Mrazek and Haggerty 1994). Studies need to be well designed and conducted. There are well-understood scientific principles that govern this. But studies also need to be grounded in reality and thus ultimately scalable if we are to make a real difference to sizable vulnerable populations. Whilst, as this book will show, the volume of work published about what interventions are effective is steadily increasing, in contrast the science and art of understanding and facilitating governments' adoption of evidence-informed policy really is in its infancy. In this area in particular we have much still to learn.

The Challenge of Evaluation

A public health approach to violence is thus focused on pragmatically making a difference. It has no slavish adherence to a fixed philosophical model and it does not require us to fully understand the basis of the programmes success. It is, at least initially, enough simply that something works and that we can get it in place on a scale commensurate with the size of the problem and at a cost realistically affordable by the responsible administration. Yet such an approach can bring a clash with standard reductionist scientific method, as the perfect experiment is rarely possible in this field. And even if it were, one would have to question what would it really tell us if its methodology was not useable at scale.

None of this is an excuse for bad science. Rather it is a reason to do studies carefully, appropriately and with an eye from the start on implementing those programmes and bits of programmes that work—and then working to understand how and why they do work, and so improving them.

However violence reduction also faces a well-recognized funding challenge. It has yet to discover (and probably never will discover) a 'magic' intervention such as the seat belt, the airbag, or the helmet that together have put road safety on the funding map. With violence reduction more imagination and a longer time perspective is needed.

The urgency for prevention in this area is no doubt in part driven by a realization of the costs involved. Some of these are obvious and direct, for example in the expensive care of the seriously wounded. But some are large and insidious. For example, the costs of caring for those with psychiatric problems as a result of assault or for those who turn to alcohol, drugs, and tobacco as self-medication in the face of domestic abuse and childhood maltreatment. There are the unseen opportunity costs such as the cancer care work or cleft palate repairs that the maxillofacial surgeons could be doing if they were not treating wounds resulting from nightclub brawls. Finally there are the societal costs: in terms of policing, justice, and jails; in terms of labour and taxes lost; and, all too often in the developing world, in terms of economic development forgone.

None of which really touches upon the most important cost of all that is the incalculable suffering imposed on those who are left behind. The family and friends of homicide victims have traditionally received little in the way of attention or support. They are encouraged to take solace from the workings of judicial systems that typically impose lifetime imprisonment or worse on perpetrators. Ironically, at which point the families of the perpetrator and those of the victim will be sharing a sense of bereavement and loss. The fact that solving a murder and imprisoning the perpetrator did not prevent the next murder was a major consideration in inspiring John Carnochan, an experienced homicide detective, to found the Scottish Violence Reduction Unit along with Karyn McCluskey in 2005. The work of this police-led unit in seeking to prevent violence through the deployment of a public health approach has inspired many in Scotland and further afield to believe that violence can be prevented. John and Karyn were themselves encouraged by the work of a small but dedicated team at WHO HQ in Geneva and by the efforts of pioneers in this field across the world. We have been very fortunate that many, perhaps most, of those pioneers have agreed to contribute to this book.

The Rationale for this Book

Which brings us to the issue of why bring this book together now and why in this format. It seems to us we are at an important and exciting time in the development of violence prevention science, policy, and practice. We have an increased recognition of the scale of the issue and a growing body of evidence about what works. We also benefit from the beginnings of an understanding of how to help administrations mobilize that evidence base and this therefore seemed the right time to pull together this collection.

The book is deliberately not a textbook of how to do violence reduction work but rather a vehicle for presenting cutting-edge global violence reduction research; an exploration of progress and challenges and a sharing of thoughts. We wish to provide a stimulus, for researchers, policy-makers, and practitioners, to work collectively to make violence a less obvious part of our shared world. Eliminating violence from global society is not possible in the way small pox was eliminated. We simply don't yet understand the underlying mechanisms well enough to come anywhere close to elimination. But, we have good reasons to believe that very substantial reductions in homicide and deliberate injury rates are entirely possible.

The book seeks to take a logical approach in its layout. After this single chapter opening section of context setting and explanation,

in which we have also explained what in practice we mean by the adoption of a public health approach to violence, there follows a series of sections of related chapters.

Section 2 (Chapters 2–11) covers the descriptive epidemiology of the problem and reminds us of the scale of the burden of morbidity and mortality that we impose on humankind by wrongly accepting the inevitability of violence.

Section 3 (Chapters 12–16) takes the argument for prioritizing this area further by laying out the consequences of violence.

Section 4 (Chapters 17–34) explores what we know about what works by looking at the published literature on evidence informed programmes to reduce violence.

Section 5 (Chapters 35–44) tackles the challenging issue of creating contexts that inhibit or prevent violence, through taking a careful look at national and international policies to reduce violence.

Section 6 (Chapters 45 and 46) seeks to summarize and review the main challenges and priorities facing researchers, practitioners, and policy-makers.

In coming together as a team to edit this volume we deliberately sought to blend a northern and southern hemisphere perspective. We have tried to reach out through contacts and in some cases cold calling eminent individuals in our field. We strived for geographic spread and were frequently frustrated by the dominance of a few northern western nations as the location of research studies. But things are changing and the work of the WHO-coordinated Violence Prevention Alliance is potentially important in facilitating research collaborations and policy development on a mutual aid basis. We are optimistic that future editions of this volume will enjoy an even more diverse authorship than that which we have been privileged to work with on this occasion. They stand ready with us to help and learn from colleagues in parts of the world where violence reduction work is still in its infancy. Together we can use scientific enquiry and shared experience to reduce global levels of violence. We hope this book helps with that important collective endeavour.

Acknowledgement

The writing of this chapter was supported in part by a grant from the University of Cape Town's Research Committee (URC) to the second author.

References

Anderson, C. A., and Bushman, B. J. (2002). Human aggression. *Annual Review of Psychology*, 53, 27–51.

Baschetti, R. (2007) Evolutionary, neurobiological, gene-based solution of the ideological 'puzzle' of human altruism and cooperation *Medical Hypotheses*, 69, 2, 2007, 241–9.

Bronfenbrenner, U. (1979). *The Ecology of Human Development: Experiments by Nature and Design*. Harvard University Press: Cambridge MA.

Bronfenbrenner, U. (1986). Ecology of the family as a context for human development: Research perspectives. *Developmental Psychology*, 22, 723–42.

Dahlberg, L. L., and Krug, E. G. (2002). Violence—a global public health problem. In: E. G. Krug, L. L. Dahlberg, J. A. Mercy, A. B. Zwi, and R. Lozano (eds), *World Report on Violence and Health*. Geneva, Switzerland: World Health Organization, pp. 1–22.

Dodge, K. A. (2008). Framing public policy and prevention of chronic violence in American youths. *American Psychologist*, 63, 573–90.

Farmer, P. (2004) An anthropology of structural violence *Current Anthropology*, 45, 3, 305–25.

Griffiths, S., Jewell, T., and Donnelly, P. (2005) Public health in practice: the three domains of public health, *Public Health*, 119, 10, 907–13.

Kessel, F., and Rosenfield, P. L. (2008). Towards transdisciplinary research: Historical and contemporary perspectives. *American Journal of Preventive Medicine*, 35, S225–34.

Krug, E. G., Dahlberg, L. L., Mercy, J. A., Zwi, A. B., and Lozano, R. (eds) (2002)., *World Report on Violence and Health*. Geneva, Switzerland: World Health Organization.

Moreno, E. (2011) The society of our 'out of Africa' ancestors (I): The migrant warriors that colonized the world. *Communicative & Integrative Biology*, 4,163–170; http://dx.doi.org/10.4161/cib.4.2.14320

Mrazek, P. J., and Haggerty, R. J. (1994). *Reducing Risks for Mental Disorders: Frontiers for Preventive Intervention Research*. Washington, DC: Institute of Medicine.

New York Times editorial Nov 24 2012 2012 http://www.nytimes.com/2012/11/25/opinion/sunday/juvenile-injustice-and-the-states.html?_r=0 (accessed 8 Jan 2014).

Pinker, S. (2011) *The better angels of our nature: why violence has declined*. London, Penguin.

Saladié, P., Huguet, R. Rodríguez-Hidalgo, A., Cáceres, I., Esteban-Nadal, M., Arsuaga, J.L., Bermúdez de Castro, J.M., and Carbonell, E. (2012) Intergroup cannibalism in the European Early Pleistocene: The range expansion and imbalance of power hypotheses *Journal of Human Evolution*, 63, 5, 682–95.

Stouthamer-Loeber, M., Wei, E., Loeber, R., and Masten, A.S. (2004). Desistance from persistent serious delinquency in the transition to adulthood. *Development and Psychopathology*, 16, 897–918.

SECTION 2

The descriptive epidemiology of violence

CHAPTER 2

Homicide

Richard Matzopoulos, Kavi Bhalla,
and James E. Harrison

Overview of Homicide

Homicide, including murder, is not only the most severe form of interpersonal violence, but it is also the measure most widely used to compare the extent of interpersonal violence across countries, cities, and regions. In this chapter, homicide refers to the causing of intentional death, or grievous injury to a person that resulted in death, at the hands of one or more other persons. This includes the criminal justice categories of murder and manslaughter, the definition and scope of which may differ between jurisdictions. There is a considerable range of estimates from international studies. The Global Burden of Disease (GBD) study suggests that there were 456,300 homicides in 2010, but higher estimates are common: 526,000–Geneva Declaration Secretariat 2011; 600,000 (World Health Organization (WHO) 2008). However, all sources concur that homicides are unevenly distributed. More than half of homicides occur in one-quarter of the world's nations representing just 18 per cent of the global population (Eisner and Nivette 2012).

Homicide is not the only relevant measure of interpersonal violence. For each violence-related death there are many non-fatal events and violent incidents spanning the violence typology from acts of sexual violence and emotional abuse to verbal threats to physical safety, but these are considerably more difficult to define and record for comparative purposes. Homicides on the other hand are recorded more routinely across several systems: e.g. in police crime statistics, in vital registration systems, and by health services. There are certainly limitations and definitional issues pertaining to each of these data sources, and these need to be considered and interpreted when deriving comparative statistics. This chapter critically examines the various sources of homicide data and synthesizes these data to provide a summary of the pattern of homicide across regions and amongst particular groups at risk. The risks for homicide, as with interpersonal violence more generally, are numerous and complex. These range from demographic factors such as age and sex and behavioural factors (notably the use of alcohol and other drugs that disinhibit violence and aggression), through to major societal and structural factors. Poverty, deprivation, and inequality are strong determinants (Butchart et al. 2004; Krahn et al. 1986; Sampson et al. 1997; United Nations Office on Drugs and Crime 2011) and urban living, with increased population density, degraded environment, overloaded infrastructure, and stretched service delivery, is associated with higher injury and homicide rates (Santos et al. 2006).

In this chapter the focus is on the demographic factors and risk factors that are directly measurable from the current sources of homicide data. The global and regional homicide estimates are provided by age, sex, and mechanism (i.e. whether by firearm, sharp force or other means) based on the homicide estimates of the GBD study (Lozano et al. 2012). While these data exclude deaths from collective violence, it is important to note the blurred boundary between deaths attributable to war, terrorism, and legal intervention and those that can be called homicide. For example, the epidemic of violence by Mexican drug gangs might be considered a form of terrorism. Similarly, some might consider recent state-sanctioned killings in the Middle East as murder or terrorism rather than as the consequence of a civil war.

A further limitation of restricting the analysis to data derived from sources describing the cause of death is the absence of certain themes familiar to the criminal justice readership. These include the characteristics of the perpetrator(s) (e.g. age, sex, and number involved), the victim–perpetrator relationship and the circumstances of the occurrence (e.g. as a result of a domestic dispute or during a robbery). However, there is no single data source that provides reliable comparative data at a regional level.

Key Sources of Homicide Data

Vital Registration

National vital registration systems that include cause of death reporting on death certificates provide an important source of information to guide public health policy and practice (Mahapatra et al. 2007) and to estimate homicide mortality (Liem and Pridemore, 2012; WHO Regional Office for Europe 2012), provided that the data are categorized appropriately and of good quality. Classification according to the International Statistical Classification of Disease and Related Health Problems (ICD) (WHO 1992) is imperative, as it provides a standardized framework for collecting and reporting mortality statistics (Mahapatra et al. 2007). This makes homicide statistics derived from death registration data more easily comparable than equivalent statistics derived from the criminal justice system. Death registration systems can also include additional information such as the age and sex of the deceased and the mechanism of homicide, which facilitates epidemiological investigations into the determinants of homicide. These data are available centrally from the WHO Mortality Database (WHOMDB), which collates official reporting from member states (WHO 2011). However, the quality of death registration data can vary substantially among countries (Mathers et al. 2005) and high-quality data are limited to high-income countries and a few others in the Caribbean, Latin America, Eastern Europe, and Central Europe. Death registration data from most countries in Africa, South Asia, and Southeast Asia are either not available or are of poor quality.

Three key aspects influence the quality of estimates derived from vital registration datasets: the completeness of the registration, the specificity of cause of death recording, and the reliability of the cause-of-death attribution. Sometimes it is feasible to adjust estimates by adjusting for completeness, and systematically reattributing deaths to specific causes. This is particularly useful when the causes of some homicides are only partly specified by the codes from the vital registration system.

Criminal Justice Data

National homicide counts are also available from the records of law enforcement and criminal justice systems. Cross-national analysis is complicated by several factors. First, the data represent crimes reported to national authorities. The reliance on completed case documentation, and frequent conflicts of interests arising from political imperatives to reduce crime rates, can result in under-reporting. Second, national legal systems may also differ substantially as to what constitutes a homicidal crime. Third, recording practices differ considerably from country to country. They may also vary within a country, particularly where more than one legal jurisdiction exists within a nation.

Despite the difficulty and limited success of cross-national comparisons (Liem and Pridemore 2012), crime data too are compiled centrally, in this case by the United Nations Office on Drugs and Crime (UNODC) in their Survey on Crime Trends and the Operations of Criminal Justice Systems (CTS). Their 2005–06 release contains data from 86 countries (United Nations Office on Drugs and Crime 2011). In contrast to death registration data, the CTS contains demographic information about offenders. Information about the method used to commit the homicide, such as by firearm or poisoning, has not been recorded except in the latest release in which a distinction is made for firearm homicides.

Verbal Autopsies

A 'verbal autopsy' involves a trained interviewer asking a deceased individual's next-of-kin, household members, friends, or healthcare workers, a series of questions about the signs and symptoms prior to death to determine the circumstances of death. In settings with very limited resources, verbal autopsies are applied in multi-centre health-monitoring initiatives such as Health and Demographic Surveillance Surveys (HDSS) that provide on-going proxy measures of a region's health information. These methods are widely used in the global health metrics community to estimate cause-specific mortality. For example, in China and India, the world's two most populous countries, vital registration systems record only a small and non-representative fraction of national deaths (Jha et al. 2006; Rao et al. 2005). Sample registration systems reporting causes of death using verbal autopsy provide information on a representative cross-section of the population (Office of the Registrar General of India in collaboration with Centre for Global Health Research 2009; Rao et al. 2005; Yang et al. 2005). Routine cross-sectional surveys such as Demographic and Health Surveys and Multiple Indicator Cluster Surveys are a largely untapped, but potentially rich, source of homicide data in low- and middle-income countries provided that explicit questions about injury events are included in survey questionnaires.

However, the validity of the verbal autopsies for the collection of information on injuries has not been established (Murray et al. 2007). The use of verbal autopsy may be particularly problematic in the event of homicides and suicides, with possibilities of non-disclosure for reasons including stigma and post-traumatic stress, or, conversely, recall of an extremely traumatic event that occurred well beyond the period defined by the study. These biases may vary considerably both across and within countries. Utility can also be limited by small sample sizes, insufficient detail about the injury event, in particular the intentionality, the infrequency of the surveys, and the limitations that apply to surveys more generally.

Health Facility Data

Information on homicides can also be obtained from data collected in hospitals and mortuaries (Bartholomeos et al. 2012). These sources are particularly important in the absence of a reliable death register. Legal requirement for inquiry or forensic investigation into the circumstances and causes of deaths by injuries can add value to mortuary data. Low- and middle-income countries with fatal injury surveillance systems or that have conducted cross-sectional studies in health facilities include Ethiopia, Ghana, Jamaica, Mozambique, and South Africa (Abdella et al. 2011; London et al. 2002; Matzopoulos 2005; Small Arms Survey 2009; Ward et al. 2002). As with data arising from vital registration and criminal justice systems, there are definitional issues pertaining to injury surveillance that need to be managed to enable comparability across settings. Surveillance systems based in health facilities often use ICD coding (or variants thereof) and others apply local policing and criminal justice categorization. Another drawback is that surveillance systems usually rely on sentinel sites that correspond with large facilities in urban areas or populous districts and regions. Nevertheless, these systems usually provide useful information about the demographic profile of the deceased as well as the injury event (e.g. the time, place, and scene of the assault) with which to inform prevention efforts.

Estimation Methods

The GBD-2010 homicide estimates in this chapter are based on the methods of the study and the collective work of the GBD Injury Expert Group convened to support that study (GBD Injury expert group 2012). The ICD-based external cause definitions of homicide used in GBD-2010 are shown in Table 2.1.

GBD-2010 included all available empirical measurements of population health that might inform estimates of fatal and non-fatal injury incidence. A project-wide process was undertaken to identify and acquire relevant data sources for all diseases. The injury expert group, in addition, published a call for data contributions in a leading academic journal (Bhalla et al. 2009), undertook reviews of published and grey literature, and initiated partnerships to acquire data from information-poor regions. A systematic review of the published estimates of the incidence of violence in low- and middle-income countries appraised the following key data sources for inclusion in the GBD-2010 estimates:

Table 2.1 ICD-based operational definition of homicides in GBD-2010

	ICD-10 codes	ICD-9 codes
Assault by all means	X85 to Y09, Y87.1	E960 to E969
Assault by firearm	X93–X95	E965.0–E965.4
Assault by sharp object	X99	E966
Assault by other and unspecified means	X85–X92, X96–X98, Y00–Y09	E960–E964, E965.5–E965.9, E967–E969

Source: data from Global Burden of Injuries, *GBD-2010*, Copyright © 2012, available from http://www.globalburdenofinjuries.org.

- Vital Registration Statistics: Cause-of-death tabulations covering many years from national vital registration system were available from many parts of the world, including from many low- and middle-income regions such as most countries in Latin America and Eastern Europe. However, the quality, completeness, and coverage of vital registration in several regions, such as Africa and South and Southeast Asia was problematic.

- Verbal Autopsies: Sample registration systems that tracked causes of death were available from several countries including India and China. In addition, data were available from the network of demographic surveillance sites including many rural settings in Africa and Asia.

- Mortuary/burial registers: Medico-legal records from mortuaries and burial permit offices were digitized from several mortuaries in Africa.

- Mortality modules from national population censuses and several large sample surveys were analysed to extract cause-of-death tables.

- Homicides reported in crime statistics were extracted from national statistical publications and from the publications of the UNODC Crime Trends Survey.

Harmonization of these data with more routine sources included the following processes:

- an assessment of completeness of mortality data sources,

- mapping across different coding schemes used in the underlying data,

- reattribution of poorly specified cause codes in mortality data,

- splitting data by sex and by GBD age groups,

- smoothing for stochastic fluctuations, and

- outlier detection.

As per the GBD-2010 method, Cause of Death Ensemble Modeling (CODEm) was used to estimate deaths from homicides and the various mechanisms disaggregated by age, sex, country, and year for all countries from 1980 to 2010. CODEm has been used extensively in the GBD-2010 project for most major causes of death. In recent studies, the CODEm model has been used to analyse maternal mortality (Hogan et al. 2010), breast and cervical cancer mortality (Forouzanfar et al. 2011), and malaria mortality (Murray et al. 2012). The CODEm methodology has been described in

detail (Foreman et al. 2012), as has its application in GBD-2010 (Lozano et al. 2012), and is based on the following three steps:

i. Numerous plausible regression-based statistical models are developed for each cause. All possible permutations of selected covariates are tested and only models where the sign on the coefficient for a covariate is in the expected direction are retained.

ii. Blend models (ensembles), or blends of these various component models, are developed.

iii. The validity of all component models and ensembles is evaluated by doing out-of-sample predictions, with the model or ensemble that performs best on such validations being selected. Model performance criteria include error in predicted death rate, trend, and validity of uncertainty estimates

Each mortality model is for a single cause of death (e.g. homicide), and the sum of the resulting estimates of cause-specific mortality may not equal a separate estimate of total deaths from all causes. Thus, deaths from specific causes are rescaled to match the all-cause envelope using a simple algorithm (Lozano et al. 2012).

Homicide Rates by Region

Estimates from the GBD-2010 indicate that homicide rates are substantially higher in certain regions of the world than others, most notably (i) Southern sub-Saharan Africa, (ii) Central Latin America, (iii) Tropical Latin American, (iv) Eastern Europe, (v) the Caribbean, and (vi) Central sub-Saharan Africa (Figure 2.1). Rates in these six regions exceed 10 per 100,000 population and account for almost half of all homicides globally (46 per cent), even though they account for just 12 per cent of the global population.

Assault by firearms and sharp objects are the two most common mechanisms of homicide, together accounting for 70 per cent of homicides globally and each is accorded its own category within the GBD study. The use of weapons (firearms and knives) accounts for much of the variability in homicide rates between regions and firearms are the most common mechanism of homicides in the regions with the highest homicide rates (Figure 2.1). Homicide by other means (i.e. not involving either firearms or sharp objects) is more evenly distributed.

Homicide by Age and Gender of Victim

Homicide peaks among young adult males aged 20–29 years and then declines steadily with increasing age (Figure 2.2). This age peak tends to be more pronounced within regions with very high homicide rates. The fewest homicides tend to be recorded among the youngest age categories, the exception being in the first month of a child's life, at which time homicide risk is greater than at any other time during childhood.

Whereas certain types of non-fatal violence may affect females more than males, such as with sexual violence, a considerable majority of homicide victims are males. The overall male-to-female ratio exceeds 4:1 mainly due to the high incidence of homicides among young adults that affects males disproportionately. Among women, it is the elderly that have a higher risk of being killed. For both sexes the elderly are a particularly vulnerable age group and are more frequently targeted than middle-aged adults.

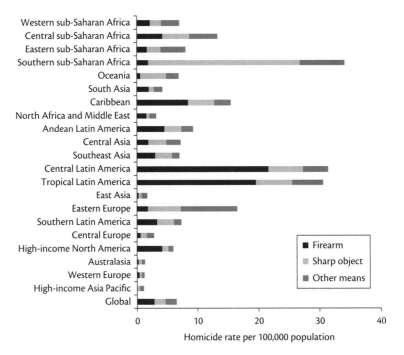

Fig. 2.1 Homicide rates by region and mechanism of death, 2010.

Source: data from Global Burden of Injuries, *GBD-2010*, Copyright © 2012, available from http://www.globalburdenofinjuries.org. Note: GBD-2010 estimates for homicides in Southern sub-Saharan Africa were strongly influenced by South Africa vital registration statistics, which provide the most complete data in the region but are a poor source for identifying mechanism of homicide. If we were to apply the estimates of the recent Injury Mortality Survey for 2009, which provides a nationally representative sample of injury deaths we expect that approximately one third of homicides in the region would be attributed to firearms(Matzopoulos et al., 2013).

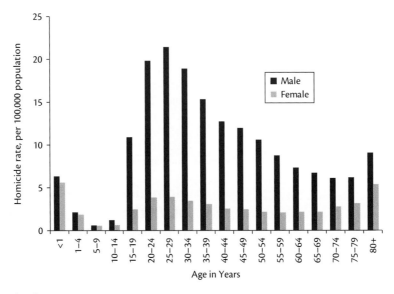

Fig. 2.2 Age-specific homicide rates (2010).

Source: data from Global Burden of Injuries, *GBD-2010*, Copyright © 2012, available from http://www.globalburdenofinjuries.org.

Homicide Trends

Notwithstanding the increase in the number of homicides, from 338,700 (95% Uncertainty Interval 245,800–416,600) in 1990 to 456,300 (354,900–610,900) in 2010, the GBD-2010 study suggests that there has been negligible change in incidence rates. The homicide rate decreased from 6.7 per 100,000 population in 1990 (4.8–8.3) to 6.5 (5.1–8.9) in 2010 (Lozano et al. 2012). Larger changes occurred at regional level with, for example, a substantial increase in South Asia and decreases in high-income North America and East Asia (Figure 2.3).

The trend analysis suggests that assaults by both firearms and sharp objects are increasing as a proportion of all homicides. Firearms alone account for 40 per cent of homicides and almost half the increase recorded in total homicides between 1990 and 2010 is attributable to the increases in the estimated number of

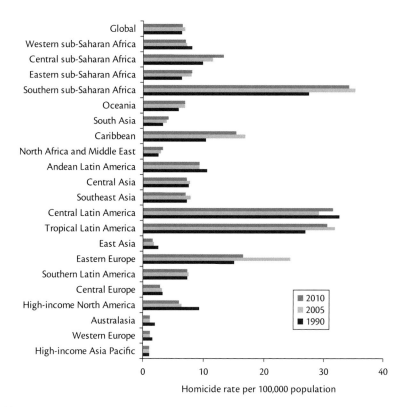

Fig. 2.3 Regional trends in homicides 1990–2010.
Source: data from Global Burden of Injuries, *GBD-2010*, Copyright © 2012, available from http://www.globalburdenofinjuries.org.

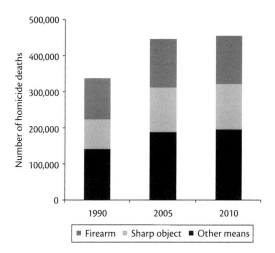

Fig. 2.4 Relationship between total homicides and mechanism-specific homicide rates.
Source: data from Global Burden of Injuries, *GBD-2010*, Copyright © 2012, available from http://www.globalburdenofinjuries.org.

firearm homicides (Figure 2.4). The male to female ratio is also more pronounced, with more than seven male firearm homicides for every female homicide.

Gaps In the Evidence: Homicide as a Global Priority

Homicide remains one of the leading causes of injury mortality. Its global ranking among leading causes of premature mortality

(i.e. years of life lost) has increased in rank from 22nd in 1990 to 20th in 2010 (Lozano et al. 2012). In two regions, Tropical Latin America and Central Latin America, it is the leading cause of premature mortality and it is among the top ten causes of premature mortality in four others: Southern sub-Saharan Africa (4th), the Caribbean and Eastern Europe (both 8th), and Andean Latin America (9th). As the homicide rate has not changed significantly over the last two decades, this change in ranking is explained in part by decreasing mortality from other major causes of premature mortality, such as maternal mortality and most communicable diseases.

The knowledge base for prevention is constantly being revised and refined, but is still drawn primarily from countries with low levels of homicide.

There are interventions that have been shown to be effective in reducing violence in low-income settings (Jewkes et al. 2008; Pronyk et al. 2006) and these should be applied to high-risk groups wherever possible. The prominence of assaults by sharp objects and firearms in particular suggests that reducing access to weaponry and lethal means, while not necessarily affecting a reduction and aggressive behaviour that leads to interpersonal violence, may at least reduce the likelihood of fatal and severe outcomes.

Development of a broader knowledge base that is more reflective of the world's regions and particularly those most affected by violence is one of three key strategies identified by Eisner and Nivette (2012) to reduce the global homicide rate to one-quarter of present levels in the next 50 years (Eisner and Nivette 2012). The current estimates indicate that just four GBD regions had rates below or close to Eisner and Nivette's target rate of approximately 1.5 per 100,000 population in 2010 (Western Europe, high-income Asia

Pacific, Australasia, and East Asia) representing approximately 20 per cent of the global population.

Not enough is known about the causes of violence and whether the known risks delineated according to ecological models in the literature are universally applicable. Eisner and Nivette (2012) recommend undertaking cross-culturally comparative longitudinal studies to provide empirical evidence on the risk and protective factors that are most relevant in different cultural, economic, and political contexts. The unequal distribution of homicide by region and the strong correlation between countries with low socio-economic status, high income inequality, and high homicide also suggest that homicide is affected by upstream and structural drivers. Societies with high levels of homicide are characterized by high state corruption, low investments in public health and education, poor state stability, ethnic, ideological or religious cleavages, and high inequality (Nivette 2011). These are not necessarily within reach of the scalable programmatic interventions that have been effective in other settings, and so the reduction of homicide in countries that are particularly affected will require a long-term multi-dimensional approach. Eisner and Nivette (2012) argue that broader institutional and societal changes should form an integral part of the broader effort to effect a reduction in homicide globally. Where homicide is unevenly distributed sub-nationally interventions should target populations experiencing the highest levels of risk.

Conclusion

The estimates in this chapter confirm the importance of homicide as a prevention priority. Substantial knowledge gaps need to be addressed if efforts to reduce homicide are to be effective. There is an over-reliance on data sourced from a few countries with reliable data. Ironically, information on homicide tends to be poorest for the countries in which this cause of death is most common. The utility for prevention of homicide estimates can be improved by including information about key risk factors, which should be routinely available, such as the role of alcohol and the victim–perpetrator relationship. Reducing violence in countries with high rates of homicide will also require research to address the information deficit pertaining to causes and interventions, as well as the concomitant investment in research and the structural reforms required to address the upstream drivers of violence.

References

Abdella, K., Bartolomeos, K., Tsegaye, F., Bhalla, K., and Abraham, J. (2011). Estimates of the burden of injuries in Ethiopia derived from all existing data sources. *Injury Prevention*, 16, A210.

Bartolomeos, K., Kipsaina, C., Grills, N., Ozanne-Smith, J., and Peden, M. (2012). *Fatal Injury Surveillance in Mortuaries and Hospitals: A Manual For Practitioners*. Geneva: World Health Organization.

Bhalla, K., Harrison, J., and Abraham, J. et al. (2009). Data sources for improving estimates of the global burden of injuries: call for contributors. *PloS Medicine*, 6, e1000001.

Butchart, A., Phinney, A., Check, P., and Villaveces, A. (2004). *Preventing Violence: A Guide to Implementing the Recommendations of the World Report on Violence and Health*. Geneva: World Health Organization.

Eisner, M., and Nivette, A. (2012). How to reduce the global homicide rate to 2 per 100,000 by 2060. In: R. Loeber and B. C. Walsh (eds.)., *The Future of Criminology*. New York: Oxford University Press, 219–28.

Foreman, K. J., Lozano, R., Lopez, A. D., and Murray, C. J. (2012). Modeling causes of death: an integrated approach using CODEm. *Population health metrics*, 10, 1.

Forouzanfar, M. H., Foreman, K. J., and Delossantos, A. M. et al. (2011). Breast and cervical cancer in 187 countries between 1980 and 2010: a systematic analysis. *Lancet*, 378, 1461–84.

Global Burden of Injuries (2012). *GBD Injury Expert Group. (2012)*. Available at http://www.globalburdenofinjuries.org [Accessed 12 November 2013]

Hogan, M. C., Foreman, K. J., and Naghavi, M. et al. (2010). Maternal mortality for 181 countries, 1980-2008: a systematic analysis of progress towards Millennium Development Goal 5. *Lancet*, 375, 1609–23.

Jewkes, R., Nduna, M., and Levin, J. et al. (2008). Impact of Stepping Stones on incidence of HIV and HSV-2 and sexual behaviour in rural South Africa: cluster randomised controlled trial. *BMJ: British Medical Journal*, 337, 391–5.

Jha, P., Gajalakshmi, V., and Gupta, P. C. et al. (2006). Prospective study of one million deaths in India: rationale, design, and validation results. *PLoS medicine*, 3, e18.

Krahn, H., Hartnagel, T. F., and Gartrell, J. W. (1986). Income inequality and homicide rates: cross-national data and criminological theories. *Criminology*, 24, 269–95.

Liem, M., and Pridemore, W. (2012). *Handbook of European Homicide Research: Patterns, Explanations, and Country Studies*. New York: Springer.

London, J., Mock, C., Abantanga, F. A., Quansah, R. E., and Boateng, K. A. (2002). Using mortuary statistics in the development of an injury surveillance system in Ghana. *Bulletin of the World Health Organization*, 80, 357–64.

Lozano, R., Naghavi, M., and Foreman, K. et al. (2012). Global and regional mortality from 235 causes of death for 20 age groups in 1990 and 2010: a systematic analysis for the Global Burden of Disease Study 2010. *Lancet*, 380, 2095–2128.

Mahapatra, P., Shibuya, K., and Lopez, A. D et al. (2007). Civil registration systems and vital statistics: successes and missed opportunities. *Lancet*, 370, 1653–63.

Mathers, C. D., Fat, D. M., Inoue, M., Rao, C., and Lopez, A. D. (2005). Counting the dead and what they died from: an assessment of the global status of cause of death data. *Bulletin of the World Health Organization*, 83, 171–7.

Matzopoulos, R. (2005). *A Profile of Fatal Injuries in South Africa, 2004: Sixth Annual Report of the National Injury Mortality Surveillance System*. Cape Town: Medical Research Council. Available at: http://www.doh.gov.za/docs/reports/2007/sec1a.pdf [Accessed 18 November 2013].

Matzopoulos, R., Prinsloo, M., Bradshaw, D., Pillay-van Wyk, V., Gwebushe, N., Mathews, S., Martin, L., Laubscher, R., Lombard, C., and Abrahams, N.*The Injury Mortality Survey: A national study of injury mortality levels and causes in South Africa in 2009*. Cape Town: South African Medical Research Council, 2013.

Murray, C. J. L., Lopez, A. D., Feehan, D. M., Peter, S. T., and Yang, G. (2007). Validation of the symptom pattern method for analyzing verbal autopsy data. *PLoS Medicine*, 4, e327.

Murray, C. J. L., Rosenfeld, L. C., and Lim, S. S. et al. (2012). Global malaria mortality between 1980 and 2010: a systematic analysis. *Lancet*, 379, 413–31.

Nivette, A. E. (2011). Cross-national predictors of crime: a meta-analysis. *Homicide Studies*, 15, 103–31.

Office of the Registrar General of India in collaboration with Centre for Global Health Research (2009). *Report on Causes of Death in India, 2001-2003*. New Delhi: Office of the Registrar General.

Pronyk, P. M., Hargreaves, J. R., Kim, J. C. et al. (2006). Effect of a structural intervention for the prevention of intimate-partner violence and HIV in rural South Africa: a cluster randomised trial. *Lancet*, 368, 1973–83.

Rao, C., Lopez, A. D., Yang, G., Begg, S., and Ma, J. (2005). Evaluating national cause-of-death statistics: principles and application to the case of China. *Bulletin of the World Health Organization*, 83, 618–25.

Sampson, R. J., Raudenbush, S. W., and Earls, F. (1997). Neighborhoods and violent crime: a multilevel study of collective efficacy. *Science*, 277, 918–24.

Santos, S. M., Barcellos, C., Sá Carvalho, M., Santosa, S. M., Barcellosa, C., and SáCarvalhob, M. (2006). Ecological analysis of the distribution and socio-spatial context of homicides in Porto Alegre, Brazil. *Health & Place*, 12, 38–47.

Small Arms Survey (2009). *Firearm-related Violence in Mozambique*. Geneva: Small Arms Survey, Graduate Institute of International and Development Studies. Available at http://www.smallarmssurvey.org/publications/by-type/special-reports.html [Accessed 18 November 2013].

United Nations Office on Drugs and Crime. (2011). *2011 Global Study on Homicide*. Vienna: UNODC.

Ward, E., Durant, T., Thompson, M., Gordon, G., Mitchell, W., and Ashley, D. (2002). Implementing a hospital-based violence-related injury surveillance system-a background to the Jamaican experience. *Injury Control & Safety Promotion*, 9, 241.

World Health Organization. (1992). *International Statistical Classification of Diseases and Related Health Problems*. Geneva: WHO. Available at http://www.who.int/classifications/icd/en/ [Accessed 18 November 2013]

World Health Organization. (2008). *The Global Burden of Disease: 2004 Update*. Geneva: WHO.

World Health Organization. (2011). *WHO Mortality Database (WHOMDB)*. Geneva: WHO. Available at http://www.who.int/healthinfo/statistics/mortdata/ [Accessed 12 November 2013].

World Health Organization Regional Office for Europe. (2012). *European Detailed Mortality Database (EDMB)*. Available at http://data.euro.who.int/dmdb/ [Accessed 12 November 2013].

Yang, G., Hu, J., Rao, K. Q., Ma, J., Rao, C., and Lopez, A. D. (2005). Mortality registration and surveillance in China: history, current situation and challenges. *Population Health Metrics*, 3, 3.

CHAPTER 3

The epidemiology of child maltreatment

Melissa T. Merrick, Beverly L. Fortson, and James A. Mercy

Introduction to the Epidemiology of Child Maltreatment

Child maltreatment is an important public health and human rights problem among low-, middle-, and high-income countries around the world (Pinheiro 2006; Runyan et al. 2002). It is associated with a host of immediate and long-term, life-long health consequences, including changes to brain architecture and development, poor physical and mental health, altered biological factors, reduced cognitive ability and educational attainment, and impaired psychosocial functioning (Felitti et al. 1998; Fortson and Mercy 2012; Leeb et al. 2008, 2011; Shonkoff et al. 2009). Although addressing the specific health outcomes of child maltreatment is crucially important, addressing the problem of child maltreatment itself, and from a public health perspective, is warranted, given the magnitude and burden it places on the health of the public.

Child Maltreatment around the World

Child maltreatment is an international problem, affecting hundreds of millions of children globally. Many of these children come to the attention of social services and other agencies while others go unrecognized altogether, making the precise international scope of the problem difficult to ascertain. Of the data that are available, problems such as single data sources, data availability and quality, cultural variations in parenting and related social norms and laws, and varied definitions among the multiple sectors addressing maltreatment limit the utility and reliability of the data. The World Health Organization (WHO 2006) found that between a quarter and a half of children report physical abuse by a caregiver, while Stoltenborgh et al. (2011) found that 12 per cent of children worldwide report sexual abuse.

The United States Centers for Disease Control and Prevention (CDC) defines child maltreatment as any act, or series of acts, of commission (abuse) or omission (neglect) by a parent or other caregiver that results in harm, potential for harm, or threat of harm to a child (Leeb et al. 2008). Brief CDC definitions for the subtypes of child maltreatment are presented in Table 3.1. Box 3.1 highlights a related area of international concern: child sexual exploitation.

Variations by Reporter/Data Source

Child maltreatment victimization rates are often based on reports from a single source which can yield varied prevalence estimates depending on the data source utilized. For example, a recent meta-analysis of the prevalence of sexual abuse around the world found that self-report studies yielded prevalence rates that were 30 times higher than rates based on official reports (Stoltenborgh et al. 2011). In 2011, U.S. state and local child protection services agencies received 3.7 million reports of maltreated children. Substantiations were made in 681,000 (9.1 per 1,000 in the population) of these cases (U.S. Department of Health & Human Services (USDHHS) 2012). However, when children are asked directly about their experiences of maltreatment, the rate in the general U.S. population is substantially higher, at a rate of 136 per 1000 children or approximately 1 in 10 U.S. children (Finkelhor et al. 2009). In addition, U.S. child protection services data indicate that young children are at highest risk for maltreatment (USDHHS 2012), yet self-report data from a national survey of violence against children indicate that rates of maltreatment are highest among 14- to 17-year-olds (Finkelhor et al. 2009). Data from official sources may also distort descriptions of the type of persons at risk and characteristics of the problem, as these also are often discordant from self-reports (e.g. Pinto and Maia 2012). In a national study of maltreatment in Kenya, less than 10 per cent of girls and boys who self-reported any type of abuse as a child reported having received any social, health, or criminal justice services (Technical Working Group, UNICEF-Kenya 2012). Consequently, studies relying on data from official sources probably underestimate the true magnitude of the problem and may not accurately reflect the groups at highest risk. Self-report surveys often provide a better estimate of the true magnitude of child maltreatment, but they, too, can be problematic due to sampling biases and problems with memory. Thus, reliance on multiple indicators and sources in the assessment and surveillance of maltreatment can lead to better estimates of its true magnitude.

Sexual Abuse Estimates

A recent meta-analysis of the prevalence of sexual abuse in Africa, Asia, Australia, Europe, North America, and South America estimated the global prevalence to be 11.8 per cent or 118 per 1000 children, based on 331 independent samples and around

Table 3.1 Brief CDC definitions of child maltreatment subtypes

Subtype of Maltreatment	Definition[1]
Physical abuse	Intentional use of physical force against a child that results in, or has the potential to result in, physical injury *Exceptions* Physical injuries to the anal or genital area or surrounding areas (e.g. anal or genital bruising or tearing; internal injuries resulting from penetration by a penis, hand, finger, or other object) that occur during attempted or completed sexual abuse, or other physical injuries that result from attempted or completed sexual abuse (e.g. bruises due to restraint, hitting, pushing) are considered sexual abuse and do not constitute physical abuse.
Sexual abuse	Any completed or attempted (non-completed) sexual act, sexual contact with, or exploitation (i.e. non-contact sexual interaction) of a child by a caregiver.
Psychological abuse	Intentional caregiver behaviour that conveys to a child that he/she is worthless, flawed, unloved, unwanted, endangered, or valued only in meeting another's needs.
Neglect	The failure to provide for a child's basic physical, emotional, or educational needs or to protect a child from harm or potential harm[2]
Failure to provide	Failure by a caregiver to meet a child's basic physical, emotional, medical/dental, or educational needs, or combination thereof.
Failure to supervise	Failure by the caregiver to ensure a child's safety within and outside the home given the child's emotional and developmental needs.

[1] For complete definitions, see Leeb, R. T et al., 2008

[2] Mitigating circumstances for failing to provide for a child's basic needs should be noted. The CDC Definitions are intended to be used in conjunction with recommended data elements for public health surveillance.

Source: Leeb, R. T., Paulozzi, L., Melanson, C., Simon, T., and Arias, I. (2008). *Child Maltreatment Surveillance: Uniform Definitions for Public Health and Recommended Data Elements, Version 1.0*. Atlanta, GA: Centers for Disease Control and Prevention, National Center for Injury Prevention and Control. Available at:http://www.cdc.gov/violenceprevention/pdf/CM_Surveillance-a.pdf [Accessed 9 August 2013].

Box 3.1 Child sexual exploitation

Child sexual exploitation can include the coercion of a child to engage in any unlawful or psychologically harmful sexual activity, commercially or otherwise; the use of children in prostitution or other unlawful sexual practices; the participation of children in pornographic performances and materials; and the solicitation of children for sexual purposes. In 2002, WHO estimated that 150 million girls and 73 million boys had experienced forced sexual intercourse or other forms of sexual violence involving physical contact (Pinheiro 2006). Millions more are likely exploited into prostitution or pornography each year. Child sexual exploitation and other forms of exploitation (e.g. the recruitment and use of children in armed conflict) are to the detriment of a child's immediate and long-term mental and physical health, education, and spiritual, moral, and social-emotional development (IOM and NRC 2013; Runyan et al. 2002). Victims of child sexual exploitation are also at increased risk for acquiring sexually transmitted infections and diseases and for having poor reproductive outcomes. Child sexual exploitation is also a violation to the human rights of child victims. Increased surveillance and research efforts are needed to better understand the magnitude and epidemiology of the often clandestine problem of child sexual exploitation around the world and to inform necessary prevention and intervention efforts.

---

10 million participants (Stoltenborgh et al. 2011). Another review documented the prevalence of sexual abuse to range up to 43 per cent for women and 60 per cent for men in 21 different countries (Pereda et al. 2009). Even for regions in which less is known about the overall prevalence, there are increasing reports of sexual abuse to child protective services agencies, suggesting that it is as much a problem in those countries as in other countries (e.g. Taiwan; Chen et al. 2012).

Other Child Maltreatment Estimates

It is difficult to compare the prevalence of physical abuse, emotional abuse, and neglect across countries given variations in cultural norms and the perception and measurement of such (Runyan et al. 2002; WHO 2006). Given that relatively little is known about how parents discipline their children, especially in low- and middle-income countries, the United Nations Children's Fund (UNICEF 2010) examined child disciplinary practices in a range of countries from 2005 to 2006. The report cites that 76 per cent of children aged 2 to 14 experienced some form of violent discipline

(physical abuse and/or emotional abuse) in the past month. The percentage of children experiencing any violent discipline ranged from 38 per cent in Bosnia and Herzegovina to almost 95 per cent in Yemen. In fact, three-quarters of the countries surveyed exceeded a rate of 70 per cent for violent discipline and half of the countries surveyed exceeded 80 per cent. Importantly, 17 per cent of children, on average, were subjected to severe forms of violent discipline (e.g. hitting the child on the head, ears, or face).

In a review specific to countries in East Asia and the Pacific region (Fry 2011), overall prevalence rates of physical abuse ranged from 10 per cent in a study of parents in China to 30.3 per cent in a study of students in Thailand. In general, prevalence rates tended to decrease as the severity of the behaviours increased. Fry (2011) also cited prevalence rates ranging from 22 to over 43 per cent for neglect, depending on the methodology and definitions employed. Lifetime prevalence of emotional abuse ranged from 31.3 per cent in the Republic of Korea to 68.5 per cent in China for representative samples.

Variations by Race and Class

Child maltreatment occurs across all social and demographic strata and no social class or family setting is immune to its public health impact (Al-Mahroos et al. 2005; Pinheiro 2006; UNICEF 2010). In most countries surveyed by UNICEF (2010), characteristics such as wealth, age of caregivers, and household size were not associated with the prevalence of physical abuse. In U.S. studies, socioeconomic status has repeatedly been linked to all forms of maltreatment; however, confounding issues severely limit the interpretation of such findings (Sedlak et al. 2010). Maker et al. (2005) noted that studies on physical abuse among Latino, Asian, and Middle Eastern families commonly use low socioeconomic status, shelter, or clinical samples, greatly restricting the generalizability of the results. While it is well accepted that factors such as poverty, unemployment, and single-parent households put children at increased risk for maltreatment, more rigorous research that fully accounts for potential confounding variables and assesses for temporality are greatly needed to fully examine associations among race, class, and maltreatment.

Risk, Protective, and Maintaining Factors

Child maltreatment is the result of a number of individual, family, and environmental factors, all of which interact at multiple levels of the social ecology (Cicchetti and Toth 2005). Researchers have long speculated that family-level contextual factors are most influential in determining child exposure to maltreatment and outcomes (Cicchetti and Lynch 1993); however, recent evidence suggests that the environment and community play a large role in maltreatment victimization and perpetration (Coulton et al. 2007; Klein 2011). Unfortunately, no single factor tells the entire story about how and why maltreatment occurs.

In research on child maltreatment, several factors have been found to increase or decrease the likelihood of victimization and perpetration, although the research has focused overwhelmingly on risk factors. Risk and protective factors for child maltreatment victimization and perpetration are outlined in Table 3.2 and discussed. In many instances, there is substantial overlap in the risk and protective factors for each subtype of maltreatment. While a history of maltreatment may serve as a risk factor, such a history does not suggest that one will go on to become a perpetrator. Thornberry et al. (2012) found that the positive association between a history of maltreatment and subsequent perpetration is based largely on methodologically weak research designs; more rigorous research had mixed results.

Sexual Abuse

Factors most commonly identified as increasing risk for sexual abuse include child age and sex, and perpetrator sex and relationship to the victim. Contrary to popular belief, perpetrators of sexual abuse are not always 'dirty old men' nor are they strangers (Deblinger et al. 2009). Approximately 85 per cent of sexual abuse cases that come to the attention of law enforcement involve a perpetrator known to the child (Finkelhor 2009). Clinical and research findings suggest that females aged 7–12 years are at the highest risk of sexual abuse (Miller-Perrin and Perrin 2007). Other factors that appear to increase risk include the presence of a stepfather in the home, inter-parental violence, and family isolation and residential mobility (Miller-Perrin and Perrin 2007). Ethnicity and socioeconomic status have not been consistently identified as risk factors for sexual abuse; sexual abuse appears to cut across all races and levels of income (Miller-Perrin and Perrin 2007).

International research on sexual abuse suggests that the most common perpetrators of sexual abuse are male family members, including fathers and brothers (Pinheiro 2006), yet in general, males and females report similar rates of sexual abuse victimization (Haj-Yahi and Tamish 2001). Rates of sexual abuse are high in some countries but children may not realize the behaviours are wrong or inappropriate as the countries lack legal protection associated with sexual abuse and/or perpetuate patriarchal attitudes suggesting that women and children are inferior (Pinheiro 2006).

Physical Abuse

Research has suggested that child sex and age are risk factors for physical abuse victimization, whereas parent age, education, and socioeconomic and marital status are risk factors for perpetration (Miller-Perrin and Perrin 2007). There was no difference in the prevalence of physical abuse exposure among boys and girls in half the countries surveyed by UNICEF (2010); however, boys were slightly more likely to be the victims of physical abuse in the remaining countries. Physical abuse increased with age, peaked at age 5–9 years, and then fell in the oldest age group. Although some research has documented a relationship between parental marital status, age, education, and socioeconomic status and physical abuse, the relationships were not consistently observed in the countries surveyed, particularly for parental marital status and age. In about half of the countries surveyed, limited education and lower household income were risk factors for physical abuse (UNICEF 2010). Pinheiro (2006) noted that children whose parents are young, single, and poor or who have inadequate social support and lack extended family support are at increased risk of maltreatment victimization. In addition, parents with poor impulse control, low self-esteem, mental health problems, and substance use are more likely to perpetrate physical abuse and neglect. In some countries (e.g. Jamaica and India), overcrowding is a risk factor for physical abuse (Hunter et al. 2000; Ricketts and Anderson 2008). Meta-analyses by Stith and colleagues (2009) found large effect sizes for the relationship between physical abuse and parent anger/hyper-reactivity, family conflict, and family cohesion.

Child Neglect

Risk and protective factors for neglect are often cited as being the same or similar to those of physical abuse; however, as noted by Stith and colleagues (2009), neglect is a very different phenomena from physical abuse. Neglect becomes less of an issue as children get older because they are less dependent on their parents over time (Pinheiro 2006). In many countries, cases of neglect are difficult to interpret because of general poor health and under-nutrition in the country as a whole. In the United States, children under the age of 4 years are particularly vulnerable to neglect (USDHHS 2012). Stith and colleagues (2009) found strong relationships between neglect and five risk factors: parent–child relationship, parent perceives child as problem, parent's level of stress, parent anger/hyper-reactivity, and parent self-esteem. Pinheiro (2006) also notes sex differences in rates of neglect, as females are seen as less 'valuable' in countries such as India, China, and Nepal. Although some research suggests that children with disabilities are at increased risk for all types of maltreatment, evidence for this association remains equivocal due to variability in research samples, key definitions, and study methodology (Leeb et al. 2012). Factors that have been associated with the perpetration of neglect include poor impulse control, low self-esteem, mental health problems, and substance use (Pinheiro 2006).

Psychological (Emotional) Abuse

In general, the risk and protective factors for emotional abuse are unclear because of its association with all types of maltreatment (Iwaniec et al. 2006). In UNICEF's (2010) survey, boys and girls aged 10–14 years were more likely than younger children

Table 3.2 Risk and protective factors for the perpetration and victimization of child maltreatment

Ecological Context	Type of Factor	Child Maltreatment Exposure	
Individual	Risk	Perpetration	• Parents' lack of understanding of children's developmental needs and parenting skills (e.g. harsh discipline, hostile caregiving) • Parents' own history of child abuse • Household substance abuse and/or mental health issues including depression • Parental characteristics such as young age, low education, single parenthood, large number of dependent children, and low income • Parental thoughts and emotions that tend to support or justify maltreatment behaviours • History of abuse/neglect of same or another child or other household criminal behaviour • Parental cognitive deficits
		Victimization	• Children younger than 4 years of age (neglect) • Boys (physical abuse) and girls (sexual abuse) in early to middle childhood • Special needs that may increase caregiver burden (e.g. physical or intellectual disabilities, mental health issues, behaviour problems, and chronic physical illnesses) • Prior victimization, experienced directly or witnessed
	Protective	Perpetration	• Parental coping (problem solving)
		Victimization	• None identified with consistent empirical support
Relationship/Family	Risk	Perpetration	• Social isolation, lack of social support as a child and in current relationship • Family disorganization, dissolution, and violence, including intimate partner violence • Parenting stress, poor parent-child relationships, and negative interactions • Non-biological, transient caregivers in the home (e.g. mother's male partner) • Large family size • Current/past family contact with social services/child welfare
		Victimization	• None identified with consistent empirical support
	Protective	Perpetration	• Supportive family environment and social networks
		Victimization	• None identified with consistent empirical support
Community	Risk	Perpetration	• Community violence and high crime rate • Concentrated neighbourhood disadvantage (e.g. high poverty and residential instability, overcrowding, high unemployment rates, high density of alcohol outlets) and poor social connections
		Victimization	• None identified with consistent empirical support
	Protective	Perpetration	• Communities that support parents and take responsibility for preventing abuse
		Victimization	• None identified with consistent empirical support
Social/Cultural	Risk	Perpetration	• Income inequalities/poverty • Cultural norms supporting the use of corporal punishment and the privacy of the family
		Victimization	• None identified with consistent empirical support
	Protective	Perpetration	• None identified with consistent empirical support
		Victimization	• None identified with consistent empirical support

to experience emotional abuse. Other research has documented higher rates of emotional abuse in older children (Pinheiro 2006). Low parental education, lack of income, and household overcrowding, as well as low social support and lack of extended family support have been associated with the perpetration of emotional abuse (Pinheiro 2006). Orphaned children are at increased risk of emotional abuse, even if they live with relatives, as are children in families in which there is partner violence (Pinheiro 2006).

Other Research

As displayed in Table 3.2, little research on the aetiology of child maltreatment exists at the outer levels of the social ecology. Of the research that is available, samples vary across studies in terms of risk. Lower rates of maltreatment are found in communities with concentrated affluence, while higher rates of victimization and perpetration are documented in communities with inadequate resources for child supervision, more concentrated socioeconomic disadvantage (e.g. income or poverty levels, low property values, unemployment, residential instability, increased child care burden), and greater racial and ethnic diversity (Coulton et al. 2007; Klein 2011). Coulton and colleagues (2007) also found that family connectedness to the community could serve as a protective factor. Other community-level factors of interest include laws and policies related to access to family planning services, alcohol availability, acceptable levels of environmental toxins, access to mental health and substance abuse treatment, and access to birth, death, and marriage registration. Policies that focus on education, child care, parental leave, healthcare, unemployment, and social security that leave children and families without economic and social safety nets may increase child maltreatment due to increased levels of family stress and social isolation (Pinheiro 2006).

Gaps in the Evidence

The availability of epidemiologic data on the magnitude, nature, and causes of maltreatment has increased dramatically across the world; however, the availability and quality of data varies. We can be much more confident about the conclusions we reach about child maltreatment in some parts of the world than others. Advances in building a collection of solid data across the world hinge on progress in several areas. First, the comparability and precision of prevalence studies should be increased by adopting more standardized measurement. Second, the use of randomly selected samples that are sufficiently large and representative to generate accurate estimates of maltreatment should be promoted. Third, the underlying limitations inherent in the various research methods employed to generate information on maltreatment should be stated explicitly so that findings are correctly interpreted and used.

In terms of research on child maltreatment risk and protective factors, this review suggests that improvements in four areas are called for. First, given that the aetiology of child maltreatment has focused overwhelmingly on risk, more research on protective factors is needed. Second, more research is needed on risk and protective factors at the community and societal levels, as the great bulk of the existing literature focuses on individual and family level factors. To better address the limitations with protective factor research, direct and buffering protective factors should be examined. Third, greater investment in longitudinal studies is critical to appropriately control for confounds and examine temporality of risk and protective factors. Finally, greater investment in cross-national research would better elucidate the contribution of community and societal level risk and protective factors for child maltreatment.

Conclusion

Despite methodological limitations and differences across studies, child maltreatment is a global phenomenon affecting millions of children. Child maltreatment and other adverse childhood experiences have both immediate and life-long health impacts. The long-term consequences of maltreatment also affect the social and economic development of a country. Fang et al. (2012) estimated lifetime costs of child maltreatment at $124 billion each year for the United States alone. In prioritizing child maltreatment prevention efforts, policymakers and healthcare professionals may mitigate the long-term consequences, thereby freeing resources and improving quality of life for millions of children and adults. Given what we know about risk and protective factors for maltreatment, promoting safe, stable, nurturing relationships and environments for children and families is essential for assuring life-long health (Centers for Disease Control & Prevention 2010). Critical to future progress will be a continued effort to improve our understanding of the prevalence, nature, and causes of child maltreatment around the world.

Author Note

The findings and conclusions in this report are those of the authors and do not necessarily represent the official position of the Centers for Disease Control and Prevention.

References

Al-Mahroos, F., Abdulla, F., Kamal, S., and Al-Ansari, A. (2005). Child abuse: Bahrain's experience. *Child Abuse and Neglect*, 29, 187–93.

Centers for Disease Control and Prevention, National Center for Injury Prevention and Control. (2010). *Safe, Stable, and Nurturing Relationships May Shield Children against Poor Health Later in Life.* Available at: http://www.cdc.gov/ViolencePrevention/pub/healthy_ infants.html [Accessed 21 November 2013].

Chen, Y., Fortson, B. L., and Tseng, K. (2012). Pilot evaluation of a sexual abuse prevention program for Taiwanese children. *Journal of Child Sexual Abuse*, 21, 621–45.

Cicchetti, D., and Lynch, M. (1993). Toward an ecological/transactional model of community violence and child maltreatment: consequences for children's development. *Psychiatry*, 56, 96–118.

Cicchetti, D., and Toth, S. L. (2005). Child maltreatment. *Annual Review of Clinical Psychology*, 1, 409–38.

Coulton, C. J., Crampton, D. S., Irwin, M., Spilsbury, J. C., and Korbin, J. E. (2007). How neighborhoods influence child maltreatment: a review of the literature and alternative pathways. *Child Abuse & Neglect*, 31, 1117–42.

Council of Europe Convention on the Protection of Children against Sexual Exploitation and Sexual Abuse, articles 18–23 (Lanzarote, 25 Nov. 2007; CETS 201). Available at: http://conventions.coe.int/Treaty/ Commun/QueVoulezVous.asp?NT=201&CL=ENG [Accessed 23 August 2013].

Deblinger, E., Thakkar-Kolar, R. R., Berry, E. J., and Schroeder, A. M. (2009). Caregivers' efforts to educate their children about child sexual abuse: a replication study. *Child Maltreatment*, 15, 91–100.

Fang, X., Brown, D. S., Florence, C. S., and Mercy, J. A. (2012). The economic burden of child maltreatment in the United States and implications for prevention. *Child Abuse and Neglect*, 36, 156–65.

Felitti, V. J., Anda, R. F., and Nordenberg, D. et al. (1998). Relationship of child-hood abuse and household dysfunction to many of the leading causes of death in adults. *American Journal of Prevention Medicine*, 14, 245–58.

Finkelhor, D. (2009). The prevention of childhood sexual abuse. *Future of Children*, 19, 169–94.

Finkelhor, D., Turner, H., Ormrod, R., Hamby, S., and Kracke, K (2009). Children's exposure to violence: a comprehensive national survey. *Juvenile Justice Bulletin*. Washington, DC: U.S. Department of Justice, Office of Justice Programs, Office of Juvenile Justice and Delinquency Prevention.

Fortson, B. L., and Mercy, J. (2012). Violence against children. In: J. M. Rippe (ed.), *Encyclopaedia of Lifestyle Medicine and Health*. Thousand Oaks, CA: Sage, pp.2818–29.

Fry, D. (2011). *A Systematic Review of Research on Child Maltreatment in the East Asia and Pacific Region: Final Report.* East Asia and Pacific Regional Office: United Nations Children's Fund.

Haj-Yahi, M. M., and Tamish, S. (2001). The rates of child sexual abuse and its psychological consequences as revealed by a study among Palestinian university students. *Child Abuse & Neglect*, 25, 1303–27.

Hunter, W., Jain, D., Sadowski, L., and Sanhueza, A. (2000). Risk factors for severe child discipline practices in rural India. *Journal of Pediatric Psychology*, 25, 435–47.

Institute of Medicine and National Research Council (IOC and NRM). (2013). *Confronting Commercial Sexual Exploitation and Sex Trafficking of Minors in the United States*. Washington, DC: The National Academies Press.

Iwaniec, D., Larkin, E., and Higgins, S. (2006). Research review: risk and resilience in cases of emotional abuse. *Child and Family Social Work*, 11, 73–82.

Klein, S. (2011). The availability of neighborhood early care and education resources and the maltreatment of young children. *Child Maltreatment*, 16, 300–11.

Leeb, R. T., Bitsko, R. H., Merrick, M. T., and Armour, B. S. (2012). Does childhood disability increase risk for child abuse and neglect? *Journal of Mental Health Research in Intellectual Disabilities*, 5, 4–31.

Leeb, R. T., Lewis, T., and Zolotor, A. J. (2011). A review of physical and mental health consequences of child abuse and neglect and implications for practice. *American Journal of Lifestyle Medicine*, 5, 454–68.

Leeb, R. T., Paulozzi, L., Melanson, C., Simon, T., and Arias, I. (2008). *Child Maltreatment Surveillance: Uniform Definitions for Public Health and Recommended Data Elements, Version 1.0.* Atlanta, GA: Centers for Disease Control and Prevention, National Center for Injury Prevention and Control. Available at: http://www.cdc. gov/violenceprevention/pdf/CM_Surveillance-a.pdf [*Accessed 9 August 2013*].

Maker, A. H., Shah, P. V., and Agha, Z. (2005). Child physical abuse: prevalence, characteristics, predictors, and beliefs about parent-child violence in South Asian, Middle Eastern, East Asian, and Latina women in the United States. *Journal of Interpersonal Violence*, 20, 1406–28.

Miller-Perrin, C. L., and Perrin, R. D. (2007). *Child Maltreatment: An Introduction*. Thousand Oaks, CA: Sage.

Pereda, N., Guilera, G., Forns, M., and Gómez-Benitob, J. (2009). The international epidemiology of child sexual abuse: a continuation of Finkelhor (1994). *Child Abuse & Neglect*, 33, 331–42.

Pinheiro, P.S. (2006). *World Report on Violence against Children*. Geneva: United Nations. Available at: http://unviolencestudy.org/ [Accessed 9 August 2013].

Pinto, R. J. and Maia, A. C. (2012). A comparison study between official records and self-reports of childhood adversity. *Child Abuse Review*, 22, 354–66.

Ricketts, H., and Anderson, P. (2008). Impact of poverty and stress on the interaction of Jamaican caregivers with young children. *International Journal of Early Years Education*, 16, 61–74.

Runyan, D., Wattam, C., Ikeda, R., Hassan, F., and Ramiro, L. (2002). Child abuse and neglect by parents and other caregivers. In: E. Krug, L. L. Dahlberg, J. A. Mercy, A. B. Zwi, and R. Lozano (eds.). *World Report on Violence and Health*. Geneva: World Health Organization, pp. 59–86.

Sedlak, A. J., Mettenburg, J., and Basena, M. et al. (2010). *Fourth National Incidence Study of Child Abuse and Neglect (NIS–4): Report to Congress*. Washington, DC: U.S. Department of Health and Human Services, Administration for Children and Families.

Shonkoff, J. P., Boyce, W. T., and McEwen, B. S. (2009). Neuroscience, molecular biology, and the childhood roots of health disparities: building a new framework for health promotion and disease prevention. *Journal of the American Medical Association*, 301, 2252–9.

Stith, S. M., Liu, T., Davies, L. C., and Boykin, E. L. et al. (2009). Risk factors in child maltreatment: a meta-analytic review of the literature. *Aggression and Violent Behavior*, 14, 13–29.

Stoltenborgh, M., van IJzendoorn, M. H., Euser, E. M., and Bakermans-Kranenburg, M. J. (2011). A global perspective on child sexual abuse: meta-analysis of prevalence around the world. *Child Maltreatment*, 16, 79–101.

Technical Working Group, United Nations Children's Fund—Kenya Country Office, U.S. Centers for Disease Control and Prevention & Kenya National Bureau of Statistics. (2012). *Violence against Children in Kenya: Findings from a 2010 National Survey*. Nairobi, Kenya: United Nations Children's Fund Kenya Country Office.

Thornberry, T. P., Knight, K. E., and Lovegrove, P. J. (2012). Does maltreatment beget maltreatment? A systematic review of the intergenerational literature. *Trauma, Violence, & Abuse*, 13, 135–52.

United Nations Children's Fund (UNICEF), Division of Policy and Practice. (2010). *Child Disciplinary Practices at Home: Evidence from a Range of Low- and Middle-income Countries*. New York: UNICEF.

U.S. Department of Health and Human Services, Administration for Children and Families, Administration on Children, Youth and Families Children's Bureau. (2012). *Child Maltreatment 2011*. Washington, DC: USDHHS. Available at: http://www.acf.hhs.gov/sites/default/files/cb/cm11.pdf [Accessed 25 August 2013].

World Health Organization (2006). *Preventing Child Maltreatment: A Guide to Taking Action and Generating Evidence*. Geneva: WHO & International Society for Prevention of Child Abuse and Neglect.

CHAPTER 4

Youth violence

Catherine L. Ward

Introduction to Youth Violence

Most violence is youth violence: violence is disproportionately committed by young people, and young people are disproportionately the victims of violence. Deaths from homicide peak in the 20–29 age group (Matzopoulos and colleagues, Chapter 3 of this volume), and prevalence of arrests for violent crime follow the well-known age–crime curve (see Figure 4.1) (Farrington 1986), as does prevalence of self-reported violence (Loeber and Hay 1997). While the age peak varies across times and locations, it is typically in the late teens through early twenties (Farrington 1986).

The regular, predictable nature of this phenomenon makes the prevention of youth violence absolutely central to any public health agenda.

Age, Gender, and Ethnicity in Youth Violence

However, it is not necessarily youth who should be the targets of intervention. While arrests for violence peak in the teens and twenties, there is an earlier peak for aggression, between ages 2 and 4 years (Tremblay and Côté 2009): as Tremblay argues in Chapter 5 of this volume, aggression in young people begins in early life, and the key question is why some desist while others follow stable or escalating trajectories.

Life-course developmental approaches identify which risk and protective factors influence desistance from, or escalation of, violence. Two typologies of the development of offending (including violent offending) dominate the literature: Loeber and Hay's (1994) delineation of three pathways to offending in boys (Figure 4.2), and Moffitt's (1993) taxonomy of adolescence-limited versus life-course persistent offending (Figure 4.3).

The three pathways described in Loeber and Hay's (1994) model are the authority conflict pathway, which starts with stubborn behaviour that escalates to authority avoidance such as truancy; the covert pathway that starts with shoplifting and lying that escalates to moderate to serious delinquency such as fraud and theft; and the overt pathway, which starts with minor aggression such as bullying and escalates to serious violence such as rape. More serious offenders are on multiple pathways simultaneously (Loeber and Hay 1994), and it appears that more frequent offenders are more likely to engage in violent acts (Piquero et al. 2012). Yet the stepwise progression implied by this model has yet to be investigated (Piquero et al. 2012), and it was developed based on a sample that did not include girls (Loeber and Hay 1994).

Moffitt's (1993) taxonomy describes a small group of offenders who start young and persist, and a majority who start offending in adolescence and then desist. Moffitt (1993) proposes that life-course persistent offenders start life with neuropsychological deficits that interact with environmental problems (such as harsh parenting) that together put them on this path, whereas adolescence-limited offenders experience a 'maturity gap' that they attempt to overcome through mimicking delinquent peers. While several typologies suggest that there are more than two groups, in general typology studies are largely consistent with

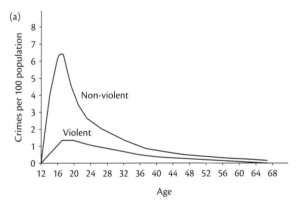

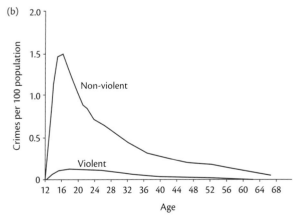

Fig. 4.1 The relation between age and crime, (a) for American males, and (b) for American females. Both graphs show the rate of arrests per 100 population for Index offences in 1982.

Reproduced from Farrington, D. P., Age and crime, *Crime and Justice*, Volume 7, pp. 189–192, Copyright © 1989, with permission from University of Chicago Press, includes data from Federal Bureau of Investigation, *Uniform Crime Reports*, 1982, US Government Printing Office, Washington DC, USA

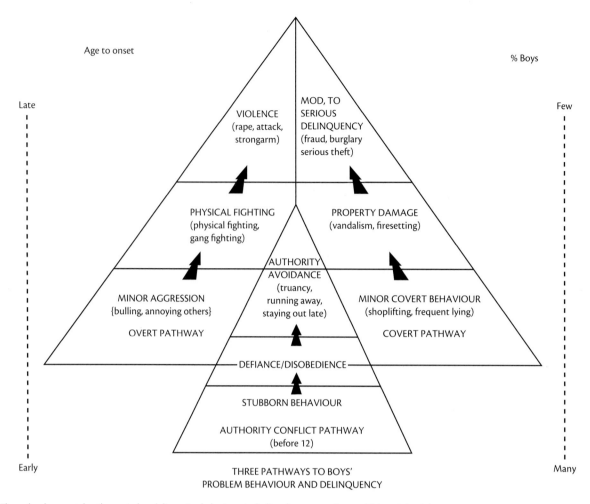

Fig. 4.2 Three developmental pathways in boys' disruptive behaviour, including the overt pathway which ends in violence

Reproduced from Loeber, R., and Hay, D., Developmental approaches to aggression and conduct problems, in M. Rutter and D. Hay (eds.), *Development through Life: A Handbook for Clinicians,* pp. 488–516, Blackwell, Oxford, UK, Copyright © 1994, with permission from John Wiley & Sons, Inc.

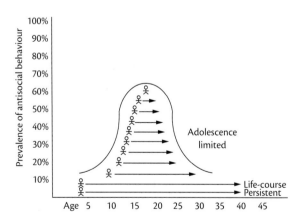

Fig. 4.3 Moffitt's (1993) illustration of the changing prevalence of participation in antisocial behaviour across the life course; the curve represents the well-known age-crime curve, while the arrows represent the participation by individuals in antisocial behaviour.

Reproduced with permission from Moffitt, T. E., Adolescence-limited and life-course persistent antisocial behavior: a developmental taxonomy, *Psychological Review,* Volume 100, Number 4, pp. 74–701, Copyright © 1993 American Psychological Association, Inc.

Moffitt's original proposal and find three or four groups: a non-violent group, a life-course persistent group, escalators, and desistors (Jennings and Reingle 2012).

More recently, Dodge and colleagues (2008) have proposed a cascade model that attempts to show how risk factors influence each other in a 'cascade' that ends in youth violence (see Figure 4.4). In this model, disadvantaged social contexts experienced early in life predict harsh and inconsistent parenting, which predicts social and cognitive deficits, which in turn predict conduct problems, which predict social and academic failure in elementary school, which predict parental withdrawal from supervision and monitoring, which predicts association with deviant peers, which ultimately predicts youth violence. This models how predictor domains interact with each other to play a causal role in aggression.

Gender plays an important role in youth violence. Girls tend to follow the same trajectories as boys, but are more likely to be on stable low-violence trajectories and less likely to be on stable high-violence ones (Piquero et al. 2012). Males tend to be involved in direct aggression, while females more in indirect or relational aggression such as gossip and social exclusion (Crick and Grotpeter 1995), which may reflect gender norms in society—but also that

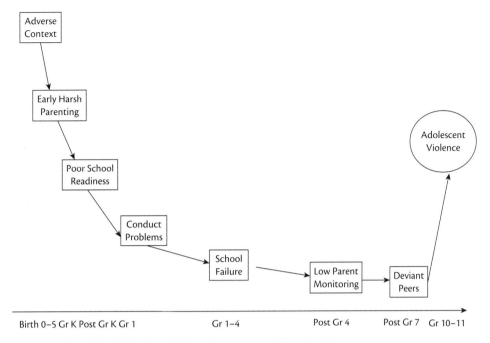

Fig. 4.4 Hypothesized dynamic cascade model explaining how risk factors interact to result in youth violence
Reproduced from Dodge, K. A. et al, Testing an idealized dynamic cascade model of the development of serious violence in adolescence, *Child Development*, Volume 79, Issue 6, pp. 1907–27, Copyright © 2008 Society for Research in Child Development, Inc., with permission from John Wiley & Sons, Inc.

gender may interact with risk and protective factors to produce different effects (Baxendale et al. 2012). For instance, although the same risk factors appear to influence the likelihood of violence in both genders (Miller et al. 2010; Odgers et al. 2008), studies that investigate poor parental support as a risk factor find the same rates across gender, but also that males are more likely to report violent behaviour (Baxendale et al. 2012). Romantic involvement appears to be a particular risk factor for girls' involvement in violence, but not for boys (Xie et al. 2011).

Ethnicity is another factor that may influence rates of violence. Studies based on several data sources from the United States show that minorities in that context are both more likely to be involved in serious, violent offending, and more likely to persist in such offending (Piquero et al. 2012). As with gender, this may reflect different levels of risk factors, or differential responses to risk factors (for instance, one study, again in the United States, found that Hispanics who reported depression were more likely to desist from violence than whites who did not report such symptoms (Reingle et al. 2013)). Racialized categories are typically proxies for advantage or disadvantage, often concentrated disadvantage (Foster 2012), and not intrinsic characteristics of people, but have not received much attention in the study of youth violence (Piquero et al. 2012).

Theoretical Approaches to Understanding Youth Violence

There are, in essence, two theoretical understandings of youth violence (Baxendale et al. 2012): social cognitive theories, and developmental pathways (or trajectory models). Social learning theories propose that violent and non-violent behavioural repertoires are learned through observational learning and through achieving rewards for certain types of behaviour; and that whether children

are violent in particular situations depends on what is happening in the situations, their construal of those events, and their sense of their own competence in responding with a particular behaviour (Anderson and Huesmann 2003). Trajectory models map the development of aggression (and desistance from aggression) over the life course. These approaches are not inconsistent with each other, and both draw on risk and protective factors to describe which individuals are more at risk of violent behaviour, or more likely to desist.

Other Risk and Protective Factors Influencing the Likelihood of Youth Violence

In essence, developmental models and risk factors explain how the potential for violence develops; situational factors explain why it occurs (Farrington 1998). For some young people—those who have no history of aggression prior to a violent incident—situational factors may be more important than developmental ones (Dahlberg and Potter 2001). Aggression is the outcome of a confluence of several situational and personological factors, the latter referring both to the individual's state of mind in the situation where violence occurs, and to a personal preparedness to carry out aggression that has developed over time (Anderson and Huesmann 2003).

Situational Risk

Motives for violence among male youth change over time, and depend on whether the young man is alone or in a group (Farrington 1998). A Canadian study revealed that in younger adolescents motives are more likely to be a search for excitement, but by the late teens and early twenties will be utilitarian (Le Blanc and Frechette 1989). A study of US youth revealed that most acts of violence were committed either for revenge or because of provocation (Agnew 1990). In the Cambridge-Somerville Youth Study, boys on their own were most likely to fight because they were provoked and angry; in groups, fights quickly became serious and occurred because neither side was willing to act in a conciliatory way and both wished to demonstrate their masculinity (Farrington 1998).

The presence of alcohol or weapons also increases the likelihood of violence (Mercy et al. 2002). Alcohol appears to function via three mechanisms: physiological disinhibition of behaviour, psychological disinhibition through expecting intoxication when drinking, and impairment of social cognition; while the presence of a weapon 'primes' violence-related cognitive structures, making them more likely to influence behaviour (Anderson and Huesmann 2003). High levels of arousal and stress also appear to disinhibit aggression (Anderson and Huesmann 2003).

Risk and Protective Factors that Influence Development

Neighbourhood Factors

Disadvantaged neighbourhoods have higher rates of youth violence (Dodge et al. 2008), although the direct effects of the neighbourhood are weak compared with those of more proximal risk factors, such as those located in the family or individual (Lynam et al. 2000). The effect of neighbourhood characteristics may also be moderated by individual characteristics: impulsive boys are at higher risk in disadvantaged neighbourhoods, whereas non-impulsive boys are at low risk regardless of neighbourhood context (Lynam et al. 2000). Further, neighbourhood disadvantage appears to be a risk factor only for boys who have many other protective factors or a balance of risk and protective factors (boys who have many proximal risk factors are not at greater risk because of neighbourhood disadvantage) (Wikström and Loeber 2000), while living in a non-deprived, non-violent neighbourhood is protective for all boys (Lösel and Farrington 2012). It is also worth noting that it is not simply poverty rates in the neighbourhood that affect youth violence but rather levels of informal social control and cohesion: social cohesion in a neighbourhood can buffer the effects of poverty (Lösel and Farrington 2012).

School Factors

Both the characteristics of the school and of the individual's attitudes towards and achievement at school play a role. A positive school climate, including support and supervision from teachers, and clear classroom rules, provides protective school characteristics (Lösel and Farrington 2012), which no doubt also play a role in fostering individual's academic characteristics. Protective characteristics of individuals include strong bonds to school, high motivation for schoolwork, and reaching higher education (Lösel and Farrington 2012). School failure, by contrast, is a risk factor; and in Dodge and colleagues' (2008) cascade model is itself predicted by other risk factors that differ by gender: in boys, school failure is predicted by early externalizing behaviour and a lack of school readiness, whereas in girls it is predicted by early problems with parents and adverse social context.

The Peer Group

As with other forms of delinquency, association with aggressive peers is a risk factor (Baxendale et al. 2012). Association with aggressive peers is associated with deficits in parental monitoring and discipline practices (Dodge et al. 2008). By contrast, peer groups that disapprove of aggression, who are non-violent, and who are religious, are protective, as is—at the other extreme—social isolation (Lösel and Farrington 2012).

Family Factors

A host of family factors increase risk for youth violence: poor parental supervision; lack of warmth in the parent–child relationship; harsh, inconsistent discipline; parental attitudes favourable to aggression; family structure (either single parent families or large families); low socioeconomic status; violence in the home; substance misuse by family members; low parental education; parental expectations of their children's school achievement; and maternal depression (Baxendale et al. 2012; Dodge et al. 2008; Duke et al. 2010 Resnick et al. 2004). Child maltreatment is a risk factor for youth violence and intimate partner violence (Duke et al. 2010; Fang and Corso 2007), and for boys to progress on the overt, covert, and authority conflict pathways (Stouthamer-Loeber et al. 2001).

These family risk factors operate by influencing child characteristics. For instance, child maltreatment and harsh discipline lead to impaired empathy and social problem-solving via emotional dysregulation, as does witnessing family violence (Dodge et al. 2008). Parenting is also a dynamic endeavour: it must shift as children mature, in response to children's behaviour, and in response to the environment. For instance, as children progress into adolescence, parental monitoring becomes particularly important, and especially so in contexts of risk (Dodge et al. 2008). On the other hand, parental monitoring is reciprocal: as adolescents become increasingly antisocial, parents tend to withdraw supervision (Dodge et al. 2008). Parenting is also influenced by other factors: for instance, family poverty may exert its effect via increasing parental distress and decreasing support, which in turn diminish effectiveness and increase coercive behaviour towards children (Dodge et al. 2008).

Protective factors have, of course, also been identified in the family. These include a positive family environment; eating dinner together; a close relationship with at least one parent; parental supervision; parental disapproval of aggression; low physical punishment; intense involvement in family activities; family role models for constructive coping; positive parental attitudes towards children's education; and medium socioeconomic status (Baxendale et al. 2012; Lösel and Farrington 2012).

Individual Characteristics

Individual characteristics that put children at risk of developing aggression can loosely be divided into two groups: those that are early indicators that a child is on an aggressive path; and those that are the intrinsic characteristics of children that put them on that path in the first place, which are in turn viewed as the expressions of underlying neurobiological vulnerabilities.

Indicators that a child is on an aggressive path include truancy, cruelty to people, and minor physical fighting (Pardini et al. 2012). These are important because the considerable continuity of externalizing behaviour problems is one of the most robust findings of developmental criminology (Dodge et al. 2008; Moffitt 1993). Intrinsic characteristics that put children on that path in the first place include depressed mood, inability to recognize emotions in others, a bias to attribute hostile intentions to others, cruelty, poor social problem-solving, poor verbal abilities, difficulty regulating emotions, impulsivity, and callous, unemotional traits (Dodge et al. 2008; Frick and Viding 2009; Loeber et al. 2012; Pardini et al. 2012).

Substance misuse (particularly alcohol) and victimization are additional risk factors frequently identified in the literature (Baxendale et al. 2012; Resnick et al. 2004). Victimization appears to be moderated by family functioning: one study found that youth in well-functioning families were less likely to be aggressive even if exposed to high levels of violence, while young people from families with low emotional cohesion and poor parenting practices were more likely to be exposed to community violence, and then to perpetrate violence themselves (Gorman-Smith et al. 2010).

Several neurobiological influences have been identified as influencing the likelihood of aggression. For instance, one of the most enduring and robust findings is that boys and men are far more likely to be aggressive than girls and women. Testosterone levels have been proposed to account for this gender difference, and it appears that circulating testosterone levels do in fact affect brain functioning, resulting in a strong reward motivation, low social sensitivity, and dampened regulation of motivational and emotional processes, which are in turn modulated by environmental and genetic risk factors that can shape behaviour on an aggressive path (Yildirim and Derksen 2012).

Other neurobiological vulnerabilities include difficult temperament and difficulties regulating attention and behaviour—early characteristics of life-course persistent offenders (Moffitt 2006). Life-course persistent offending appears to be highly heritable (56–70 per cent), as do both reactive and proactive aggression (Piquero et al. 2012), adding strength to an argument in favour of a role for genes in creating these temperamental vulnerabilities to aggression. Indeed, serotonin and dopamine are neurotransmitters implicated in aggression (serotonin for its role in self-control and dopamine for its role in the brain's reward system), and genes appear to affect levels of these hormones, their biological effects, and the rate at which they are produced, released, and reabsorbed (Pavlov et al. 2012).

Yet genetic vulnerabilities must interact with the environment to achieve expression as aggression (Pavlov et al. 2012). For instance, in the presence of protective factors, the behavioural endophenotypes induced by testosterone can be prosocial traits (such as leadership) rather than aggression (Yildirim and Derksen 2012). Further, the exact nature of the gene–environment relationship is not clear. Some risk factors viewed as environmental (for instance, harsh, cold parenting) may be evoked by heritable temperament (irritable children may elicit harsh discipline from parents); and genetic differences in sensitivity to the environment may also play a role in which children take an aggressive path (Baxendale et al. 2012; Frick and Viding 2009).

Loeber and Pardini (2008) note that there are four assumptions underlying a genetically deterministic view: (i) that there is stability in the individual differences in neurobiological factors underlying aggression—yet aggression changes over the life-course; (ii) that there are neurobiological origins to the mechanisms that give rise to aggression—yet there is as yet very little agreement on what those underlying mechanisms are; (iii) that the development of aggression can be explained to some extent by environmental factors—yet it is unclear what role neurobiological factors

play (beyond environmental factors) in either the escalation to or desistance from violence; (iv) societal rates of violence shift over time, and the relationship to neurobiological factors is not clear. They offer two further points for consideration: that behavioural dysregulation is proposed as the chief marker for neurobiological factors, yet in prospective studies it is not a good predictor of aggression; and, further, that there is evidence that aspects of temperament can be changed, so there is doubt as to whether neurobiological factors are immutable (Loeber and Pardini 2008).

Relatively less attention has been paid to protective factors than to risk factors, and often these are the reverse of risk factors. For instance, callous, unemotional traits put young people at risk for aggression—because they are less likely to experience arousal in response to distress in others—while anxiety and distress at the negative effects of one's behaviour on others is protective (Frick and Viding 2009). Other protective factors include above-average intelligence, low impulsivity, easy temperament, low attention deficit hyperactivity disorder, anxiety, shyness, prosocial attitudes (positive attitudes towards family and school; non-aggression-prone social cognitions and beliefs), academic achievement, older mother at birth of first child, good relations with peers, positive relationships with parents and other adults, religiosity, and, in addition, some biological factors: high heart rate and high monoamine oxidase A activity (Loeber et al. 2009; Lösel and Farrington 2012; Resnick et al. 2004).

The relationship between risk and protective factors is key in predicting outcomes. The probability of violence decreases in a dose–response relationship as protective factors increase (Lösel and Farrington 2012), but there are also subtleties. For instance, the influence of several risk factors differs by age (Pardini et al. 2012): for boys enrolled in the Pittsburgh Youth Study, low peer delinquency is a protective factor for aged 15–18 years and for boys aged 13–14 years with serious conduct problems; a negative attitude towards delinquency is protective for age 13–14 years; and a low perceived likelihood of being caught and high levels of neighbourhood disorder are risk factors for age 15–18 years. It is key that developmental models specify how risk and promotive factors shift in their influence over development; exposure to different risk domains increases as children age, and while some persist in their influence others increase or decrease (Loeber et al. 2009). In addition, most risk factors appear to emerge at birth, in preschool years, and in elementary school, with fewer risk factors emerging in adolescence; this implies that the interventions prior to adolescence are likely to be most effective (Loeber et al. 2009).

Risk and Protective Factors Influencing Desistance

Protective factors that keep children from taking a violent pathway are of course important, but factors that promote desistance from violence are equally important. Despite much evidence that desistance happens for most, if not all, offenders, this area is not well understood (Walker et al. 2013).

Gaps in the Evidence

Gaps in the evidence base for youth violence arise both through problems in methods used in studies, and in the content areas that are addressed.

From a methods perspective, there are three main problems. First, the field has relatively few longitudinal studies, especially those that continue beyond adolescence. This has several effects: it is difficult to separate associations between variables from causal relationships (Baxendale et al. 2012), and it is also difficult to understand the different influences of different risk and protective factors over the age-span and on different groups, nor can we understand desistance (Baxendale et al. 2012; Broidy et al. 2003; Jennings and Reingle 2012). Second, the field is dominated by school-based surveys, but these may exclude the most violent as they are also the adolescents who are least likely to be at school; and third, measures of violence are often only a part of broader measures of delinquency, making it hard to distinguish influences on violence (Baxendale et al. 2012).

These problems in methods are echoed by gaps in the content of research. Prime amongst these gaps is the study of protective factors, and how they operate both to prevent children from taking an aggressive pathway in the first place and how they operate to promote desistance from aggression (Loeber and Pardini 2008; Piquero et al. 2012; Walker et al. 2013). Many of the same risk and protective factors that influence violence also influence the development of other problems, including other forms of delinquency and internalizing disorders; we have yet to understand how different outcomes result from the same risk factors (Loeber and Pardini 2008). In a similar vein, it is well established that violent offenders are frequent offenders, but which risk factors distinguish non-violent offenders from violent ones is also yet to be identified (Piquero et al. 2012). Nor do we yet understand how risk and protective factors influence

each other, although some attempts have been made to understand the different influences of different risk and protective factors for different ages, different ethnic groups, and different genders (Baxendale et al. 2012; Dodge et al. 2008; Reingle et al. 2013). Even so, the development of violent offending in girls needs far more investigation (Baxendale et al. 2012). Finally, neurobiological understandings of vulnerability to becoming aggressive, including the influence of genes and how these interact with the environment, is an area in its infancy (Loeber and Pardini 2008).

Conclusion

The prevention of youth violence is key to efforts to prevent violence, since most violence is in fact youth violence. Current models suggest that most risk factors emerge in the early years (Loeber et al. 2009), making that the most strategic time to intervene. But equally it is clear that different risk and protective factors come into play at different ages, so that (i) opportunities for intervention continue throughout the life span (Dodge et al. 2008), and (ii) a developmental approach to prevention is crucial. Intervention studies can assist in further specifying which risk and protective factors are most influential at what ages (Loeber et al. 2009).

Acknowledgement

Writing this chapter was supported in part by a grant from the University of Cape Town's Research Committee (URC).

References

Agnew, R. (1990). The origins of delinquent events: an examination of offender accounts. *Journal of Research in Crime and Delinquency, 27,* 267–94.

Anderson, C. A., and Huesmann, L. R. (2003). Human aggression: a social-cognitive view. In: M. A. Hogg and J. Cooper (eds.), *The Sage Handbook of Social Psychology.* Thousand Oaks, CA, Sage Publications, Inc., pp. 296–323.

Baxendale, S., Cross, D., and Johnston, R. (2012). A review of the evidence on the relationship between gender and adolescents' involvement in violent behavior. *Aggression and Violent Behavior, 17,* 297–310.

Broidy, L. M., Tremblay, R. E., and Brame, B. et al. (2003). Developmental trajectories of childhood disruptive behaviors and adolescent delinquency: a six-site, cross-national study. *Developmental Psychology, 39,* 222–45.

Crick, N. R., and Grotpeter, J. K. (1995). Relational aggression, gender and social-psychological adjustment. *Child Development,* 66, 710–22.

Dahlberg, L. L., and Potter, L. B. (2001). Youth violence: developmental pathways and prevention challenges. *American Journal of Preventive Medicine, 20,* 3–14.

Dodge, K. A., Malone, P. S., and Greenberg, M. T. (2008). Testing an idealized dynamic cascade model of the development of serious violence in adolescence. *Child Development, 79,* 1907–27.

Duke, N. N., Pettingell, S. L., McMorris, B. J., and Borowsky, I. W. (2010). Adolescent violence perpetration: associations with multiple types of adverse childhood experiences. *Pediatrics, 125,* e778–86.

Fang, X., and Corso, P. S. (2007). Child maltreatment, youth violence, and intimate partner violence: developmental relationships. *American Journal of Preventive Medicine, 33,* 281–90.

Farrington, D. P. (1986). Age and crime. *Crime and Justice, 7,* 189–250.

Farrington, D. P. (1998). Predictors, causes and correlates of male youth violence. *Crime and Justice, 24,* 421–75.

Foster, D. (2012). Gender, class, 'race', and violence. In: C. L. Ward, A. v. d. Merwe, and A. Dawes (eds), *Youth violence: Sources and Solutions in South Africa.* Cape Town, South Africa: UCT Press, pp. 23–51.

Frick, P. J., and Viding, E. (2009). Antisocial behavior from a developmental psychopathology perspective. *Development and Psychopathology, 21,* 1111–31.

Gorman-Smith, D., Henry, D. B., and Tolan, P. H. (2010). Exposure to community violence and violence prepetration: the protective effects of family functioning. *Journal of Clinical Child & Adolescent Psychology,* 33, 439–49.

Jennings, W. G., and Reingle, J. M. (2012). On the number and shape of developmental/life-course violence, aggression, and delinquency trajectories: A state-of-the-art review. *Journal of Criminal Justice, 40,* 472–89.

Le Blanc, M., and Frechette, M. (1989). *Male Criminal Activity from Childhood through Youth.* New York, N.Y.: Springer-Verlag.

Loeber, R., Burke, J. D., and Pardini, D. A. (2009). Development and etiology of disruptive and delinquent behavior. *Annual Review of Clinical Psychology,* 5, 291–310.

Loeber, R., and Hay, D. (1994). Developmental approaches to aggression and conduct problems. In: M. Rutter and D. Hay (eds.). *Development through Life: A Handbook for Clinicians.* Oxford, U.K.: Blackwell, pp.488–516.

Loeber, R., and Hay, D. (1997). Key issues in the development of aggression and violence from childhood to early adulthood. *Annual Review of Psychology,* 48, 371–410.

Loeber, R., Menting, B., and Lynam, D. R. et al. (2012). Findings from the Pittsburgh Youth Study: cognitive impulsivity and intelligence as predictors of the age-crime curve. *Journal of the American Academy of Child & Adolescent Psychiatry,* 51, 1136–49.

Loeber, R., and Pardini, D. A. (2008). Neurobiology and the development of violence: common assumptions and controversies. *Philosophical Transactions: Biological Sciences, 363,* 2491–503.

Lösel, F., and Farrington, D. (2012). Direct protective and buffering protective factors in the development of youth violence. *American Journal of Preventive Medicine,* 43, S8-S23.

Lynam, D. R., Caspi, A., Moffitt, T. E., Wikström, P. O., Loeber, R., and Novak, S. (2000). The interaction between impulsivity and neighborhood context on offending: the effects of impulsivity are stronger in poorer neighborhoods. *Journal of Abnormal Psychology,* 109, 563–74.

Mercy, J. A., Butchart, A., Farrington, D., and Cerdá, M. (2002). *Youth violence.* In: E. G. Krug, L. L. Dahlberg, J. A. Mercy, A. B. Zwi and R. Lozano (eds), *World Report on Violence and Health.* Geneva, Switzerland: World Health Organization, pp.23–56.

Miller, S., Malone, P. S., and Dodge, K. A. (2010). Developmental trajectories of boys' and girls' delinquency: sex differences and links to later outcomes. *Journal of Abnormal Child Psychology,* 38, 1021–32.

Moffitt, T. E. (1993). Adolescence-limited and life-course persistent antisocial behavior: a developmental taxonomy. *Psychological Review,* 100, 674–701.

Moffitt, T. E. (2006). Life-course persistent versus adolescence-limited antisocial behaviour. In D. Cicchetti and D. J. Cohen (eds), *Developmental Psychopathology.* New York, N.Y.: Wiley, pp. 571–98.

Odgers, C. L., Moffitt, T. E., and Broadbent, J. M. et al. (2008). Female and male antisocial trajectories: from childhood origins to adult outcomes. *Development and Psychopathology, 20,* 673–716.

Pardini, D. A., Loeber, R., Farrington, D., and Stouthamer-Loeber, M. (2012). Identifying direct protective factors for nonviolence. *American Journal of Preventive Medicine,* 43, S28–40.

Pavlov, K. A., Chistiakov, D., and Chekhonin, V. P. (2012). Genetic determinants of aggression and impulsivity in humans. *Journal of Applied Genetics,* 53, 61–82.

Piquero, A. R., Carriaga, M. L., Diamond, B., Kazemian, L., and Farrington, D. P. (2012). Stability in aggression revisited. *Aggression and Violent Behavior,* 17, 365–72.

Piquero, A. R., Jennings, W. G., and Barnes, J. C. (2012). Violence in criminal careers: a review of the literature from a developmental life-course perspective. *Aggression and Violent Behavior,* 17, 171–9.

Reingle, J. M., Jennings, W. G., Lynne-Landsman, S. D., Cottler, L. B., and Maldonado-Molina, M. M. (2013). Towards an understanding of risk and protective factors for vioence among adolescent boys and men: a longitudinal analysis. *Journal of Adolescent Health,* 52, 493–8.

Resnick, M. D., Ireland, M., and Borowsky, I. W. (2004). Youth violence perpetration: what protects? What predicts? Findings from the National Longitudinal Study of Adolescent Health. *Journal of Adolescent Health,* 35, 424.e1–10.

Stouthamer-Loeber, Loeber, M. R., Homish, D. L., and Wei, E. (2001). Maltreatment of boys and the development of disruptive and delinquent behavior. *Development and Psychopathology,* 13, 941–55.

Tremblay, R., and Côté, S. M. (2009). Development of sex differences in physical aggression: the maternal link to epigenetic mechanisms [comment]. *Behavioral and Brain Sciences,* 32, 290–1.

Walker, K., Bowen, E., and Brown, S. (2013). Psychological and criminological factors associated with desistance from violence: a review of the literature. *Aggression and Violent Behavior,* 18, 286–99.

Wikström, P. O., and Loeber, R. (2000). Do disadvantaged neighborhoods cause well-adjusted children to become adolescent delinquents? A study of male juvenile serious offending, individual risk and protective factors, and neighborhood context. *Criminology,* 38, 1109–42.

Xie, H., Drabick, D. A. G., and Chen, D. (2011). Developmental trajectories of aggression from late childhood through adolescence: similarities and differences across gender. *Aggressive Behavior,* 37, 387–404.

Yildirim, B. O., and Derksen, J. J. L. (2012). A review on the relationship between testosterone and life-course persistent antisocial behavior. *Psychiatry Research*, 200, 984–1010.

CHAPTER 5

Developmental origins of physical aggression

Richard E. Tremblay

An Introduction to Developmental Origins of Physical Aggression

This chapter describes the state of knowledge on the development of physical aggression from early childhood to adulthood. Unravelling the developmental origins of physical aggression has been important to understand (i) when and why humans start using physical aggression; (ii) why some humans suffer from chronic physical aggression; (iii) how to prevent the development of this disorder which causes much distress to the aggressors and their victims; (iv) why situational prevention of aggression is important at all ages and in all cultures.

Longitudinal studies of large population samples were needed to understand the developmental origins of physical aggression. These studies had to start as close as possible to birth and they generally tracked the putative causal factors, correlates, and outcomes. Considering the distress and financial cost of physical violence among humans, there are surprisingly few longitudinal studies that have tried to chart the development of physical aggression from birth onwards. This lack of attention to physical aggression from the early years onwards appears to be the result of a long-held belief that humans start to use physical violence during late childhood and early adolescence as a result of social learning (e.g. Bandura 1977; Zimbardo 2007).

The conclusion of the United States Academy of Science Panel on Understanding Violent Behaviour created in the late 1980s is a good example of the social learning perspective for aggressive behaviour:

> Modern psychological perspectives emphasise that aggressive and violent behaviours are learned responses to frustration, that they can also be learned as instruments for achieving goals, and that the learning occurs by observing models of such behaviour. Such models may be observed in the family, among peers, elsewhere in the neighbourhood, through the mass media...(Reiss and Roth 1993, p. 7).

Similarly, the 2002 World Health Organization report on violence concluded:

> The majority of young people who become violent are adolescent-limited offenders who, in fact, show little or no evidence of high levels of aggression or other problem behaviours during their childhood (Krug et al. 2002, p. 31).

This social learning view of the development of antisocial behaviour was very clearly described more than two centuries ago by Jean-Jacques Rousseau (1762/1979). The first phrase of his book on child development and education, *Émile*, makes the point very clearly: 'Everything is good as it leaves the hands of the Author of things; everything degenerates in the hands of man' (p. 37). A few pages later he is still more explicit and appears to be writing the agenda for twentieth-century research on the development of violent behaviour: 'There is no original sin in the human heart, the how and why of the entrance of every vice can be traced' (p. 56). Rousseau's strong stance was in clear opposition to Hobbes (1647/1998), who, a century earlier, described infants as selfish machines striving for pleasure and power, and declared:

> It is evident therefore that all men (since all men are born as infants) are born unfit for society; and very many (perhaps the majority) remain so throughout their lives, because of mental illness or lack of discipline...Therefore man is made fit for Society not by nature, but by training (p. 25).

This Hobbes–Rousseau debate concerning the developmental origin of antisocial behaviour has far-reaching consequences, not only for child development investigators and educators, but also for political scientists, philosophers, and policymakers. Because the underlying debate is clearly grounded in our views of human nature, it is not surprising that investigators are likely to prefer the 'origin of aggression' that best fit their view of human nature, and their political commitment. However, since most political philosophers appear to agree that society must be built on the natural tendencies of man, it is surprising that research on the early developmental origins of violence has not been a priority for the social sciences.

There is no doubt that physical aggression is a crucial component of human's behavioural heritage. Our ancestors needed to be skilled in the art of physical aggression to eat, to defend themselves against predators, to compete for mating, to protect their brood, and to acquire resources. However, like all other social animals, humans need to learn to use aggression sparingly because physically aggressive encounters can be fatal, and lack of self-control among social animals leads to social exclusion.

Because the life of citizens in developed countries today is very rarely dependent on physical aggression, we easily forget that the life of our ancestors was, in the words of Hobbes, 'solitary, poor, nasty, brutish and short' (Hobbes 1651/1999, p. 110). Historical analyses of homicide rates indicate that physical violence has systematically and substantially decreased among European citizens over the past 500 years (Eisner 2003). Homicides in European cities decreased from 40 to 1 per 100,000 citizens per year. We can conclude with Elias (1939) that the civilizing process has brought numerous advantages to humans, although, surprisingly, we often look back nostalgically to our primitive nature. Interestingly, the estimated rate of 'homicide' among our closest non-human relatives, chimpanzees, is 261 per 100,000 (Wrangham et al. 2006).

What is 'Physical Aggression'?

The simplest way to define 'physical aggression' is to follow the ethological approach and list the physical aggressions in agonistic encounters (Restoin et al. 1985). However, it is difficult to make a complete list of the multitude of means humans invented to physically hurt other humans. Examples of the most basic physical aggressions should be sufficient to make the concept clear: hitting, slapping, kicking, biting, pushing, grabbing, pulling, shoving, beating, twisting, choking. Some scales use terms such as fighting and bullying to summarize these behaviours. Threatening to physically aggress, use of objects and weapons to aggress is also included in the definition used by ethologists. In a playful context these behaviours are defined as playful aggression. For example, the Olympic Games reward humans who are best at the basic war-like behaviours of a 2-year-old: run, throw, hit, push, pull, etc. Thus an agonistic interaction context is needed to conclude that the behaviour is a physical aggression.

Chronic physical aggression can be defined as a tendency to use physical aggressions significantly more frequently than the large majority of a birth cohort over many years. Thus repeated assessments over many years (longitudinal studies) of random samples of a population birth cohort are needed to estimate the prevalence of chronic physical aggression during specific developmental periods. Such studies provide an opportunity to assess the different developmental trajectories of physical aggression in a population and estimate the proportion of individuals on a chronic trajectory (Nagin and Tremblay 1999).

In contrast, occasional physical aggression can be defined as the use of physical aggression at a rate that corresponds to the rate of a relatively large number of members in a population cohort. As will be described, the rate of physical aggression for the majority of members in a birth cohort varies substantially with age and subgroups of occasional physical aggression can be identified. However, risk factors that discriminate between chronic and occasional physical aggression are easier to identify than risk factors that discriminate subgroups of occasional physical aggression.

Development of Physical Aggression During Early Childhood

Studies of physical aggression during infancy have clearly shown that humans start to use physical aggression towards the end of the first year after birth when they have acquired the motor coordination to push, pull, hit, kick, etc. (Hay et al. 2011; Tremblay et al. 1999). The first population birth cohort to study the developmental trajectories of physical aggression from infancy onwards was the Québec Longitudinal Study of Child Development (Tremblay et al. 1999, 2004). Figure 5.1 illustrates the results of the physical aggression developmental trajectory analyses from 17 to 60 months with this birth cohort (Côté et al. 2007). We can see that half of the children are in the middle trajectory of physical

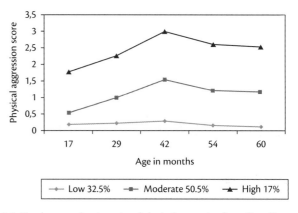

Fig. 5.1 Developmental trajectories of physical aggression from 17 to 60 months. Reproduced with permission from Côté, S. M. et al., The role of maternal education and non-maternal care services in the prevention of children's physical aggression, *Archives of General Psychiatry*, Volume 64, Issue 11, pp. 1305–12, Copyright © 2007 American Medical Association. All rights reserved.

aggression frequency, a third are on a low trajectory, while 17 per cent are on a high trajectory. Based on the earlier definition, we can consider the high trajectory as a chronic physical aggression trajectory and the two others as occasional physical aggression trajectories, while taking into account that the frequencies of aggressions varies depending on age.

These analyses are based on prospective repeated assessments of physical aggressions reported by mothers over many years. From this perspective developmental trajectories should be a better estimate of a chronic behaviour problem than an assessment at a given point in time, even if that assessment attempts to reconstruct past behaviour. Longitudinal data have shown that within a year mothers do not recall the age of onset of their children's physical aggressions (Tremblay 2000). In a clinical study of boys between 7 and 12 years of age, the mean age of physical aggression onset reported by parents was 6.75 years (Frick et al. 1993). Retrospective information collected in the Pittsburgh Youth Study (Loeber and Stouthamer-Loeber 1998) compared to prospective data is a good example of the problem with retrospective dating of physical aggression onset. The subjects ($N = 503$) represented the Pittsburgh public schools' male eighth graders and were close to 14 years old (mean age = 13.8; SD = 0.80) at the first data collection. The cumulative age of onset of physical aggressions reported by the mothers and the boys at that first data collection indicated that by age 5 years less than 5 per cent of the boys had initiated use of physical aggressions and almost no one had initiated fighting. In sharp contrast, the prospective data represented in Figure 5.1 on physical aggression from 17 months after birth indicate that children who do not initiate physical aggression before 3 years of age are extremely rare. These prospective studies suggest that the peak frequency in use of physical aggression for most humans is somewhere between 2 and 4 years of age (see Figure 5.2 and NICHD Early Child Care Research Network 2004). The recall problem suggests that retrospective assessments of children or adolescents cannot identify the age of onset and developmental trajectories of physical aggression use or of chronic physical aggression (chronic physical aggression). Hence the conclusion reached by the World Health Organization report on Violence (Krug et al. 2002) as previously cited needs to be updated.

Developmental Trajectories of Physical Aggression after Early Childhood

The developmental trajectories of physical aggression after early childhood have now been studied in many different cultures. From these studies we can expect between 7 per cent and 11 per cent of elementary school children to be on a chronic physical aggression trajectory (Broidy et al. 2003; Campbell et al. 2010; Nagin and Tremblay 1999). That percentage tends to be higher for preschool children (Côté et al. 2007; Tremblay et al. 2004) and lower for adolescents (Brame et al. 2001). This decrease in chronic physical aggression cases with age corresponds to the general decrease in frequency of physical aggression with age after the peak in early childhood (see Figure 5.2 from Tremblay and Côté 2009).

Most children use physical aggression during the preschool years, but most children also learn to use alternatives to physical aggression with age, and this applies to a number of chronic cases during early childhood and preadolescence (Nagin and Tremblay 1999). In fact there is good evidence that the learning process to gain control over physical aggression continues throughout adulthood (Sampson and Laub 2003).

Crime records from the middle ages to modern times suggest that this phenomenon is not new. The likelihood of committing a homicide and most other crimes has always decreased from late adolescence and early adulthood to old age (Eisner 2003). Trajectories of physical aggression covering different age periods (early childhood to childhood, childhood to adolescence, adolescence to adulthood) also indicate that chronic physical aggression very rarely onsets after early childhood (NICHD Early Child Care Research Network 2004; van Lier et al. 2009).

Outcomes of Chronic Physical Aggression Trajectories During Childhood

Longitudinal studies of physical aggression trajectories during childhood have been used to study how well they predict future outcomes such as school performance, social adjustment, mental health, and violent behaviour. The first longitudinal study to describe developmental trajectories of physical aggression from school entry to adolescence (Nagin and Tremblay 1999) reported that boys on a teacher-rated high trajectory of physical aggression from 6 to 15 years of age were at highest risk of self-reported violence as well as other forms of delinquency at 17 years of age, even after having controlled for hyperactivity and oppositional behaviour. The chronically aggressive boys were also at highest risk of school drop-out. A study which used six longitudinal studies from Canada, New Zealand, and the United States (Broidy et al. 2003) reached the same conclusion for male adolescent violent delinquency, but not for female adolescent violent delinquency. The authors attributed the sex difference in prediction to the fact that the prevalence of female adolescent violent delinquency was too low. However, a later analysis of one of the female samples (Fontaine et al. 2008) reported that elementary school girls who were on a chronic physical aggression trajectory combined with a chronic hyperactivity trajectory were more likely than others to report physical and psychological aggression towards intimate partners by age 21 years. They were also more likely to report early pregnancy, welfare assistance, nicotine use problems, and low educational attainment. A more recent analysis of a population sample of males and females (Pingault et al. 2013) reported that the 9.5 per cent of children on a high physical aggression trajectory between 6 and 12 years, according to mother and teacher rating, represented 28.2 per cent of all those who had a criminal record by age 24 years. In addition, they represented 45.9 per cent of all recorded criminal charges and 57.4 per cent of the violence charges. Therefore, children on a high trajectory of physical aggression during elementary school are not only more likely to have a criminal record but also to have more criminal charges. There is evidence that the criminal outcomes of childhood physical aggression during adolescence and adulthood are preceded by a large range of negative social and academic outcomes by the end of elementary school for boys and girls (Campbell et al. 2010).

Early Risk Factors and Prevention of Chronic Physical Aggression Trajectories

Sex of the child is one of the most important risk factors for chronic physical aggression. When children start using physical aggression at the end of the first year after birth there are no significant differences in frequency of physical aggressions between boys and

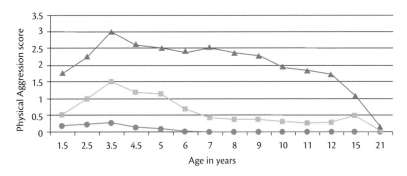

Fig. 5.2 Trajectories of physical aggression from infancy to adulthood.

Reproduced from Tremblay, R. E. and Côté, S. M., Development of sex differences in physical aggression: the maternal link to epigenetic mechanisms, *Behavioral and Brain Sciences*, 32, Volume 32, Issue 3–4, pp. 290–1, Copyright © 2009, with permission from Cambridge University Press, <http://dx.doi.org/10.1017/S0140525X09990200>.

girls (Hay et al. 2011); however, the differences appear soon after and increase until adolescence (e.g. Côté 2007). Between 10 and 15 years of age boys are close to 20 times (OR = 18.84) more at risk than girls of being on a chronic physical aggression trajectory (van Lier et al. 2009).

Twin studies have become important tools to understand the contributions of environmental and genetic factors in the development of human characteristics, including aggression. However, to date there appears to be only one longitudinal study that used a large sample of twins from infancy onwards to study the contributions of genetic and environmental factors in the development of aggression. The study reported that 19 months after birth 58 per cent of the variance in frequency of physical aggression rated by mothers could be attributed to genetic contributions and 42 per cent to common environmental contributions (Dionne et al. 2003). Physical aggression at 72 months after birth was rated by kindergarten teachers and genetic contribution to variance in frequency was estimated to be 66 per cent with 34 per cent attributed to common environmental factors (van Lier et al. 2007).

Although these results suggest a substantial contribution of genetic factors in the use of physical aggression from infancy to school entry, environmental factors are also very important. The developmental trajectories of physical aggression previously described indicate that the environmental conditions are essential to learn alternatives to physical aggression during early childhood. Studies of physical aggression trajectories during early childhood with singletons have identified the following types of environmental risk factors: (i) Maternal characteristics, including life style and mental health; (ii) family characteristics; (iii) maternal parenting; (iv) child characteristics (Campbell et al. 2010; Côté et al. 2006; Hay et al. 2011; NICHD Early Child Care Research Network 2004; Tremblay et al. 2004).

Maternal and family characteristics are key for planning preventive interventions because they can be used to identify pregnant women at risk of having children on a chronic physical aggression trajectory (e.g. Olds et al. 1998). The maternal characteristics identified include mothers' young age at birth of their child, mothers' smoking during pregnancy, mothers' antisocial behaviour during adolescence, mothers' depression, and mothers' low level of education. Family characteristics include low income, family dysfunction, and the presence of siblings. High-risk maternal parenting behaviours include mothers' hostile–coercive–harsh parenting and lack of sensitivity. Finally, as expected, boys were found to be at higher risk than girls of being on the chronic physical aggression trajectory.

It is important to note that these studies of environmental risk factors were not done in the context of a genetically informative design (e.g. twin studies or sibling studies), hence we do not know to what extent the significant environmental risk factors are correlated or interact with genetic factors (Szyf et al. 2009). Nonetheless, the environmental risk factors identified by these studies can be used to identify at-risk groups for preventive experiments. Such experiments are useful to test the effectiveness of the interventions as well as test causal hypotheses (Tremblay 2003). Maternal and family characteristics are especially key for early preventive interventions because they can be used to identify at-risk pregnant women (e.g. Olds et al. 1998).

The challenge for the future is to integrate preventive experiments within genetically informative longitudinal studies of risk factors. The discovery of environmental effects on gene expression (epigenetics) is providing the tools to meet this challenge (Tremblay 2010).

The term 'epigenetic' refers to the mechanisms which programme genes and can change gene function without modifying gene sequence, mainly through changes in DNA methylation and chromatin structure. This programming is responsive to environmental effects, especially during foetal and early post-natal development. Thus, environments can impact phenotypes through their chemical impact on programming of gene function (Szyf et al. 2009). Epigenetic effects are well known in cancer research and have recently been shown to possibly explain the obesity epidemic and behaviour regulation (Meaney and Szyf 2005; Szyf et al. 2009).

Epigenetic studies focus specifically on the physical effects of the environment on gene expression at a given moment in time. The classic example for effects of neglectful environments comes from an experimental study of maternal behaviour in rats which showed that rat pups insufficiently licked by their mothers in the days following birth (i.e. neglected) have increased methylation of the gene encoding the glucocorticoid receptor in the hippocampus, resulting in reduced expression (Weaver et al. 2004). The study further showed that this gene methylation effect had downstream effects on the hypothalamic–pituitary–adrenal axis, which regulates stress responses in the body.

Epigenetic mechanisms are especially important because they provide a powerful explanation for early maternal and family effects on the development of physical and mental health problems, including chronic physical aggression. Furthermore, DNA methylation changes over time can be used as markers of environmental effects during development, including assessment of preventive and corrective intervention effects.

This discussion of early risk factors has shown that trajectories of chronic physical aggression are specifically related to maternal characteristics: maternal age at first pregnancy, history of behaviour problems, education, smoking, depression, coercive parenting, etc. This can easily be understood from the traditional environmental perspective: a poor early environment has an impact on the developing foetus and infant. Mother characteristics turn out to be more important risk factors than father characteristics because the former carry the child in their womb during foetal life and are more involved in care giving during early childhood. However, the exact bio-psycho-social mechanisms linking poor quality environment to disorganized behaviour remain unclear, to say the least.

The epigenetic story provides a basic mechanism that has the advantage of being parsimonious, testable, and promising for prevention. The most fascinating aspect of this mechanism is that it provides an environmentally based explanation of intergenerational transmission for physical and mental disorders which involves genes but is not genetically transmitted. These mechanisms are still far from being clearly understood, but they provide a challenging alternative perspective to the traditional gene vs. environment and gene–environment interaction hypotheses.

The first epigenetic study of children with chronic physical aggression (Wang et al. 2012) used subjects from the longitudinal study of boys living in low socio-economic environments described previously (Nagin and Tremblay 1999; Tremblay et al. 1994). Blood was collected from two groups of the boys when they were 27 years old to assess DNA methylation patterns (in monocytes and T cells) of the serotonin transporter (5-HT). The first group included boys who were on a high trajectory of physical aggression during childhood. The second group included boys who were on a normal trajectory of physical aggression. Brain imaging of serotonin synthesis was also obtained from the same boys around age 27 years. We found that chronic physical aggression during childhood was associated with increased DNA methylation in specific CpG sites in monocytes and T cells of the serotonin transporter gene. Interestingly, we also found associations between measures of serotonin synthesis in the brain and differential DNA methylation in T cells and monocytes in the same CpG sites that revealed association with chronic physical aggression during childhood. These findings are the first evidence of the association between environmentally related differences in DNA methylation in white blood cells and *in vivo* measures of 5-HT in the living human brain. Experimental studies with rats and monkeys which started at birth (e.g. Weaver et al. 2004) are suggesting that the associations between DNA methylation and aggression observed in humans were caused by perinatal environmental effects.

Conclusions

The available data on the development of physical aggression from early childhood to adulthood lead to the following conclusions: (i) the vast majority of humans have used physical aggression; (ii) the vast majority of humans also learn with age to use means of solving problems other than the use of physical aggression; (iii) some need more time than others to learn; (iv) females learn more quickly than males; (v) by adolescence not much more than 5 per cent of males can be considered cases of chronic physical aggression, while female cases are exceptional; (vi) most of the chronic physical aggression cases during adolescence were on a chronic physical aggression trajectory since early childhood; (vii) since most humans used physical aggression and learned alternatives during childhood, most adults are at risk of using physical aggression if in a given situation it appears to be the 'best' solution to the problem. Thus, to continue to reduce the incidence of physical aggression among humans, societies need to implement effective situational preventive strategies as well as effective early preventive interventions of chronic physical aggression. The latter preventive approach will benefit from our new understanding of environmental effects on gene expression during pregnancy and early childhood.

References

Bandura, A. (1977). *Social Learning Theory*. Englewood Cliffs, NJ: Prentice Hall Inc.

Brame, B., Nagin, D. S., and Tremblay, R. E. (2001). Developmental trajectories of physical aggression from school entry to late adolescence. *The Journal of Child Psychology and Psychiatry*, 42, 503–12.

Broidy, L. M., Nagin, D.S., and Tremblay, R. E. et al. (2003). Developmental trajectories of childhood disruptive behaviors and adolescent delinquency: a six site, cross national study. *Developmental Psychology*, 39, 222–45.

Campbell, S. B., Spieker, S., Vandergrift, N., Belsky, J., and Burchinal, M. (2010). Predictors and sequelae of trajectories of physical aggression in school-age boys and girls. *Development and Psychopathology*, 22, 133–50.

Côté, S. M. (2007). Sex differences in physical and indirect aggression: a developmental perspective. *European Journal of Criminal Policy Research*, 13, 183–200.

Côté, S. M., Boivin, M., and Nagin, D. S. et al. (2007). The role of maternal education and non-maternal care services in the prevention of children's physical aggression. *Archives of General Psychiatry*, 64, 1305–12.

Côté, S. M., Vaillancourt, T., LeBlanc, J. C., Nagin, D. S., and Tremblay R. E. (2006). The development of physical aggression from toddlerhood to pre-adolescence: a nation wide longitudinal study of Canadian children. *Journal of Abnormal Child Psychology*, 34, 71–85.

Dionne, G., Tremblay, R., Boivin, M., Laplante, D., and Pérusse, D. (2003). Physical aggression and expressive vocabulary in 19 month-old twins. *Developmental Psychology*, 39, 261–73.

Eisner, M. (2003). Long-term historical trends in violent crime. In: M. Tonry (ed.), *Crime and Justice: A Review of Research*. Chicago, IL: University of Chicago Press, pp. 83–142.

Elias, N. (1939). *The Civilizing Process: The History of Manners*. New York, N.Y.: Blackwell Publishing.

Fontaine, N., Carbonneau, R., and Barker, E. D., et al. (2008). Girls' hyperactivity and physical aggression during childhood and adjustment problems in early adulthood. *Archives of General Psychiatry*, 65, 320–8.

Frick, P. J., Lahey, B. B., and Loeber, R. et al. (1993). Oppositional defiant disorder and conduct disorder: a meta-analytic review of factor-analyses and cross-validation in a clinic sample. *Clinical Psychology Review*, 13, 319–40.

Hay, D. F., Mundy, L., and Roberts S., et al. (2011). Known risk factors for violence predict 12-month-old infants' aggressiveness with peers. *Psychological Science*, 22, 1205–11.

Hobbes, T. (1647/1998). *De Cive: On the Citizen*. New York, NY: Cambridge University Press.

Hobbes, T. (1651/1999). *Leviathan*. Renascence Editions, University of Oregon. Available at: https://scholarsbank.uoregon.edu/xmlui/bitstream/handle/1794/748/leviathan.pdf?sequence=1 [Accessed 19 November 2013].

Krug, E. G. Dahlberg, L. L Mercy, J. A., Zwi, A. B., and Lozano, R. (2002). *World Report on Violence and Health*. Geneva: World Health Organization. Available at: http://www.who.int/violence_injury_prevention/violence/world_report/en/ [Accessed 19 November 2013].

Loeber, R., and Stouthamer-Loeber, M. (1998). Development of juvenile aggression and violence. Some common misconceptions and controversies. *American Psychologist*, 53, 242–59.

Meaney, M. J., and Szyf, M. (2005). Maternal care as a model for experience-dependent chromatin plasticity? *Trends in Neurosciences*, 28, 456–63.

Nagin, D., and Tremblay, R. E. (1999). Trajectories of boys' physical aggression, opposition, and hyperactivity on the path to physically violent and nonviolent juvenile delinquency. *Child Development*, 70, 1181–96.

NICHD Early Child Care Research Network (2004). Trajectories of physical aggression from toddlerhood to middle school: predictors, correlates, and outcomes. *SRCD Monographs*, 69, 1–146.

Olds, D., Henderson, C. R. Jr, and Cole, R. et al. (1998). Long-term effects of nurse home visitation on children's criminal and antisocial behavior: 15-year follow-up of a randomized controlled trial. *Journal of the American Medical Association*, 280, 1238–44.

Pingault, J.-B., Côté, S. M., Lacourse, E., Galera, C., Vitaro, F., and Tremblay, R. E. (2013). Childhood hyperactivity, physical aggression and criminality: a 19 year prospective population-based study. *PLoS One*, 8, 1–7.

Reiss, A. J., and Roth, J. A. (1993). *Understanding and Preventing Violence*. Washington, DC: National Academy Press.

Restoin, A., Montagner, H., and Rodriguez, D. et al. (1985). Chronologie des comportements de communication et profils de comportement chez le jeune enfant. In: R. E. Tremblay, M. A. Provost, and F. F. Strayer (eds), *Ethologie et Développement de L'enfant*. Paris: Editions Stock/Laurence Pernoud, pp. 93–130.

Rousseau, J.-J. (1762/1979). *Emile or On Education*. New York: Basic Books.

Sampson, R. J., and Laub, J.H. (2003). Life-course desisters? Trajectories of crime among delinquent boys followed to age 70. *Criminology*, 41, 555–92.

Szyf, M., Weaver, I., Provencal, N., McGowan, P. O., Tremblay, R. E., and Meany, M. J. (2009). Epigenetics and behaviour. In: R. E. Tremblay, M. A. G. van Aken, and W. Koops (eds), *Development and Prevention of Behaviour Problems: From Genes to Social Policy*. Sussex, United Kingdom: Psychology Press, pp. 25–59.

Tremblay, R. E. (2000). The origins of youth violence (ISUMA). *Canadian Journal of Policy Research*, 1, 19–24.

Tremblay, R. E. (2003). Why socialization fails? The case of chronic physical aggression. In: B. B. Lahey, T. E. Moffitt, and A. Caspi (eds), *Causes of Conduct Disorder and Juvenile Delinquency*. New York: Guilford Publications, pp. 182–224.

Tremblay, R. E. (2010). Developmental origins of disruptive behaviour problems: The 'original sin' hypothesis, epigenetics and their consequences for prevention. *Journal of Child Psychology and Psychiatry*, 51, 341–67.

Tremblay, R. E. and Côté, S. M. (2009). Development of sex differences in physical aggression: the maternal link to epigenetic mechanisms [comment]. *Behavioral and Brain Sciences*, 32, 290–1.

Tremblay, R. E., Japel, C., and Perusse, D. et al. (1999). The search for the age of 'onset' of physical aggression: Rousseau and Bandura revisited. *Criminal Behavior and Mental Health*, 9, 8–23.

Tremblay, R. E., Nagin, D. S., and Séguin, J. R. et al. (2004). Physical aggression during early childhood: trajectories and predictors. *Pediatrics*, 114, e43–50.

Tremblay, R. E., Pihl, R. O., Vitaro, F., and Dobkin, P. L. (1994). Predicting early-onset of male antisocial-behavior from preschool behavior. *Archives of General Psychiatry*, 51, 732–39.

van Lier, P., Boivin, M., and Dionne, G. et al. (2007). Kindergarten children's genetic vulnerabilities interact with friends' aggression to promote children's own aggression. *Journal of the American Academy of Child and Adolescent Psychiatry*, 46, 1080–7.

van Lier, P. A., Vitaro, F., Barker E. D., Koot, H. M., and Tremblay R. E. (2009). Developmental links between trajectories of physical violence, vandalism, theft, and alcohol-drug use from childhood to adolescence. *Journal of Abnormal Child Psychology*, 37, 481–92.

Wang, D., Szyf, M., and Benkelfat, C. et al. (2012). Peripheral SLC6A4 DNA methylation is associated with in vivo measures of human brain serotonin synthesis and childhood physical aggression. *PLoS ONE*, 7, 1–8.

Weaver, I. C., Cervoni, N., and Champagne, F. A. et al. (2004). Epigenetic programming by maternal behavior. *Nature Neuroscience*, 7, 847–54.

Wrangham, R. W., Wilson, M. L., and Muller, M. N. (2006). Comparative rates of violence in chimpanzees and humans. *Primates*, 47, 14–26.

Zimbardo, P. G. (2007). *The Lucifer Effect: Understanding How Good People Turn Evil* New York, N.Y.: Random House.

CHAPTER 6

The epidemiology of intimate partner violence

Heidi Stöckl, Karen Devries, and Charlotte Watts

Introduction to the Epidemiology of Intimate Partner Violence

Violence against women in its many forms has been recognized as a highly prevalent human rights and public health issue (García-Moreno and Stöckl 2009). Over the last 20 years there has been a recognizable increase in the research on the prevalence of violence against women, especially intimate partner violence.

While the number of studies on the prevalence of intimate partner violence and its social costs and long-term effects, such as child maltreatment and economic costs, has increased over the past decade, there has been less research on the health effects of exposures to different forms of intimate partner violence (Krug et al. 2002). Existing literature nevertheless suggests that intimate partner violence might lead to a wide range of potential health effects, including physical, sexual, reproductive, and mental health problems. The pathways linking intimate partner violence with adverse health outcomes are known to be both direct, through injuries resulting from the violent acts, and indirect, through increased stress, reduced mobility, and limited access to resources and healthcare. For example, sustained and acute elevated stress levels, often an immediate and long-term consequence of intimate partner violence, have been linked to cardiovascular disease, hypertension, gastrointestinal disorders, chronic pain, and the development of insulin-dependent diabetes (Miller 1998). In addition, some women also try to manage the stress and trauma caused by intimate partner violence through the use of alcohol, prescription medication, tobacco, or other drugs (Campbell 2002). Intimate partner violence is therefore of critical importance, not only in its own right, but also in terms of its long-term implications for the burden of disease.

This chapter presents an overview of the body of scientific data on the prevalence of intimate partner violence experienced by women and its risk and protective factors, providing additional information on intimate partner violence during pregnancy and intimate partner homicide.

Intimate Partner Violence around the World

The 1993 Declaration on the Elimination of Violence against Women defined violence against women as;

any act of gender-based violence that results in, or is likely to result in, physical, sexual or psychological harm or suffering to women, including threats of such acts, coercion or arbitrary deprivation of liberty, whether occurring in public or in private life (United Nations General Assembly 1993).

Intimate partner violence, as one form of violence against women, has been defined as physical, sexual, emotional, or economic abuse, including controlling behaviour committed by an intimate partner. The definition of intimate partner also includes same-sex partners. While emotional abuse, often defined as being humiliated, insulted, intimidated or threatened and controlling behaviours (including not being allowed to see friends or family) is also known to significantly impact the well-being and health of women (Coker et al. 2000; Jewkes 2010), a lack of agreement on standard definitions and measures means that the evidence for this particular form of intimate partner violence is still patchy. Most of the existing research on intimate partner violence is therefore still focused on physical and sexual intimate partner violence.

Intimate partner violence surveys commonly measure physical violence through asking participants if they have ever (life-time prevalence), or in the last year, experienced at least one act of physical violence. Acts of physical violence typically listed range from being slapped or pushed to being choked or having a gun, knife, or other weapon used on them. Acts of sexual violence often capture experiences such as being physically forced to have sexual intercourse to being forced to do something sexual that they found humiliating or degrading.

The 2012 Global Burden of Disease study included intimate partner violence as a risk factor for poor health in women (Devries et al. 2013; Lim et al. 2013). Estimates for men were not computed because of a lack of global data about health effects. In brief, to estimate the global prevalence rates for women, a systematic review of the existing literature was conducted; inclusion criteria were representative population-based studies with prevalence estimates for intimate partner violence among ever-partnered women aged 15 years or older; these criteria identified 250 studies. In addition, analyses of four major multi-site surveys that included questions on intimate partner violence were conducted. In total, data from 141 studies in 81 countries were entered into a random effects meta-regression that was fitted to produce prevalence estimates for all Global Burden of Disease regions and age groups, as well as global estimates. These estimates for intimate partner violence were corrected for differences in definitions of violence, time periods of measurement, severity of violence, and whether a study was national or sub-national. The global prevalence of lifetime exposure to physical or sexual intimate partner violence, or both, among all ever-partnered women worldwide, established by the Global Burden of Disease study, was 30.0 per cent (95 per cent CI 27.8 per cent to 32.2 per cent) (Devries et al. 2013).

Variations by Region

Regional breakdowns of the prevalence of intimate partner violence showed that the prevalence was highest in the WHO (World Health Organization) Southeast Asian, Eastern Mediterranean, and African regions. In these three regions, approximately 37 per cent of ever-partnered women reported that they had experienced intimate partner violence at some point in their life. In the Americas approximately 30 per cent of women reported lifetime experiences of intimate partner violence, while the prevalence was around 25 per cent in all other regions (see Table 6.1 for details) (Devries et al. 2013).

Variations by Age

A further variation is the prevalence rates of intimate partner violence among ever-partnered women across different age groups. The findings in Table 6.2 show that prevalence rates only vary slightly by age, with young women having nearly the same exposure rates to intimate partner violence as older women (Devries et al. 2013). This suggests that intimate partner violence commonly starts early in women's relationships.

Intimate Partner Violence during Pregnancy

Because of its health consequences for both the mother and the unborn child, research on intimate partner violence in the last decade has paid special attention to the time of pregnancy. Three multisite surveys—the Demographic and Health Survey (DHS Survey) (Devries et al. 2010), the International Violence against Women Survey (Devries et al. 2010), and the WHO Multicountry Study on domestic violence against women (WHO Study) (García-Moreno et al. 2005) investigated the prevalence of physical intimate partner violence in different countries. The three

Table 6.1 Percentage prevalence of lifetime experiences of physical and/or sexual violence from a partner by WHO region

WHO Region	Prevalence (%)	95% Confidence Intervals
High-income countries	23.2	20.2–26.2
Africa	36.6	32.7–40.5
Americas	29.8	25.8–33.9
Eastern Mediterranean	37.0	30.9–43.1
Europe	25.4	20.9–30.0
Western Pacific	24.6	20.1–29.0
Southeast Asia	37.7	32.8–42.6
Global	26.4	23.6–29.3

Source: data from Devries, K. M. et al., The global prevalence of intimate partner violence against women, *Science*, Volume 340, Number 6104, pp. 1527–8, Copyright © 2013 American Association for the Advancement of Science. All Rights Reserved.

Table 6.2 Intimate partner violence: global prevalence by age group among ever-partnered women

Age Group	Prevalence (%)	95% Confidence Intervals
15–19	24.2	21.5–26.9
20–24	26.8	24.3–29.3
25–29	27.8	25.3–30.3
30–34	26.8	24.3–29.2
35–39	25.8	22.5–29.1
40–44	27.9	23.0–32.7
45–49	25.1	22.6–27.6
50–54	27.1	19.9–34.4
55–59	20.1	10.4–29.9
60–64	21.4	11.0–31.9
65–69	19.1	14.4–23.8

Source: data from Devries, K. M. et al., The global prevalence of intimate partner violence against women, *Science*, Volume 340, Number 6104, pp. 1527–8, Copyright © 2013 American Association for the Advancement of Science. All Rights Reserved.

surveys found the lifetime prevalence of physical intimate partner violence during pregnancy to range between 1 per cent in urban Japan to 28 per cent in rural Peru; with the majority of surveys estimating a prevalence between 4 and 12 per cent (Devries et al. 2010; García-Moreno et al. 2005). In these surveys higher prevalence rates emerged in Latin American and African countries, with lower rates reported in the surveyed European and Asian countries (Devries et al. 2010).

The WHO Study on domestic violence against women further found that intimate partner violence during pregnancy is often conducted with the clear aim to also harm the unborn baby, as between 23 per cent (rural Tanzania) and up to 52 per cent (rural Peru) of women who experienced physical intimate partner violence during pregnancy reported that their partner punched or kicked them in the abdomen (García-Moreno et al. 2005).

In addition to population-based surveys, numerous surveys have been conducted in antenatal care clinics around the world for which no representative data are available. These surveys yield substantially higher rates. For example, a systematic review of antenatal care studies from Africa found prevalence rates of 23–40 per cent for physical, 3–27 per cent for sexual, and 25–49 per cent for emotional, intimate partner violence during pregnancy (Shamu et al. 2011).

Intimate Partner Homicide

Another way of capturing intimate partner violence is to examine its most serious outcome—homicide. The Global Burden of Disease study also estimated the prevalence of intimate partner homicide across the world. In addition to a systematic literature review, it also consisted of a survey of relevant homepages of country statistics offices, Ministries of Justice, Home offices, or Police Headquarters of the 169 WHO listed countries. If no information was found, the respective agencies were contacted via email. In total 227 different studies and statistics were found, capturing 1,122 estimates across 66 countries from 1982 to 2011 (Stöckl et al. 2013).

Findings of this study suggest that the overall median percentage of homicides committed by an intimate partner is above 13 per cent, with a median above 38 per cent for female homicides having been perpetrated by an intimate partner while the median proportion for men was 6 per cent. Given the high number of homicides (approximately 20 per cent) for which the victim–offender relationship is not known, it can be assumed that the results presented are conservative and that the true prevalence is much higher (Stöckl et al. 2013).

Regional differences emerged as well. One of the most striking differences was the relatively high number of studies on intimate partner homicide in high-income countries and the lack of information, especially on male intimate partner homicide, in other regions of the world. The overall median percentage of intimate partner homicides among murdered women was above 58 per cent in the Southeast Asia region, above 40 per cent in high-income countries and the African region, and above 38 per cent in the Americas. Percentages were lower in the Western Pacific region with 19 per cent, the lower and middle-income European region with 20 per cent, and the Eastern Mediterranean region with 14 per cent (Stöckl et al. 2013).

Among male homicides, the overall median percentage of intimate partner homicide was highest in high-income countries with more than 6 per cent, the African region with 4 per cent, and the lower and middle income European Region with more than 3 per cent. In all other regions the median percentages were less than 2 per cent (Stöckl et al. 2013).

Risk, Protective, and Maintaining Factors

This section provides an overview of the evidence for factors associated with intimate partner violence, relying chiefly on risk factor analyses using multi-country surveys of low, middle, and high income settings in Africa, Asia, Europe, Australia, and America. These studies include analyses based on the WHO Study (Abramsky et al. 2011), the DHS Survey (Hindin et al. 2008), the World Safe study (Jeyaseelan et al. 2004), and a macro analysis of more than 50 countries (Kaya and Cook 2010).

The risk, protective, and maintaining factors for intimate partner violence are presented by the strength of existing evidence. Risk and protective factors that have been measured with agreed and standardized measures and that received support across a number of settings are presented before factors that are built on less conclusive support.

Several important methodological limitations issues have to be taken into account when interpreting these risk and protective factors. As most risk and protective factor analyses on intimate partner violence are based on cross-sectional survey data it is often impossible to distinguish if certain associations are outcomes of, causes of, or merely associated with, intimate partner violence. Also, risk for violence is multi-causal and probabilistic rather than deterministic. Having a certain risk factor therefore only means that a person is more likely to experience intimate partner violence, not that every person with that risk factor will experience intimate partner violence. Apart from examining the influence of individual risk factors for intimate partner violence,

more needs to be understood about the influence of risk factors combined within one woman for her risk of intimate partner violence. A distinction also needs to be made between individual risk and protective factors, and population-based factors, as, for example, individual levels of drinking might increase a particular woman's risk of intimate partner violence, while population-based drinking levels might be irrelevant to her specific risk of experiencing intimate partner violence. Unless stated otherwise, the risk and protective factors outlined in this chapter refer to individual and not population-based analyses. Last, while there might be a connection between a risk factor and intimate partner violence, the association may in reality be indirectly through an unmeasured factor associated with both intimate partner violence and the measured risk factor, rather than the direct association of the two.

Alcohol

Men's alcohol use and abuse has been identified as a clear risk factor by a number of studies worldwide, including the WHO Study (Abramsky et al. 2011), the DHS Survey (Hindin et al. 2008), and the World Safe study (Jeyaseelan et al. 2004), as well as two systematic reviews investigating its association (Foran and O'Leary 2008; Gil-Gonzalez et al. 2006). A recent systematic review of longitudinal studies has also shown a relationship between women's alcohol use and intimate partner violence victimization (Devries et al. 2014). Several pathways may explain the connection between alcohol abuse and intimate partner violence. One potential pathway is that alcohol abuse and intimate partner violence are associated because of other factors related to both drinking and intimate partner violence, such as young age or low socioeconomic status. Another potential pathway builds on the knowledge that alcohol abuse is detrimental for relationship quality as it promotes counterproductive argument styles and aggressive or violent responses, in addition to the higher levels of aggression alcohol use causes due to inference with cognitive abilities (DeMaris et al. 2004; Klostermann and Fals-Stewart 2006).

Childhood Experiences of Violence

Another risk factor that emerged in nearly all countries of the WHO Study and the DHS Survey (Abramsky et al. 2011; Hindin et al. 2008), and which has also been verified by several longitudinal studies in high-income countries (Fergusson et al. 2006; Moffitt and Caspi 1999), is women's and their partner's experiences of abuse during childhood. Experiences of childhood abuse can range from corporal punishment, child sexual abuse, to witnessing parental violence. In more than 10 of the sites the WHO multi-country study the risk for intimate partner violence was especially high when both the woman and her partner were abused in childhood (Abramsky et al. 2011). Social learning theory suggests several connections between childhood experiences of abuse and intimate partner violence. One connection is that children model parental behaviour—children who observe their parents dealing with difficult situations through violence on a regular basis are more likely to perceive violence as an effective conflict solving strategy, and they might lack alternative models of conflict solution. Another connection is that experiences of violence disrupt children's attachment process which impairs their ability to distinguish between love and violence (Renner and Slack 2006). Both connections can influence these children's later choice of partners, and they may be more likely to choose violent partners (Tolan et al. 2006).

Unfavourable Gender and Violence Norms and Attitudes

Despite the difficulties in measurement, unfavourable gender attitudes, especially those that entail being supportive of wife beating, emerged as another clear risk factor for intimate partner violence, in the WHO Study (Abramsky et al. 2011), in the DHS Survey (Hindin et al. 2008), and in a representative analysis of eight African countries (Andersson et al. 2007). Underlying explanations for these associations can be derived from feminist and gender role theories, which maintain that the patriarchal nature of society promotes violence against women by socializing women and men into predefined roles. While women are often educated to be nurturing and understanding, men are socialized to be successful and dominant breadwinners (Fernández 2006). Intimate partner violence can occur if men feel threatened in their role by their partner's demands or gains of more equality, and if they feel their authority, masculinity or control is diminished (Jewkes et al. 2003). Ideas of empowerment and liberal behaviour might thereby increase levels of violence for women whose surroundings consider these ideas or behaviour as deviant and punishable, or in relationships where women have a higher status in society than their partner. This implies that until full gender equality is achieved, women who behave traditionally are in less danger of experiencing intimate partner violence, since they behave according to their roles and do not challenge masculine identities (Pallitto and O'Campo 2005).

Relationship Status and Quality

Relationship status and quality is measured by several indicators, the most prominent being marital status, relationship duration, or number of children. While a few studies, including a few sites in the WHO study (Abramsky et al. 2011), found higher rates of intimate partner violence among cohabiting women, other population-based studies established that short relationship duration or relationship dissatisfaction increases women's risk of experiencing intimate partner violence (Karamagi et al. 2006; Stöckl et al. 2011). Social exchange theory explains these associations with its claim that intimate partner violence occurs when partners believe that the costs of violence are lower than the expected rewards, such as increased power and dominance. Potential costs include the reduction in relationship quality and the chance that the abused will retaliate, call the police, or end the relationship (Williams 1992). Abusive partners perceive these costs as smaller if they are sure of their dominant physical, psychological, and economic position in the relationship or if they are less committed to the relationship, marked by cohabiting status or short relationship duration. In addition, it has been argued that cohabiting couples are more likely to have arguments about the boundaries of their relationships, which can lead to stress and trigger violence (Gelles 2007).

Children can be both a risk and a protective factor for intimate partner violence. Children might be perceived as a risk factor if they tie women to an abusive partner economically or through the belief that it is important for children to grow up with a father under any circumstance. However, children can also improve relationships by encouraging appropriate behaviour in front of them and by reducing couples' social isolation through connecting parents to schools, neighbours, and broader social networks (Hoffman et al. 1994).

Education, Employment, and Age

As with children, women's education can be both a risk and a protective factor for intimate partner violence. In the WHO study and the DHS survey, women's, and especially both women's and their partner's, higher levels of education versus low or no levels of education were protective against intimate partner violence, as was women's employment and low income (Abramsky et al. 2011; Hindin et al. 2008). Furthermore, countries with high female secondary school enrolment and countries with high female labour force participation in non-agricultural sectors also had lower prevalence rates of last-year physical intimate partner violence (Kaya and Cook 2010). However, there are also some studies, for example a national representative survey study from Germany, which found that high levels of education increased women's risk of experiencing intimate partner violence (Stöckl et al. 2011).

These associations are best explained by the resource and the relative resource theories. These theories claim that abusive partners use violence because other resources, including education, employment, job prestige, income, or community standing, are unavailable to them or fail to allow them to achieve dominance and power in their relationships (Goode 1971). The protective aspects of education and employment against intimate partner violence for women include the increased access to wider social networks, information, and support women receive in the pursuit of higher levels of education, and the resultant improved confidence and bargaining position in their relationship. However, in societies with rigid gender roles and in relationships where the woman commands more of these resources than their partners, they might also serve as risk factors for intimate partner violence (McMullan 2007).

Closely linked to the argument on education and employment is young age as a risk factor for intimate partner violence, as couples who form a union early are more likely to have early pregnancies and more children, which in turn increases their likelihood to suffer employment instability and financial difficulties (DeMaris et al. 2004). Young age has been found to be associated with intimate partner violence in a number of countries (Abramsky et al. 2011; Hindin et al. 2008).

Women's Social and Wider Surroundings

While there is a clear theoretical explanation for the influence of women's social and wider surroundings for intimate partner violence, there are few tangible measures and empirical studies providing support for them. Factors that are frequently investigated suggest that living in an urban or rural area is significantly associated with intimate partner violence, for example in Uganda and South Africa (Jewkes et al. 2003; Karamagi et al. 2006), and that having a partner who is involved in fights with other men or women's experience of non-partner violence, increase women's risk of intimate partner violence (Abramsky et al. 2011; Stöckl et al. 2011); in Germany, women's social isolation is a risk factor for increased intimate partner violence (Stöckl et al. 2011). Explanations for how intimate partner violence is linked to women's social and wider surroundings are provided by social disorganization theory. This theory claims that neighbourhoods with a positive sense of community and strong social networks have lower rates of intimate partner violence as residents share common values and exert social control upon each other (Almgren 2005). Neighbourhood surveillance and social cohesion not only prevent couples from solving their disputes violently, and provide comfort, encouragement, and financial help to deal with difficult situations, they also reduce stress by lowering crime rates and antisocial behaviour in the neighbourhood (DeMaris et al. 2004).

Gaps in the Evidence

Understanding of intimate partner violence has increased substantially over the last few years, with numerous prevalence studies drawing on population-based surveys covering most of the globe. There are also an increasing number of analyses conducted in different countries that show that many risk and protective factors are similar across the world, while also highlighting important regional and local differences. These studies are important for developing targeted interventions. What is still missing, however, is a deeper understanding of the developmental pathways that connect early negative childhood experiences to women's experiences of intimate partner violence in their later life, especially in respect to how different risk and protective factors interact and combine to increase a woman's risk or resilience to intimate partner violence. While there have been several studies in high-income countries, there is still a lack of longitudinal evidence from middle and low-income countries. Pathways may differ across diverse economic and cultural contexts, where social norms and meanings attached to women's social roles and gendered patterns of behaviour are not necessarily the same as in high-income regions.

References

Abramsky, T., Watts, C., and Garcia-Moreno, C. et al. (2011). What factors are associated with recent intimate partner violence? Findings from the WHO multi-country study on women's health and domestic violence. *BMC Public Health*, 11, 109.

Almgren, G. (2005). The ecological context of interpersonal violence from culture to collective efficacy. *Journal of Interpersonal Violence*, 20, 218–24.

Andersson, N., Ho-Foster, A., Mitchell, S., Scheepers, E., and Goldstein, S. (2007). Risk factors for domestic physical violence: national cross-sectional household surveys in eight southern African countries. *BMC Women's Health*, 7, 11.

Campbell, J. C. (2002). Health consequences of intimate partner violence. *Lancet*, 359, 1331–6.

Coker, A. L., Smith, P. H., Bethea, L., King, M. R., and Mckeown, R. E. (2000). Physical health consequences of physical and psychological intimate partner violence. *Archives of Family Medicine*, 9, 451–57.

Demaris, A., Benson, M. L., Fox, G. L., Hill, T., and Van Wyk, J. (2004). Distal and proximal factors in domestic violence: a test of an integrated model. *Journal of Marriage and Family*, 65, 652–67.

Devries, K. M., Kishor, S., Johnson, H., et al. (2010). Intimate partner violence during pregnancy: analysis of prevalence data from 19 countries. *Reproductive Health Matters*, 18, 158–70.

Devries, K. M., Mak, J. Y. T., García-Moreno, C., et al. (2013). The global prevalence of intimate partner violence against women. *Science*, 340, 1527–8.

Devries, K. M., Child, J. C., Bacchus, L. J., et al. (2014). Intimate partner violence victimization and alcohol consumption in women: a systematic review and meta-analysis. *Addiction* 109, 379–91.

Fergusson, D. M., Boden, J. M., and Horwood, L. J. (2006). Examining the intergenerational transmission of violence in a New Zealand birth cohort. *Child Abuse & Neglect*, 30, 89–108.

Fernández, M. (2006). Cultural beliefs and domestic violence. *Annals of the New York Academy of Sciences*, 1087, 250–60.

Foran, H. M., and O'Leary, K. D. (2008). Alcohol and intimate partner violence: a meta-analytic review. *Clinical Psychology Review*, 28, 1222–34.

García-Moreno, C., Jansen, H., Ellsberg, M., Heise, L., and Watts, C. (2005). *WHO Multi-Country Study on Women's Health and Domestic Violence against Women*. Geneva, Switzerland: World Health Organization.

García-Moreno, C., and Stöckl, H. (2009). Protection of sexual and reproductive health rights: addressing violence against women. *International Journal of Gynecology & Obstetrics*, 106, 144–7.

Gelles, R. (2007). Exchange theory. In: N. Jackson (ed.), *Encyclopedia of Domestic Violence*. New York and London: Routledge, pp. 302–5.

Gil-Gonzalez, D., Vives-Cases, C., Alvarez-Dardet, C., and Latour-Pérez, J. (2006). Alcohol and intimate partner violence: do we have enough information to act? *The European Journal of Public Health*, 16, 278–84.

Goode, W. (1971). Force and violence in the family. *Journal of Marriage and the Family*, 33, 624–36.

Hindin, M. J., Kishor, S., and Ansara, D. L. (2008). *Intimate Partner Violence among Couples in 10 DHS Countries: Predictors and Health Outcomes*. Calverton, MD, U.S.A.: Macro International Incorporated.

Hoffman, K. L., Demo, D. H., and Edwards, J. N. (1994). Physical wife abuse in a non-Western society: an integrated theoretical approach. *Journal of Marriage and the Family*, 131–46.

Jewkes, R. (2010). Emotional abuse: a neglected dimension of partner violence. *The Lancet*, 376, 851–2.

Jewkes, R. K., Levin, J. B., and Penn-Kekana, L. A. (2003). Gender inequalities, intimate partner violence and HIV preventive practices: findings of a South African cross-sectional study. *Social Science and Medicine*, 56, 125–34.

Jeyaseelan, L., Sadowski, L. S., and Kumar, S. et al. (2004). World studies of abuse in the family environment–risk factors for physical intimate partner violence. *Injury Control and Safety Promotion*, 11, 117–24.

Karamagi, C. A., Tumwine, J. K., Tylleskar, T., and Heggenhougen, K. (2006). Intimate partner violence against women in eastern Uganda: implications for HIV prevention. *BMC Public Health*, 6, 284.

Kaya, Y., and Cook, K. J. (2010). A cross-national analysis of physical intimate partner violence against women. *International Journal of Comparative Sociology*, 51, 423–44.

Klostermann, K. C., and Fals-Stewart, W. (2006). Intimate partner violence and alcohol use: exploring the role of drinking in partner violence and its implications for intervention. *Aggression and Violent Behavior*, 11, 587–97.

Krug, E., Dahlberg, L., Mercy, J., Zwi, A., and Lozano, R. (2002). *World Health Report on Violence and Health*. Geneva, Switzerland: World Health Organization.

Lim, S. S., Vos, T., Flaxman, A. D., and Danaei, G. et al. (2013). A comparative risk assessment of burden of disease and injury attributable to 67 risk factors and risk factor clusters in 21 regions, 1990–2010: a systematic analysis for the Global Burden of Disease Study 2010. *Lancet*, 380, 2224–60.

McMullan, E. (2007). Education as a risk factor for domestic violence. In: N. Jackson (ed.), *Encyclopedia of Domestic Violence*. New York and London: Routledge, pp. 267–70.

Miller, A. H. (1998). Neuroendocrine and immune system interactions in stress and depression. *Psychiatric Clinics of North America*, 21, 443–63.

Moffitt, T. E., and Caspi, A. (1999). *Findings about Partner Violence from the Dunedin Multidisciplinary Health and Development Study*. Washington DC: U.S. Department of Justice, Office of Justice Programs, National Institute of Justice.

Pallitto, C. C., and O'Campo, P. (2005). Community level effects of gender inequality on intimate partner violence and unintended pregnancy in Colombia: testing the feminist perspective. *Social Science & Medicine*, 60, 2205–16.

Renner, L. M., and Slack, K. S. (2006). Intimate partner violence and child maltreatment: understanding intra-and intergenerational connections. *Child Abuse & Neglect*, 30, 599–617.

Shamu, S., Abrahams, N., Temmerman, M., Musekiwa, A., and Zarowsky, C. (2011). A systematic review of African studies on intimate partner violence against pregnant women: prevalence and risk factors. *PloS ONE*, 6, e17591.

Stöckl, H., Devries, K., and Rotstein, A. et al. (2013). The global prevalence of intimate partner homicide: a systematic review. *Lancet*, 382, 859–65.

Stöckl, H., Heise, L., and Watts, C. (2011). Factors associated with violence by a current partner in a nationally representative sample of German women. *Sociology of Health & Illness*, 33, 694–709.

Tolan, P., Gorman-Smith, D., and Henry, D. (2006). Family violence. *Annual Review of Psychology*, 57, 557–83.

United Nations General Assembly. (1993). Declaration on the Elimination of Violence against Women, Article 1. (20 Dec. 1993; A/RES/48/104).

Williams, K. R. (1992). Social sources of marital violence and deterrence: testing an integrated theory of assaults between partners. *Journal of Marriage and the Family*, 620–29.

CHAPTER 7

Prevalence of non-partner sexual violence: a review of global data

Naeemah Abrahams, Karen Devries, Charlotte Watts, Christina Pallitto, Max Petzold, Simukai Shamu, and Claudia García-Moreno

Introduction to the Prevalence of Non-Partner Sexual Violence

Sexual violence is recognized as a human rights violation with profound public health impact and huge health and social consequence (Jewkes et al. 2002). The terms 'sexual violence', 'rape', and 'sexual abuse' encompass a broad range of forms of violence which have been defined in the World Health Organization's *World Report on Violence and Health* as:

> any sexual act, attempt to obtain a sexual act, unwanted sexual comments or advances, or acts to traffic, or otherwise directed, against a person's sexuality using coercion, by any person regardless of their relationship to the victim, in any setting, including but not limited to home and work (Jewkes et al. 2002, p. 149).

It is universally accepted that gender power inequality in society is the most important social force behind the problem of sexual violence (Jewkes 2002; Jewkes et al. 2011). These include prevalent notions of male sexual entitlement and male rights to use rape as punishment as has been shown in studies of sexual violence perpetrators (Jewkes et al. 2011; Wood et al. 2008). In addition, a culture of tolerance to sexual violence against women is reflected in, and reinforced by, the lack of seriousness with which the crime is treated by some members of the community, police, parts of the criminal justice system, and policymakers (Seedat et al. 2009).

The study of sexual violence can be approached in a number of different ways, including how it happens over the lifespan (e.g. female genital mutilation, child sexual abuse, rape in marriage); the context in which it happens (e.g. within intimate relations, date rape, sexual abuse at school, sexual harassment within work settings, and incest within family settings); and by perpetrator type (intimate partners and non-intimate partners). Non-partner perpetrators include strangers, acquaintances, friends, colleagues, peers, teachers, neighbours, police, military personnel, and family members such as fathers, brothers, uncles, cousins, and step relations. It might be asked why one should analyse rape by perpetrator since research shows that non-partner sexual violence has much in common with intimate partner sexual violence (Plichta and Falik 2001; Tjaden and Thoennes 2006), sharing some of the same risk factors, and also having similar health and social impact to that described in Chapter 6 (Plichta and Falik 2001; Tjaden 2006). However, there are also important differences between the two phenomena, including different population prevalence levels, and different impacts on health. The differences in population prevalence may suggest different drivers, such as varying levels of gender inequality, masculinities emphasizing heterosexual performance, community tolerance in the form of acceptance of male sexual entitlement for different forms of violence, and general levels of specific types of community violence such as gang violence. In addition, there may be different factors that influence reporting, with stigma of intimate partner rape and non-partner rape being different and therefore influencing reporting and help seeking differently (Abrahams and Mathews 2013). In addition, data suggest stranger rapes are more violent and can more often involve weapons, leading to greater physical injury, while those by known perpetrators may be less violent but the betrayal of trust may have a larger impact on mental health (Culbertson et al. 2001; Jones et al. 2004; Temple et al. 2005). Other differences include the period of abuse and when the sexual violence occurs: within an intimate partnership it often occurs over a long period, accompanied by controlling behaviour by the perpetrator, a pattern which may not be present in non-partner sexual violence. In addition, all forms of child sexual abuse can be considered non-partner sexual violence. It is also recognized that women can perpetrate violence against men within intimate relationships as well as in non-intimate partner relationships. Our focus in this analysis however is on the more common form of violence, that is violence against women by men.

This chapter presents the results of a systematic review and meta-analysis of existing data on the population prevalence of non-partner sexual violence reported by women from the age of 15 years. This review was done as part of the work for the Global Burden of Disease Study, to contribute to the quantification of the burden of disease and injury attributed to interpersonal violence (Murray et al. 2012). In addition, this analysis of global data will contribute to the recent call from United Nations bodies for better data to assist in the development of prevention interventions and for scaling up responses (United Nations 2013).

Methods

A global review of population-based prevalence estimates of non-partner sexual violence against women 15 years and older was undertaken, involving both peer-reviewed and grey literature. A systematic search was made of the following databases: the Cochrane Library, Medline, PubMed, Embase, CINAHL, British Nursing Index, Science Direct, British Medical Journal, Wiley InterScience, Health Management Information Consortium; social sciences databases (International Bibliography of Social Sciences, PsychINFO, Web of Science), and international databases (ADOLEC, Global Health, African Healthline, LILACS, Index Medicus of the Eastern Mediterranean, Southeast Asian, and Western Pacific Regions, Medcarib, Popline). Articles published from 1 January 1998 to 31 December 2010 were included. The search was updated to include studies and reports from 1 January 2011 to end 31 December 2011. We also hand-searched citations and requested experts to suggest other materials.

We also made contact with the authors and the data managers of large studies dedicated to violence against women. We requested data disaggregated by age and sex on non-partner sexual violence from the authors of the International Violence against Women Survey (IVAWS) (eight countries) (Johnson et al. 2008); the World Health Organization Multi Country Study (WHO-MCS) on Women's Health and Domestic Violence (Garcia-Moreno et al. 2005) (ten countries); Demographic and Health Surveys (DHS) (eight countries) (DHS 2007); Gender Alcohol and Culture International Study (GENACIS) (16 countries) (GENACIS 2007); the Centres for Disease Control Reproductive Health Surveys (CDC RHS) (two countries) (CDC), and Crime Victimization Surveys across the globe (no relevant estimates) (ICVS).

We included representative population-based studies with estimates of non-partner sexual violence. We considered including non-population-based studies in regions where data were limited, but did not find any to include. We included data on women aged 15 years and older on both lifetime and current (past year) exposure to non-partner sexual violence. We recognize that sexual violence between the ages of 15 and 18 years is also considered child sexual abuse, but the lower age range of 15 years is commonly used in intimate partner violence estimates, and we therefore used the lower age limit of 15 years for this analysis.

Because we were interested in sexual violence perpetrated by all perpetrators other than intimate partners, that is strangers, acquaintances, friends, family members, colleagues, teachers, police, military personnel, etc., we excluded studies where the analysis combined intimate and non-intimate perpetrators (e.g. International Crime Victimization Surveys). We accepted any author definition of sexual violence (i.e. rape and any other form of sexual violence), and excluded studies that combined sexual and non-sexual violence in the analysis (e.g. combined sexual and physical). Unlike the measurement of intimate partner violence, most studies that we reviewed used a single, general question, to ask women about their experiences of non-partner sexual violence.

One of the most common questions was: 'Were you ever forced to have sex or to perform a sexual act when you did not want to with someone other than your partner'. Narrow definitions were used by a few individual studies and these measured specific acts such as '. . . ever touched sexually against your wishes' (Ackard and Neumark-Sztainer 2003). We also looked at whether prevalence estimates were based on a single or multiple non-partner perpetrators, and included the estimate for combined perpetrators (if available) to ensure consistency, as most studies did not ask separate questions for different types of non-partner perpetrators.

We screened the abstracts and extracted the data into an EpiData database. For our meta-analysis we required prevalence and uncertainty estimates, including the numerator, denominator, and design effect for studies with clustered sampling. Information on methodological variables that could assist in the identification of potential biases and assist with the assessment of the quality of the studies was extracted. We extracted information on whether the perpetrator data were analysed as a single or a combination of perpetrators; how sexual violence was defined; the exposure period, for example ever or current (last year); study sites (national/regional/urban/rural); whether the study was part of a larger data set, if the questionnaire was derived from the questionnaire used in the WHO multi-country study on Women's Health and Domestic Violence; and whether fieldworkers received special training in how to ask about violence sensitively, and to respond appropriately if respondents became distressed.

Meta-Regression Models

We used random effects meta-regression in Stata 12.1 to produce both an adjusted and unadjusted prevalence model and produced summary prevalence estimates for all Global Burden of Disease regions. We did not calculate estimates by age group because of limited data on specific age groups. The standard deviation of the prevalence was calculated as the value of the upper limit of the 95 per cent confidence interval divided by 1.96. If no standard deviation or no confidence interval was reported, the Wilson method was used to estimate the confidence limits based on the prevalence data.

We controlled for covariates in the models and these were selected based on previous knowledge. Prior to model fitting, covariates were checked for correlation to avoid multi-collinearity. The covariates were whether the study was a national study, if the study was dedicated to violence against women, if the study measured lifetime violence or past year violence, if a broad definition of sexual violence was used, and if the study measured single perpetrators or combined different non-partner perpetrators. To obtain a global estimate, the regional estimates were weighted by region population sizes of women aged 15–49 years for the year 2010.

Results

We identified 7,231 abstracts/records for screening. The main reasons for exclusion were incorrect study design (non-population-based studies), studies focused on partner violence, or analysis combined perpetrators or type of violence (Figure 7.1). 189 records/abstracts were identified for full text screening, and after assessment 77 studies covering 56 countries were included, producing 412 estimates from women

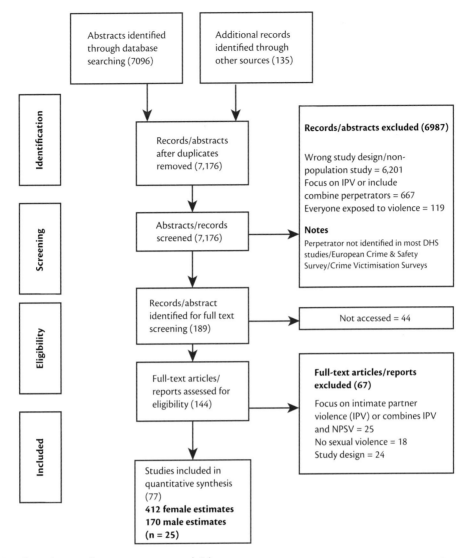

Fig. 7.1 Flowchart of review of prevalence studies on non-partner sexual violence.

15 years and older. Table 7.1 presents key characteristics of the 412 estimates. Data were available from all the Global Burden of Disease study regions with four regions (Asia Pacific, high income; North Africa/Middle-East; Europe, Eastern; sub-Saharan Africa, Central) having less than six estimates each. Only one estimate was found for the sub-Saharan African Central region (Democratic Republic of Congo) (Johnson et al. 2010) with eight regions having estimates from only one country. The regions with the largest proportions of estimates were Europe, Western (58 estimates) followed by sub-Saharan Africa, East (43 estimates). Six conflict setting countries contributed population estimates (Liberia, Timor-Leste (Timor East), Democratic Republic of the Congo, Kosovo, Philippines, and Sri Lanka), with the studies in Africa focussing on capturing conflict related sexual violence.

More than half (59.7 per cent) of the estimates were derived from dedicated violence against women studies, and a similar proportion was from nationally representative samples (53.8 per

cent). The majority of estimates measured lifetime non-partner sexual violence (81.8 per cent), combined perpetrators (93.7 per cent), and used a single question to capture any forced sexual act (91.5 per cent). Globally, 7.2 per cent (95 per cent CI 5.3–9.1) of women experienced non-partner sexual violence (Table 7.2). There were variations across the regions and the prevalence ranged from 3.3 per cent (95 per cent CI 0–8.3) in Asia, South, to 21 per cent (95 per cent CI 4.5–37.5) in sub-Saharan Africa, Central. Regions with high prevalence were sub-Saharan Africa, Central and Southern as well as Australasia. The wide confidence interval in the sub-Saharan Africa, Central region is most likely due to this being based on a single estimate. Regions with lower estimates were Asia South, Asia Southeast, and North Africa/Middle East.

The Asia Pacific high-income region had a considerably higher estimate than the other four Asian regions, while Eastern Europe had a much lower prevalence than the other two European regions. Similarly among the Latin American regions, the

Table 7.1 Characteristics of the 412 non-partner sexual violence prevalence estimates among females included in systematic review

	No of estimates	% of estimates	Countries
Asia Pacific, High Income	5	1.21	Japan
Asia, Central	9	2.18	Kazakhstan
Asia, East	14	3.4	Hong Kong
Asia, South	20	4.85	India, Bangladesh
Asia, Southeast	36	8.74	Philippines, Timor-Leste (Timor East), Maldives, Thailand, Sri Lanka,
Australasia	25	6.07	New Zealand, Australia
Caribbean	9	2.18	Belize
Europe, Central	38	9.22	Czech Republic, Poland, Serbia and Montenegro, Kosovo
Europe, Eastern	5	1.21	Lithuania, Ukraine, Azerbaijan
Europe, Western	58	14.08	Switzerland, Spain, Isle of Man, Sweden, Kingdom of Great Britain and Northern Ireland, Denmark, Finland, Germany,
Latin America, Andean	16	3.88	Peru
Latin America, Central	32	7.77	Costa Rica, Nicaragua, Jamaica
Latin America, Southern	14	3.4	Uruguay, Argentina
Latin America, Tropical	19	4.61	Brazil
North Africa/Middle East	4	0.97	Turkey
North America, High income	26	6.31	United States of America, Canada
Oceania	6	1.46	Samoa, Kiribati
Sub-Saharan Africa, Central	1	0.24	DRC
Sub-Saharan Africa, East	43	10.44	Uganda, Ethiopia, Mozambique, United Republic of Tanzania, Kenya, Malawi, Zambia
Sub-Saharan Africa, Southern	12	2.91	Namibia, South Africa, Zimbabwe,
Sub-Saharan Africa, West	20	4.85	Liberia, Sierra Leone, Burkina Faso, Ghana
Conflict settings	36	8.74	Liberia, Timor-Leste (East Timor), Democratic Republic of the Congo, Kosovo, Philippines, Sri Lanka

Adapted from *The Lancet*, Abrahams, N et al, Global prevalence of non-partner sexual violence: a systematic review, 12 February 2014, DOI: 10.1016/S0140-6736(13)62243-6, Copyright © 2014 World Health Organization, with permission from Elsevier.

southern region had a much lower prevalence, and among the sub-Saharan African regions the western regions also had a considerably lower estimate than the other three African regions. We present a forest plot of both the adjusted and unadjusted estimates (Figure 7.2) and similar results are found with all the confidence intervals of the unadjusted estimates overlapping with those of the adjusted estimates.

Rates of Non-Partner Sexual Violence Identified

The analysis has shown that, globally, 7.2 per cent of all women had experienced non-partner sexual violence. Levels above 15 per cent were found in four regions: Australasia; Latin America Andean; sub-Saharan Africa, Central, and sub-Saharan Africa, South, while the lowest estimates were found for Asia, South, and North Africa/Middle East.

This is the first time that global and regional estimates of non-partner sexual violence have been calculated based on a comprehensive systematic review. Generally, higher prevalence estimates were found for regions with more data points, except

for sub-Saharan Africa, Central, for which a single conflict setting country (Democratic Republic of the Congo) provided the estimate for this region and this is the highest estimate found in our review. With the exception of this region, lower prevalence was found for regions with fewer data. The findings confirm that non-partner sexual violence is widespread. The regional variations may reflect true variations but may also be linked to the availability of data, levels of disclosure, and the context of sexual violence such as war related sexual violence, although sexual violence does not occur in every armed conflict (Cohen et al. 2013). Sexual violence is highly stigmatized in most settings and this affects disclosure, with fear of being blamed and lack of perceived support from families, friends, and services leading to under-reporting (Abrahams et al. 2013; Kelly et al. 2005), and influencing help seeking and recovery (Moore and Farchi 2011).

The estimates found in this review are therefore most likely underestimates, and this is confirmed by more recent population studies on male perpetration. South Africa was the first country to publish population-based perpetration results where non-partner and partner rape was disaggregated; this showed

Table 7.2 Unadjusted and adjusted prevalence estimates of non-partner sexual violence by global regions: (adjusted for national study, combination of perpetrators and training of fieldworkers)

	Unadjusted prevalence % (95% CI)	Adjusted prevalence % (95% CI)
Global	8.9 (7.9–9.8)	7.2 (5.3–9.1)
Asia Pacific, High Income	16.7 (9.1–24.4)	12.2 (4.2–20.2)
Asia, Central	2.5 (0–8.6)	6.4 (0–13.0)
Asia, East	5.3 (0.9–9.6)	5.8 (0.1–11.6)
Asia, South	4.4 (0.5–8.2)	3.3 (0–8.3)
Asia, Southeast	6.0 (3.2–8.8)	5.2 (0.9–9.6)
Australasia	13.5 (10.2–16.9)	16.4 (11.5–21.4)
Caribbean	1.2 (0–6.8)	10.3 (3.7–16.9)
Europe, Central	9.6 (6.7–12.0)	10.7 (6.1–15.3)
Europe, Eastern	1.1 (0–8.3)	6.9 (0–14.1)
Europe, Western	7.8 (5.6–10.0)	11.5 (7.2–15.7)
Latin America, Andean	16.6 (12.5–20.7)	15.3 (10.1–20.5)
Latin America, Central	9.3 (6.3–12.4)	11.8 (7.3–16.4)
Latin America, Southern	1.9 (0–6.6)	5.8 (0.3–11.4)
Latin America, Tropical	8.3 (4.5–12.1)	7.6 (2.6–12.7)
North Africa/Middle East	4.0 (0–1.0)	4.5 (0–12.7)
North America, High Income	8.1 (5.0–11.4)	13.0 (9.0–16.9)
Oceania	14.2 (7.5–20.9)	14.8 (7.4–22.2)
Sub-Saharan Africa, Central	29.5 (11.9–47.1)	21.0 (4.5–37.5)
Sub-Saharan Africa, East	12.0 (9.4–14.6)	11.4 (7.3–15.6)
Sub-Saharan Africa, Southern	21.0 (16.0–25.9)	17.4 (11.4–23.3)
Sub-Saharan Africa, West	6.0 (2.2–9.8)	9.1 (4.8–13.2)

Reprinted from *The Lancet*, Abrahams, N. et al., Global prevalence of non-partner sexual violence: a systematic review, 12 February 2014, DOI: 10.1016/S0140-6736(13)62243-6, Copyright © 2014 World Health Organization, with permission from Elsevier.

that non-partner rape was more common than intimate partner rape (21.4 per cent raped a woman who was not a partner; 14.3 per cent raped a current or ex-partner) (Jewkes et al. 2012). This was followed by studies conducted in the Asia and the Pacific regions with the UN Multi-country Cross-sectional Study on Men and Violence: the results on non-partner rape from interviews with 10,178 men showed that single perpetrator rape prevalence varied between 4 and 41 per cent across the nine sites (Jewkes et al. 2013). Men's exaggeration of perpetration in these studies has been considered as a possible explanation for the discrepancy between men and women's reported rates, but comparing the prevalence reported by women in the same populations shows that women invariably report lower prevalence of victimization across the different sites in South Africa and the Asia-Pacific, implying male rates of perpetration are not exaggerated but that women under-report victimization (Machisa et al. 2011; Jewkes et al. 2013).

Gaps in the Evidence

The review had limitations. The study was largely constrained by the limited availability of quality population-based data. Eight regions had data from only one country, and many countries did not have any population-based data at all. This is reflected in the wide uncertainty bounds in the regional estimates. The highest prevalence in this review was found for the sub-Saharan, Central region (21 per cent), but this is based on a single estimate from the eastern region of the Democratic Republic of the Congo, which explains the wide uncertainty (Johnson et al. 2010). This estimate was derived from a study that focused on conflict-related sexual violence, perpetrated by combatants during the past 16 years of conflict (Johnson et al. 2010), with great detail given to identifying types of perpetrators. It is worth noting that conflict-affected settings provide major challenges in the execution of population-based surveys and obtaining a representative sample may be difficult due to logistical and security issues. In addition, many conflicts are localized to specific parts of a country and data from national studies may not reflect the situation of specific, conflict-affected sites fully. A recent report on wartime sexual violence from Cohen et al. (2013) warns of the many misconceptions related to sexual violence in conflict and how much remains unknown because of the lack of data.

Although more than 50 per cent of the 412 estimates were derived from dedicated violence against women studies, the focus in most of these studies was on intimate partner violence, and the measure of non-partner sexual violence was most often based on a single question. This single question is not in-line with current recommendations on violence-related surveys, which are to ask about experience of behaviourally specific acts. In addition, the lack of information on the range of perpetrators of sexual violence is an important limitation. Other study limitations include the inability to conduct age-disaggregated analysis, which made it impossible to calculate age-specific estimates. In addition, we included in our review studies that interviewed women aged 15 years and older, who reported their experiences of sexual violence since age 15. We did this in order to make a distinction with child sexual abuse. However, young women in the age group 15–18 years, who report having experienced non-partner sexual violence could also be considered, by some legal definitions, to have experienced child sexual abuse, so these two categories are not mutually exclusive. We also did not include men as victims, although this is increasingly recognized as an issue needing attention. Population level data are also limited for men.

In spite of the limitations, this review demonstrates that sexual violence is a common experience in the lives of many women. Sexual violence, irrespective of perpetrator, violates the human rights of victims and has a profound and enduring impact on their lives. Studies have shown that sexual violence can lead to short- and long-term health consequences. There is increasing evidence of the health effects following exposure to non-partner sexual violence, in particular mental health problems including depression, anxiety, and alcohol use disorders (Hankin et al. 1999; Kimerling et al. 2007; Plichta and Falik 2001), which is similar to that found for intimate partner violence. Furthermore, any one form of sexual violence increases the risk for other forms of violence, with many child sexual abuse studies showing an increased risk for later victimization (Dunkle et al. 2004; Fang and Corso 2007; Fergusson

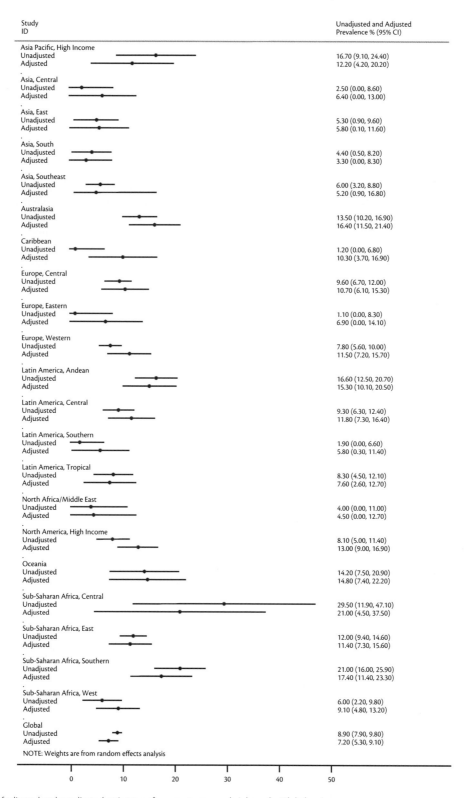

Study ID	Unadjusted and Adjusted Prevalence % (95% CI)
Asia Pacific, High Income	
Unadjusted	16.70 (9.10, 24.40)
Adjusted	12.20 (4.20, 20.20)
Asia, Central	
Unadjusted	2.50 (0.00, 8.60)
Adjusted	6.40 (0.00, 13.00)
Asia, East	
Unadjusted	5.30 (0.90, 9.60)
Adjusted	5.80 (0.10, 11.60)
Asia, South	
Unadjusted	4.40 (0.50, 8.20)
Adjusted	3.30 (0.00, 8.30)
Asia, Southeast	
Unadjusted	6.00 (3.20, 8.80)
Adjusted	5.20 (0.90, 16.80)
Australasia	
Unadjusted	13.50 (10.20, 16.90)
Adjusted	16.40 (11.50, 21.40)
Caribbean	
Unadjusted	1.20 (0.00, 6.80)
Adjusted	10.30 (3.70, 16.90)
Europe, Central	
Unadjusted	9.60 (6.70, 12.00)
Adjusted	10.70 (6.10, 15.30)
Europe, Eastern	
Unadjusted	1.10 (0.00, 8.30)
Adjusted	6.90 (0.00, 14.10)
Europe, Western	
Unadjusted	7.80 (5.60, 10.00)
Adjusted	11.50 (7.20, 15.70)
Latin America, Andean	
Unadjusted	16.60 (12.50, 20.70)
Adjusted	15.30 (10.10, 20.50)
Latin America, Central	
Unadjusted	9.30 (6.30, 12.40)
Adjusted	11.80 (7.30, 16.40)
Latin America, Southern	
Unadjusted	1.90 (0.00, 6.60)
Adjusted	5.80 (0.30, 11.40)
Latin America, Tropical	
Unadjusted	8.30 (4.50, 12.10)
Adjusted	7.60 (2.60, 12.70)
North Africa/Middle East	
Unadjusted	4.00 (0.00, 11.00)
Adjusted	4.50 (0.00, 12.70)
North America, High Income	
Unadjusted	8.10 (5.00, 11.40)
Adjusted	13.00 (9.00, 16.90)
Oceania	
Unadjusted	14.20 (7.50, 20.90)
Adjusted	14.80 (7.40, 22.20)
Sub-Saharan Africa, Central	
Unadjusted	29.50 (11.90, 47.10)
Adjusted	21.00 (4.50, 37.50)
Sub-Saharan Africa, East	
Unadjusted	12.00 (9.40, 14.60)
Adjusted	11.40 (7.30, 15.60)
Sub-Saharan Africa, Southern	
Unadjusted	21.00 (16.00, 25.90)
Adjusted	17.40 (11.40, 23.30)
Sub-Saharan Africa, West	
Unadjusted	6.00 (2.20, 9.80)
Adjusted	9.10 (4.80, 13.20)
Global	
Unadjusted	8.90 (7.90, 9.80)
Adjusted	7.20 (5.30, 9.10)

NOTE: Weights are from random effects analysis

Figure 7.2 Forest plot of adjusted and unadjusted estimates of non-partner sexual violence by Global regions.

Reprinted from *The Lancet*, Abrahams, N et al, Global prevalence of non-partner sexual violence: a systematic review, 12 February 2014, DOI: 10.1016/S0140-6736(13)62243-6, Copyright © 2014 World Health Organization, with permission from Elsevier.

et al. 1997), and more recently the link between harsh childhoods and adult perpetration (Jewkes et al. 2010; Mathews et al. 2011).

Conclusion

This first global review of the prevalence of non-partner sexual violence has shown that one in 14 women globally has been sexually assaulted by someone other than a partner, since the age of 15. For reasons described here, including the stigma and blame attached to sexual violence, this is likely to be an underestimate. The psychological effects of sexual violence and the high prevalence confirm that it is a pressing health and human rights concern, requiring serious attention. There are important data gaps, and the further standardization of research tools and methods would improve future measurement and monitoring. The review highlights the need for countries to have their own population-level data on the levels of sexual violence by different perpetrators to understand the magnitude of the problem, to better understand the main risk factors, and to develop appropriate policies and responses, including both comprehensive sexual assault services and primary prevention interventions. Reducing gender-based violence and building gender equality is a global challenge and an important development goal for governments across the world. Addressing and preventing non-partner sexual violence is a critical aspect of achieving this goal.

Acknowledgement

Data in the chapter are from *The Lancet*, Abrahams, N. et al, Global prevalence of non-partner sexual violence: a systematic review, 12 February 2014, DOI: 10.1016/S0140-6736(13)62243-6, Copyright © 2014 World Health Organization and World Health Organization, *Global and regional estimates of violence against women: prevalence and health effects of intimate partner and non-partner sexual violence,* World Health Organization, Geneva, Switzerland, Copyright © 2013, available from http://www.who.int/reproductivehealth/publications/violence/9789241564625/en/index.htm

References

Abrahams, N. R. J., and Mathews, S. (2013). Depressive symptoms after a sexual assault among women, understanding victim-perpetrator relationship and the role of social perceptions. *African Journal of Psychiatry*, 16, 288–93.

Ackard, D. M., and Neumark-Sztainer, D. (2003), Multiple sexual victimizations among adolescent boys and girls: prevalence and associations with eating behaviors and psychological health. *Journal of Child Sexual Abuse*, 12, 17–37.

CDC. *Centre for Disease Control and Prevention Reproductive Health Surveys*. United States: Centre for Disease Control and Prevention. Available at: http://www.cdc.gov/reproductivehealth/Global/surveys.htm [Accessed 12 November 2013].

Cohen, D. K., Hoover Green, A., and Wood, E. J. (2013), Wartime sexual violence misconceptions, implications and ways forward. *Special Report 323*, 2–15. Washington, DC: United States Institute of Peace.

Culbertson, K. A., Vik, P. W., and Kooiman, B. J. (2001). The impact of sexual assault, sexual assault perpetrator type, and location of sexual assault on ratings of perceived safety. *Violence against Women*, 7, 858–75.

DHS, M. (2007). *Liberia Demographic and Health Survey 2007*. Measure DHS. Available at http://www.measuredhs.com/Data/ [Accessed 12 November 2013]

Dunkle, K., Jewkes, R., and Brown, H.C. et al. (2004). Prevalence and patterns of gender-based violence and revictimization among women attending antenatal clinics in Soweto, South Africa. *American Journal of Epidemiology*, 160, 230–9.

Fang, X., and Corso, P. S. (2007). Child maltreatment, youth violence, and intimate partner violence: developmental relationships. *American Journal of Preventive Medicine*, 33, 281–90.

Fergusson, D. M., Horwood, L. J., and Lynskey, M. T. (1997). Childhood sexual abuse, adolescent sexual behaviors and sexual revictimization. *Child Abuse & Neglect*, 21, 789–803.

Garcia-Moreno, C., Jansen, H., Elssberg, M., Heise, L., and Watts, C. (2005), *WHO Multi Country Study on Women's Health and Domestic Violence against Women*. Geneva, Switzerland: WHO.

Genacis. (2007). *Gender, Alcohol and Culture: An International Study (GENACIS)*. Available at http://www.genacis.org/ [Accessed 02 July 2011].

Hankin, C. S., Skinner, K. M., Sullivan, L. M., Miller, D. R., Frayne, S., and Tripp, T. J. (1999). Prevalence of depressive and alcohol abuse symptoms among women VA outpatients who report experiencing sexual assault while in the military. *Journal of Traumatic Stress*, 12, 601–12.

IVCS. *International Victim Crime Survey*. Available at: http://www.unicri.it/services/library_documentation/publications/icvs [Accessed 12 November 2013].

Jewkes, R. (2002). Intimate partner violence: causes and prevention. *Lancet*, 359, 1423–29.

Jewkes, R. K., Dunkle, K., Nduna, M., Jama, P. N., and Puren, A. (2010). Associations between childhood adversity and depression, substance abuse and HIV and HSV2 incident infections in rural South African youth. *Child Abuse and Neglect*, 34, 833–41.

Jewkes, R., Fulu, E., Roselli, T., and Garcia-Moreno, C. (2013). Prevalence and risk factors for non-partner rape perpetration: findings from the UN multi-country cross-sectional study on men and violence in Asia and Pacific. *The Lancet Global Health*, 1, e208–e18.

Jewkes, R., Nduna, M., Shai, N. J., and Dunkle, K. (2012). Prospective study of rape perpetration by young South African men: incidence & risk factors. *PLoS ONE*, 7, e38210.

Jewkes, R., Sen, P., and Garcia-Moreno, C. (2002). Sexual violence. In: E. Krug, I. I. Dahlberg, J. A Mercy, A. B. Zwi, and R. Lozano (eds). *World Report on Violence and Health*. Geneva: World Health Organization, pp. 148–81

Jewkes, R., Sikweyiya, Y., Morrell, R., and Dunkle, K. (2011). Gender inequitable masculinity and sexual entitlement in rape perpetration South Africa: findings of a cross-sectional study. *PloS ONE*, 6, e29590.

Johnson, H., Ollus, N., and Nevala, S. (2008). *Violence against Women. An International Perspective*. New York: Springer.

Johnson, K., Scott, J., and Rughita, B. et al. (2010). Association of sexual violence and human rights violations with physical and mental health in territories of the Eastern Democratic Republic of the Congo. *JAMA*, 304, 553–62.

Jones, J. S., Wynn, B. N., Kroeze, B., Dunnuck, C., and Rossman, L. (2004). Comparison of sexual assaults by strangers versus known assailants in a community-based population. *American Journal of Emergency Medicine*, 22, 454–9.

Kelly, L., Lovett, J., and Regan, L. (2005). *A Gap or a Chasm? Attrition in Reported Rape Cases*, London: Home Office Research, Development and Statistics Directorate.

Kimerling, R., Gima, K., Smith, M.W., Street, A., and Frayne, S. (2007). The veterans health administration and military sexual trauma. *American Journal of Public Health*, 97, 2160–6.

Machisa, M., Jewkes, R., Lowe Morna, C., and Rama, K. (2011). The war @ home: preliminary findings of the Gauteng Gender Violence Prevalence Study. Gauteng Gender Links. Available at: http://www.genderlinks.org.za/article/the-war-at-home—gbv-indicators-project-2011-08-16 [Accessed 12 November 2013]

Mathews, S., Jewkes, R., and Abrahams, N. (2011). 'I had a hard life': exploring childhood adversity in the shaping of masculinities among men who killed an intimate partner in South Africa. *British Journal of Criminology*, 51, 960–77.

Moore, A., and Farchi, M. (2011). Is rape-related self blame distinct from other post traumatic attributions of blame? A comparison of severity and implications for treatment. *Women & Therapy*, 34, 447–60.

Murray, C. J. L., Ezzati, M., and Flaxman, A. D., et al. (2012). GBD 2010: design, definitions, and metrics. *The Lancet*, 380, 2063–6.

Plichta, S. B., and Falik, M. (2001). Prevalence of violence and its implications for women's health. *Women's Health Issues*, 11, 244.

Seedat, M., Van, N. A., Jewkes, R., Suffla, S., and Ratele, K. (2009). Violence and injuries in South Africa: prioritising an agenda for prevention. *Lancet*, 374, 1011–22.

Temple, J. R., Weston, R., and Marshall, L. L. (2005). Physical and mental health outcomes of women in nonviolent, unilaterally violent, and mutually violent relationships. *Violence and Victims*, 20, 335–59.

Tjaden, P., and Thoennes, N. (2006). *Extent, Nature and Consequences of Rape Victimization: Findings from the National Violence Against Women Survey*. Washington, DC: US Dept. of Justice, Office of Justice Programs, National Institute of Justice.

United Nations (2013). The elimination and prevention of all forms of violence against women and girls: agreed conclusions. In: *Commission on the Status of Women. Report on the 57th Session*. New York: United Nations. Available at: http://www.un.org/ga/search/view_doc.asp?symbol=E/2013/27&referer=http://www.un.org/womenwatch/daw/csw/57sess.htm&Lang=E [Accessed 12 November 2013]

Wilson, E. B. (1927). Probable inference, the law of succession, and statistical inference. *Journal of the American Statistical Association*, 22, 209–12.

Wood, K., Lambert, H., and Jewkes, R. (2008). 'Injuries are beyond love': physical violence in young South Africans' sexual relationships. *Medical Anthropology: Cross Cultural Studies in Health and Illness*, 27, 43–69.

CHAPTER 8

Male-on-male violence: A leading cause of death around the world

Francesco Mitis and Dinesh Sethi

Introduction to Male-on-Male Violence

The purpose of the chapter is to describe the burden of physical violence occurring in males, some risk factors associated with being a male victim, and propose policy action ahead. The main focus will be on males aged 15–59 years as victims of male violence.

Globally, an estimated 535,000 people are murdered every year. These data from vital registration systems show that 83 per cent of these deaths are in males (World Health Organization 2011), and 89 per cent occur during their economically active years (15–59 years). Interpersonal violence in males is therefore not only a leading cause of premature death, but of economic loss to society. The majority (73 per cent) of homicides occur in men aged 15–44 years. For those aged 15–29 years, interpersonal violence is the second leading cause of deaths and the 5th leading cause of death in those aged 30–44.

Homicides Committed by Males

Vital registration information records data on homicide victims, but not on their perpetrators. Data on perpetration are not routinely available disaggregated by age, sex, and other characteristics, and are difficult to compare across countries. Such data need to be obtained from the justice sector and are dependent on police recording. Most high-income countries (HIC) collect data on perpetrators and routinely store information on perpetrator age, weapons used, and relationship with the victim. However, only few countries have detailed linked data on both victim and perpetrator characteristics. An example, from the United States of America for the period 2000–2009, reported that for one-to-one homicides, 90 per cent of perpetrators were male. Sixty-four per cent of the murders involved male-on-male violence, 26 per cent involved male on female, 7 per cent involved female on male violence, and 3 per cent involved female on female. Ninety per cent of males were murdered by males, and this picture has been predominant in spite of the reduction in homicide rates (United Nations Office on Drugs and Crime 2011). A global study showed that in ten countries of the Americas, 96 per cent of the perpetrators were male (86 per cent of victims were male), in four Asian countries,

86 per cent of perpetrators and 62 per cent of victims were male, whilst in 20 European countries the figures were 88 per cent and 65 per cent respectively. The proportion of male perpetrators is higher in countries with higher homicide rates.

For the purposes of this chapter, the proportion of 90 per cent has been applied to derive estimates of male-on-male homicides. Globally it is thus estimated that 358,000 males aged 15–59 years were murdered by males (WHO 2011). Ninety-five per cent of these occurred in low- and middle-income countries, with 33 per cent in the WHO Americas Region (AMRO), 30 per cent in WHO African Region (AFRO), 19 per cent in WHO Southeast Asia Region (SEARO), 8 per cent in WHO Western Pacific Region (WPRO), 7 per cent in WHO European Region (EURO), and 3 per cent in WHO Eastern Mediterranean Region (EMRO) (Member States constituting the WHO Regions are described in the Global Burden of Disease Study, WHO 2011).

Globally rates are highest in young people aged 15–29 years with 21.1 deaths per 100,000 population followed by people aged 30–44 years (19.0 per 100,000) and are lowest in children under 15. The highest mortality rates were in males aged 15–29 years in the low- and middle-income countries of AMRO followed by AFRO (Figure 8.1), with the lowest rates in the HIC of WPRO and EURO.

When comparing male homicide rate ratios by WHO Region and country income, then EURO has the highest rate ratios (Figure 8.2). This is because Western Europe has some of the safest countries in the world in contrast to Eastern Europe, with a 51-fold difference between the country with the highest homicide rate compared to the lowest one (WHO Regional Office for Europe 2013). EMRO appears to be the most homogeneous region in terms of differential mortality. These differences show the potential gains that could be made in premature mortality from male homicides if all countries achieved the lowest observed rates. In this way it is estimated that 336,000 deaths or 94 per cent of male homicide deaths could be avoided.

Trends in Male Homicides

In EURO the highest homicide rates are reported in the Commonwealth of Independent States (CIS). The dissolution of Soviet Union and the social, economic, and political transition was associated with deregulation, increased alcohol and weapons

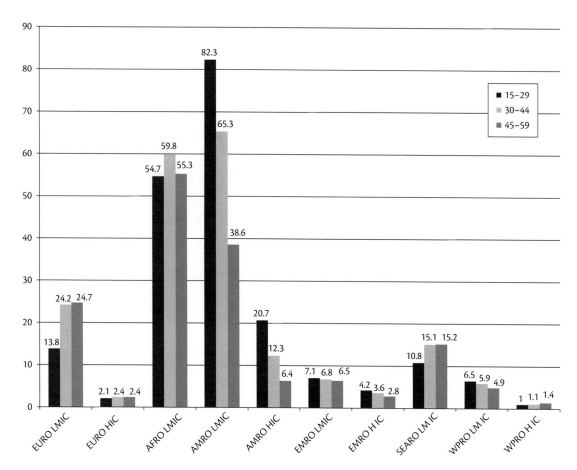

Fig. 8.1 Mortality rates in males by age and country income level in different WHO regions.
Source: data from World Health Organization, *Global burden of disease: Disease and injury regional estimates* [online database], World Health Organization, Geneva, Switzerland, Copyright
© 2011, available from http://www.who.int/healthinfo/statistics/mortality/en/index2.html

availability, weaker enforcement, and the loss of social support networks. This resulted in steep increases in homicides in the early 1990s (McKee 2000, Sethi et al. 2006), as demonstrated in the CIS; this has been followed by the recent large falls in homicide rates (Figure 8.3). In contrast, rates in the European Union (EU) have shown a steady downward trend.

It is not possible to assess trends in many other regions because of incomplete data. For example in AFRO only three countries (Lesotho, Mauritius, and South Africa) have provided three or more years of consecutive data (UNODC 2011). In AMRO, homicide rates have been variable (Gawrisewski et al. 2012); large declines have been observed in the United States of America in the last 15 years while rates in Southern America fell since 2002 to level out in recent years (De Souza et al. 2012). A steep increase of rates has been reported in the Caribbean Region since the 1990s and in Central America since the mid-2000s, due to increases in drug trafficking-related violence while in Asian countries mortality due to homicides has been declining (UNODC 2011).

Non-fatal Assaults

Homicides represent only the most visible and extreme outcomes of male violence. Outcomes will be influenced by factors such as firearm use, intoxication of perpetrators and victims, intervention by bystanders, and the speed and quality of emergency services.

Many assaults require emergency medical attention requiring prolonged hospital stays. It is estimated that for every fatality, there are 20 assaults requiring hospital admissions and hundreds requiring emergency department care (Krug et al. 2002). Routine hospital information is incomplete in most countries and rarely links victims and perpetrators. Scattered information is instead provided by some studies (Cassell et al. 2011). Not all cases of violence present to hospital or are ascertained by health professionals, and so may only be detected through population surveys. In the absence of such studies, the scale of non-fatal violence may be underestimated in many countries.

There are few multi-country standardized surveys of violence in males. An exception is the Health Behaviour in School Aged Children study, conducted in 38 countries, which describes a higher prevalence of male violence (Currie et al. 2012). These show that the average prevalence of bullying in schools in 15-year-old boys is 16 per cent (ranging from 4 to 36 per cent) and being bullied is 10 per cent (3–25 per cent). In contrast the average for girls is 7 per cent.

Risk Factors

There is no single risk factor which can explain a violent behaviour but, instead, a range of complex interacting factors that can be understood by way of the ecological model which takes into

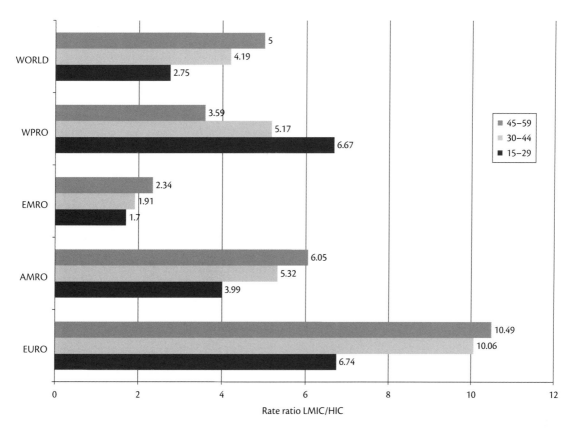

Fig. 8.2 Male homicide rate ratios comparing low- and middle-income to high-income countries for different age groups and WHO regions.*

*SEARO and AFRO excluded because they have no high-income countries.

Source: data from World Health Organization, *Global burden of disease: Disease and injury regional estimates* [online database], World Health Organization, Geneva, Switzerland, Copyright © 2011, available from http://www.who.int/healthinfo/statistics/mortality/en/index2.html

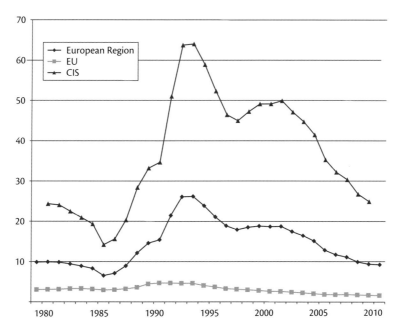

Fig. 8.3 Mortality among males aged 30–44 due to homicides in WHO European Region.*

*The historical subgroupings of the EU until 2007 and the CIS until 2006 are used. For CIS this consists of: Armenia, Azerbaijan, Belarus, Georgia, Kazakhstan, Kyrgyzstan, Republic of Moldova, Russian Federation, Tajikistan, Turkmenistan, Ukraine, and Uzbekistan.

Source: data from World Health Organization Regional Office for Europe, *Mortality indicators by 67 causes of death, age and sex (HFA-MDB)* [online database], WHO Regional Office for Europe, Copenhagen, The Netherlands, Copyright © 2013, available from http://data.euro.who.int/hfamdb/.

consideration risk factors, and their interaction, at individual, relational, community, and societal level (Krug et al. 2002). The bulk of the literature comes from the Americas, Europe, and the Western Pacific Region as well as studies from South Africa. Few results were found from the Middle East and South Asia.

Community and Society Level

The inequalities in mortality rates described between countries also exist within countries, with the poorest segments of the population more at risk throughout the world. The Commission on Socioeconomic Determinants of Health (CSDH) has brought renewed attention to the plight of the socioeconomically deprived, reporting that inequalities in health are increasing (CSDH 2008) and this is true of interpersonal violence in many countries. A recent review from Europe found consistent associations between material deprivation and increased risk of assault (Laflamme et al. 2009). From the United Kingdom, the risks of admission for assaults in males increased exponentially with increasing quintiles of neighbourhood deprivation, with the odds of 5.5 times higher in the poorest quintile than in the richest. In males aged 17–19 years, violence accounted for 20 per cent of the entire gap between wealthiest and poorest quintiles in all-cause emergency hospital admissions (Bellis et al. 2011). In Scotland the social gradient for homicides was studied for the period 1980–2005. The death rate among men aged 20–59 in routine occupations was nearly 12 times the higher managerial and professional occupations. In addition to that, men under 65 living in the most deprived areas had a death rate due to assault 31.9 times that of those living in the least deprived quintile (Leyland and Dundas 2010). In the Russian Federation a study was conducted to evaluate the association between socioeconomic changes and homicides in a transitional society between 1991 and 2000. Results found a strong association showing increases in homicides rates in regions with the highest unemployment and reported lower homicides in regions with more privatization (Pridemore and Kim 2007). A more recent European multi-country study (Stickley et al. 2012) assessed socioeconomic inequalities in homicide mortality in 12 European countries and reported that inequalities in education influenced homicide rates in men aged 35–64 years. In Europe, (Sethi et al. 2010) strong associations were found for youth violence for social inequalities and deprivation, the availability of alcohol and weapons, the presence of an illicit drug trade, concentrations of poverty, and cultural norms, school, and institutional environments that condone violence.

Studies from the Unites States report that gang violence typically occurs more frequently in the poorest socioeconomic groups. Non-fatal weapon-related injuries showed a very steep socioeconomic gradient and there was an increased risk of homicide deaths associated with residence in neighbourhoods with lower socioeconomic status (Krieger et al. 2003). Youth homicides were eight times higher in the most deprived group compared to their most affluent counterparts (Singh et al. 2013). The recent decline in homicide rates have been attributed to a proportionately greater decrease in male homicide rates in the deprived urban areas, attributed to a decline in the use of crack and cocaine and successful urban development and preventive policies targeting deprived neighbourhoods (UNODC, 2011).

In Brazil, several studies reported higher homicide rates in areas with concentrated slums and lower rates in areas with higher incomes and educational levels (Santos et al. 2006; Viana et al. 2011). A similar observation from Colombia noted that 93 per cent of the victims of homicides between 1980 and 2007 were male, and mainly from lower socioeconomic strata (Franco et al. 2012). A recent study analysed the characteristics of homicides in Latin American countries, to show that countries with higher homicide rates had higher proportions of urbanized population and rates of poverty. The highest homicide rates were observed in countries with the highest disparities in urban concentrations of poverty (Briceño-Leon et al. 2008).

A multi-country study of eight nations, covering four continents, found that homicide rates were generally higher in areas with lower per capita income and higher unemployment rates (Lester 2001). Links between economic growth, income inequality, and violence have been demonstrated by multi-country studies (Fajnzylber et al. 1999). Reports from Central America and Latin America demonstrate increased levels of violence in association with poverty, corruption, and social change (UNODC 2007).

Weapons used in assaults and homicides vary; while in Europe homicides are generally committed by the use of sharp objects or physical force (Sethi et al. 2010), firearms are more commonly used in the Americas, where the proportion of homicides using firearms is 74 per cent compared to a world average of 42 per cent (108 countries). In many Latin American countries firearm availability and use is linked to criminal activity, street crime, and drug trafficking. Data from 45 cities in developing countries suggest that assaults by firearm are strongly associated with gun availability (UNODC 2011).

The relationship between alcohol availability and homicides among youth has been studied in the largest 91 U.S. cities. After adjusting for other potential confounders, a strong association was found between alcohol outlet density and homicide rates for youth aged 13–17 and 18–24 (Parker et al. 2011). A study conducted in Canada is consistent with these findings (Ray et al. 2008). Earlier pub closing times resulted in a reduction in 37 per cent of night-time assaults in comparison with a control locality (Kypri et al. 2011). Conversely a study in Colombia demonstrated that extended licensing hours was associated with increased risk of homicides (Sánchez et al. 2011).

Relational Level

Risk factors for male violence include family structure such as young single-parent families or very large families, lack of parental support, having a poor relationship with parents and carers, being associated with delinquent peers, and being involved in gang activities. In the U.S. a study showed that having another or female guardian living in the household decreased the risk of weapon carrying (Sethi et al. 2010). Poor supervision of children has been demonstrated to be a good predictor of violence in youth (McCord 1979), while living in single-parent families was found to be a risk factor for developing aggressive behaviours. It has been suggested that this may be due to a failure to learn non-violent means of conflict resolution (Sethi et al. 2010). Having delinquent friends as a risk factor for youth violence was also reported from Peru (Perales and Sogi 1995). Involvement with gangs is primarily a male phenomenon. Results from various studies from around the world indicate an association between gang involvement and violent behaviour (Krug et al. 2002).

Individual Level

There are numerous risk factors that have been clearly demonstrated to increase the likelihood of being at risk of violence. These include younger age; mental and behavioural characteristics such as hyperactivity and attention deficit disorders, depression, poor behavioural control, sensation-seeking, low self-esteem, impulsiveness; low academic achievement; having experienced violence in the past; and alcohol and street drug use (Krug et al. 2002). In many countries victims are very similar to perpetrators and tend to be young males living in poor urban areas, and from minority groups (Menard 2002). Previous victimization as a risk factor for perpetration of violence has been described in several countries (Shaffer and Ruback 2002).

In South Africa interpersonal violence accounted for 42.8 per cent of the injury DALYs (Disability-Adjusted Life Years) attributed to alcohol in males (Schneider et al. 2007) while in Australia the influence of alcohol use on rates of violence in males aged 30–44 was 8.9 times higher in the indigenous versus the general population (Calabria et al. 2010). A one-litre increase in per capita consumption was followed by an 8 per cent increase in male homicide rates and a 6 per cent increase in male homicide rates (Ramstedt 2011).

The Bureau of Justice from the United States of America reported that in 2004 nearly a third of state and a quarter of federal prisoners committed their offence under the influence of drugs and that 18 per cent committed their crime to obtain money for drugs (Mumola and Karberg 2006).

Gaps in the Evidence

While much is known about male-on-male violence, there are key gaps in our knowledge. For instance, data on non-fatal violence are scarce. There is much to be gained from well-designed studies using standardized instruments and from data linkage between hospital and police data (Sethi et al. 2010). Rather more fundamentally, the question as to why males are more likely to be victims and perpetrators of violence needs to better understood.

Conclusion

To conclude, males are much more likely than females to be victims of fatal and serious assaults. Ninety per cent of this violence is perpetrated by other males. There are large inequalities across the globe but the highest homicide rates are among younger men in low- and middle-income countries of the Americas and Africa.

There are well described risk factors for male violence and these include socioeconomic deprivation, large urban concentrations of poverty, an illicit drug trade, the availability of weapons and alcohol, poor parenting, lower educational achievement, and previous exposure to violence. Males who live in poorer material and social conditions are more likely to engage in risk taking behaviour such as consuming more alcohol, taking illicit drugs, carrying weapons, and using violence as a means of addressing conflict (Sethi et al. 2010). Maltreatment and other adverse experiences in childhood will have far reaching impacts on male violence, both through these health harming behaviours and their impact on the intergenerational transmission of violence (Sethi et al. 2013).

Much policy attention has been given to areas of violence such as child maltreatment and intimate partner violence, but little attention has been given to the area of preventing males becoming victims of violence. There is a need to address the root causes of such violence. This requires addressing the structural factors that contribute to societal and community level risk factors and investing in preventive approaches throughout the life course (Krug et al. 2002). Other areas that need attention are reducing access to weapons, modifying bullying in schools and the workplace, making drinking and urban environments safer, and addressing cultural norms that support violence in males. Further, there is a lack of support services for boys and men that should be made more accessible and equitable.

Implementing such programmes requires multi-sectoral approaches and stronger governance within the health sector to coordinate such responses. The prevention of violence needs to be integrated into health, educational, and social policies and requires high level government backing to ensure that sufficient resources are devoted to prevention, support services, and research. Opportunities for such policy integration across the sectors need to be exploited, such as that proposed by, *Health 2020: A European Policy Framework Supporting Action across Government and Society for Health and Well-being* (WHO Regional Office for Europe 2012). An adequate societal response also requires an investment in well trained personnel who are focused on violence prevention (WHO 2007).

References

Bellis, M. A., Hughes, K., Wood, S., Wyke, S., and Perkins, C. (2011). National five-year examination of inequalities and trends in emergency hospital admission for violence across England. *Injury Prevention*, 17, 319–25.

Briceño-Leon R., Villaveces, A., and Concha-Eastman, A. (2008). Understanding the uneven distribution of the incidence of homicide in Latin America. *International Journal of Epidemiology*, 37, 751–7

Calabria, B., Doran, C. M., Vos, T., Shakeshaft, A. P., and Hall, W. (2010). Epidemiology of alcohol-related burden of disease among Indigenous Australians. *Australian and New Zealand Journal of Public Health*, 34, S47–51.

Cassell, E., Reid, N., Clapperton, A., Houy-Prang, K., and Kerr, E. (2011) Assault-related injury among young people aged 15-34 years that occurred in public places: deaths and hospital-treated injury. *Hazard* Victorian Injury surveillance Unit, available from http://www.iec.monash.edu.au/miri/research/research-areas/home-sport-and-leisure-safety/visu/hazard/haz73.pdf, accessed 1 May 2013.

Commission on Social Determinants of Health. (2008). Closing the gap in a generation: health equity through action on the social determinants of health.*Final Report of the Commission on Social Determinants of Health*. Geneva: World Health Organization.

Currie, C., Zanotti, C., and Morgan, A. et al. (2012). *Social Determinants of Health and Well-being among Young People. Health Behaviour in School-aged Children (HBSC) Study: International Report from the 2009/2010 Survey.* Copenhagen: WHO Regional Office for Europe.

de Souza, E. R., de Melo, A. N., Franco, S. A., Alazraqui, M., and González-Pérez, G. J (2012). Estudo multicêntrico da mortalidade por homicídios em países da América Latina [Multicentric study of deaths by homicide in Latin American countries]. *Ciência & Saúde Coletiva*, 17, 3183–93.

Franco, S. et al. (2012). [Deaths by homicide in Medellin, 1980–2007]. *Cien Saude Colet*, 17, 3209–18.

Fajnzylber, P., Lederman, D., and Loayza, N. (1999). *Inequality and Violent Crime*. Washington, D.C., World Bank.

Gawryszewski, V.P. et al. (2012). Homicídios na região das Américas: magnitude, distribuição e tendências, 1999–2009 [Homicides in the Americas region: magnitude, distribution and trends, 1999–2009]. *Ciência & Saúde Coletiva*, 17, 3171–82.

Kypri, K. et al. (2011). Effects of restricting pub closing times on night-time assaults in an Australian city. *Addiction* 106, 303–10.

Krieger, N. et al. (2003). Monitoring socioeconomic inequalities in sexually transmitted infections, tuberculosis, and violence: geocoding and choice of area based socioeconomic measures—the public health disparities geocoding project (US). *Public Health Report* 118, 240–60.

Krug, E. et al. (2002). *World Report on Violence and Health*. Geneva. World Health Organization.

Laflamme, L. et al. (2009). *Addressing the Socioeconomic Safety Divide: A Policy Briefing*. Geneva: WHO Regional Office for Europe.

Lester, D. (2001). Regional studies of homicide: a meta-analysis.*Death Studies* 25, 705–8.

Leyland, A.H. and Dundas, R. (2010). The social patterning of deaths due to assault in Scotland, 1980–2005: population-based study. *Journal of Epidemiology and Community Health* 64, 432–9.

McCord, J. (1979). Some child-rearing antecedents of criminal behavior in adult men. *Journal of Personality and Social Psychology* 37, 1477–86.

McKee, M. et al. 2000. Health policy-making in central and eastern Europe: why has there been so little action on injuries? *Health Policy and Planning* 15, 263–9.

Menard, S. (2002). Short and long term consequences of adolescent victimization. *Youth Violence Research Bulletin*. Avaialble from https://www.ncjrs.gov/pdffiles1/ojjdp/191210.pdf.

Mumola, C.J., and Karberg, J.C. (2006). Drug use and dependence, State and federal prisoners, 2004. Bureau of Justice Statistics. Special report. Washington, DC: US Department of Justice.

Parker, R. N. et al. (2011). Alcohol availability and youth homicide in the 91 largest US cities, 1984–2006. *Drug and Alcohol Reviews* 30, 505–14.

Perales, A., and Sogi, C. Conductas violentas en adolescentes: identificaio´n de factores de riesgo para diseño de programa preventivo. [Violent behaviour among adolescents: identifying risk factors to design prevention programmes.] In: C. Pimentel Sevilla (ed.), *Violencia, familia y niñez en los sectores urbanos pobres.* [*Violence, the family and childhood in poor urban sectors.*] Lima, Cecosam, 1995, 135–54.

Pridemore, W. A., and Kim, S.W. (2007). Socioeconomic change and homicide in a transitional society. *Sociol Q*, 24 (48), 229–51.

Ramstedt, M. (2011). Population drinking and homicide in Australia: a time series analysis of the period 1950–2003. *Drug and Alcohol Reviews*, 30:466–72.

Ray, J. G. et al. (2008). Alcohol sales and risk of serious assault. *PLoS Medicine*, 13(5), e104.

Sánchez, A. L. et al. (2011). Policies for alcohol restriction and their association with interpersonal violence: a time-series analysis of homicides in Cali, Colombia. *International Journal of Epidemiology* 40, 1037–46.

Santos, S.M., Barcellos, C., and Sá Carvalho, M. (2006). Ecological analysis of the distribution and socio-spatial context of homicides in Porto Alegre, Brazil.*Health Place*, 12, 38–47.

Schneider, M. et al. (2007). South African Comparative Risk Assessment Collaborating Group. Estimating the burden of disease attributable to alcohol use in South Africa in 2000. *South African Medical Journal* 97(Pt 2), 664–72.

Sethi, D. et al. (2006). Reducing inequalities from injuries in Europe. *Lancet*, 368:2243–50.

Sethi, D. et al. (2010). *European Report on Preventing Violence and Knife Crime among Young People.* Copenhagen: WHO Regional Office for Europe.

Sethi, D. et al. (2013). *European Report on Preventing Child Maltreatment.* Copenhagen: WHO Regional Office for Europe.

Shaffer, J., and Ruback, R. (2002). Violent victimization as a risk factor for violent offending among juveniles. *Juvenile Justice Bulletin*, available from https://www.ncjrs.gov/pdffiles1/ojjdp/195737.pdf.

Singh, G. K. et al. (2013). All-Cause and Cause-Specific Mortality among US Youth: Socioeconomic and Rural-Urban Disparities and International Patterns. *Journal of Urban Health* 90(3), 388–405.

Stickley, A. et al. (2012). Socioeconomic inequalities in homicide mortality: a population-based comparative study of 12 European countries. *European Journal of Epidemiology* 27:877–84.

United Nations Office on Drugs and Crime. (2011). *Global Study on Homicide. Trend, Contexts, Data.* Vienna: UNODC.

UNODC. (2007). *Crime and Development in Central America. Caught in the Crossfire.* Vienna: UNODC.

Viana, L.A. et al. (2011). Social inequalities and the rise in violent deaths in Salvador, Bahia State, Brazil: 2000–2006. *Cad Saude Publica*, 27(Suppl. 2):S298–308.

World Health Organization. *Preventing Injuries and Violence: A Guide for Ministries of Health.* Geneva: WHO, 2007.

World Health Organization. (2011). *Global Burden of Disease. Disease and Injury Regional Estimates* [online database]. Geneva: WHO. http://www.who.int/healthinfo/statistics/mortality/en/index2.html, accessed 5 June 2013.

World Health Organization Regional Office for Europe. (2012). *Health 2020: A European Policy Framework Supporting Action across Government and Society for Health and Well-being.* Copenhagen: WHO Regional Office for Europe.

World Health Organization Regional Office for Europe. (2013). *Mortality Indicators by 67 Causes of Death, Age and Sex (HFA-MDB)* [online database]. Copenhagen: WHO Regional Office for Europe. http://data.euro.who.int/hfamdb/, accessed 5 June 2013.

CHAPTER 9

The epidemiology of elder abuse

Bridget Penhale and Isabel Iborra

Introduction to the Epidemiology of Elder Abuse

Elder abuse is not a modern-day phenomenon (Stearns 1986). Historical studies have shown that even in some ancient literary works there are depictions of behaviours that today would be described as abuse (Rheinharz 1986). However, it was not until the twentieth century that researchers, professionals, and policymakers began to pay attention: firstly to child abuse (in the 1960s), then to domestic violence (in the 1970s), and finally to the abuse and neglect experienced by older people (in the 1980s). The problem itself was first identified by a group of doctors in the United Kingdom in the 1970s, who coined the original term *granny battering* (Baker 1975), and by the end of the decade the term *elder abuse* appeared (Bennett et al. 1997).

This latest 'discovery' in the area of family violence is still relatively unknown within society today. Because of this, so far the area lacks the wealth of scientific evidence to back it up, which the other areas—minors and younger adult women—have been able to develop (Bazo 2004; Bennett et al. 1997). There is also general agreement among experts that levels of abuse and negligence are set to increase globally in future due to specific demographic changes which are resulting in an ageing population (particularly a decrease in infant mortality and increase in life expectancy; Iborra et al. 2013). In a recent report on elder abuse published by the World Health Organization (WHO), it is estimated that by 2050 one-third of the population will be aged 60 and over, and this ageing population will be likely to result in more older people at risk of mistreatment (Sethi et al. 2011).

Conceptual Clarification

Definition of Elder Abuse

Elder abuse is a complex problem and as such is difficult to define. There is no universally accepted definition which takes into account all the different aspects of violence and abuse that must necessarily be included (Penhale et al. 2000). Some definitions mainly focus on *family violence*, others on the maltreatment occurring in care homes, and others on *social abuse*, meaning the types of administrative abuse that deprive an older person from receiving the adequate basic services needed for their welfare. Although in other areas social abuse may align with institutional abuse, in relation to elder abuse institutional abuse has a specific meaning concerning particular institutional settings, such as care homes and hospitals. It is clear therefore that full agreement concerning terminology does not yet exist for elder abuse. Yet although it may not be essential to have a universal definition, it is vital for researchers to have a clear and precise definition of the term so they can work within standard criteria.

One of the first definitions of elder abuse was developed by the American Medical Association in 1987; this included physical abuse, psychological abuse, sexual abuse, and neglect of an elderly person by their caregiver as well as acts or omissions that either harm or threaten harm to the well-being and/or health of an older person (p. 966).

In 2002, INPEA—the international organization, which has in recent years been promoting studies and actions against this type of violence—offered a further definition, adapted from the definition developed by the United Kingdom charity Action on Elder Abuse. This definition was ratified by WHO in the Toronto Declaration (WHO/INPEA 2002, p. 3). Here, elder abuse was defined as:

> A single or repeated act, or lack of appropriate action, occurring within any relationship where there is an expectation of trust, which causes harm or distress to an older person. It can be of various forms: physical, psychological/emotional, sexual, financial, or simply reflect intentional or unintentional neglect.

Types of Elder Abuse and their Consequences

The majority of authors concur that there are five main types of elder abuse (Iborra 2008).

Physical Abuse

Physical abuse is any voluntary act that causes or may cause physical harm or injury to the elderly person.

Some examples of this type of abuse are hitting, burning, and shaking. It is important to note that this type of abuse also includes physical and chemical restraints. The most frequent consequences of physical abuse are bruises, broken bones, burns, and other physical injuries. Death may also occur, either as a result of severe assault or suffocation, or as the result of the severity of injuries sustained from the physical attack(s) on the person.

Psychological or Emotional Abuse

Psychological abuse is any act (normally verbal) or any attitude that causes or may cause psychological and/or emotional harm to the elderly person. Examples of this type of abuse include behaviours that insult, terrorize, humiliate, or threaten individuals, and actions that deprive the person of love and security. Especially relevant in the psychological abuse of older people are the threats that are meted out, the most common being those of abandonment and institutionalization, which are often designed and used to intimidate individuals.

The main consequences of this type of abuse are depression, anxiety, fear, and sadness. Longer-term effects such as suicidal thoughts and post-traumatic stress disorder may occur in those individuals who experience many years (or even decades) of abuse, such as older women who experience intimate partner violence throughout their relationships and that may endure in later life (Penhale and Porritt 2011). Psychological violence is usually confined to language—both verbal acts and those accompanied by physical gesture—but the consequences usually affect the victim's cognitive, emotional, and behavioural functioning. Psychological abuse is the most prevalent type of abuse found in the majority of existing studies and very often occurs alongside and at the same time as other types of abuse.

Neglect

Neglect is the failure to meet one's obligations in caring for an elderly person, or to fail to carry out specific actions or engage in appropriate care tasks. Separate definitions do not usually appear for neglect, which is often considered almost as a sub-type of abuse. It is also generally acknowledged as being either intentional or unintentional. Neglect often involves withholding or depriving the individual of his/her basic needs, such as adequate nutrition, hydration and hygiene, access to medication, heating, and other necessities of daily life. This category does not generally include situations of self-neglect, although in some countries such as the United States and Israel self-neglect is included as a type of elder abuse, particularly in relation to service responses. Abandonment is one of the most extreme forms of neglect.

Typical consequences of this type of abuse may be malnutrition, dehydration, poor hygiene, and pressure ulcers. In the most extreme situations, death may also occur, usually as a result of severe malnutrition or dehydration, or the body's inability to recover from major and often-extensive pressure ulcers.

Financial Abuse

Financial abuse is the illegal or non-authorized use of an elderly person's financial resources or property.

It includes the use, misuse, or abuse of the elderly person's property, finances, or affairs, including coercion concerning the signing of legal and financial documents.

Major consequences are the inability to pay for services or bills, and a resultant deterioration in standards of living and quality of life. Elders have traditionally been considered, and indeed they still are, at risk of suffering this kind of abuse, particularly if they live in isolated situations and where they may be viewed as 'easy targets'. Women who experience abuse at the hands of their partners are the other group that appear to be particularly vulnerable to this type of abuse as the control exercised by their partners may extend to enforced economic dependence.

Sexual Abuse

Sexual abuse is any non-desired physical contact where the elderly person is used as a means by which the aggressor obtains sexual stimulation or gratification. Examples include fondling; oral, anal or vaginal penetration with objects, fingers, or the penis; sexual

harassment; forcing the person to perform sexual acts on the aggressor or to look at (or watch) pornographic material.

Among the consequences for victims it is very common to find trauma in the genital, breast, mouth, and anal areas; sexually transmitted diseases; or distressed behaviour. The last one may be particularly likely as a result of witnessing or being forced to view explicit material.

In short, each type of abuse is determined by certain, specific behaviours with different consequences for each victim. Concerning the most extreme consequence—the death of the victim—this is mainly the result of two types of abuse: physical abuse and neglect. Whilst some progress has been made in several countries in developing service responses, particularly in relation to physical abuse, it is important to emphasize that withholding the basic needs of a dependent elderly person over lengthy periods can result in their death (through extreme malnutrition or dehydration, for instance). Furthermore, improvement in quality standards in care settings, which contain a focus on abuse and neglect, is not yet either universally applied or accepted as necessary.

Table 9.1 lists the range of behaviours associated with each type of abuse along with their main consequences. It is important to stress that, apart from the specific effects of each type of abuse, victims may also present with psychological problems (such as depression or anxiety) whatever the type of abuse, and the emotional consequences of abuse may last for very long periods of time (Table 9.1).

Prevalence of Elder Abuse

The first research studies into the prevalence of elder abuse took place in Australia, Canada, China, the United States, Norway, and Sweden in the late 1980s; these were then followed by Brazil, Chile, India, Israel, Japan, the UK, South Africa, and other European countries in the 1990s (Wolf et al. 2002). The first research studies in Spain came later (Bazo 2001). If we take into account that there has only been three decades of dedication to this area of study, it should come as no surprise to discover the overall scarcity of studies into the incidence and prevalence of elder abuse.

Moreover, investigating elder abuse is prone to a series of difficulties. Firstly, elderly people are often very reluctant to report cases of abuse. Even in cases where abuse has been detected, many older people do not recognize it as such and/or refuse to report it because of the nature of their relationship with the aggressor/abuser and often ambivalent features of such relationships. Secondly, due to certain features of old age (such as illnesses, skin peculiarities, and so forth) it is sometimes very difficult to distinguish the signs of abuse from those of a possible illness or health condition.

Even when these problems are addressed in studies in this area, there is an added difficulty, which must be overcome: the comparability of data. Each existing study has tended to use a different definition of abuse, investigates different categories or types of abuse, applies different methods, and even uses different cut-off ages when defining the sample (of elderly people). These divergences mean that it is incredibly difficult to compare the results from different studies and therefore the possibility for results to be generalized is very much reduced.

Nevertheless, Table 9.2 lists the prevalence of each type of abuse found in the main existing studies carried out nationally in diverse countries. It is also important to add here that the WHO

Table 9.1 Examples and consequences of different types of abuse

Type of abuse	Examples	Examples of consequences
Physical Abuse	Beating, slapping, burning, pushing, shaking.	Scratches, injuries, contusions, marks, bruises, fractures, dislocations, abrasions, burns, hair loss.
Emotional Abuse	Rejecting, insulting, terrorizing, isolating, shouting, blaming, humiliating, intimidating, threatening, ignoring, depriving of affection.	Depression, anxiety, despair, sleep disorders, loss of appetite, fear, confusion, low mood and self-esteem, suicidal thoughts.
Neglect	Withholding basic necessities (nutrition, hydration, hygiene, weather-appropriate clothing, health or social care), abandonment.	Malnutrition, dehydration, inadequate hygiene, hypothermia or hyperthermia, pressure ulcers.
Financial Abuse	Appropriation, utilization or misappropriation of the elderly person's money or property, forging of signatures, forcing elders to sign documents (contracts or wills).	Inability to pay bills, lack of services, eviction, decrease in standard of living.
Sexual Abuse	Fondling or kissing, penetration, humiliation, harassment, forced to watch pornographic material.	Emotional distress, trauma of the genitals, breasts, mouth, anal area; sexually transmitted diseases, bite marks.

Reproduced with kind permission from Iborra I., *Elder Abuse in the Family in Spain*, Queen Sofía Centre, Valencia, Spain, Copyright © 2008.

Table 9.2 Types and levels of abuse by country (in percentages)

	Physical and sexual abuse	Psychological abuse	Neglect	Financial abuse	Total
Australia (Kurrle et al. 1992)	2.1	2.5	1.4	1.1	4.6
Canada (Podnieks 1989)	0.5	1.4	0.4	2.5	4
Ireland (Naughton et al. 2010)	0.55	1.2	0.3	1.3	2.2
Israel (Eisikovits et al. 2004)	2	8	18	6.6	
Spain (Iborra 2008)	0.2	0.3	0.3	0.2	0.8
United Kingdom (O'Keeffe et al. 2007)	0.4	0.4	1.1	0.7	2.6
United States (Pillemer and Finkelhor 1988)	2.0	1.1	0.4	–	3.2

Reproduced with kind permission from Iborra I., **Elder Abuse in the Family in Spain**, Queen Sofía Centre, Valencia, Spain, Copyright © 2008.

estimates that between 4 and 6 per cent of the elderly have suffered some kind of abuse at the hands of family members (Wolf et al. 2002). Additionally, a further recent WHO report confirms that the prevalence of elder maltreatment in the community is about 3 per cent and may be as high as 25 per cent for older people with high support needs (Sethi et al. 2011).

The latest study dealing with elder abuse, the ABUEL study (ABuse and health among ELderly in Europe), which undertook research in seven EU countries (German, Greece, Italy, Lithuania, Portugal, Spain, and Sweden), found a reported prevalence of 19.4 per cent of mental abuse, 2.7 per cent of physical abuse, 0.7 per cent of sexual abuse, and 3.8 per cent of financial abuse (Soares 2010).

Risk Factors for Elder Abuse

Risk factors for violence include any feature that makes a person vulnerable to perpetrating or experiencing violent behaviour. The fact that a person may have risk factors does not necessarily imply that they will go on to abuse others; it simply means that they have a higher probability of being involved in those behaviours than people without those factors present. It also means that the index

of suspicion of professionals should be higher in order to be aware of the increased possibility that violence might occur. No single factor explains why some individuals behave violently toward others or why violence is more prevalent in some communities than in others (Krug et al. 2002). Applying the ecological model (Bronfenbrenner 1979) is helpful to understanding violence as the complex interplay of individual, relationship, community, and social factors (Krug et al. 2002).

Individual Factors

The first level of the Ecological Model focuses on the characteristics in the individual, which increase the likelihood of their being either a victim or a perpetrator of violence. In addition to biological and demographic factors, it includes other factors such as impulsivity, substance abuse, and a prior history of aggression and abuse.

◆ **Gender:** There appears to be a close consensus in the literature that it is women who suffer from the more severe cases of physical and emotional abuse, as well as its being women who are the principal victims of sexual abuse (Pillemer and Finkelhor 1988), but with the levels of neglect being similar for both sexes.

When considering the gender of perpetrators, several studies have found a higher prevalence of male as opposed to female abusers. However, there is an increasing tendency to differentiate this data depending on the type of abuse perpetrated. Authors following this line of investigation confirm that women tend to be more responsible in cases of neglect, while men are more likely to be responsible for the more extreme and severe forms of abuse as well as physical and sexual abuse (Iborra and Penhale 2011).

◆ *Age of victim*: The risk of abuse increases with age. Many studies have found higher levels of abuse in people over the age of 75, especially in cases of neglect and financial abuse (Iborra and Penhale 2011).

◆ *Victim's dependence or disability*: Maltreatment rates increase with dependency, disability or with declining health status (Iborra and Penhale 2011). Certain questions related to disability—such as changes in expectations, decreased functional capacity, and ignorance of the effects of illness on cognition—may serve to increase the risk of certain types of abuse (Bazo 2002).

◆ *Dementia*: Several different studies have found higher levels of abuse in older people with cognitive problems. People with Alzheimer's disease or dementia in particular are three times more likely to suffer abuse compared to the general population (Iborra and Penhale 2011). One factor to take into account is that research carried out on people with dementia has shown that aggressive behaviour on the part of the older person (or that which is viewed as provocative by the other party) may trigger a violent response from the carer (Pillemer and Suitor 1992).

◆ *Psychopathology*: A number of studies have found that depression, suicidal thoughts, and feelings of unhappiness, shame or guilt are common among victims (Bonnie and Wallace 2003; Muñoz 2004).

In relation to the perpetrators of maltreatment against older people, studies (of which there are few) show that such individuals are more likely to have psychological problems (especially depression) and substance-abuse problems than those carers with no (known) history of abusive behaviour (Cooney and Mortimer 1995; González et al. 2005; Lachs and Pillemer 1995; Pillemer 2005; Wolf and Pillemer 1989). The abuse of psychoactive substances, and especially alcohol dependence, among perpetrators has been closely associated with situations of continued and severe maltreatment, specifically in cases of physical abuse. There may also be links with financial abuse in order to provide the means to maintain lifestyles involving substance misuse.

◆ *Aggressor's financial problems*: A review of studies carried out by the WHO showed that financial difficulties on the part of a perpetrator are a major risk factor for elder maltreatment (Krug et al. 2002).

Relationship Factors

The second level of the Ecological Model explores how close social relationships—with peers, intimate partners, and family members—may increase the risk of violent victimization and the perpetration of violence.

◆ *Stress*: Several studies have highlighted the importance of the perception of stress and burnout syndrome as predictors for the presence of elder maltreatment (Coyne and Reichman 1993; Steinmetz 1990). It is however apparent that there is no direct causal relationship between care-giving, stress, and maltreatment. The latest research in this area seems to point to the type of relationship prior to the abuse as possibly being an important predictive factor for maltreatment (Wolf et al. 2002).

◆ *Financial dependence of the aggressor*: In many cases perpetrators are financially dependent on the victim for their accommodation, maintenance, transport, and other costs (Iborra and Penhale 2011). Perpetrators may also have financial problems due to difficulties in relation to substance misuse.

◆ *Living conditions*: According to different studies, living alone reduces the risk of maltreatment, whereas living with a family member is a risk factor for becoming a victim of violence (Pillemer 1988, 2005; Pillemer and Suitor 1992). Living alone may, however, be a risk factor for certain types of abuse such as financial abuse and exploitation (O'Keeffe et al. 2007)

Community Factors

The third level of the Ecological Model examines the community contexts in which social relationships are embedded, such as workplaces and neighbourhoods. This level deals with factors affecting the community at large, such as poor, deprived areas, high levels of job insecurity and unemployment, poor levels of social support, and weak social systems.

◆ *Social isolation*: Social isolation is a characteristic risk factor for domestic violence in families. Elderly victims of maltreatment generally have fewer social contacts. It is also common for victims to live alone with the perpetrator, who is often their sole caregiver (Pillemer 2005). In addition, some research studies have suggested that perpetrators also have problems with social relationships and are more isolated (Cooney and Mortimer 1995; González et al. 2005).

◆ *Lack of social support*: A number of studies show that abusive carers lack the social support to assist them with their care-giving tasks (Iborra and Penhale 2011). The available data indicate that the importance of the lack of social support as a risk factor may be related to the presence of burnout in carers, the extremely high levels of need among victims, and to social isolation, among other issues.

Social Factors

The fourth and final level of the Ecological Model examines the wider societal factors that influence rates of violence. Included here are those factors which create a climate in which there is an acceptance of violence, those that lower inhibitions against violence, and those that create and sustain gaps between different segments of society. Wider societal factors include cultural norms that support violence as an acceptable way to resolve conflicts, or the presence of certain cultural attitudes and traditions such as ageism and sexism, which may influence the development and maintenance of violence towards certain groups or individuals, in this case older people and perhaps in particular older women.

- *Ageism:* Butler coined the term 'ageism' in 1969 to refer to a process by which people are systematically stereotyped for the mere fact of being old, in the same way as racism and sexism act in reaction to the colour of a person's skin or gender. The term was first used in an article in the *Washington Post* and later further defined (Butler and Lewis 1973; Bytheway 1995). In this respect, ageism may act as a major category, serving as a societal or cultural backdrop in which elder maltreatment is accepted and permissible (Penhale et al. 2000).

- *Violent culture:* Culture is believed to play a very important role in spreading violent behaviour. Tolerance of violence within society may be reflected in the media, in the acceptance of certain behaviours towards disabled people or the way that nations resolve conflicts. This acceptance or normalization of violence permeates daily activities and may contribute to the manifestation of violence.

Protective Factors

When considering risk factors we also need to take into account protective factors, which might help an individual to withstand the potentially adverse effects of risk factors. Such characteristics and variables improve an individual's resilience, increase resistance to the particular risk factor, and generally strengthen the individual against the undesirable event or disorder from happening. Although research in relation to older people's resilience and protective factors is lacking, some have been identified (Mowlam et al. 2007):

- relationship norms and personal values, with those reporting more positive relationships and values having an improved capacity to withstand abuse

- social and community connectedness, with those who are more socially connected reporting less harmful effects of abuse

- religious beliefs, where individuals with strong beliefs report an improved ability to withstand the more negative effects of abuse and violence

- living alone, bereavement, and fear of being alone interact more negatively so that those who live alone or who are bereaved show less resistance to harmful effects of abuse

- health, where good reported health appears to strengthen the individual's resistance to the harmful effects

- previous life experiences, where positive prior experiences are a beneficial support

- personality and personal qualities, and

- specific tactics in the form of coping strategies developed and used to deal with the maltreatment (once this occurs).

Research that fully explores the nature of protective factors has so far been lacking and more research is needed in this area. This is of particular relevance in relation to identification of those factors that might be influential in preventing elder abuse from occurring.

Conclusion

Elder abuse is a complex and multi-faceted problem, covering a broad continuum. In view of this, it appears unlikely that one single risk factor could account for the majority of situations of elder abuse. As previously indicated, the reasons why the situation has occurred and the risk factors associated with this are likely to be an interaction of several factors, largely depending on specific circumstances. It is therefore important to explore and determine the nature of such factors and possible co-existing interactions. Although research during the past two decades has provided some evidence relating to the nature and extent of elder abuse, there is not yet any definite consensus about prevalence, or which risk factors are of prime importance in the genesis and perpetuation of situations of elder abuse and neglect. And as noted, one of the main limitations within much of the research has been the use of different definitions and methodologies, which has limited the extent of any comparability. Elder abuse is a serious social problem with prevalence rates that vary across different cultures and countries; there is a need, on an international basis, for more standardized definitions, research instruments (such as screening tools), and methods in order to further determine the nature of the problem and to develop appropriate responses to it.

References

American Medical Association (1987) Report of the council of scientific affairs of the AMA: elder abuse and neglect, *Journal of American Medical Association (JAMA)*, 257, 966–71.

Baker, A. A. (1975). Granny battering. *Modern Geriatrics*, 5, 20–4.

Bazo, M. T. (2001). Negligencia y maltrato a las personas ancianas en España. *Revista Española de Geriatría y Gerontología*, 36, 8–14.

Bazo, M. T. (2002). Diversas manifestaciones de la violencia familiar. *Alternativas. Cuadernos de Trabajo Social*, 10, 213–9.

Bazo, M. T. (2004). Perfil de la persona mayor víctima de violencia. In: J. Sanmartín (ed.). *El Laberinto de la Violencia*. Barcelona: Ariel, pp. 219–27.

Bennett, G., Kingston, P., and Penhale, B. (1997). *The Dimensions of Elder Abuse: Perspectives for Practitioners*. London: MacMillan.

Bonnie, R., and Wallace, R. (2003). *Elder Maltreatment: Abuse, Neglect, and Exploitation in an Aging America*. Washington, D.C.: The National Academies.

Bronfenbrenner, V. (1979). *The Ecology of Human Development: Experiments by Nature and Design*. Cambridge: Harvard University Press.

Butler, R., and Lewis, M. (1973) *Aging and Mental Health*. St. Louis, M.O.: Mosby.

Bytheway, B. (1995). *Ageism*. Buckingham: Open University Press.

Cooney, C., and Mortimer, A. (1995). Elder abuse and dementia: a pilot study. *International Journal of Social Psychiatry*, 4, 276–83.

Coyne, A., and Reichman, W. (1993). The relationship between dementia and elder abuse. *American Journal of Psychiatry*, 150, 643–6.

Eisikovits, Z., Winterstein, T., and Lowenstein, A. (2004). *The National Survey on Elder Abuse and Neglect in Israel*. Haifa: University of Haifa.

González, J. A., Flórez, F. J., González, A., García, D., and Salgado, A. (2005). Malos tratos al anciano. In: T. Sánchez (ed.), *Maltrato de Género, Infantil y de Ancianos*. Salamanca: Universidad Pontificia de Salamanca, pp. 105–19.

Iborra, I. (2008). *Elder Abuse in the Family in Spain*. Valencia: Queen Sofía Centre.

Iborra, I., and Penhale, B. (2011). Risk factors. In: D. Sethi, S. Wood and F. Mitis et al. (eds), *European Report on Preventing Elder Maltreatment*. Denmark: World Health Organization, pp. 29–42.

Iborra, I., García, Y., and Grau, E. (2013). Spain. In: A. Phelan (2013). *International Perspectives on Elder Abuse*. London: Routledge, pp. 168–87.

Krug, E., Dahlberg, L., Mercy, J., Zwi, A., and Lozano, R. (2002). *Report on Violence and Health*. Geneva: World Health Organization.

Kurrle, S. E., Sadler, P. M., and Cameron, I. D. (1992). Patterns of elder abuse. *Medical Journal of Australia*, 155, 150–3.

Lachs, M. S., and Pillemer, K. (1995). Abuse and neglect of elderly persons. *New England Journal of Medicine*, 332, 437–43.

Mowlam, A., Tennant, R., Dixon, J., and McCreadie, C. (2007). *UK Study of Abuse and Neglect of Older People: Qualitative Findings*. London: National Centre for Social Research.

Muñoz, J. (2004). *Personas Mayores y Malos Tratos*. Madrid: Ediciones Pirámide.

Naughton, C., Drennan, J., and Treacy, M. P. et al. (2010). *Abuse and Neglect of Older People in Ireland. Report on the National Study of Elder Abuse and Neglect*. Dublin: National Centre for the Protection of Older People.

O'Keeffe, M., Hills, A., and Doyle, M. et al. (2007). *UK Study of Abuse and Neglect of Older People. Prevalence Survey Report*. London: National Centre for Social Research and King's College London.

Penhale, B., Parker, J., and Kingston, P. (2000). *Elder Abuse. Approaches to Working with Violence*. Birmingham: Venture.

Penhale, B., and Porritt, J. (2011). *Intimate Partner Violence and Older Women: UK National Report*. Sheffield: University of Sheffield.

Pillemer, K. (2005). Factores de riesgo del maltrato de mayores. In: I. Iborra (ed.), *Violencia Contra Personas Mayores*. Barcelona: Ariel, pp. 69–85.

Pillemer, K., and Finkelhor, D. (1988). The prevalence of elder abuse: a random sample survey. *Gerontologist*, 28, 51–7.

Pillemer, K., and Suitor, J. (1992). Violence and violent feelings: what causes them among family caregivers. *Journal of Gerontology*, 47, S165–72.

Podnieks, E. (1989). *National Survey on the Abuse of the Elderly in Canada*. Ottawa: Ryerson Polytechnic Institute.

Rheinharz, S. (1986). Loving and hating one's elders: twin themes in legend and literature. In: K. Pillemer and R. Wolf (eds). *Elder Abuse: Conflict in the Family*. Dover, MA: Auburn House, pp. 25–48.

Sethi, D., Wood, S., and Mitis, F. et al. (2011), *European Report on Preventing Elder Maltreatment*. Denmark: World Health Organization.

Soares, J. (2010). *Abuse and Health in Europe*. Kaunas: Lithuanian University of Health Sciences Press.

Stearns, P. (1986). Old age family conflict: the perspective of the past. In: K. Pillemer and R. Wolf (eds). *Elder Abuse: Conflict in the Family*. Dover, MA: Auburn House, pp. 3–24.

Steinmetz, S. K. (1990). Elder abuse: myth and reality. In: T. H. Brubaker (ed.), *Family Relationships in Later Life. 2nd ed.* Newbury Park, CA: Sage, pp. 193–211.

WHO/INPEA (2002). *Missing Voices: Views of Older Persons on Elder Abuse*. Geneva: World Health Organization.

Wolf, R., Daichman, L., and Bennett, G. (2002). Abuse of the elderly. In: E. G. Krug, L. L. Dahlberg, J. A. Mercy, A. B. Zwi and R. Lozano (eds), *World Report on Violence and Health*. Geneva: World Health Organization, pp. 133–58.

Wolf, R., and Pillemer, K. (1989). *Helping Elderly Victims: The Reality of Elder Abuse*. New York: Columbia University Press.

CHAPTER 10

Beyond convention: anthropology, drugs, and violence

Jorja Leap

Introduction to Beyond Convention: Anthropology, Drugs, and Violence

Over time, 'the usual suspects', including criminologists, psychologists, and sociologists, have examined the relationship between drugs and violence. Yet, as the problems engendered by this relationship endure, it is necessary to consider new perspectives, including those offered by anthropologists. With its emphasis on cultural context and rigorous use of participant observation, anthropology offers a multi-layered and nuanced view of street-level drug dealing, use, and impact.

This chapter offers an ethnographic account of the complex relationship between violence and drugs, focusing on the street level. It combines participant observation and life history interviews into themes that have emerged from over 12 years of fieldwork in Los Angeles, California, focused on active and former gang members and their families who exist in violent but well-established communities. Illegal drugs comprise a powerful thread that weaves its way through everyday life in these communities; because of this, residents talk openly about the social problems created by 'dope'. Gang members interviewed during this research proved articulate and knowledgeable, and their voices created a narrative history that illuminated the relationship between violence and street drugs, including drug sales and the surrounding code of conduct, collateral damage, trauma, and self-medication. Beyond this, individual life histories provided a window into how race, culture, and gender further affect the drugs and violence dynamic.

The relationship between drugs and violence is often portrayed as one of individual impulsivity accompanied by random, erratic behaviour. In fact, this interaction is much more complicated and layered. Drug abuse and violent behaviour is frequently pre-meditated and strategic, based on issues of economic need, group enforcement, self-medication, and long-term trauma.

Ethnographic Approach

For the past two decades, there have been detailed qualitative examinations of the culture of drug networks and their role in community life. Researchers, acting as participant observers, have added depth and complexity to findings concerning the relationship between drugs and violence. Bourgois' (1996) seminal work, *In Search of Respect: Selling Crack in El Barrio*, offered anthropological insight into the Puerto Rican immigrant community in East Harlem, New York, where marginalized individuals struggled with poverty, revealing that drugs provided opportunities for social advancement within a context of violence and fear. More recent ethnographies have built upon this work. Both Venkatesh (2008) and Contreras (2012) embedded themselves in the daily lives of gang members and the surrounding community, illuminating not only the intersection of drugs and violence, but also the impact of poverty, family violence, gender, age, education, trauma, access to services, and more. Similarly Leap (2012) and Phillips (2012) both employed an ethnographic approach to depict the tensions between families, gang members, and law enforcement. From an unusual perspective, Moskos (2008) collected ethnographic data during his year-long employment as a police officer in Baltimore, Maryland, which informed his belief that street drugs should be legalized in order to better control violence. From another perspective, Boyle (2010) provided an ethnographic account of his two decades as a priest working with gang-involved youth in East Los Angeles, California.

These ethnographies portray the socio-economic and political systems that impact marginalized neighbourhoods while detailing individual struggles for survival, economic stability, personal attachment, and security. Each tells a story of communities being left behind, where meaningful programmes and interventions remain incomplete or altogether absent. As participant observers, these researchers and authors analyse individual experiences influenced by neighbourhood rituals and drug dealing practices that unfold alongside the competing forces of violence and community stability.

Life Histories and Autobiographies

Using a qualitative methodology strongly related to ethnography, anthropologists have developed the study of individuals through the documentation of the 'life history'. The collection and analysis of life histories has proven helpful to researchers interpreting cultural change and deviance and their respective consequences over time. The approach is highly phenomenological, designed to enable an individual to 'tell the story' of his or her life to better understand personal identity, the surrounding community, and the impact of individual and cultural transformation. This approach requires researchers to compile life narratives during multiple interviews conducted over a long time periods, in each individual's own words, using open-ended questions. Despite its efficacy in other settings, there has been little anthropological research on gang and/or criminal life histories that might include information about the relationship between drugs and violence. This is surprising given these individuals' pronounced desire to recount their life histories during fieldwork and in the ever-increasing number of autobiographies by former gang members, including well-known works by Rodriguez (1993, 2011) and Scott (1993) as well as newer autobiographies by Williams (2004), Sanchez (2000, 2003), Morris (2008), and the account of one woman (Brown 2006).

Ethnographic Setting and Preliminary Findings

In 2002, I began informal observations of the behaviours, rituals, and social practices of active and former gang members in gang-impacted communities throughout Los Angeles County. Los Angeles County is characterized by urban sprawl: there is no city centre and no single violent community. Work conducted by the Los Angeles Mayor's Office and the Advancement Project identified 14 'hot spots' where there was a concentration of violence and crime. Based on my initial research and a network of relationships that afforded me extensive contacts and credibility in these communities, I ultimately chose to work within one hot spot: Watts in South Los Angeles. Within Watts, three housing developments— Jordan Downs, Nickerson Gardens, and Imperial Courts—are recognized as the scene of some of the most entrenched gang crime in Los Angeles. These developments or 'projects' as they are commonly known, have long been acknowledged as 'ground zero' for gang activity in Los Angeles.

Historically, most residents in the Watts 'projects' have been African-American although in recent years (Medina 2012) the population has shifted to include Mexicans and Central Americans. My on-going work in Watts was augmented with extensive observations throughout South Los Angeles and the Los Angeles Harbour Area. Through this work, several facets of the relationship between drugs, gang activity, and violence began to emerge. To further examine this relationship, I conducted fieldwork and interviews with former gang members at several gang intervention agencies including Homeboy Industries, Toberman Community Center, and Communities in Schools. This work, combined with 100 individual life histories I collected over a ten-year period, revealed a portrait of distinct yet interrelated aspects of the street drug trade, the occurrence and practice of violence, and the lives of individuals and families affected by their interaction.

Violence and Relationships

From the onset it was apparent that violence inevitably accompanied street drug activity, or as one gang member explained, 'Ya can't have slangin' [drug dealing] without goin' bangin' [engaging in gang-related violence]'. This inter-relationship most frequently involved individuals who knew one another and had committed acts of violence against one another over prolonged periods of time, primarily through gang activity. Additionally, street violence was reinforced within family systems. Elevated rates of street drug sales and related crime were accompanied by equally high rates of child abuse and domestic violence. Finally, firearms, up to and including automatic weapons, were readily available to children, adolescents, and young adults who routinely carried them. All of this created an atmosphere of instability and eminent violence. As one gang member explained, 'Drugs is easy, guns is easy—what isn't easy is keepin' it all cool, keepin' it under control'.

Gang and community rituals further fostered the interaction between drugs and violence through relational practices involving inclusion, exclusion, and humiliation.

Most common is the initiation ritual of being 'jumped in' to gang membership, which involves being beaten and humiliated by multiple gang members. Another practice occurs through the ritual display of hand signs. These signs portray allegiance to the gang along with demonstrating disrespect for enemy, rival gangs; they are a barometer of inclusion and exclusion. Gang hand signs comprise incendiary non-verbal behaviour, particularly when a hand sign is demonstrated or 'thrown' at a rival gang member. This behavioural ritual, also referred to as 'set tripping' typically provokes conflict and violence.

Individuals are expected to 'put in work' for the neighbourhood (a synonym for gang), which includes dealing drugs and meting out punishment to those who have operated outside sanctioned drug networks, or who have breached the gang code of conduct regarding territory and business practices. The value of inclusion and the wish to avoid exclusion serve as effective social controls; specific individuals are excluded from any sort of drug dealing or distribution, particularly drug addicts who are deemed unreliable. Trust is central to gang and community life with personal and collective reputations always 'in play'. Individuals are 'down for the hood' or 'stand-up', all phrases signalling unconditional loyalty and allegiance to the gang. An informal street network constantly communicates information, spreading rumours and gossip about territorial feuds, who is obedient, and who is not functioning in accordance with gang norms and expectations. The most damaging rumours and dangerous labels involve accusations of serving as an informant for law enforcement. Accusations based on suspicion and weak evidence may result in withdrawal, suspending any access to street drugs, and cutting off gang ties. In more extreme cases, when an individual has been discovered 'snitching', there is violent retaliation that may include homicide. However, such retaliation is neither monolithic nor automatic. Instead, violence is often filtered through several critical factors, most notably race, culture, and gender.

Race and Culture

For decades, Southern California communities have been held hostage by a street culture characterized by violent conflicts involving African-American (black) and Mexican (brown) gangs. These conflicts have both intra-racial and inter-racial dimensions, fuelled by drugs, territory, and women. Long-term gang rivalries have been further complicated by the recent influx of Central American gangs that have added new and more lethal elements to the 'game'—a term used to connote street drug trade. One gang member observed, 'It's always gonna be on between blacks and browns. But MS-13–it's a different game. They're gonna kill their brother if they've got it like that'.

Racial and cultural tensions surrounding drug dealing and territory are further amplified by generational differences. There are currently Mexican gangs in East Los Angeles whose providence encompasses five generations and African-American gangs tracing their lineage back three generations. Older individuals frequently discuss how younger drug dealers and gang members, 'just comin' up' do not abide by traditional rules. One 'OG', or Original Gangster, lamented:

> It's different now. These youngsters don't got any respect for the neighborhood. They do what they wanna do. We put the neighborhood first—these youngsters put themselves first. And they go blastin' anyone—sometimes they'll blast someone from their own hood!

Gender

Historically, men used drugs to fuel violence while women used drugs to recover from violence (Atkinson et al. 2009). Now both genders play non-traditional roles in the drug–violence dynamic. In the past, women were only peripherally involved, if they participated at all, serving as accessories to drug dealing that operated through men. This has changed for multiple reasons. First, lesbians and transgender females have increasingly assumed higher profile roles in African-American and Latino gangs. Traditionally, homophobic gang members have rejected gay men but now describe lesbians as 'part of the hood'. Additionally, women—both gay and straight—have assumed active roles in neighbourhood life, serving as drug dealers, shooters, and in some very limited cases, shot callers or leaders. One former gang member chronicled the changes:

> Women just used to bein' baby mamas had their men get locked up, they needed money. Then they got into it, some of them became shooters—it was part of the game. Pretty soon these girls—women— were rollin' up and shootin' people. They put in work for the hood, they got jumped in and everything.

This was reinforced in the memories of a female former gang member who recalled:

> I had my first baby when I was 14—and my baby's daddy got locked up. What the fuck was I gonna do—I needed money, I kinda caught up that way and I started slangin'. I learned to use a gun too—in case anyone fucked with me.

In the past, women in gang-infested communities either became the victims of sexual violence and/or they suffered from drug abuse. However, as they assumed increasingly active roles in street-level crime and violence, recent research reveals that, their rates of gang membership have begun to dramatically increase (Wolf and Gutierrez 2012). Despite these trends, many male gang members remain reluctant to afford women either full status or the full consequences of participation in the drugs and violence dynamic. Several men insisted, 'I could never shoot a woman— she's someone's mama'.

Street Dealing

Drug dealing represents both a business enterprise and a source of employment for marginalized individuals. As street drug

networks have grown, so has the need for rules, structure, and consequences, with the threat of violence used as a source of order and enforcement. One former shot caller tersely explained, 'Business has always gotta be tight'. On-going ethnographic observation revealed that violence is used strategically to enforce rules regarding business practices, drug dealing territories, and punishment for disloyalty. One former gang member explained:

> I knew sometimes when someone was comin' into my territory, rollin' up to my corner, they gotta be put in their place. If they set up in your territory—you gotta protect your business.

Violence is strategically employed to keep business 'in order'. Several individuals described preventing their employees from setting up competing drug enterprises. 'Ya gotta stay in control of your people', one gang member offered, 'you give em' enough but not so much that they can start their own thing'.

Alongside monitoring employees, commercial territory must be protected. Most conversations invariably returned to the subject of territory or 'turf'. While gangs mark geographic areas with graffiti, territory is important beyond the issue of neighbourhood reputation. Drug dealing operations on different streets or parks are carefully guarded by gangs using violence to protect their turf and business. It is also notable that with increasing organization and higher profit stakes, violence becomes more focused, strategic, and effective, less random and impulsive. It also becomes more lethal and divorced from gang activity. However, this type of focus only evolves after years of drug dealing and criminal operations. As one former gang member commented, 'It's big business, you gotta be organized—no more gangbanging, just profits and consequences'.

All street drug trade concentrates on completely avoiding another danger: law enforcement. During quieter nights of observation with limited street activity, a former gang member explained, 'These are the nights the cops patrol. Everyone knows it and goes inside'. Aside from such general caution, there are specific sanctions against shooting at or killing police officers. One gang member warned, 'If you shoot a cop, they're gonna be up your ass—the cops won't stop til they've gotcha—they're as bad as gangsters'.

In contrast, both African-American and Latino gangs invoke explicit sanctions regarding the use of violence against snitches. During fieldwork, individuals offered multiple cautionary tales of snitches who 'got plugged' or 'got their tongues cut off', or 'got their nuts cut off'. Drug dealers invariably feared that a snitch or informant would endanger both their network and their lives. One individual, carefully talking in 'hypotheticals', described what he would do 'if someone in my crew was a snitch. I gotta bring a hammer down on their head'. With further discussion it emerged he meant a literal hammer. 'Sometimes a gun's too fast, painless— you gotta make a snitch feel the pain. Just speakin' theoretically'.

Individuals also described another area in which sanctions operated: becoming addicted to one's own product. 'It's no good. You can't shoot straight if you're high', a former shot caller observed. Addicts were viewed as incapable of rational business decision-making, posing a threat to the game, their families, and themselves. Another former gang member explained how drug abuse and eventual addiction proved to be a turning point:

> Everyone told me, don't try cocaine. I thought I could control it. Pretty soon I was snortin' and smokin' all of my product. I burned

summa my people and they came after me. I was doin' crazy stuff. I was stealin' stuff and sellin' stuff and poundin' anyone who came after me. I almost shot onna my best friends. But I wound up in prison—which was the best thing that coulda happened to me because my life finally turned around.

Collateral Damage: Violence as a Side Effect

The violence surrounding street drug dealing often results in what many refer to as 'collateral damage'—the unintended consequences suffered by those not directly involved. One gang member explained, 'It's no good when ya get civilians involved. It might be someone's mama or someone's baby who gets killed. That's deep'. When random violence affects the uninvolved and the unintended, the results are often disastrous. In informal discussions, a former gang member recalled the response when a child was mistakenly killed:

> Even though it was an accident, y'know [gang] got a green light. That means that someone in the neighborhood that killed the youngster gotta die to pay for the youngster's death. It's street justice, ya can't stop it.

Along with this threat of street justice, collateral damage inevitably brought an overwhelming response from law enforcement. 'It's already intense, but if a kid gets killed', a gang member whistled to himself, 'the police, they everywhere'.

Drug-related violence is not restricted to the street; instead it spills into family relationships. Domestic violence and child abuse are long-noted side effects of the disinhibiting properties of street drugs. In their life histories, men and women both detailed pasts filled with domestic violence and child abuse. From both informal discussions and formal interviews that formed part of the Watts ethnography as well as in life histories collected from other sites, every single individual without exception reported experiencing childhood abuse—whether physical, sexual, or some form of neglect, much of it linked to drug use and addiction. Several women described incidents of sexual abuse that they attributed to drugs or alcohol. One woman recalled, 'My stepdad would get high and didn't know what he was doing and he'd rape me over and over', while another woman connected drugs to sexual abuse:

> You just knew in my family when the men were using, you were gonna get it—they would force themselves on someone, usually me. My momma used to say, it's not really your daddy so it doesn't matter. My momma had boyfriends and when she wasn't there they would make me do stuff—sexual stuff—or they said they'd kill me.

Another woman, who had been an active gang member until she became addicted to methamphetamine, described how, 'When I turned 13 my mom and dad started selling me to get money to do more drugs'.

While reported sexual abuse was more prevalent among women, drug-related physical abuse was common among both males and females. In a sample of 50 former gang members' life histories at Homeboy Industries' gang intervention programme, 48 men and women reported multiple instances of physical abuse, all linked with the use of alcohol or drugs (Franke and Leap 2010). The two individuals who did not experience physical abuse reported that their parents were severe heroin addicts and, in the words of one,

'got so high they never even knew what was goin' on. I raised myself, I wish they woulda disciplined me'.

Individuals expressed two distinct opinions of child abuse. Sexual abuse was labelled 'sick', 'fucked up', 'perverted', and 'the worse thing you could do to someone'. In contrast, physical abuse was viewed as normative and a socially acceptable form of discipline with individuals insisting, 'I gotta beat my kid once in a while', and 'My daddy beat me and I came up okay'. The problems child abuse engendered did not stop with the abuse itself. Both active and former gang members feared children's protective services. Many had been placed in foster care as children and as adults they worried that children's services would remove children from their homes. In the Homeboy sample of 50, seven individuals currently had children placed with relatives or in foster homes while two women had successfully managed to regain custody of their children.

Alongside child abuse, domestic violence was strongly linked with substance abuse for both men and women. However, as women's roles in gang life evolve, so has their participation in domestic violence: they are frequently perpetrators as well as victims. This holds true for lesbian as well as heterosexual relationships. Several women specifically described beating up their partners and men's accounts confirmed these reports. 'I'm scared of one of my baby mamas when she's high', one former gang member confessed. 'Don't give out my name but lemme tell you when she gets drunk, she could beat up anyone'. Another gang member described how he and his former girlfriend beat one another up, saying, 'When we got high, we kinda took turns'. Individuals invariably linked the use of drugs and alcohol with increasing domestic violence. Several individuals who possessed a reputation of being dangerous when intoxicated discussed their often unsuccessful efforts at both sobriety and anger management. One explained, 'I don't know what happens, if I get high I can't control myself. That's why I go to meetings every night and stay sober. I get too fuckin' crazy otherwise'.

Drugs were divided into two major types: those that would exacerbate violence and those that fostered passivity. Cocaine and its most addictive form, crack, have been linked with violent behaviours since the 1980s (Fryer et al. 2013; Grogger and Willis 2000). Since the 1990s, crystal meth, a highly addictive form of psychoactive stimulant methamphetamine, also known as meth, crystal, ice, or glass, has been associated with destructive violence (Hinkes-Jones 2011). A former gang member offered, 'These kids shoot it up, stay up four or five days putting in work, and then they want to beat up everyone, kill everyone, they lose complete control'. Heroin and marijuana were not related to violence but meth and alcohol were viewed as 'dangerous'. When taken in combination these latter substances were described as 'bad' and 'they will fuck you up like you don't know'. Almost everyone agreed with one gang member's assessment that 'bud [marijuana] is not something you're gonna worry about—you just chill out behind it', with a former gang member claiming, 'It's better for someone to smoke a little bud—they're just gonna be coo'. But if they drink or smoke glass—fugget it. It's baaaaaaad'.

Individuals maintained that the crimes they committed to fund addiction including burglary, robbery, petty theft (usually shoplifting), forgery, and in some cases, prostitution, rarely turned violent. One woman insisted, 'I didn't do crimes to hurt a victim—I usually got charged with property crimes', while another man, a chronic heroin addict admitted, 'I was usually too out of it—high or waiting to get high—to do anything violent'. Nevertheless, there was consensus that some drug use—specifically cocaine and methamphetamine—often led to violent and impulsive acts. One gang member observed, 'Crack, cocaine, yeh, I don't wanna get close to anyone up on that'.

Self-medication

Ethnographic observation and interviews revealed one more unintended and profound consequence of street-level drugs and violence. The majority of individuals interviewed described their need for drugs to deal with the impact of violence on their lives. Drugs were not recreational; instead they served as a form of self-medication. One woman provided a succinct rationale for her reliance on drugs, insisting, 'If I didn't take them I'd be screaming 24/7'. Individuals described lives fraught with depression, reporting a cluster of symptoms associated with post-traumatic stress disorder. Detailing his struggles after attempting to leave gang life, one man explained:

> You can leave it physically but it's still inside of you. You feel scared alla the time—someone is gonna get you, someone is gonna shoot you, someone is gonna break into your place in the middle of the night. So you take a little something to sleep at night. Then you take a little something to get through the day. Then you take something more. You do it to stay calm, you do it to forget, you do it to keep thoughts out of your mind.

His account was not unusual. Most individuals described symptoms that included shortness of breath, insomnia, intrusive and repetitive thoughts, nightmares, and flashbacks. Additionally, every woman and the majority of men in the sample reported seeking mental health services at gang intervention and public health agencies. At these sites, individuals frequently saw a psychiatrist who prescribed anti-anxiety medication and/or anti-depressants to help deal with the long-term psychiatric after effects of violence. One former gang member observed, 'First, I'm on heroin, now I'm on anti-depressants. What's the difference—I feel like I'm on drugs all the time'. This cycle often has negative consequences. One former gang member was an addict who cycled between heroin and antidepressants; when he stopped taking drugs altogether he would become emotionally and physically de-regulated, abusing his wife and children. His violence and drug use created a situation of chronic instability that never resolved, embodying the unintended consequences of the drugs and violence dynamic.

For many, the relationship between violence, drugs, and trauma is often further complicated by involvement with the criminal justice system. In both prison and jail, drugs are readily available and violence is an on-going reality. Both men and women sentenced to long or repeated periods of incarceration experience chronic mental health problems and a deepened need for self-medication. Recognizing this reality, in 2000, California's Proposition 36 redefined drug addiction as a public health issue. As a result, first offenders found guilty of non-violent drug possession are no longer incarcerated but instead sentenced to drug rehabilitation programs.

Drugs and Violence: the Final Paradox

Multiple lessons can be drawn from the examination of ethnographic data and the life histories of individuals who have been involved in street-level drug trade, substance, and violence. While drugs intersect with violence on a daily—even hourly—basis, this is only part of the story. Individuals also use drugs to self-medicate, anaesthetizing themselves against myriad psychological struggles including childhood trauma, post-traumatic stress disorder, chronic depression, and involvement with the criminal justice system. No single race or gender possesses an exclusive claim to such problems—men and women of every ethnicity have been exposed to repeated violence and trauma. Women, long characterized as victims, have become increasingly involved in drug dealing and drug-related violence. To further complicate matters, the involved actors may be both perpetrators and victims—intimidating others in their struggle to deal with the long-term trauma that has haunted their lives. Invariably, these divided identities coupled with violent activity lead to long-term impacts on community and government resources: dead children, murderous retaliation, fragmented families, long-term incarceration, and social instability.

Future practice and policy aimed at breaking the connection between drugs and violence at the street-level must consider the life courses of the individuals and communities involved. There is a need to understand the impact of trauma and the collateral damage from drug-related violence. Most importantly, there is a need to draw upon the strengths and desires of communities that long to be free of both drugs and violence. One former gang member best summarized this reality, observing, 'We all want the same things—a good place to live, better lives for our kids, and to be able to sleep at night and not worry if you're gonna live to see the next day'.

Acknowledgements

The author gratefully acknowledges the assistance of Mark Leap and Karrah Lompa, M.S.W., during the writing of this chapter.

References

Atkinson, A., Anderson, Z., Hughes, K., Bellis, M.A., Sumnall, H., and Syed, Q. (2009). *Interpersonal Violence and Illicit Drugs*. United Kingdom: Centre for Public Health Liverpool John Moores University/World Health Organization Collaborating Centre for Violence Prevention.

Bourgois, P. (1996). *In Search of Respect: Selling Crack in El Barrio*. Cambridge: Cambridge University Press.

Boyle, G. (2010). *Tattoos on the Heart: The Power of Boundless Compassion*. New York: Free Press.

Brown, C. (2006). *A Piece of Cake: A Memoir*. New York: Crown Press.

Contreras, R. (2012). *The Stickup Kids: Race, Drugs, Violence and the American Dream*. Berkeley: University of California Press.

Franke, T., and Leap, J. (2010). *Homeboy Industries Evaluation Report*. Haynes Foundation.

Fryer R., Heaton P., Levitt S., and Murphy K. (2013). Measuring crack cocaine and its Impact. *Economic Inquiry*, 51, 1651–81.

Grogger, J., and Willis, M. (2000). The emergence of crack cocaine and the rise in urban crime rates. *Review of Economics and Statistics*, 82, 519–29.

Hinkes-Jones, L. (2011). How the plummeting price of cocaine fueled the nationwide drop in violent crime. *The Atlantic Cities*. Available at: http://www.theatlanticcities.com/jobs-and-economy/2011/11/cocaine-plummeting-price-nationwide-drop-violent-crime/474/ [Accessed 13 November 2013].

Leap, J. (2012). *Jumped in: What Gangs Taught Me about Violence, Drugs, Love and Redemption*. Boston: Beacon Press.

Medina, J. (2012). In years since the riots, a changed complexion in South Central. *New York Times*, 24 April 2012.

Morris, D. J. (2008). *War of the Bloods in My Veins: A Street Soldier's March Towards Redemption*. New York: Scribner.

Moskos, P. (2008). *Cop in the Hood: My Year Policing Baltimore's Eastern District*. Princeton: Princeton University Press.

Phillips, S. (2012). *Operation Fly Trap: L.A. Gangs, Drugs and the Law*. Chicago: The University of Chicago Press.

Rodriguez, L. (1993). *Always Running: La Vida Loca: Gang Days in L.A.* New York: Touchstone.

Rodriguez, L. (2011). *It Calls You Back*. New York: Touchstone.

Sanchez, R. (2000). *My Bloody Life: The Making of a Latin King*. Chicago: Chicago Review Press.

Sanchez, R. (2003). *Once a King, Always a King: The Unmaking of a Latin King*. Chicago: Chicago Review Press.

Scott, K. (1993). *Monster: The Autobiography of an L.A. Gang Member*. New York: Grove Press.

Substance Abuse and Crime Prevention Act of 2000 (Proposition 36). United States: California Secretary of state.

Venkatesh, S. (2008). *Gang Leader for a Day*. New York: The Penguin Press.

Williams, S. T. (2004). *Blue Rage, Black Redemption: A Memoir*. New York: Touchstone.

Wolf, A., and Gutierrez, L. (2012). It's about time: prevention and intervention services for gang affiliated girls. *The California Cities Gang Prevention Network*, Bulletin 26.

CHAPTER 11

The geographic, socioeconomic, and cultural determinants of violence

Vania Ceccato

Introduction to the Geographic, Socioeconomic and Cultural Determinants of Violence

Violence is defined by the World Health Organization as the intentional use of physical force or power, threatened or actual, against a person, or against a group or community that either results in or has a high likelihood of resulting in injury, death, psychological harm, maldevelopment, or deprivation (WHO 2002). In this chapter, the focus is on places where violence (the criminal act against a person, ranging from assault to lethal violence) is high, both in absolute and relative terms. In the United States, cities such as New Orleans and Detroit have in recent times experienced homicides rates above 50 per 100,000, but none of these cities reached rates found in some Latin American cities, such as Juarez, in Mexico (148 per 100,000 inhabitants), or Maceió, in Brazil (135 per 100,000 inhabitants). In South Africa, although the murder rate has decreased significantly from 68 per 100,000 people in 1995–1996, it is still high at 31 per 100,000 inhabitants (2011/2012) compared to the global homicide rate of 8 per 100,000.

The interesting question that arises from this disparate group of high violence neighbourhoods across the world, Detroit, United States, Rio de Janeiro, Brazil or Cape Town, South Africa, is do they have anything in common? And they do appear to share some characteristics. In addition to institutional neglect and environmental injustice, these areas are populated by individuals who suffer from long-term deprivation and poor health often related to bad environmental conditions. However, degrees of poverty and variations in levels of institutional neglect are considered insufficient to explain why these areas are more violent than others. Although environmental criminology has since the early twentieth century made attempts to interpret the links between violence and socioeconomic conditions, it is still an empirical question as to whether social processes operate in a similar way across different places and countries.

The objective of this chapter is to make a contribution to this knowledge base by reviewing explanations for violence (levels and patterns), drawing from principles of criminological theories that are supported by evidence from Northern American and European cities as well as from cities of the Global South.

Explaining Violence

Violence is often caused by a combination of determinants or 'triggers'. A number of these 'triggers' are discussed in this chapter, paying attention to the ecological characteristics that determine the contexts where violence takes place (e.g. geographic, socioeconomic, cultural, and life style). These explanations for violence should be considered as complementary rather than competing with each other.

Demography and Socioeconomic Conditions

Demographic composition, particularly gender and age, is known to be good predictor of the level of violence, especially in deprived areas. The highest homicide rates, both in terms of victimization but also perpetration relate to young males (Fox and Piquero 2003; Salla et al. 2012). Social factors are also important. Social disorganization theory links many forms of delinquency and crime with the presence of weak, informal social controls (Shaw and McKay 1942; Kornhauser 1978; Bursik Grasmick 1993) triggered by housing mobility, weak social ties, and poor normative social structures. High homicide rates are a sign of severe social disorder (Wilson and Kelling 1982). But even in less chaotic communities young men growing up in areas with high violence rates tend to have less access to jobs and less exposure to conventional role models. In addition there are fewer working-class and middle-class households to serve as buffers against the effects of uneven and poor economic conditions (Krivo and Peterson 1996). Some argue that the effect of poverty *per se* in generating violence is not as important as the impact of relative deprivation (Burton et al. 1994). The fact that a group is relatively deprived in comparison with others provides the conditions for conflict and violence.

Changes in institutions also directly affect the supply and demand for jobs, schools, and health care across the country. Rapid change may weaken social control and it can generate *anomic conditions* (e.g. Merton 1938; Agnew 1992) that are characterized by a breakdown or absence of social norms and values, and create favourable conditions for crime. Inequality in the distribution of resources can motivate individuals towards crime. Some of these motivated individuals would overcome blocked opportunities through theft/robbery, or express frustration about their incapacity to reach these resources, through violence. An unanswered question is whether violence in anomic conditions is a result of a search for improvement of material conditions only. The distinctive features of high-crime cities perhaps provide some clues. In British cities, Hancock (2001) describes such areas as having a neglected built environment that is characterized by; poorly designed and poorly maintained housing, a lack of natural surveillance, an abundance of empty properties, a lack of public facilities, and the presence of environmental hazards. There may be visible signs of gang activity, drug dealing, truancy, and young people hanging around the streets with little in the way of purposeful activity. Some of these features are also found in high-crime areas of cities of the Global South, such as Rio de Janeiro or São Paulo, but they tend to be magnified by social inequality, organized crime, and poor governance (see e.g. Caldeira 2000; Ceccato et al. 2007). In São Paulo the geography of homicides coincides with that of the infant mortality. Figure 11.1 exemplifies the fact that one may survive poor living conditions as a child but may not free oneself from the clutches of criminogenic conditions that lead to early death.

Ceccato et al. (2007) suggest that the geographical variation in homicide has been shown to be related to areas of poverty, but also to central areas where people concentrate for leisure and entertainment, including pockets of drug-related activity where illegal firearms are easily available. These underlying conditions in cities such as São Paulo are indicative of institutional neglect,

which means that basic public services and infrastructure fail to attend citizens equally; even if they exist, they are not accountable. In such circumstances, violence becomes a means of imposing social control by dominant members of the group (Black 1984). Moreover, in social contexts like this, where there is little or no access to dispute-resolution structures (for example, small claims courts,) or to agents of dispute mediation (e.g. lawyers or legitimized community representatives), violence may be seen as the only possible means by which to solve a problem. Kubrin and Weitzer (2003) suggest that police practices may also play an important role as generators of violence (Zaluar 2012). As in any other large city, disadvantaged areas in São Paulo or Stockholm have criminogenic conditions that make conflicts and violence part of everyday life. These are long lasting and triggered by disputes over scarce resources or repression by the Police (Chevigny 1999), or simply by the presence of weapons on the streets or other crimes, such as drug-related offences (Ceccato et al. 2007).

European and American criminology research has revealed strong associations between structural and cultural factors and violent crime at the intra-urban level (for a review, see Heitmeyer and Hagan 2003). Sampson and Wilson (1995) assess structural and cultural factors in explaining violence, arguing that low residential quality creates social isolation and a concentration of the disadvantaged. This leads to cultural adaptations that undermine the social control that is fundamental to deter crime.

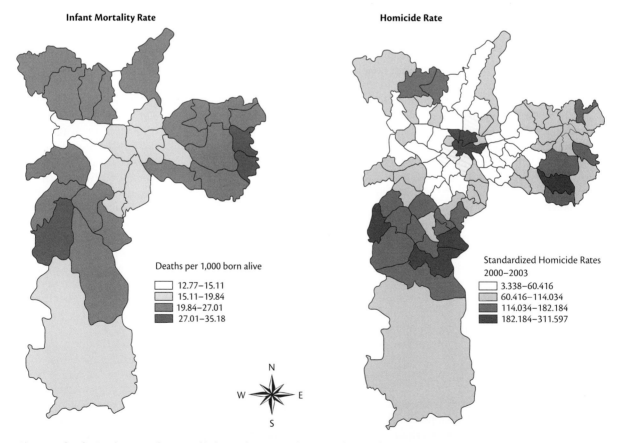

Fig. 11.1 Almost perfect fit? Deaths at age of 1 year and by homicide in São Paulo municipality, Brazil.

Source: data from Fundação Seade, data on infant mortality registered by public health authorities in São Paulo municipality, 1998 and Secretaria de segurança publica de São Paulo, data on homicides registered by police authorities in São Paulo municipality, 2006.

The Culture of Violence

Cultural differences in values, norms, and beliefs held by members of groups or subgroups are seen as important in explaining variations in rates of violence, particularly in the United States (Messner and Rosenfeld 1999). The core idea is that some subcultures provide greater normative support for violence than others in upholding values such as honour (for an extensive review of cultural and sub-cultural theories of homicides, see Corzine et al. 1999). In the United States, the evidence for this subculture of violence is the concentration of high rates of murder that have characterized the south from its earliest settlement through to the beginning of the twenty-first century. The existence of profound differences in levels of violence between ethnic groups is however a controversial field (Farrington et al. 2003) but has been suggested to be part of the explanation for large regional differences in homicide rates elsewhere. In contemporary Estonia, for instance, Russians make up a significant part of the population who are both victims and perpetrators in cases of homicide. Salla et al. (2012) suggest, however, that culture alone does not explain high homicide rates among Russians in Estonia. They suggest that deadly violence in Estonia is related to mechanisms linking long-term socioeconomic deprivation to social exclusion, combined with hazardous drinking patterns. The groups of perpetrators and victims of homicide largely coincide geographically in Estonia: they are males, middle-aged, Russian-speaking, unemployed and poorly educated, either from Tallinn or from economically deprived areas of north-east Estonia, such as Ida-Viru County. Figure 11.2 shows that despite the fact that overall homicide rates in Estonia are falling, the rates in Ida-Viru County remain almost as high as national rates from the early years of Estonia's post-independence period.

One of the criticisms of studies that explore ethnic or cultural explanations of violence is the fact that it is not always possible to untangle structural factors from cultural ones (Parker 1989; Kilsztajn et al. 2003). Structural conditions such as poverty and/or inequalities are sources of regional disparity, and it is argued that

accounting for these features would alone explain the regional variations in the prevalence of violence. At an intra-urban level, in Rio de Janeiro for instance, high-crime areas are characterized by open violence among young males, daily sounds of gun shots and extensive connections between everyday crime, drug dealing and ready access to illegal weapons (Chevigny 1999; Zaluar 2012)—in other words a culture of violence that goes beyond poverty.

In a culture of violence, the importance of shared values is perhaps important to legitimize violence between groups (e.g. between members of opposing gangs) but also perhaps to free them from other more positive societal constraints, for example family, religious, or community networks. And, indeed, Bursik and Grasmick (1993) argue for the importance of such networks in preventing and reducing violence.

From Social Cohesion to Collective Efficacy

Evidence shows how social cohesion at the neighbourhood level (in other words, high levels of social trust and co-operation between citizens for mutual benefit) can lead to fewer criminogenic conditions (Rosenfeld et al. 2001). Whilst social cohesion and civil engagement have less often been analysed in North American and Western European cities, it is argued here that in developing countries their positive role cannot be taken for granted. Zaluar (2012), for example, shows how entangled forms of power take over existing community and religious organizations in shanty towns, called 'favelas' in Rio, Brazil. The development of new forms of illegal business has infiltrated slum areas and makes them into gateways for criminal organizations. Trafficking gangs dominate some 'favelas' whilst drug lords restrict dweller and government agent movements in others. This development has come together with armed mobs and militias. In these war-like conditions, young males are the most common victims of homicides.

Such communities could be argued to be highly cohesive, albeit in a dysfunctional and fear-driven manner. And so it is perhaps not social cohesion alone that leads to civic engagement and reduced

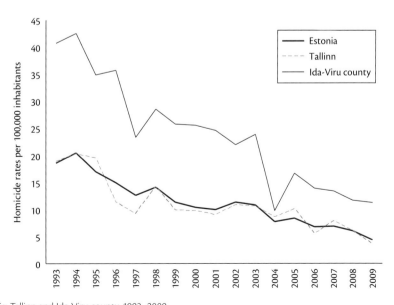

Fig. 11.2 Homicide rates in Estonia, Tallinn and Ida-Viru county, 1993–2009.
Source: data from *Statistics Estonia*, Tallinn, Estonia, Copyright © Statistics Estonia 2014 available from http://pub.stat.ee/px-web.2001/I_Databas/Social_Life/07Justice_and_security/03Crime/03Crime.asp and data from the National Police Board, Estonia.

violence. Another school of thought devotes more attention to individual agency rather than the need for sharing common values, as a prerequisite for social cohesion. Collective efficacy is the group-level term used by Sampson et al. (1997) to refer to the situation where there are shared expectations within the group and a willingness to engage in processes of social control for the common good. Sampson et al. (1997) suggest that action to restrict crime does not necessarily require strong local social ties or associations. Collective action may take place where personal ties and social networks are weak. What is important is a willingness to intervene on behalf of the common good, for instance, by engaging in activities that improve overall safety of the neighbourhood (e.g. actions combating drug and alcohol addictions that may lead to violence).

The Addiction–Violence Link

Goldstein (1985) provides insight into the dynamics of the drug homicide linkage. This author suggests three ways in which drug consumption and drug trafficking may causally be related to violence. The first kind of violence is psycho-pharmacological caused by the properties of the drug itself. The second is economic–compulsive violence motivated by the need or desire to obtain drugs, and the third is systemic violence, which is associated with traditionally aggressive patterns of interaction within the system of drug distribution and use. Baumer et al. (1998) confirm that areas in the United States with higher levels of crack cocaine use have higher homicide rates as well as higher levels of other offences. The presence of alcohol and the availability of weapons (Felson and Messner 1996) and drugs increase the likelihood that certain types of confrontational interaction escalate into a killing. More recently, Lipton et al. (2013) found that the presence of alcohol outlets, drug possession, and trafficking arrests were predictive of violent crime. In cities with strong links between drug trafficking and violence, such as in São Paulo, 'revenge' is the most common reason behind multiple murders (*chacinas*). It is believed that drug trafficking employs more than 20,000 couriers (*aviõezinhos*), the majority of whom are adolescents between 10 and 16 years of age, often coming from poor families. The chance of being arrested is small and traffickers have no difficulty in recruiting them to deliver drugs—a task that often leads to violence and death (Ceccato et al. 2007). These authors suggest that unlike in Rio de Janeiro, where drug-selling points are concentrated in the hills and managed by a few 'drug barons', in São Paulo the selling points seem to be widely scattered over the city and are managed by hundreds of small traffickers, not only in poor neighbourhoods but also in central areas where many drug-selling points are concentrated.

Mobility and The Role of the Environment on Violence

Most theories of urban criminology have so far concentrated either on the neighbourhood conditions of crime location or on where offenders live, missing a great deal of information on people's whereabouts over time in the city. This missing information is vital for understanding why an individual decides to commit a crime, for instance violence. In Wikström et al. (2010), the interaction between individuals' crime propensity and their exposure to criminogenic environments was empirically tested using a group of young people. Although not limited to violence alone, findings showed that those who spend more time in criminogenic environments (e.g. being unsupervised with peers in neighbourhoods

with a poor collective efficacy) tend to be more frequently involved in acts of crime. Wikström et al. (2010, p. 81) note, however, that:

> this relationship depends on the young person's crime propensity. Having a crime-averse morality and strong ability to exercise self-control appears to make young people situationally immune to influences from criminogenic settings, while having a crime-prone morality and poor ability to exercise self-control appears to make young people situationally vulnerable to influences from criminogenic settings.

The importance of situational conditions for violence has long being pointed out in international literature. Land use shapes the flows of human routine activities and affects the number of interactions that are criminologically relevant and which could lead to offences (Cohen and Felson 1979). In São Paulo, most homicides may happen close to the victim's home but outdoors (Ceccato 2005), particularly in city centres. City centres tend be violent places regardless of the time of the year because they concentrate land uses that attract activities that may lead to crime and violence, with bars, restaurants, entertainment, and cultural and sport activities. Another, perhaps complementary explanation for temporal variations in violence is suggested by theories that link ambient conditions to aggression. This assumption, as will be discussed, is based on the idea that changes in the weather, or extremes of weather, function as 'stressors' leading to violent behaviour.

The Weather–Aggression Explanation

The general aggression model (Anderson et al. 2000) suggests that weather, and particularly temperature, heightens physiological arousal and leads to aggressive thoughts and, in certain cases, violence. Individuals who are highly sensitive to changes in the weather might exhibit behavioural or mood changes, leading to violence. Although poorly studied, this assumption is not new. Quételet (1842) in his nineteenth-century study suggested that the greatest number of crimes against a person is committed during summer and the fewest during winter. Since then, researchers have found new empirical evidence on how crime levels vary over time and space. Some relate these temporal differences to the direct impact of weather on behaviour whilst others associate them indirectly, via variations and changes in people's routine activity over time but also may interact with individual's socioeconomic conditions. A recent study from St Louis, United States, shows that neighbourhoods with higher levels of social disadvantage are likely to experience higher levels of violence as a result of anomalously warm temperatures resulting from climate change. Mares (2013) indicates that 20 per cent of the most disadvantaged neighbourhoods are predicted to experience over half of the climate change-related increases in cases of violence.

Most of the literature from the Northern hemisphere indicates that more violent crimes occur on hot days (e.g. Hakko 2000; Rotton and Frey 1985). An exception is the study by Ceccato (2005), which shows that for São Paulo, temperature has an influence on violence rates, but it is not the only factor. Findings show stronger evidence that changes in people's routine activity during the summer has more effect on violence than weather variables alone. Homicides take place when most people have time off, particularly during vacations (hot months of the year), evenings and weekends, which indicates the importance of changes in routine activity, from structured (e.g. home–work–home) to unstructured ones Figure 11.3 shows seasonal differences in clusters of violence by season both in Stockholm, Sweden, and São Paulo, Brazil.

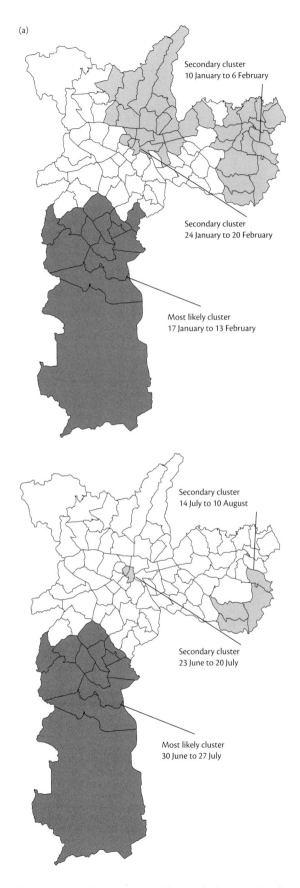

(a)

Secondary cluster
10 January to 6 February

Secondary cluster
24 January to 20 February

Most likely cluster
17 January to 13 February

Secondary cluster
14 July to 10 August

Secondary cluster
23 June to 20 July

Most likely cluster
30 June to 27 July

Fig. 11.3 Clusters of homicides in a tropical city, (a) São Paulo, Brazil, 2000–2002, and clusters of violence in a Scandinavian city, (b) Stockholm, Sweden, 2006–2008.
Reprinted from Uittenbogaard, A., and Ceccato, V., Space-time clusters of crime in Stockholm, Sweden. Review of European Studies, Volume 4, pp. 148–56, Copyright © 2012 Canadian Center of Science and Education, licenced under the Creative Commons Licence 3.0 and *Journal of Environmental Psychology*, Volume 25, Issue 3, Ceccato, V., Homicide in São Paulo, Brazil: assessing spatial-temporal and weather variations, pp. 249–360, Copyright © 2005, with permission from Elsevier, www.sciencedirect.com/science/journal/02724944.

(b)

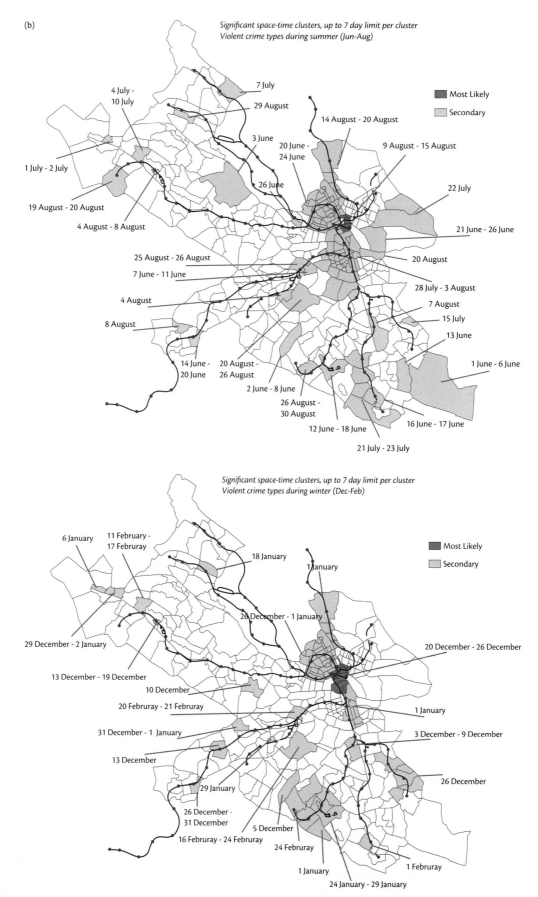

Fig. 11.3 continued.

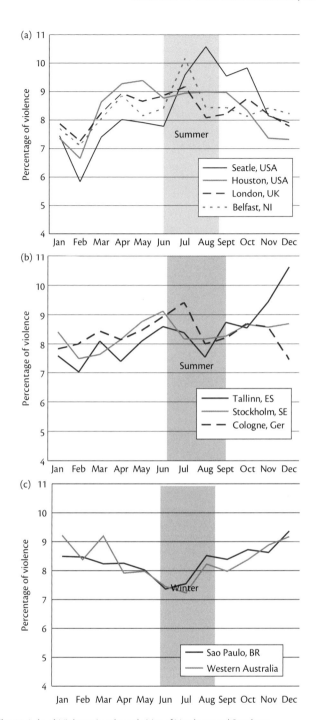

Fig. 11.4 (a–c) Violence in selected cities of Northern and Southern Hemispheres, by months of the year, 2011.

Source: data from Cologne Police Department, *Cases of violence: Police Dispatch Data, 2010 and 2011*, Copyright © 2012. The data includes cases of homicide, assault and aggravated assault, excluding cases of rape and robbery. For Cologne, the data excludes homicides but they are relatively few in relation to the total violence..

Figure 11.3 shows that although the location of primary clusters is similar and stable between summer and winter (dark blue), the concentration of violence increases in size during vacation time (summer) and shrinks afterwards (winter) for secondary clusters (light blue), when people get back to structured activities. SaTScan produces types of clusters in this mode: primary clusters (the most

likely ones), that is clusters that are least likely to be due to chance and secondary clusters (the weak ones according to their likelihood ratio test statistic). Secondary clusters means that while it is possible to pinpoint the general location of a cluster, its exact boundaries must remain uncertain (Kulldorff 2013). In the case of Stockholm, secondary clusters shrink in the winter but not in the city centre, where an expansion of the primary clusters is noticed, particularly around Christmas time (20–26 December). These two examples indicate that poor and/or central neighbourhoods are more likely to have high levels of homicide, regardless of the time of the year, while in other areas violence varies based on changes in weather and/or routine activity

Figure 11.4 shows levels of violence in selected cities in 2011 from both Northern and Southern hemispheres. Violence is greater in the summer months than in the winter, but at higher latitudes, such as Tallinn and Stockholm, the pattern seems to be fairly stable over the year, that is it does not show the same variation as cities in the Southern hemisphere, in the United States, or the United Kingdom. Regardless of latitude, changes in people's routine activity (for instance, from structured activities, such as going to work or school, to unstructured activities, such as leisure, travelling, participating in festivals, drinking) constitute a reasonable explanation, but not perhaps the only one, for changes in violence levels over the year. Although the data used here are limited to a 1-year dataset, it is indicative of the importance of geographical and temporal differences in causation of violence. This evidence does not take other factors (such as alcohol consumption) into account that, together with seasonal variations of human activities, are expected to affect violence levels over time. The potential relationship between violence, changes in routine activity, and alcohol consumption still remains an empirical question. And that relationship may, for example, explain the apparent pre-Christmas upturn in violence in Tallinn.

Gaps in the Evidence

The difference in nature and magnitude of violence faced by cities in developing countries demands particular consideration as to whether the research and theories discussed in this article are adequate for interpreting situations where violence is particularly high, such as in cities like Rio or Cape Town. They may not be adequate, but they have been used for decades in theoretical benchmarking to tackle problems in cities of the Global South. In cities like Rio, the source of violence is not only imposed by external organized crime, but in some cases, it is local rulers and service providers that determine the tone for crime and violence, simply because the State is not present. In other cases, police are repressive and corrupt. What is social control in such areas? Or is it better to say, for whom is social control? In these areas, 'safety' is built on the basis of fear of mafia-like social networks; so are social disorganization principles of any use in these settings? The importance of considering the context of violence is fundamental also for finding ways of tackling it. This calls for the need for comparative and policy oriented research that looks for specific causes of violence, which are so far missing in the international literature. Policy and actions may maximize their chances of successfully combating violence if they rely on knowledge that stems from the contexts to which they actually apply. Temporal and geographical patterns of violence across countries and latitudes reflect weather and routine activity changes over time—a fact that should not be neglected in future research or when defining policy interventions.

Conclusions

This chapter seeks to show that violent areas share a number of commonalities, such as having populations that suffer from long-term deprivation, institutional neglect, and poor health conditions. However these factors alone cannot explain why certain areas are more violent than others. The international literature has long suggested a number of possible explanations for high levels of violence other than those discussed, ranging from the role of social networks, individuals' life styles and cultures, as well as the importance of the environment in affecting individual routine activity over time and space. Despite these developments, future research should devote time to assess why violence tends to be concentrated at particular areas and times. The interaction between environmental, demographic, and socioeconomic factors in the causation of violence needs further investigation.

Acknowledgements

The author thanks a number of colleagues that have provided data for this study: from Germany, Dietrich Oberwittler, from Estonia, Andri Ahven, from Brazil, Secretaria de Segurança Publica de São Paulo, from Western Australia, Michael Townsley and national police records websites from the UK and the United States.

References

Anderson, C. A., Anderson, K. B., Dorr, N., De Neve, K. M., and Flanagan, M. (2000). Temperature and aggression. In: M. P. Zanna (ed.) *Advances in Experimental Social Psychology.* New York: Academic Press, pp. 33–133.

Agnew, R. (1992). Foundation for a general strain theory. *Criminology, 30,* 47–87.

Baumer, E., Lauritsen, J. L., Rosenfled, R, and Wright, R. (1998). The influence of crack cocaine on robbery, burglary, and homicide rates: a cross-city, longitudinal analysis. *Journal of Research in Crime and Delinquency*, 35, 316–40.

Black, D. (1984). Social control as a dependent variable. In: D. Black (ed.), *Toward a General Theory of Social Control.* Orlando: Academic Press, pp. 1–26.

Bursik, R. J., and Grasmick, H. G. (1993). *Neighbourhoods and Crime.* New York: Lexington.

Burton, J. R., Cullen, F. T., Evans, T. D., and Dunaway, R. G. (1994). Reconsidering strain theory: operationalization, rival theories and adult criminality. *Journal of Quantitative Criminology,* 35, 213–39.

Caldeira, T. P. R. (2000). *City of Walls: Crime, Segregation and Citizenship in São Paulo.* Berkeley, CA: University of California Press.

Ceccato, V. (2005). Homicide in São Paulo, Brazil: assessing spatial-temporal and weather variations. *Journal of Environmental Psychology,* 25, 249–360.

Ceccato, V., Haining, R., & Kahn, T. (2007). The geography of homicide in São Paulo, Brazil. *Environment and Planning A,* 39, 1632–53.

Chevigny, P. (1999). Defining the role of the police in Latina America. In: J. Mendez, G. O'Donell amd P. S. Pinheiro (eds), *The (Un)rule of Law and the Underprivileged in Latin America.* Notre Dame: Notre Dame University Press, pp. 49–70.

Cohen, L. E., and M. Felson. (1979). Social change and crime rate trends: a routine activity approach. *American Sociological Review,* 44, 588–608.

Corzine, J., Corzine, L. H., and Whitt, H. P. (1999) Cultural and subcultural theories of homicide. In: M. D. Smith and M. A. Zahn (eds), *Homicide: A Sourcebook of Social Research.* London: Sage, pp. 42–58.

Farrington, D. Loeber, R., and Southamer-Loeber, M. (2003). How can the relationship between race and violence be explained? In D. F. Hawkins (ed.), *Violent Crime: Assessing Race and Ethnic Differences.* Cambridge: Cambridge University Press, pp. 213–37.

Felson, R., and Messner, S. F. (1996). To kill or not to kill? Lethal outcomes in injurious attacks. *Criminology* 34, 519–45.

Fox, J. A., and Piquero, A. R. (2003). Deadly demographics: population characteristics and forecasting homicide trends. *Crime and Delinquency*, 49, 339–59.

Goldstein J. C. (1985), The drugs-violence nexus: a tripartite conceptual framework. *Journal of Drug Issues,* 14, 493–506.

Hakko, H. (2000). Seasonal variation of suicides and homicides in Finland. PhD dissertation. Oulu, Finland: Department of Psychiatry, University of Oulu; Department of forensic psychiatry, University of Kuopio.

Hancock, L. (2001). *Community Crime and Disorder: Safety and Regeneration in Urban Neighbourhoods.* Basingstoke: Palgrave Press.

Heitmeyer, W., and Hagan, J. (2003) *International Handbook of Violence Research.* Dordrecht: Kluwer.

Kilsztajn S., Rossbach A., Carmo N., Sugahara L., and Souza, L. B. (2002) Vítimas Fatais da Violência e Mercados de Drogas na Região Metropolitana de São Paulo. LES/PUCSP, São Paulo.

Kulldorff, M. (2013) SaTScan User Guide. Available at http://www.satscan. org/techdoc.html [Accessed 28 December 2013].

Kornhauser, R. (1978). *Social Sources of Delinquency.* Chicago: University of Chicago Press.

Krivo, L. J., and Peterson, R. D. (1996). Extremely disadvantaged neighborhoods and urban crime. *Social Forces,* 75, 619–50.

Kubrin, C. E., and Weitzer, R. (2003) Retaliatory homicide: concentrated disadvantage and neighbourhood culture. *Social Problems,* 50, 157–80.

Lipton, R., Yang, X., Braga, A. A., Goldstick, J., Newton, M., and Rura, M. (2013). The geography of violence, alcohol outlets, and drug arrests in Boston. *American Journal of Public Health,* 103, e8.

Mares, D. (2013). Climate change and levels of violence in socially disadvantaged Neighbourhood groups. *Journal of Urban Health,* 90, 768–83.

Merton, R. (1938). Social structure and anomie. *American Sociological Review* 3, 672–82.

Messner, S., and Rosenfeld, R. (1999). Social structure and homicide: theory and research. In: M. D. Smith, and M. A. Zahn (eds), *Homicide: A Sourcebook of Social Research.* London: Sage, pp. 27–34.

Parker, R. N. (1989). Poverty, subculture of violence, and type of homicide. *Social Forces,* 67, 983–1007.

Quetelet, A. J. (1842). *A treatise on man and the development of his faculties. A fascism. (Reproduction of the English translation of 1842).* Gainesville, Florida: Scholar's Facsimiles and Reprints.

Rosenfeld, R., Messner, S. F., and Baumer, E. P. (2001). Social capital and homicide. *Social Forces,* 80, 283–309.

Rotton, J., and Frey, J. (1985). Air pollution, weather, and violent crimes: concomitant time series analysis of archival data. *Journal of Personality and Social Psychology,* 49, 1207–20.

Salla, J., Ceccato, V., and Ahven, A. (2012). Homicide in Estonia. In: M. Liem and W. A. Pridemore (eds), *Handbook of European Homicide Research.* Dordrecht, Heidelberg, New York, London: Springer, pp. 421–35.

Sampson, R. J., and Wilson, W. J. (1995). Toward a theory of race, crime and urban inequality. In: J. Hagan and R. D. Peterson (eds), *Crime and Inequality.* Stanford: Stanford University Press, pp. 37–57.

Sampson, R. J., Raundenbush, S. W., and Earls, F. (1997). Neighborhoods and violent crime: a multilevel study of collective efficacy. *Science,* 277, 918–24.

Shaw, C. R., and McKay, H.D. (1942). *Juvenile Delinquency and Urban Areas.* Chicago: University of Chicago Press.

Uittenbogaard, A., and Ceccato, V. (2012). Space-time clusters of crime in Stockholm, Sweden. *Review of European Studies,* 4, 148–56.

World Health Organization (2002) World report on violence and health. Available at: http://www.who.int/violence_injury_prevention/violence/world_report/en/ [Accessed 19 February 2013].

Wikström, P. O. H., Ceccato, V., Hardie, B., and Treiber, K. (2010). Activity fields and the dynamics of crime advancing knowledge about the role of the environment in crime causation. *Journal of quantitative criminology,* 26, 55–87.

Wilson, J. Q., and Kelling, G. L. (1982). Broken windows. *Atlantic Monthly,* 249, 29–38.

Zaluar, A. (2012). Turf war in Rio de Janeiro: youth, drug traffic, guns and hyper-masculinity. In V. Ceccato (ed.), *The Urban Fabric of Crime and Fear.* Dordrecht, Heidelberg, New York, London: Springer, pp. 217–36.

SECTION 3

The consequences of violence

CHAPTER 12

The consequences of violence: assessing the health burden of violence

Megan Prinsloo, Debbie Bradshaw, and Ian Neethling

Introduction to Assessing the Health Burden of Violence

The most widely recorded data source for violence is mortality statistics (see Matzopoulos et al., this volume). However, the majority of violence appears to be non-fatal and results in injuries, with victims having an increased risk of psychological and behavioural problems, including depression, alcohol abuse, anxiety, suicidal behaviour, and reproductive health problems (World Health Organization (WHO) 2002a). The consequences of violence therefore have enormous impact on individuals' health, as well as considerable social and economic impact.

It is therefore essential to measure the impact of violence to inform public health actions. This chapter describes the commonly used classifications and indicators for measuring the health impact of violence, highlighting international standards and measurement tools, and extending previous reviews. It also reports on the recently published 2010 Global Burden of Disease (GBD) estimates of health burden resulting from interpersonal violence (Murray et al. 2012), and the methods used for estimating its health impact, when considered as a risk factor.

Classifications for Mortality, Morbidity, and Functional Disability

In order to measure the health burden of violence, clear definitions and classifications of the types of violence, and of the health impacts, are essential. The *World Report on Violence and Health* (WHO 2002a) proposed a typology which divides violence into three broad categories: self-directed violence, interpersonal violence, and collective violence. Based on the setting, the victim–perpetrator relationship and possible motives for the violence, the three broad categories are then further divided into seven subtypes of violence, including suicidal behaviour and self-abuse; family and intimate partner violence (including child and elder abuse), and community violence among acquaintances/strangers. Also included in the typology is the nature of violent acts, which can be physical, sexual, psychological, or involve deprivation or neglect.

The International Classification of Diseases and Related Health Problems (ICD) is used to classify causes of death, morbidity, and injury (WHO 2008). Unnatural deaths are grouped on the basis of intent and manner of the death (assault, self-harm, legal intervention and war, accidents, and intent undetermined/unknown) and the specific external cause (strangulation, firearm, blunt object, etc.). In addition, the ICD can be used to classify the nature of the injuries (fracture of the skull, injury to eyes, etc.).

The *World Report on Disability* states that 'disability' is the umbrella term for impairments, activity limitations, and participation restrictions, and refers to the 'interaction between persons with impairments and attitudinal and environmental barriers that hinder their full and effective participation in society on an equal basis with others' (WHO 2011, p. 4). The International Classification of Functioning (ICF) provides a framework for measuring health and disability at individual and population levels and has been endorsed by the WHO for use as the international standard to describe and measure health and disability (54th World Health Assembly 2001). The ICF is structured through two lists: a list of body functions and structure and a list of domains of activity and participation. A list of environmental factors is also included in the ICF, since functioning and disability of an individual usually occurs in a context (WHO 2002b), and it is recommended that this be adopted as a universal framework to provide a common framework for reliable, comprehensive national and international data on disability (WHO 2011).

Measurement of Health Impact

Hendrie and Miller (2004) reviewed four types of measures of injury burden, including mortality- and morbidity-related indices, composite indices of morbidity and mortality, and costs. In addition, there is an emerging field of measurement of the impact of injuries relating to physical impairment/functional disability and health related quality of life (Polinder et al. 2010).

Mortality-Related Indices

The principal resource for quantifying the burden of injuries is counts of absolute numbers of injury deaths in a population during a specific time period, and ranking how these relate to other causes of death. Mortality data represent the most severe outcomes of injury and are the most consistently recorded data source for the consequences of injuries in many countries. Thus an annual homicide rate has become the most widely used measure of the health impact of violence.

Morbidity-Related Indices

Morbidity is measured by the incidence of non-fatal outcomes of injury in a population, as well as the severity of the consequent trauma. Incidence can be measured using administrative data such as the number of injury-related hospital admissions, emergency department presentations, hospital outpatient attendances, and general practice consultations. Several scales and scoring systems have been developed to record the severity of non-fatal injury. These methods for determining injury severity have been based on the type and anatomical distribution of injury, the physiological response to injury, or both (see Table 12.1 for a summary, some of which have been adapted from Peden, 1998a,b). They all require a clinical assessment by a clinician, nurse, or paramedic.

Physical Impairment/Functional Disability

An individual assessment of disability is often required for the affected person to receive disability benefits. These tend to use medical criteria and may under-represent some domains of functioning. However, measurement of disability or the severity

of injuries at population level informs policy and programme decision-makers about the magnitude of the problem and how to remove disabling barriers and improve services (WHO 2011). It is therefore necessary to have instruments that can measure all domains of functioning.

Polinder and colleagues (2010) have highlighted the need for sound epidemiological data on the incidence, severity, and duration of the functional consequences of injuries to make valid estimates of the years lived with disability due to injuries. This field of measurement is still emerging, with numerous health-related quality of life (HRQL) instruments such as the Medical Outcome Short Form-36 (SF-36) (Ware and Sherbourne 1992) and the European Quality of Life instrument-5 dimensions (EQ 5-D) (The EuroQol Group 1990). The EQ-5D is a brief scale that incorporates dimensions of mobility, self-care, usual activities, pain and discomfort, anxiety, and depression. The Health Utility Index (HUI) (Feeny et al. 1995; Horsman et al. 2003) classifies the health status/functional capacity of each individual at a point in time. The HUI3 classification system includes eight attributes: vision, hearing, speech, ambulation, dexterity, emotion, cognition, and pain.

In a review of studies that measured HRQL among injured populations for the period 1995–2005, Polinder and colleagues (2010) found a lack of consensus on HRQL instruments and study designs. Guidelines have been developed to conduct follow-up studies to measure injury-related disability across countries (Van

Table 12.1 Measures of severity

Anatomical scores	**Abbreviated Injury Scale: AIS (Committee on Medical Aspects of Automotive Safety 1971)**
	• AIS assigns a six-digit numerical code and a severity score to each injury description
	• First digit classifies over 2000 injury descriptors into one of 9 body regions: head, face, neck, thorax, abdomen, spine, upper extremities, lower extremities, external
	• This is followed by the type of anatomical structure, two digits for the specific anatomical structure or nature of the injury; and the level of injury within a body region and anatomical structure
	• The seventh digit is the AIS score: 1 (minor injury severity) to 6 (max injury/possibly lethal)
	• Example: 110604.**2**= head, whole area, skin, major laceration, **moderate severity**
	Injury Severity Score: ISS (Baker et al. 1974)
	• Anatomically based ordinal scale, ranging from 1 (minor severity) to 75 (most severe)
	• To compute: the nine AIS body regions are grouped into six (head/neck, face, chest, abdominal/pelvic contents, extremities/pelvic girdle and external)
	• ISS = **sum of squares of highest AIS severity scores** for three different body regions
	• Except if: any single body region has AIS=6 (max severity), then ISS=75
	• An ISS >15= severe injury
	• If severity cannot be determined: AIS=9 and ISS=99 (cannot be calculated)
	• A simpler method, but only takes the worst injury in a region (cannot accommodate many injuries in one body region)
	• Example:
	• Fractured left femoral shaft (AIS code 851814.**3**) and a compound fracture of right tibial shaft (AIS code 853422.**3**)
	• **ISS=9** (only one injury can be used as they both occur in the same body region (lower limb))
	New Injury Severity Score: NISS (Osler et al. 1997)
	• NISS=**sum of squares of three most severe AIS injuries**, regardless of body region
	• Easier to use than the ISS and more representative of injury severity
	• Example:
	• Fractured left femoral shaft (AIS code 851814.**3**) and a compound fracture of right tibial shaft (AIS code 853422.**3**)
	• **NISS= 18** (both limb injuries can be used in the calculation)

Table 12.1 continued

Physiological scores	**Glasgow Coma Scale: GCS (Teasdale and Jennett 1974)**
	• A serial monitoring system of the progress of head injured patients; monitors changes in levels of consciousness.
	• Is based upon:
	eye opening (maximum score of 4)
	verbal response (maximum score of 5) and
	motor response (maximum score of 6)
	• Each response is given a number and the GCS is expressed by summation of the figures
	• Lowest score is 3 (no response to commands or stimuli) and highest is 15
	Revised Trauma Score: RTS (Yates 1990)
	• A functional score (assesses impact of injury on body function), usually used in combination with anatomical scores
	• Summarizes the functioning of circulation (*systolic blood pressure*), respiration (*respiratory rate*), and central nervous system (*GCS*) to determine injury severity
	• Scores range from zero (impaired functioning) to 12 (normal functioning)
	• Can be used in emergency units or on inpatients to monitor progress
	Injury Impairment Scale: IIS (Joint Committee on Injury Scaling 1994)
	• Coding system which predicts amount of functional loss at 1 year post injury
	• Based on the AIS; each of the 1,320 injury descriptions in the 1990 revision of AIS were assigned an IIS score instead of an injury severity code
	• Scores range from 0 (normal function) to 6 (impairment level prevents any useful function)
Combination scores	**Paediatric Trauma Score: PTS (Tepas et al. 1987)**
	• A triage tool as well as a predictor of mortality
	• Scores six parameters: weight, airway, systolic blood pressure, central nervous system, fractures, wounds
	• Each parameter is assessed and scored as follows:
	+2 (no injury or non-life threatening)
	+1 (minor injury or potentially life-threatening)
	−1 (life-threatening)
	• Scores range between −6 and 12
	• A trauma score of ≤8 indicates significant mortality risk
	Trauma Score and Injury Severity Score: TRISS (Boyd et al. 1987)
	• Assesses probability of survival, taking into account patient's age and mechanism of injury
	• Is a complex computation, mostly used by researchers and managers in auditing trauma units
	Kampala Trauma Score: KTS (Kobusingye and Lett 2000)
	• Patient age, number of serious injuries, systolic blood pressure, respiratory rate, neurological status are recorded
	• Scores range from 5 (most severe) to 16 (least severe)

Source: data from Committee on Medical Aspects of Automotive Safety, Rating the severity of tissue damage: I. the abbreviated scale, *Journal of American Medicine*, Volume 215, Number 2, pp. 277–80, Copyright © 1971 American Medical Association; Baker, S. P. et al., The injury severity score: a method for describing patients with multiple injuries and evaluating emergency care, *Journal of Trauma*, Volume 14, Issue 3, pp. 187–96, Copyright © 1974; Osler, T. et al., A modification of the injury severity score that both improves accuracy and simplifies scoring, *Journal of Trauma, Injury, Infection and Critical Care*, Volume 43, Issue 6, pp. 922-6, Copyright © Williams & Wilkins 1997; Teasdale, G., and Jennett, B., Assessment of coma and impaired consciousness, *The Lancet*, Volume 304, Issue 7872, pp. 81–4, Copyright © 1974; Yates, D. W., ABC of major trauma: scoring systems for trauma, *British Medical Journal*, Volume 301, Issue 6760, pp. 1090–4, Copyright © 1990; Tepas, J. J. et al., The pediatric trauma score as a predictor of injury severity in the injured child, *Journal of Pediatric Surgery*, Volume 22, Issue 1, pp. 14–8, Copyright © 1987 Published by Elsevier Inc.; Boyd, C. R., Evaluating trauma care: the TRISS method, *Journal of Trauma*, Volume 27, Issue 4, pp. 370–8, Copyright © 1987; Kobusingye, O. C., and Lett, R. R., Hospital-based trauma registries in Uganda, *Journal of Trauma*, Volume 48, Issue 3, pp. 498–502, Copyright © 2000 Lippincott Williams & Wilkins, Inc; Peden, M., Injury severity scoring made easy: part I, *Trauma Review*, Volume 6, Issue 1, pp. 10–11, Copyright © 1998 and Peden, M, Injury severity scoring made easy: part II, *Trauma Review*, Volume 6, Issue 1, pp. 11–12, Copyright © 1998.

Beeck et al. 2007), but have not yet been implemented. Rigorous evaluation and comparison of the instruments are needed, but in the meantime the EuroSafe Group advises that a combination of the EQ-5D and the HUI be used, because of its suitability, ease of use, and no cost, with assessments at 1, 2, 4, and 12 months after injury (Van Beeck et al. 2007).

The WHO Disability Assessment Schedule (WHODAS) has been developed to provide a standardized tool to measure health and disability across cultures at population level or in clinical practice, applying the ICF framework. It captures the level of functioning in six domains of life: cognition, mobility, self-care, getting along/interacting, life activities, and participation (Ustun et al. 2010). The reliability and validity of the instrument still need to be assessed.

Composite Morbidity and Mortality-Related Indices

Summary measures of population health or time-based measures are composite indices that combine information on the burden of injury from mortality and morbidity into a single measure. They include the effects of illness on both the quantity and quality of life. Disability Adjusted Life Years (DALYs) and Quality Adjusted Life Years (QALYs) are the most widely used approaches. The DALY is a time-based measure that combines both fatal and non-fatal burden, by combining years of life lost due to mortality (YLL) and years lived with disability (YLD), taking into account the severity and duration of the disability (Murray et al. 2012). The severity weights for YLDs range between zero (indicating perfect health), to one (indicating death). A QALY, however, is a year of life adjusted for its quality, where a year lived in perfect health is equal to one and the loss of a year of life is equal to zero QALYs. A year in less than full health is discounted by a quality-weighting factor (for instance, HUI scores) between zero and one, depending on the extent of loss of quality of life. The burden of injury is then measured as the sum of loss of QALYs due to mortality and morbidity (Hendrie and Miller 2004).

Costs

Costs associated with the incidence or prevalence of a particular condition can also be used to express the burden of injury as a single measure (Segui-Gomez and MacKenzie 2003). Comprehensive costs take into account the burden of all costs of injury, that is health system costs, other direct resource costs, productivity losses, and the loss of quality of life (Miller 2000). Specific subsets of costs that are commonly reported are health system costs and monetary or human capital costs (which are the sum of all costs, except loss of quality of life). One advantage of reporting costs as a measure of burden of injury is that it is easily understood by politicians and the media; but expressing the value of certain components of the burden of injury in monetary terms is difficult and assumptions have to be made, which can compromise the validity of these estimates (Hendrie and Miller 2004; see Corso and Taylor, this volume, for a discussion of the economic costs associated with violence).

Data Sources for Measuring the Burden of Violence

Data for measuring the health impact of violence may come from routine surveillance or health facility data, or from surveys and census; Table 12.2 lists various data sources.

Global Burden of Disease: Interpersonal Violence Statistics

The latest GBD study for 2010 has developed estimates of the DALYs for 291 causes of disease and injuries in 21 regions globally, using an extensive network of expert groups, additional data, and much more complex modelling approaches than was possible in the first GBD study (Murray et al. 2012). The 2010 GBD study has calculated YLLs based on a new standardized life expectancy at each age and does not use age weighting or discounting. It has also replaced incidence of disease with prevalence for the calculation of YLDs and has re-scaled the disability weights by using empirical data about the valuation of different health states through several surveys (Salomon et al. 2012). In addition, the 2010 GBD study reports on the 20-year trends in the burden of disease since 1990 using the new DALY measure.

DALYs for interpersonal violence have shown no change from 370 per 100,000 in 1990 to 371 per 100,000 in 2010. However, DALYs due to assault by sharp objects and firearms increased by 14.3 per cent and 4.1 per cent respectively (Murray et al. 2012), whereas assault by other means decreased by 13.9 per cent. In 2010, firearms accounted for 43.3 per cent of the interpersonal violence burden and sharp objects accounted for 27.5 per cent.

The DALYs estimated for interpersonal violence among males was more than four times the rate for females in 2010 (Figure 12.1). The interpersonal violence DALYs for both males and females

Table 12.2 Attributes of different data sources to measure the health impact of violence

Data source	Metric	Strength	Weakness
Mortality			
Vital statistics: death certificates	Death counts Mortality rates	Established protocols; completed by pathologists. Centralized database. Provides information on age, sex, manner, and external cause of death.	Limited information on injury event and requires further investigation on how the death occurred. Subject to erroneous coding, incomplete counts, and lack of specific detail. Not always available in resource-limited settings.
Post mortem/autopsy reports	Death counts Mortality rates	Provides full detail on injury death; completed by pathologists.	Quality varies across countries/regions. Often not computerized. Not readily available in low- and middle-income countries.
Police reports	Death counts Mortality rates	Details circumstances surrounding the death.	Under-reporting of incidents leads to under-counting. May have misreporting of incidents. Legal intervention or violence during arrest for other crimes not always recorded. Computerized data not always available.
Population/community based surveys	Death counts	Population-based.	Limited information available, unless the focus is specific to violence.
Verbal autopsy interviews	Death counts	Population-based information in settings with limited forensic services.	Subject to recall-bias and misinterpretation of death by interviewee.

Table 12.2 continued

Data source	Metric	Strength	Weakness
Morbidity			
Trauma registries, outpatient data, General Practitioner registries, and Emergency Department Surveillance Systems	Counts of health-care utilization	Information on individuals can be collected routinely, but may need modification to indicate whether the treatment was for injury and the cause of injury.	Quality of data will depend on the interest of management in such data; may be difficult to sustain in resource-limited settings. Limited to cases that sought medical attention and will reflect access to health care. Requires further investigation into patient records for detail on the nature and causes of injury.
Hospital discharge data	Counts of health-care utilization	Information on individual and injury characteristics available. Can be used to estimate incidence of severe non-fatal violence related injuries.	May require further investigation into patient records for detail on the nature and cause of injury. Population catchment area not always defined.
Retrospective record reviews	Non-fatal injury rates Injury severity scores	Detail on nature of injury and external cause of violence available from patient records. Severity scores of injuries can be calculated. Can be population-based if geographic information is collected.	Record reviews can be time-consuming and tracing of records is dependent on hospital filing system. Limited to routinely collected information, and to moderate to severe injuries where treatment was sought.
Population based surveys	Non-fatal injury rates	Population based.	Self-reported
Physical impairment/Functional disability			
Census data	Counts and rates of disability	A short set of standardized questions have been developed by the Washington Group.[*] Population-based. Socio-economic data available. Can provide trend data.	Usually limited to a few questions on disability with the cause of disability generally not recorded. Self-reported.
Population-based surveys of injuries (cross-sectional)	Health related quality of life, functional ability, health utility	Range of instruments, e.g. SF-36, EQ-5D, Health Utilities Index (HUI), WHO-DAS, can be used. Instruments available for retrospective measurement of pre-injury health status.	Accurate data on functional outcome measurements mostly lacking for developing countries. Data sources usually not comparable to enable an in-depth understanding of health-related quality of life experiences of injured individuals. Reliability and validation of instruments requires further research.
Longitudinal studies of injured populations	Duration and health state utilities to indicate functional impact of injuries	Individual-reported information on health states can be used to quantify health utilities and calculate YLDs and QALYs. Guidelines on study methods have been developed by EuroSafe.	Resource intensive, mostly lacking for developing countries. Reliability and validation of instruments required.
Composite morbidity and mortality-related indices			
Burden of Disease estimates	DALYs and QALYs	Combines information on mortality, morbidity, and injury outcomes to represent injury burden comprehensively. Long-term impact of injury also included.	Intensive data requirements; the number of assumptions for the calculation of DALYs and QALYs.

[*]Center for Disease Control, *Washington Group on Disability Statistics*, available from http://www.cdc.gov/nchs/washington_group/wg_background.htm

Source: data from Hendrie, D., and Miller, T. R., Assessing the burden of injuries: competing measures, *International Journal of Injury Control and Safety Promotion*, Volume 11, Issue 3, pp. 193–9, Copyright © 2004; Polinder, S. et al., A systematic review of studies measuring health-related quality of life of general injury populations, *BMC Public Health*, Volume 10, p. 783, Copyright © 2010; Segui-Gomez, M., and Hyder, A., *Mortality and Morbidity*, Bloomberg School of Public Health, Johns Hopkins University, Baltimore, USA, Copyright © 2011, available from http://ocw.jhsph.edu/index.cfm/go/viewCourse/course/burdenofinjuries/coursePage/lectureNotes/; and Segui-Gomez, M., and MacKenzie, E. J., Measuring the public health impact of injuries, *Epidemiologic Reviews*, Volume 25, Issue 1, pp. 3–19, Copyright © 2003.

were dominated by YLLs, an indication of premature mortality, across all ages. YLDs are calculated by multiplying the number of non-fatal injuries with the duration and disabling effect of the injury, whereas YLLs are calculated by multiplying the number of deaths at a particular age with an idealized age. The comparatively low YLDs may be due to the relatively quick recovery from non-fatal injuries and the relatively young age of mortality from interpersonal violence, which results in higher YLLs than mortality in older ages. Another reason for the low YLD estimate might be the lack of data on the long-term impact of violence and in part by the YLDs being prevalence-based for the 2010 estimates. The age-profile for the interpersonal violence DALYs follows a similar pattern for males and females, with a peak in the 20–24 year age group followed by a steady decrease in older ages.

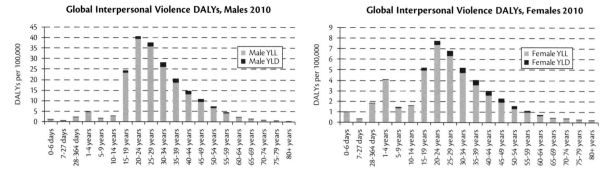

Fig. 12.1 Global DALYs* for interpersonal violence by age and sex, 2010.

*Note the difference in scale for DALYs between males and females.

Authors calculations based on data from *Global Burden of Disease Study 2010 (GBD 2010) Results by Cause 1990-2010*, Institute for Health Metrics and Evaluation, University of Washington, USA, Copyright © 2014, available from http://ghdx.healthmetricsandevaluation.org/record/global-burden-disease-study-2010-gbd-2010-results-cause-1990-2010.

The three regions with the highest DALY rate for interpersonal violence (Figure 12.2) were Southern sub-Saharan Africa (1,934 per 100,000), Central Latin America (1,662 per 100,000), and Tropical Latin America (1,618 per 100,000). Interpersonal violence was among the leading causes of death and disability in these regions. In contrast, the regions with the lowest rates were high-income countries in the Asia Pacific region (54 per 100,000), Western Europe (71 per 100,000), and Australasia (81 per 100,000); interpersonal violence was not among the leading causes of death and disability for these regions. Figure 12.2 also shows that DALY rates for interpersonal violence increased for nine of the 21 regions between 1990 and 2010, with the highest increase (55 per cent) in

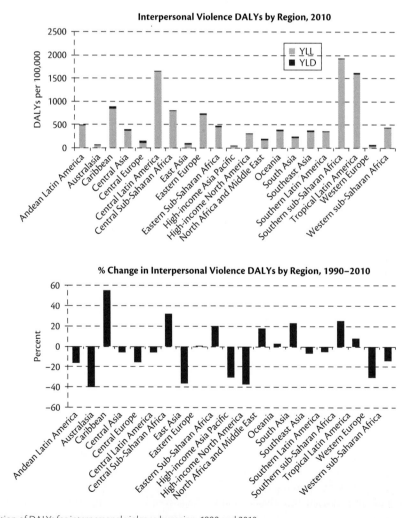

Fig. 12.2 YLL and YLD composition of DALYs for interpersonal violence by region, 1990 and 2010.

Authors calculations based on data from *Global Burden of Disease Study 2010 (GBD 2010) Results by Cause 1990-2010*, Institute for Health Metrics and Evaluation, University of Washington, USA, Copyright © 2014, available from http://ghdx.healthmetricsandevaluation.org/record/global-burden-disease-study-2010-gbd-2010-results-cause-1990-2010.

the Caribbean. The largest decrease occurred in the Australasian region (40.5 per cent).

Violence as a Risk Factor

The 2002 WHO Health Report (WHO 2002c) quantified the burden attributable to 22 selected risk factors considered modifiable. In this report, the attributable fraction of a disease or injury due to the risk factor was calculated based on the strength of the relationship between the risk factor and the incidence of a particular disease or injury based on the relative risk, and the prevalence of the exposure to the risk factor in the population (Ezzati et al. 2002). Childhood sexual abuse, a component of interpersonal violence, was included as one of the quantified risk factors. The recently published (Lim et al. 2012) comparative risk factor assessment for the 2010 GBD has quantified 67 risk factors, but also failed to include interpersonal violence because of a lack of sufficient epidemiological evidence of the causal effects. Watts and Cairncross (2012) note that this undermines the utility of the study for priority setting, and call for quality epidemiological data on the impact of interpersonal violence, but also suggest that comparative assessments include estimates with an indication of the uncertainty.

In contrast, the South African Comparative Risk Factor Assessment for 2000 (Norman et al. 2007a) estimated the burden of interpersonal violence as one of 17 risk factors that were considered. Despite the dearth of full information about the longer-term consequences of interpersonal violence, Norman et al. (2010) attempted to estimate the direct and indirect health outcomes, adopting the WHO framework of the type and nature of violence and identifying the health consequences from work done by Andrews et al. (2004) and Vos et al. (2006), as shown schematically in Figure 12.3. Following unsafe sex, interpersonal violence was identified as the second leading modifiable risk factor in South Africa, accounting for 8.4 per cent of the DALYs (Norman et al. 2007b). This was considered to be an underestimate.

Conclusion

Measuring the health burden of violence is challenged by definitional issues and limited data sources. Standard classifications, indicators, and tools need to be used more widely and the strengths of different data sources need to be considered in developing appropriate surveillance systems.

Modelling strategies have been applied to fill the information gap at a global level. Recent GBD estimates highlight that much of the health burden arises from premature mortality with a strong age and gender pattern affecting young males. The GBD estimates likely understate the extent of non-fatal burden. Furthermore, they do not consider the long-term health consequences by considering violence as a modifiable risk factor. Nonetheless, the GBD study highlights the high burden experienced in sub-Saharan Africa and Central and Tropical Latin America and low rates in the Asia Pacific, Western Europe, and Australasia regions, indicating considerable regional variations which should be utilized to understand the determinants of violence.

Acknowledgements

We thank Rosana Norman and Michelle Schneider, who developed the framework for estimating the health impact of interpersonal violence with Debbie Bradshaw.

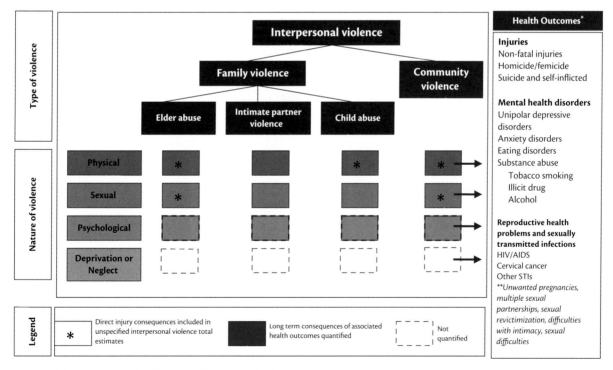

Fig. 12.3 Framework for estimating the health impact of interpersonal violence.

References

54th World Health Assembly (2001). *International Classification of Functioning, Disability and Health*. WHA 54.21. Geneva: World Health Organization.

Andrews, G., Corry, J., Slade, T., Issakidis, C., and Swanston, H. (2004). Child sexual abuse. In: M. Ezzati, A. D. Lopez, A. Rodgers, and C. J. L. Murray ((eds), *Comparative Quantification of Health Risks: Global and Regional Burden of Disease Attributable to Selected Major Risk Factors*. Geneva: World Health Organization, pp. 1851–940.

Baker, S. P., O'Neill, B., Haddon, W., and Long, W. B. (1974). The injury severity score: a method for describing patients with multiple injuries and evaluating emergency care. *Journal of Trauma*, 14, 187–96.

Boyd, C. R., Tolson, M. A., and Copes, W. S. (1987). Evaluating trauma care: the TRISS method. *Journal of Trauma*, 27, 370–8.

Committee on Medical Aspects of Automotive Safety (1971). Rating the severity of tissue damage: I. the abbreviated scale. *JAMA*, 215, 277–80.

Ezzati, M., Lopez, A., Rodgers, A., Vander Hoorn, S., and Murray, C. (2002). Selected major risk factors and global and regional burden of disease. *Lancet*, 360, 1347–60.

Feeny, D., Furlong, W., Boyle, M., and Torrance, G. W. (1995). Multi-attribute health status classification systems. Health Utilities Index. *Pharmacoeconomics*, 7, 490–502.

Hendrie, D., and Miller, T. R. (2004). Assessing the burden of injuries: competing measures. *International Journal of Injury Control and Safety Promotion*, 11, 193–9.

Horsman, J., Furlong, W., Feeny, D., and Torrance, G. (2003). The Health Utilities Index (HUI®): concepts, measurement properties and applications. *Health Quality Life Outcomes*, 1, 54.

Joint Committee on Injury Scaling (1994). *Injury Impairment Scale: 1994.* Illinois: Association for the Advancement of Automotive Medicine.

Kobusingye, O. C., and Lett, R. R. (2000). Hospital-based trauma registries in Uganda. *Journal of Trauma*, 48, 498–502.

Lim, S. S., Vos, T., and Flaxman, A. D. et al. (2012). A comparative risk assessment of burden of disease and injury attributable to 67 risk factors and risk factor clusters in 21 regions, 1990–2010: a systematic analysis for the Global Burden of Disease Study 2010. *Lancet*, 380, 2224–60.

Miller, T. R. (2000). Assessing the burden of injury: progress and pitfalls. In: D. Mohan and G. Tiwari (eds), *Injury Prevention and Control*. New York: Taylor and Francis, pp. 49–70.

Murray, C. J. L., Vos, T., and Lozano, R. et al. (2012). Disability-adjusted life years (DALYs) for 291 diseases and injuries in 21 regions, 1990–2010: a systematic analysis for the global burden of disease study 2010. *Lancet*, 380, 2197–223.

Norman, R., Bradshaw, D., and Schneider, M. et al. (2007a). A comparative risk assessment for South Africa in 2000: towards promoting health and preventing disease. *South African Medical Journal*, 97, 637–41.

Norman, R., Matzopoulos, R., Groenewald, P., and Bradshaw, D. (2007b). The high burden of injuries in South Africa. *Bulletin of the World Health Organization*, 85, 695–702.

Norman, R., Schneider, M., and Bradshaw, D. et al. (2010). Interpersonal violence: an important risk factor for disease and injury in South Africa. *Population Health Metrics*, 8, 32.

Osler, T., Baker, S. P., and Long, W. (1997). A modification of the injury severity score that both improves accuracy and simplifies scoring. *Journal of Trauma, Injury, Infection and Critical Care*, 43, 922–6.

Peden, M. (1998a). Injury severity scoring made easy: part I. *Trauma Review*, 10–11.

Peden, M. (1998b). Injury severity scoring made easy: part II. *Trauma Review*, 11–12.

Polinder, S., Haagsma, J. A., and Belt, E. et al. (2010). A systematic review of studies measuring health-related quality of life of general injury populations. *BMC Public Health*, 10, 783.

Salomon, J. A., Vos, T., and Hogan, D. R. et al. (2012). Common values in assessing health outcomes from disease and injury: disability weights measurement study for the global burden of disease study 2010. *Lancet*, 380, 2129–43.

Segui-Gomez, M., and Hyder, A. (2011). *Mortality and Morbidity*. Bloomberg School of Public Health, Baltimore: Johns Hopkins University. Available at: http://ocw.jhsph.edu/index.cfm/go/viewCourse/course/burdenofinjuries/coursePage/lectureNotes/ [Accessed 30 November 2012].

Segui-Gomez, M., and MacKenzie, E. J. (2003). Measuring the public health impact of injuries. *Epidemiologic Reviews* 25, 3–19.

Teasdale, G., and Jennett, B. (1974). Assessment of coma and impaired consciousness. *Lancet*, 304, 81–4.

Tepas, J. J., Mollitt, D. L., Talbert, J. L., and Bryant, M. (1987). The pediatric trauma score as a predictor of injury severity in the injured child. *Journal of Pediatric Surgery*, 22, 14–8.

The EuroQol Group (1990). EuroQol: a new facility for the measurement of health-related quality of life. *Health Policy*, 16, 199–208.

Ustun, T. B., Kostanjsek, N., Chatterji, S., and Rehm, J. (2010). *Measuring Health and Disability. Manual for WHO Disability Assessment Schedule 2.0*. Geneva: World Health Organization Press.

Van Beeck, E. F., Larsen, C. F., Lyons, R. A., Meerding, W. J., Mulder, S., and Essink-Bot, M. L. (2007). Guidelines for the conduction of follow-up studies measuring injury-related disability. *Journal of Trauma*, 62, 534–50.

Vos, T., Astbury, J., and Piers, L. S. et al. (2006). Measuring the impact of intimate partner violence on the health of women in Victoria, Australia. *Bulletin of the World Health Organization*, 84, 739–44.

Ware, J. E., and Sherbourne, C. D. (1992). The MOS 36-item Short-Form Health Survey (SF-36): I. Conceptual framework and item selection. *Medical Care*, 30, 473–83.

Watts, C., and Cairncross, S. (2012). Should the GBD risk factor rankings be used to guide policy? *Lancet*, 380, 2060–1.

World Health Organization (WHO) (2002a). *World Report on Violence and Health: Summary*. Geneva: WHO.

World Health Organization (2002b). *Towards a Common Language for Functioning, Disability and Health (ICF)*. Geneva: WHO.

World Health Organization. (2002c). *World Health Report. Reducing Risks, Promoting Healthy Life*. Geneva: WHO. Available at: http://www.who.int/whr [Accessed 12 February 2013].

World Health Organization (2008). *International Statistical Classification of Diseases and Related Health Problems—tenth revision. Volume 2*. Geneva: WHO.

World Health Organization (2011). Understanding disability. In: A. Officer and A. Posarac (eds), *World report on disability 2011*. Geneva: WHO, pp. 3–16.

Yates, D. W. (1990). ABC of major trauma: scoring systems for trauma. *British Medical Journal*, 301, 1090–4.

CHAPTER 13

The consequences of violence: mental health issues

Susan Hawkridge, Astrid Berg, and Soraya Seedat

Introduction to Violence-Related Mental Health Issues

In this chapter, we consolidate evidence on the epidemiology and phenomenology of mental health problems associated with violence exposure and provide some guidance on the clinical assessment and management of these sequelae. As a point of departure, it is important to note that a delicate interplay exists between violence exposure and psychopathology. This interplay needs to be understood in terms of (i) the heterogeneity of responses in children and adults to the same violent event; (ii) the frequent occurrence of multiple rather than isolated psychiatric problems following single or repeated violence-related incidents; and (iii) the impact of different types of violence over the life course in shaping psychopathology and modifying developmental trajectories, in combination with other factors (e.g. genetic or environmental factors) (Cerdá et al. 2012).

Interpersonal violence and health are inextricably linked: violence is associated with the onset, duration, and recurrence of psychiatric disorders, and individuals with pre-existing psychiatric disorders are prone to violent victimization. Direct and indirect costs, especially indirect impacts on health-related quality of life, reduced job opportunities, and community participation are considerable (Matzopoulos et al. 2008).

Violence in general, and interpersonal violence in particular, is associated with a high burden of disease. It is notable that the Global Burden of Disease Study 2010 (Murray et al. 2013) ranked interpersonal violence as the 27th leading cause globally of disability-adjusted life years, ahead of asthma, hypertensive heart disease, and alcohol and drug use disorders.

Over the past two decades there has been a proliferation of studies on the long-term psychopathological outcomes of interpersonal violence. Much of this research has been conducted in high-income countries, yet the burden of psychiatric disorders attributable to violence continues to be significantly higher in low middle income countries (LAMIC) (Dahlberg and Krug 2002).

Epidemiology of the Mental Health Effects of Violence

Exposure to community violence, school violence, childhood physical, psychological and sexual abuse, and adult interpersonal violence (IPV) has consistently been associated with depression, post-traumatic stress disorder (PTSD), other anxiety disorders, and substance use disorders as well as increased sexual risk behaviour (Kessler et al. 2010, Norman et al. 2012). Existing research collectively shows that direct experience of violence, as well as witnessing of violence, in the home environment and at school, are more likely to be associated with psychopathology than community exposure to violence (Cerdá et al. 2012; Ribeiro et al. 2009). In addition, cumulative exposure to different forms of violence is a contributor to higher levels of psychopathology than is an acute, single-incident exposure. The timing of violence exposure appears to be important in that there is growing evidence that experiencing abuse and maltreatment during critical periods of neurodevelopment can lead to changes in brain structure and function that increase vulnerability to mental health problems. Gender is another consideration, given that many studies (though not all) find that the relationship between early exposure to violence and adult negative health outcomes is stronger for women than it is for men (Olofsson et al. 2012). A number of other factors may confound or mediate the association between early violence and later psychopathology, as well as confound the association between later exposure to violence and subsequent psychopathology (Cerdá et al. 2012). This includes individual level factors (e.g. genetics, temperament, IQ, personality), family factors (parental loss, low socioeconomic status, poor parent–child relationships), and environmental factors (e.g. poverty, crime, alcohol, and drug abuse) (Matzopoulos et al. 2008).

Childhood and adolescence are critical developmental periods when the effects of exposure to interpersonal violence may be particularly damaging and pervasive. A number of theories have been posited as explanations for the relationship between early violent experiences and adult mental disorders. First, early childhood violence exposure can activate stress-responsive systems, including the hypothalamic–pituitary–adrenal (HPA) axis, sympathetic nervous system, and neurotransmitter systems, that collectively have resultant negative mental health effects on those affected. Second, past experience of violence is a significant risk factor across the lifespan for future violence victimization. Cumulative adversities across the early lifespan, when coupled with repeated stressful experiences in adulthood, may result in perturbations of the HPA axis and aberrations in the response of the immune system that can persist with widespread effects on mental health trajectories. Third, early traumatic life events may be associated with biological changes at the level of the genome (i) in the form of gene alterations in the HPA axis and immune system, and (ii) as epigenetic 'marks'.

These 'marks' (i.e. modifications in gene expression without a change in the DNA sequence), specifically involving genes underlying stress and immune regulation, may operate in mediating the association between early adverse events and long-term negative health outcomes (Bick et al. 2012). Thus, early adversity can change the functioning of the genes that we inherit at birth. In contrast to the relative stability of gene sequences, epigenetic mechanisms (e.g. the switching off of certain genes), are to some extent modified by environmental influences. Lastly, the same violence exposure can result in heterogeneity of psychopathological responses.

In population-based studies, violence has most often been studied in the context of PTSD. Compared with other (non-violent) traumatic events, violence-related traumatic events have been associated with the highest risk for PTSD.

Community Violence Exposure

Children who witness violence in their communities are at increased risk of PTSD, depression, anxiety, and substance abuse compared with unexposed children (Aisenberg and Herrenkohl 2008). Repeated and chronic exposure to community violence, as either a witness or a victim, can lead to aggressive behaviour and school failure. The mental health impact of community violence (e.g. the development of PTSD and depression) may, however, be affected by (i) type of exposure (e.g. being robbed at knifepoint and stabbed may have a more detrimental impact than being threatened with violence), (ii) physical proximity to the event, (iii) previous traumatic exposures and losses, (iv) developmental stage of the child, and (v) parental support (Aisenberg and Herrenkohl 2008). It has been suggested that parenting capacity may be a mediator of later outcomes in children with community violence exposure, in that parents who are themselves traumatized by violence may be less capable of responding appropriately to the needs of a violence-exposed child.

While community violence is often thought of as distinct from other types of violence, it commonly overlaps with domestic violence and exposure to multiple types of violence. Exposure to multiple types of violence over the life course is linked to an increased risk of, and more severe, psychopathology (Cerdá et al. 2012). Additionally, there is limited evidence that domestic violence may moderate (and worsen) the relationship between community violence and poor outcomes in children.

Childhood Violence Exposure

Childhood maltreatment encompasses sexual abuse, physical abuse, emotional abuse, and neglect. Converging evidence from the fields of epidemiology and neurobiology indicates that repetitive and/or severe abuse during critical periods of childhood brain development can impair, often permanently, the structure and activity of multiple brain circuits and major neuroregulatory systems with profound and lasting neurobehavioral consequences (Garner and Shonkoff 2012, Rikfin-Graboi et al. 2009). This supports the need for clinicians to increase efforts to detect and treat common psychiatric disorders in physically, sexually, and emotionally abused and neglected children. Children who

experience sexual or physical abuse have an elevated risk for the onset and persistence of mood, anxiety, substance use, and childhood behavioural disorders compared with children who have no abuse history (Widom et al. 2007). There is evidence to suggest that the age of onset of maltreatment may have some bearing on the type of outcome. An earlier onset has been shown to predict more symptoms of anxiety and depression in adulthood, while a later onset has been shown to be predictive of more behavioural problems in adulthood (Kaplow and Widom 2007). This may, in turn, have implications for targeting interventions aimed at preventing adult psychopathology. A recent meta-analysis found fairly robust evidence for a causal relationship with a number of health outcomes that included depressive disorders, anxiety disorders, eating disorders, suicide attempts, drug use, risky sexual behaviour, and sexually transmitted infections (Norman et al. 2012).

Intimate Partner Violence

It is plausible that the relationship between intimate partner violence (IPV) and mental disorder is a bidirectional one, although the limited numbers of longitudinal studies make inferences about causality and temporality problematic. IPV more commonly afflicts women and includes physical, sexual, or psychological harm by a current or former spouse or intimate partner (World Health Organization [WHO] 2010).

There is consistent evidence that both men and women with all types of mental disorder have a higher prevalence and increased odds of experiencing IPV and other domestic violence (which includes violence by non-intimate family members), compared to individuals without a mental disorder (Trevillion et al. 2012). This is more than a sevenfold increased risk for individuals with PTSD and a fourfold increased risk for individuals with other anxiety disorders.

IPV also results in poor mental and physical health. In a review of 75 studies of IPV and health outcomes in women, IPV was found to be associated, across studies, with a wide range of mental health problems, most commonly depression, PTSD, anxiety, suicidality and self-harm, subjective psychological distress, and sleep disturbances (Dillon et al. 2013).

The more frequent and/or sustained the exposure to IPV, the more severe the psychopathology, especially with regards to PTSD, depression, anxiety, and suicidality. Domestic violence also impacts on children's mental health. Studies in LAMIC point to a range of internalising and externalising problems, as well as suicidal ideation (Ribeiro et al. 2009).

Other Violence Exposure

A review by Benjet in 2010 focused on adversities that are more peculiar to low-income countries, namely violence due to armed conflict, female genital mutilation, child labour, and orphanhood due to AIDS, and found high rates of mental disorder (PTSD and depression) compared with unexposed youth. In children living in conflict zones, rates of PTSD ranged from 20 to 62 per cent and rates of depression from 20 to 24 per cent. Among former child soldiers rates of PTSD and depression were even higher (35–97 per cent and 53 per cent, respectively). AIDS orphans represent another vulnerable group where bullying, stigma, and poverty may mediate the association with poor mental health outcomes (Cluver et al. 2010).

Developmental Understandings of Risk/Resiliency Factors for Mental Health Outcomes in Violence-Exposed Individuals

Hidden Traumas in Infancy

In infants experienced threat is related to the caregiver's affects and availability rather than necessarily an actual physical threat (Schuder and Lyons-Ruth 2004). If the external regulating function which the caregiver provides and on which the young infant is dependent is not functioning, this increases the level of stress experienced by the young child. Maternal withdrawal as seen with postnatal depression is known to have a long-lasting effect on the young child (Grace et al. 2003). Such children are vulnerable to later stressful life events. Conversely, secure attachment acts as a buffer against later negative life events as the foundations have been laid for coping with novelty and stress (Schore 2001).

Intimate Partner Violence

Violence in the home inevitably signifies relational trauma which is usually not a single event, but cumulative and embedded in family relationships. Exposure to abuse during the formative years sets the stage for later responses to violence, particularly if the source of threat is the parent or a familiar figure. Instead of the parent being a base for security and comfort in which closeness can be sought, the child is driven to avoid a source of danger. Lower-cost behavioural strategies, namely searching out the attachment object, are not possible in these situations; thus higher-cost endocrine responses come into play. This means an increase in catecholamines and corticotropin-releasing factor (CRF), a physiological situation which may persist and make the person susceptible to on-going up-regulated stress responses (Rifkin-Graboi et al. 2009). This 'toxic stress' disrupts the architecture of the developing brain and plays a powerful role in influencing behavioural, educational, economic, and health outcomes decades later (Garner et al. 2012).

Community Violence

Community violence has been shown to impact strongly on children (Ward et al. 2012).

For the young child the impact is partly through the effect the violence has on parenting behaviour. Young children are dependent on their parents for regulation of emotions, and parents who themselves become frightened may not have the capacity to contain, soothe, and regulate the distress in their child, thus enhancing the high-cost endocrine response. Preschoolers exposed to traumatic events look to their parents not just for emotional comfort, but also for mental processing of the event. There is evidence that the symptoms of young children in such situations are predicted by their mother's psychological functioning (Lieberman and Van Horn 2004).

For the older child observational learning and role modelling assume greater importance and they may either identify with the aggressor themselves, or conversely withdraw and become inhibited. Such children are then sensitized to reacting to future violence with internalizing and/or externalizing behaviours.

Clinical Presentation and Assessment of Psychiatric Sequelae of Exposure to Violence

Some individuals present directly to the mental health care system as witnesses to, victims of, or even perpetrators, of violence. Others may present to mental health care facilities with psychiatric symptoms which are only revealed to have their roots in violent events on careful investigation. In addition, many who present with general medical complaints may be suffering from the sequelae of chronic stress related to discrete or continuous exposure to violence. Systematic inquiry specifically concerning exposure to violence, either past or current, should be part of the assessment of every patient presenting to any health facility. Early trauma has also been strongly associated with increased rates of schizophrenia, reactive attachment disorder, eating disorders, personality disorders, substance abuse, and suicide attempts (Heim et al. 2010) and it has been found that the age of traumatization may affect the type of later psychopathology, in that abuse between the ages of 3 and 5 years is associated more with later depressive symptomatology and between the ages of 9 and 11 years with PTSD (Andersen et al. 2008).

Attachment Disorders

Severely pathological caregiving in infancy, including exposure to violence, often at the hands of caregivers, may give rise to reactive attachment disorder (RAD). Children with RAD may be inhibited or disinhibited in their social interactions. In addition, disorganized–disorientated insecure attachment confers a vulnerability to PTSD (Schore 2002). Children diagnosed with disinhibited-type RAD may be particularly vulnerable to victimization.

Disruptive Behaviour Disorders

Any child presenting with a disruptive behaviour disorder (attention deficit/hyperactivity disorder, oppositional defiant disorder, or conduct disorder) as well as adults presenting with antisocial behaviour, should be screened for exposure to violence. A recent study of the link between victimization and street crime found that one of the origins (though by no means the only one) of adolescent involvement in crime may be fathers who use violence against their children. Subsequent victimization by others may become normalized, and, together, these experiences may decrease adolescents' sensitivity to risk and danger, thus facilitating involvement in criminal activity (Frederick et al. 2013).

Cognitive Disorders

Traumatic brain injury as a result of violence can result in cognitive impairment, either generalized (intellectual disability or dementia), or specific (e.g. executive dysfunction or short-term memory impairment) (Capehart and Bass 2012). The assessment and management of individuals with cognitive impairment and comorbid trauma-related pathology can be complex, and multidisciplinary involvement is usually needed.

Substance Use Disorders

The association between exposure to violence and substance use disorders is well established and appears to be mediated by cumulative trauma, depression, and anxiety disorders, especially PTSD

(Douglas et al. 2010). Individuals may present with a substance use disorder, or with medical complications of substance use.

Psychotic Disorders

A link has recently been proposed between childhood exposure to trauma and increased risk for schizophrenia (Matheson et al. 2013). Patients with a diagnosis of schizophrenia should be assessed for exposure to violence as well as comorbid trauma-related diagnoses.

Mood Disorders

There is robust evidence for an increased vulnerability to depression in victims of violence, and some indication that depression in victims of violence is more likely to be non-responsive to treatment (Kaplan and Klinetob 2000).

Anxiety and Stress-Related Disorders

Posttraumatic Stress Disorder

This may be acute or chronic, and usually presents with symptoms related to re-experiencing, alterations in cognitions and mood, avoidance, or hypervigilance (American Psychiatric Association (APA) 2013). Diagnosis may be difficult in very young children whose verbal ability may limit symptom expression, and conditions such as developmental/complex traumatic syndromes should be considered. The DSM-5 now includes a preschool subtype for children 6 years of age and younger that is more developmentally sensitive and behaviourally focused (APA 2013). Appropriate evaluation and diagnosis of traumatized young children may require specialized child mental health professionals.

Generalized Anxiety Disorder

There is evidence that vulnerability to anxiety disorders is conferred by early exposure to violence. In one study, females who were victims of violence in both childhood and adulthood received a diagnosis of generalized anxiety disorder significantly more often (23.3 per cent vs. 2.9 per cent) than women not exposed to violence (Roberts et al. 1998).

Panic Disorder

Panic disorder may co-occur with PTSD, or may present independently post trauma. There is some evidence that post-traumatic panic symptoms may predict later PTSD in the first year following exposure (Adams et al. 2011).

Social Phobia

Individuals presenting with social withdrawal or other avoidant behaviour may be misdiagnosed with social phobia, when more thorough questioning may elicit evidence of PTSD-related avoidance (Handley et al. 2009). In addition, a history of childhood maltreatment has been found in 70 per cent of a sample presenting clinically with the generalized subtype of social anxiety disorder (Simon et al. 2009).

Separation Anxiety Disorder

Preschool children exposed to violence may present with separation anxiety disorder. In one study, 65 per cent of preschool children meeting criteria for PTSD following exposure to IPV and additional traumatic events were also found to have new onset separation anxiety as a trauma-related symptom (Graham-Bermann et al. 2012).

Personality Disorders

In a large epidemiological study, childhood adversity was highly prevalent among individuals with personality disorders, and most consistently associated with schizotypal, antisocial, borderline, and narcissistic personality disorders (Afifi et al. 2011).

The Clinical Management of Victims of Violence

Basic principles in clinical management that hold across the age ranges are, firstly, the ensuring of physical safety of the victim, and, secondly, ensuring the presence of a significant other, or attachment figure, to be available to the individual. In case of intra-familial violence this may pose a challenge as often the person trusted by the victim is in fact the perpetrator. A child can only be protected if his/her allegations are taken seriously by the non-abusing parent or another adult. An urgent assessment of the child's family situation is required and cessation of unsupervised contact between child and alleged abuser should be implemented immediately.

The approach to treatment is characterized by the following goals and mechanisms (Lieberman and Van Horn 2004):

(i) Encouraging a return to normal development, adaptive coping, and engagement with present activities and future goals—for example, youth who were the victims of xenophobic violence were explicit in their wish to return to school even while displaced.

(ii) Fostering a realistic response to threat: the experience of trauma impairs the ability to appraise realistically cues to danger and safety, leading to inappropriate responses.

(iii) Maintaining regular levels of affective arousal: the traumatic stress response of numbing, avoidance, and hyper-arousal interfere with the ability to rely on others for help. Daily routines and structured activities aid self-regulation. Infants, toddlers, and preschoolers require the help of the caregiver to achieve affect self-regulation. It is thus of equal importance to attend to the caregiver's emotional state. This is particularly so for children under the age of 2 years in whom the memory of the trauma is pre-verbal and often more related to the effect the violence had on the caregivers.

(iv) Building reciprocity in intimate relationships: A traumatic event may impair the trust that existed in the parent (in the case of child victims) and in others and it may take time and effort before this trust restored. Parents often feel guilty at having failed to protect their child and this may in turn affect the emotional support they can give their child.

(v) Normalization of the traumatic response: traumatic responses can lead to fears of being 'crazy' or 'bad' in both children and adults. These universal reactions may need to be explicitly validated and legitimized.

(vi) Placing the traumatic experience in perspective: a balance needs to be achieved for both adults and children between the trauma that happened and living that has to go on. Although the debriefing model has shown conflicting results (van Emmerik et al. 2002), the ability to create a narrative around the traumatic event has been shown to improve post-traumatic symptoms (Ruf et al. 2010).

Various treatment modalities have been found to be effective (American Academy of Child and Adolescent Psychiatry 2010):

(i) rauma-focused psychotherapies delivered by trained and experienced psychotherapists should be considered first-line treatments for children and adolescents with Posttraumatic Stress Disorder. The focus should not only be on symptom improvement but also on enhancing functioning and resiliency and a return to the pre-event developmental trajectory.

Cognitive-behavioural therapies provide stress management skills and are aimed at providing mastery over trauma reminders. Psychodynamic trauma-focused psychotherapies aim to promote self-coherence and healthy development. In younger children these therapies focus on the parent–child relationship, but for older children this type of therapy provides an opportunity to mobilize more mature cognitive capacities by objectifying and explaining symptoms and trauma reminders. For adolescents and adults such unstructured sessions may open up a space in which an internal locus of control which has been lost during the trauma can be regained.

(ii) In some cases referral to child psychiatric services may be needed for consideration of adjunctive psychopharmacology.

Conclusion and Recommendations

The mental health outcomes of exposure to violence are overwhelmingly negative, pervasive, persistent, and costly to both health-care systems and society in general. A history of current or prior exposure to violence should be sought in all individuals presenting to mental health-care facilities. Careful history taking and mental state examination will help to elicit contributions made by violence to mental ill health and facilitate holistic management of psychiatric disorders. Prevention of the mental health sequelae of exposure to violence may be the single most effective intervention in terms of public health and societal well-being. Of particular importance is the need to give attention to the mental state and parenting capacity of caregivers of children who are exposed to violence.

References

Adams, R. E., and Boscarino, J. A. (2011). A structural equation model of perievent panic and posttraumatic stress disorder after a community disaster. *Journal of Traumatic Stress*, 24, 61–9.

Afifi, T. O., Mather, A., and Boman, J. et al. (2011). Childhood adversity and personality disorders: results from a nationally representative population-based study. *Journal of Psychiatric Research*, 45, 814–22.

Aisenberg, E., and Herrenkohl, T. (2008). Community violence in context: risk and resilience in children and families. *Journal of Interpersonal Violence*, 23, 296–315.

American Psychiatric Association (2013). *Diagnostic and Statistical Manual of Mental Disorders* 5th ed. Washington, D.C.: American Psychiatric Press.

American Academy of Child and Adolescent Psychiatry. (2010). Practice parameter for the assessment and treatment of children and adolescents with posttraumatic stress disorder. *Journal of the American Academy of Child Adolescent Psychiatry*, 49, 414–30.

Andersen, S. L., Tomada, A., Vincow, E. S., Valente, E., Polcari, A., and Teicher, M. H. (2008). Preliminary evidence for sensitive periods in the effect of childhood sexual abuse on regional brain development. *Journal of Neuropsychiatry and Clinical Neurosciences*, 20, 292–301.

Benjet, C. (2010). Childhood adversities of populations living in low-income countries: prevalence, characteristics, and mental health consequences. *Current Opinion in Psychiatry*, 23, 356–62.

Bick, J., Naumova, O., and Hunter, S. et al. (2012). Childhood adversity and DNA methylation of genes involved in the hypothalamus-pituitary-adrenal axis and immune system: whole-genome and candidate-gene associations. *Development and Psychopathology*, 24, 1417–25.

Capehart, B. and Bass, D. (2012). Review: managing posttraumatic stress disorder in combat veterans with comorbid traumatic brain injury. *Journal of Rehabilitation Research and Development*, 49, 789–812.

Cerdá, M., Digangi, J., Galea, S., and Koenen, K. (2012). Epidemiologic research on interpersonal violence and common psychiatric disorders: where do we go from here? *Depression and Anxiety*, 29, 359–85.

Cluver, L., Bowes, L., and Gardner, F. (2010). Risk and protective factors for bullying victimization among AIDS-affected and vulnerable children in South Africa. *Child Abuse and Neglect*, 34, 793–803.

Dahlberg, L. L., and Krug, E.G. (2002). Violence: a global public health problem. In: E. G. Krug, L. L. Dahlberg, J. A. Mercy, A. B. Zwi, and R. Lozano (eds.). *World Report on Violence and Health*. Geneva, Switzerland: World Health Organization, pp. 1–21.

Dillon, G., Hussain, R., Loxton, D., and Rahman, S. (2013). Mental and physical health and intimate partner violence against women: a review of the literature. *International Journal of Family Medicine*, 2013: 313909. doi: 10.1155/2013/313909

Douglas, K. R., Chan, G., and Gelernter, J. et al. (2010). Adverse childhood events as risk factors for substance dependence: partial mediation by mood and anxiety disorders. *Addictive Behaviors*, 35, 7–13.

Frederick, T. J., McCarthy, B., and Hagan, J. (2013). Perceived danger and offending: exploring the links between violent victimization and street crime. *Violence and Victims*, 28, 16–35.

Garner, A. S., and Shonkoff, J. P. (2012). Early childhood adversity, toxic stress, and the role of the pediatrician: translating developmental science into lifelong health. *Pediatrics*, 129, e224–31.

Grace, S. L., Evindar, A., and Stewart, D. E. (2003). The effect of postpartum depression on child cognitive development and behavior: a review and critical analysis of the literature. *Archives of Women's Mental Health*, 6, 263–74.

Graham-Bermanns, S. A., Castor, L. E., Miller, L. E., and Howell, K. H. (2012). The impact of intimate partner violence and additional traumatic events on trauma symptoms and PTSD in preschool-aged children. *Journal of Traumatic Stress*, 25, 393–400.

Handley, R. V., Salkovskis, P. M., Scragg, P., and Ehlers, A. (2009). Clinically significant avoidance of public transport following the London bombings: travel phobia or subthreshold posttraumatic stress disorder? *Journal of Anxiety Disorders*, 23, 1170–6.

Heim, C., Shugart, M., Craighead, W. E., and Nemeroff, C.B. (2010). Neurobiological and psychiatric consequences of child abuse and neglect. *Developmental Psychobiology*, 52, 671–90.

Kaplan, M. J., and Klinetob, N.A. (2000). Childhood emotional trauma and chronic posttraumatic stress disorder in adult outpatients with treatment-resistant depression. *Journal of Nervous and Mental Disease*, 188, 596–601.

Kaplow, J. B., and Widom, C. S. (2007). Age of onset of child maltreatment predicts long-term mental health outcomes. *Journal of Abnormal Psychology*, 116, 176–87.

Kessler, R. C., McLaughlin, K. A., and Green, J. G. et al. (2010). Childhood adversities and adult psychopathology in the WHO World Mental Health Surveys. *British Journal of Psychiatry*, 197, 378–85.

Lieberman, A. F., and Van Horn, P. (2004). Assessment and treatment of young children exposed to traumatic events. In: J. D. Osofsky (ed.), *Young Children and Trauma: Intervention and Treatment*. New York and London: The Guilford Press, pp. 111–38.

Matheson, S. L., Shepherd, A. M., Pinchbeck, R. M., Laurens, K. R., and Carr, V. J. (2013). Childhood adversity in schizophrenia: a systematic meta-analysis. *Psychological Medicine*, 43, 225–38.

Matzopoulos, R., Bowman, B., Butchart, A., and Mercy, J. A. (2008). The impact of violence on health in low- to middle-income countries. *International Journal of Injury Control and Safety Promotion*, 15, 177–87.

Murray, C. J., Vos, T., and Lozano, R. et al. (2013). Disability-adjusted life years (DALYs) for 291 diseases and injuries in 21 regions, 1990-2010: a systematic analysis for the Global Burden of Disease Study 2010. *Lancet*, 15, 2197–223.

Norman, R. E., Byambaa, M. De, R., Butchart, A., Scott, J., and Vos, T. (2012). The long-term health consequences of child physical abuse, emotional abuse, and neglect: a systematic review and meta-analysis. *PLoS Med*, 9, e1001349.

Olofsson, N., Lindqvist, K., Shaw, B. A., and Danielsson, I. (2012). Long-term health consequences of violence exposure in adolescence: a 26-year prospective study. *BMC Public Health*, 12, 411.

Ribeiro, W. S., Andreoli, S. B., Ferri, C. P., Prince, M., and Mari, J. J. (2009). Exposure to violence and mental health problems in low and middle-income countries: a literature review. *Revista Brasileira de Psiquiatria*, 31, S49–57.

Rifkin-Graboi, A., Borelli, J. L., and Enlow, M. B. (2009). Neurobiology of stress in infancy. In: C. Zeanah (ed.), *Handbook of Infant Mental Health*. 3rd ed. New York and London: The Guilford Press, pp. 59–79.

Roberts, G. L., Lawrence, J. M., Williams, G. M., and Raphael, B. (1998). The impact of domestic violence on women's mental health. *Australian and New Zealand Journal of Public Health*, 22, 796–801.

Ruf, M., Schauer, M., Neuner, F., Catani, C., Schauer, E., and Elbert, T. (2010). Narrative exposure therapy for 7- to 16-year olds: a randomized controlled trial with traumatized refugee children, *Journal of Traumatic Stress*, 23, 437–45.

Schore, A. N. (2001). Effects of a secure attachment relationship on right brain development, affect regulation, and infant mental health. *Infant Mental Health Journal*, 22, 7–66.

Schore, A. N. (2002). Dysregulation of the right brain: a fundamental mechanism of traumatic attachment and the psychopathogenesis of posttraumatic stress disorder. *Australian and New Zealand Journal of Psychiatry*, 36, 9–30.

Schuder, M. R., and Lyons-Ruth, K. (2004). Hidden trauma in infancy. Attachment, fearful arousal, and early dysfunction of the stress response system. In: J. D. Osofsky (ed.). *Young Children and Trauma: Intervention and Treatment*. New York, London: The Guilford Press, pp. 69–104.

Simon, N. M., Herlands, N. N., and Marks, E. H. et al. (2009). Childhood maltreatment linked to greater symptom severity and poorer quality of life and function in social anxiety disorder. *Depression and Anxiety*, 26, 1027–32.

Trevillion, K., Oram, S., Feder, G., and Howard, L. M. (2012). Experiences of domestic violence and mental disorders: a systematic review and meta-analysis. *PLoS One*, 7, e51740.

Van Emmerik, A. A., Kamphuis, J. H., Hulsbosch, A. M., and Emmelkamp, P. M. (2002). Single session debriefing after psychological trauma: a meta-analysis. *Lancet*, 49, 414–30.

Ward, C. L., van der Merwe, A, and Dawes, A. (2012). *Youth violence: Sources and Solutions in South Africa*. Cape Town: UCT Press.

Widom, C. S., DuMont, K. and Czaja, S. J. (2007). A prospective investigation of major depressive disorder and comorbidity in abused and neglected children grown up'. *Archives of General Psychiatry*, 64, 49–56.

World Health Organization. (2010) *Preventing Intimate Partner Violence and Sexual Violence against Women: Taking Action and Generating Evidence*. Geneva, Switzerland: World Health Organization.

CHAPTER 14

Violence, police, and criminal justice systems

Robin S. Engel and Jeffrey E. Clutter

Introduction to Violence, Police, and Criminal Justice Systems

Violence is a problem that has myriad causes and dauntingly intricate solutions. Despite these complexities, many democratic societies for centuries have relied nearly exclusively on the formal processing of the criminal justice system (CJS) as the primary response for handling violence (Moore et al. 1994). Until very recently, however, CJSs in many societies were poorly equipped to do more than simply respond to violence by identifying, prosecuting, and punishing offenders. Typically, CJSs are reactionary and primarily responsible for processing criminal cases. These systems attempt to fulfil the dual goals of ensuring that the accused's individual rights are preserved while seeking to distribute justice and punishment. However, they often neglect the structural conditions that might optimize violence prevention efforts. As a result, violence extols a significant burden on CJSs around the world. Although citizens rely on these agencies to lead violence prevention efforts, they are often unable to do so effectively and efficiently. However, recent advances in theory, practice, scientific principles, and partnerships demonstrate that CJSs can be more effective in reducing violence.

We begin our chapter by describing the inherent problems for the CJS in reducing violence in democratic countries, with a specific focus on the police. We limit our discussion to interpersonal violence, defined as 'threatened or actual use of physical force against a person or a group that either results or is likely to result in injury or death' (Mercy et al. 1993, p. 8). We describe the structural problems, limited resources, and underdevelopment of working partnerships that inhibit problem solving and violence reduction efforts. Thereafter, we consider in greater depth the specific issues and correlates of violence that make it especially resistant to efforts of CJSs. We describe the trend toward conceptualizing violence as a public health concern, and discuss law enforcement's role within this framework. We also describe the recent movement in CJSs towards evidence-based practices, with police effectiveness as a specific example. We conclude with a description of promising approaches that combine empirical evidence about effective policing approaches with the creation of strategic partnerships across multiple stakeholders. Ultimately, we argue that police specifically, and CJSs more generally, are now better equipped to promote and implement data-driven, evidence-based solutions to reduce violence.

Problems with Traditional CJS Responses to Violence

The frequency of violence places an enormous burden on both the victims of violence and the social institutions dealing with consequences of violence. In many countries the CJS, and more specifically the police, are the sole entities responsible for handling violence. Given that police are often perceived as the frontline response to violence, they are also expected to prevent violence in all forms (Moore et al. 1994). A number of factors exist, however, that hinder the efforts of the police and the larger CJSs worldwide to reduce violence. These factors include the reactionary style of the criminal justice process, cultures of violence, political and system-wide issues, resource constraints, and impediments to working with other external agencies.

In democratic societies, CJSs are typically designed to respond to criminal events, and thus the majority of their processes are reactionary: the process begins as a reaction to a criminal event. Rather than proactively identifying would-be offenders and preventing possible criminal activity, the majority of their efforts are spent responding to crimes after they occur—investigating the events, identifying and processing offenders, and distributing appropriate sanctions. The end goal in a reactionary CJS is to process offenders through the system and provide societal and individual justice. Although many CJSs across developed nations have become very efficient at this process, the sheer volume of criminal activity, and violence in particular, hinders a CJS's ability to do anything more than process offenders. Yet little evidence exists that this type of reactive processing can help significantly reduce the amount of crime (Goldstein 1990; Moore et al. 1994).

An additional constraint on CJSs is the manpower and financial burden associated with addressing violence. Preventative efforts to reduce violence are deemed too costly for individual jurisdictions because their limited resources are spent responding to crime and disorder and processing criminals. Further, the global economic crisis of the late 2000s has led to significant reductions in resources available for CJS agencies. Unfortunately, this has resulted in some police agencies reverting even further to reactionary styles of policing and criminal processing. They forgo the additional expenses for proactive, preventative approaches that pay large dividends in the long term, but often require significant investment in the short term.

Another factor that impairs CJSs from preventing violence is the varying cultural aspects correlated with violence globally. In every society, there are variations in the norms and narratives of violent behaviours that are considered acceptable. For example, it has been noted that violence is highly correlated with disenfranchised groups, especially low-income, minority youth (Wilson 1987). This acceptance of violence as a normal life-function has created a subculture of violence that directly contradicts the non-violent cultural norms of the rest of society (Anderson 1999). Traditional police responses are not well suited to address violence in communities with varying neighbourhood norms that encourage violent behaviour. As a result, traditional deterrence approaches are not effective for populations where interaction with the CJS is viewed as simply a cost of involvement in a criminal lifestyle that actually enhances individuals' street credibility and status (Kennedy 1997).

Other forms of cultural differences also limit the effectiveness of police and the CJS in reducing violence. As noted by Galtung (1990), there are three types of violence to consider: (i) direct violence, including acts of physical and verbal aggression; (ii) structural violence that exists when social powers prevent some members of society from obtaining their basic needs; and (iii) cultural violence that exists when aspects of individuals' cultures are used to legitimize forms of direct and structural violence. While police agencies and CJSs are specifically designed to respond to direct violence, they are inhibited from addressing structural and cultural violence by their very association with government entities. Structural violence is embedded within social structures and institutions, and stems from those in power infringing on the basic rights of others through racism, sexism, ethnocentrism, and classism. Cultural violence stems from aspects of human principles and beliefs, such as religion or political ideology. As a result, some violent acts are deemed acceptable by the government, citizens, or even CJS officials themselves. Changing cultural norms of violence is often beyond the intended scope and capabilities of the police and the CJS.

Other potential problems that increase the burden of violence on police and CJSs involve political and governmental concerns, including system sustainability and corruption. Both relate directly to governments' abilities to control crime. The sustainability of CJSs is particularly problematic for governments of developing nations, as they cannot easily cope with increasing crime levels, which often accompany development (Arthur and Marenin 1995; Harrendorf et al. 2010). Relative to developed countries, these governments typically spend much less on their CJS (Farrell and Clark 2004), and most of it is allocated primarily to police rather than prosecution, courts, and corrections (Shaw et al. 2000). Unfortunately, policing strategies are often ineffective in reducing crime (National Research Council 2004).

Forms of corruption also plague CJSs around the world, ranging from individual acts by criminal justice agents, to widespread corruption throughout entire governmental structures, which can foster violence. While corruption is incredibly difficult to measure, Transparency International's Corruption Perception Index indicates that almost 70 per cent of countries scored in the corrupt range (Transparency International 2012). Corruption reduces legitimacy of police and other criminal justice actors in the eyes of the public. When citizens perceive law enforcement officials as illegitimate, they are less likely to cooperate and comply with laws (Tyler 1990).

Finally, the lack of internal and external effective partnerships with CJSs intensifies the burden of violence on police and other CJS agencies. Internally, agencies within CJSs often work in silos and fail to communicate timely, useful information to help control violence. While technological advances in data collection and storage provide CJS agencies with the ability to collect and maintain vast amounts of data, the sharing of this information is constrained by both informal and formal barriers, including legal restrictions, political influences, and the inflexibility of many organizational structures and working cultures. For example, Gil-García et al. (2004) described four mechanisms that hinder CJS agencies from sharing information: (i) 'turf issues' and resistance to change; (ii) information technology and data incompatibility; (iii) organization diversity and multiple goals; and (iv) environmental and institutional complexity. As a result, CJSs are often inefficient at processing and sharing information regarding patterns of criminal activity and offenders that could be used for prevention efforts.

CJS agencies also routinely fail to establish effective partnerships with other governmental, business, non-profit, community, and academic entities. The lack of effective partnerships is only partially due to the inherent problems of working with CJS agencies. Given that CJSs are viewed by the public as the primary responders to violence, there is less emphasis and scrutiny placed on the response of other governmental agencies and social institutions to reduce violence. Since the development of 'modern' democratic policing and CJSs in the mid-1800s, many countries have relied on structured, organized approaches to handle violence, spearheaded by the formal enforcement arm of the government. More recently, the notion of violence as a public health issue has gained momentum (Mercy et al. 1993; Moore et al 1994). Specifically, the idea that violence is preventable through comprehensive and coordinated efforts with the public health sector has grown in popularity.

Reconceptualization of Violence as a Public Health Priority

For several decades, attempts have been made to redefine violence as a public health crisis rather than simply a criminal justice concern (Moore et al. 1994). In the 1980–1990s, public health officials noted the staggering health-related consequences and costs associated with criminal violence (Mercy et al. 1993). In addition, public health researchers and practitioners believed their analytical and operational approaches for controlling disease epidemics could also be applied to prevent criminal violence (Moore et al. 1994). It was suggested that applying epidemiological techniques commonly used in the public health field to identify specific risk factors that increase the likelihood of violence could complement the criminal justice focus on deterrence and control of violent offenders (Moore et al., 1994; World Health Organization [WHO] 2002).

The hallmark of the public health approach is that it is an interdisciplinary and evidence-driven approach emphasizing (i) thorough understanding of the problem; (ii) investigation of causes and potential solutions; (iii) developing prevention techniques; (iv) implementing the techniques across settings; and (v) evaluating the costs and benefits of various approaches (WHO 2002). The key feature that distinguishes the public health approach from the traditional legal approach (e.g. incarceration, and 'get tough' policies) is its emphasis on prevention. While not a panacea, such an approach provides a flexible means of addressing violence at multiple levels of aggregation (e.g. local, national, global). Two decades ago, Moore and his colleagues noted that:

> in all likelihood, society's main line of attack on criminal violence will continue to come from the nation's criminal justice agencies…their efforts can usefully be aided, however, by a partnership with those in public health. (1994, p. 171)

While the public health perspective of violence prevention continues to build momentum, we demonstrate that CJSs are now better positioned to assist in the fight against violence.

How Correlates of Violence Impact Prevention Efforts

Police and other criminal justice agents around the world are faced with a daunting task when trying to prevent violence, based in part on the organizational, political, and economical impediments previously noted. Yet the root causes of violence also make it extremely difficult for criminal justice agencies to systematically reduce violence. Many other societal ills are highly correlated with (and in some instances, causative of) violence. These other societal problems—poverty, illiteracy, disease, injury, child abuse, poor housing, low education, unemployment, etc.—are linked to violence, yet remain beyond the scope of most CJSs. For years, CJS officials have simply accepted the notion that because of these correlates of violence, the problem was too big to solve and therefore, violence was inevitable. Yet, one of the most helpful tools in violence prevention is social scientific evidence regarding the correlates of violence. Research findings from around the world have demonstrated consistently that violence is concentrated in a number of ways. Understanding and responding to these identified patterns can result in significant reductions in crime and violence (National Research Council 2004).

First, evidence suggests that violent crime is highly correlated with a number of additional health and social problems (WHO 2002), and these tend to cluster by individuals, groups, and geographic areas. The *World Report on Violence and Health* (2002) categorizes the causes of violence within a four-level ecological model: individual, relationship, community, and societal. Individual causes include biological and demographic factors that predispose people to violent behaviour. Relationship-based causes occur when one's family and/or friends are themselves violent, thus predisposing that person to violent behaviour. Community factors include violent contexts where relationships are rooted, including schools, workplaces, and neighbourhoods. Finally, societal factors that influence violence include cultural norms, government policies, and social inequality. Specific risk factors for violent offending and victimization can be identified within each category, and these risk factors tend to cluster (Sampson and Lauritsen 1994).

In addition, there is a large body of evidence that demonstrates violence is highly concentrated in time and space, and further that there is a high concentration of violence among particular individuals and groups, both as victims and offenders (Eck et al. 2005). The vast majority of violent incidents occur within a relatively small number of places; both quantitative and qualitative evidence suggests that violence is concentrated in these small 'hot spots' that tend to remain constant over time (Weisburd et al. 2004). Further, research has demonstrated that geographic violence hot spots range in size from as large as entire neighbourhoods to as small as individual places and single street segments (Eck et al. 2005).

Likewise, a small, highly-concentrated group of the overall population in any geographic area is often responsible for an overwhelming majority of the violence, while an equally small percentage of the population is disproportionately victimized (Farrell and Pease 1993). Often, violent offenders congregate in groups, gangs, or other forms of violent social networks. For example, a study of homicides in Cincinnati, OH, demonstrated that 74 per cent of the homicides in the city involved gang members as either victims or suspects even though gang members represented less than half of 1 per cent of the city's population (Engel et al. 2013). The evidence surrounding the repeat phenomena of violent victimization—repeat locations, repeat victims, repeat suspects—is quite clear. Research from around the world, including from the United States, Great Britain, Australia, and the Netherlands, has shown that most crime involves repeat victims with approximately 2 per cent of potential targets experiencing 50 per cent of all crimes (Grove and Farrell 2012). Greater understanding of these patterns can enhance opportunities for CJS officials to reduce violence through focused use of limited resources to maximize benefits.

These types of crime and violence concentrations are problems that can be addressed by police and CJSs. Identification of hot spots through data analyses allows CJS agencies to allocate resources to those places, people, and groups known to be associated with the majority of violence. Analyses of reported crimes, traffic stops, pedestrian stops, calls for service, and other official law enforcement contact with individuals or places can be used to systematically identify problem areas and problem people for more efficient allocation of resources. Further, tracking violence patterns using social network analysis and investigatory techniques using social media significantly adds to the amount of actionable information. If these data sources were combined with other official data from the CJS, health system, social services, schools, etc., strong prediction models could be developed and used for more effective prevention efforts.

Promising Approaches to Reduce Violence

In the last two decades, police agencies in the United States, United Kingdom, Australia, Canada, and elsewhere have begun the transition from using traditional reactive approaches to evidence-based and data-driven approaches. Some innovative policing approaches have demonstrated significant reductions in crime and violence. In the early 2000s, the National Research Council (NRC) in the United States convened the Committee to Review Research on Police Policy and Practices to review the available research regarding policing (NRC 2004). Early studies from the 1970s to the early 1980s demonstrated that the prevailing policing strategies of the time (e.g. random motorized patrol, rapid response to calls for service, foot patrols, police staffing levels, investigative work, etc.) did not significantly reduce crime. This led to an initial crisis in policing, followed by a period of tremendous change and innovation (NRC 2004).

The NRC (2004) categorized the predominant policing strategies from 1980 to 2000 using a fourfold typology classification scheme based on the diversity of approaches used by police agencies and the level of focus given to specific problems. The first dimension (diversity of approaches) refers to the content of the police strategies and tactics that are used, ranging from traditional approaches to more innovative approaches that 'expand the toolbox of policing'. The second dimension represents the level of focus or targeting activities of the police, ranging from focused on specific places or individuals, to more generalized approaches. Using these two criteria, the NRC classified policing strategies as (i) Standard Model (mostly law enforcement approaches with low level of focus); (ii) Community Policing (wide array of approaches with low level of focus); (iii) Problem-Oriented Policing (wide array of approaches with high level of focus); and (iv) Focused Policing (mostly law enforcement approaches with high level of focus). The Standard Model of policing was the operational norm for most democratic police agencies during the twentieth century. Police administrators attempted to solve crime problems reactively by using a limited number and type of potential responses, including quick response time and random patrolling. As these approaches proved to be ineffective at reducing crime, police administrators and scholars developed more innovative approaches (Figure 14.1).

The NRC reviewed the available evidence and concluded that these four categories of policing strategies varied dramatically in effectiveness (measured in terms of crime and violence reduction). They concluded that traditional policing strategies under the Standard Model demonstrated little or no evidence of effectiveness. Likewise, they reported that strategies under the Community Policing Model generated only weak to moderate evidence of effectiveness. In contrast, strategies classified as Problem Oriented Policing produced moderate to strong evidence of effectiveness. Finally, strategies characterized as Focused Policing ranged in levels of effectiveness from weak to strong based on the specific tactics used; more recent evidence demonstrates that focused policing strategies can have a significant crime prevention benefits (Braga and Weisburd 2012). The NRC recommended

the use and expansion of problem-oriented and focused policing strategies to reduce crime and violence. These police strategies may be further improved by including theoretical frameworks that attempt to explain crime problems and criminal behaviour, including routine activity theory, crime pattern theory, rational choice perspectives, and situational crime prevention.

Of the specific policing strategies and tactics reviewed, the most promising for violence reduction are hot spot policing and focused deterrence approaches. As previously described, hot spots can be readily identified through data analyses that identify patterns or trends across areas. Typically, once these geographic areas are identified, police officials used different tactics to saturate those areas with increased law enforcement efforts. The specific tactics used in these locations vary in their intensity, perceived equity, and effectiveness. In general, however, increased law enforcement focus in violence hot spots has demonstrated reductions in violence with little displacement (Braga 2001). An important consideration, however, is that some aggressive policing tactics concentrated in specific areas can lead to poor police-community relations and questions of police legitimacy (Rosenbaum 2006). Further, these approaches are resource intensive, and the reductions in crime and violence appear to be short term and/or are difficult to sustain.

Another promising approach to reduce violence includes focused deterrence strategies. First used in Boston, Massachusetts during the mid-1990s, this type of approach has proven successful in multiple cities (Braga and Weisburd 2012; Engel et al. 2013). These initiatives use a 'pulling levers' strategy to identify and directly communicate consequences for violence to at-risk gang members (Kennedy 1997). They are based on the presumption that a majority of violent offenses are committed by a small number of individuals who are often organized (to some degree) in groups or gangs. This strategy specifically narrows the focus of law enforcement to those at the highest risk to become either a victim or perpetrator of violence, adding legitimacy to the approach. The use of collective accountability is a central theme of many focused deterrence strategies, and is based on the presumption that individuals are at least loosely organized in groups (Kennedy 1997). Another underlying assumption is that while violent acts are often perpetrated by individuals, they are rooted in a group dynamic. It is believed that the majority of violence associated with gang members is based on respect issues related to the norms and narratives of the street (Anderson 1999; Kennedy 1997).

The effectiveness of these strategies is based on the presumption that group pressure and support, if handled properly, can be key mechanisms for reducing violence. To effectively reduce violence, consistent and sustained communication of the non-violence message to gang members by practitioners, social service providers, and community members is critical (Braga and Weisburd 2012). Deterrence theory suggests that individuals must clearly understand that the risks and benefits associated with their behaviours have changed in order to produce actual behavioural change (Nagin 1998). Additionally, it is expected that the group structure will play a role in both communicating the message regarding the changes in sanction risk, as well as establish new behavioural standards in the offender social network based on these changes. During face-to-face offender notification meetings, members of violent gangs are told that the violence must stop, that there will be group consequences if it does not, and that the community will

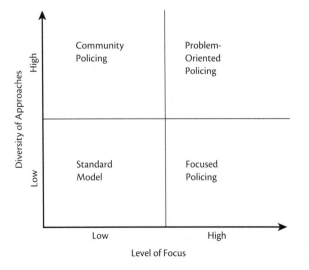

Fig. 14.1 Dimensions of police strategies.
Adapted with permission from National Research Council, *Fairness and Effectiveness in Policing: The Evidence*, National Academies Press, Washington, D.C., USA, Copyright © 2004.

support these consequences (Braga and Weisburd 2012; Engel et al. 2013). Violent gang members are also provided with streamlined social service assistance for all who want it. Versions of this type of focused policing strategy have demonstrated significant reductions in gang-related homicides ranging from 34-63 per cent (Braga and Weisburd 2012).

In addition to these focused policing strategies, renewed effort has been placed on risk identification and post-adjudication rehabilitation of individuals, particularly in the United States and Canada. Andrews and colleagues (1990) developed three principles of classification that are necessary for effective treatment of offenders: (i) risk; (ii) need; and (iii) responsivity. The risk principle requires that the amount and type of service an offender receives matches their risk of reoffending; those with the highest risk for recidivism should receive the highest levels of services. The need principle necessitates the focusing of treatment on specific criminogenic needs. Last, the responsivity principle dictates that specific cognitive-behavioural treatment be used in order to take full advantage of the intervention. These principles have led to a number of highly validated instruments that assess potential risk for offenders in order to successfully place them in rehabilitation programs. When an offender is properly classified and the appropriate rehabilitation program is successfully delivered, practitioners can generally expect a 10 per cent reduction in recidivism compared to no treatment being provided (Andrews and Bonta 2006).

Conclusion

While numerous violence reduction efforts have been implemented over the years, recent evidence suggests that law enforcement agencies can more effectively reduce violence when focused policing strategies are combined with robust, coordinated partnerships across multiple stakeholders including public health.

While police–community partnerships have been the focus of law enforcement agencies implementing community policing since the 1980s and the development of police–academic partnerships is growing (Engel and Henderson 2014), less attention has been given to sustained, comprehensive law enforcement partnerships with public health groups. Evidence suggests that previous criminal justice and public health partnerships have reduced traffic-related injuries resulting from driving under the influence of drugs or alcohol, and failure to use safety restraints (Dinh-Zarr et al. 2001; Shults et al. 2001). These criminal justice–public health collaborations, however, are often short-term responses to narrowly defined problems, rather than comprehensive sustained partnerships across systems. As criminal justice agencies around the world continue to develop community and academic partnerships, more emphasis should be placed on developing collaborations with the public health field as well.

Clearly, history has demonstrated that CJSs around the world are not equipped to handle the violence problem alone, and that now the importance of framing the problem of violence a public health priority is well recognized (WHO 2002). It is essential, however, that criminal justice agencies employ evidence-based strategies to become good partners for public health entities. CJSs are often reactive entities designed to process and punish offenders, with several inherent features that make handling violence especially difficult. Until very recently, CJS agencies lack the capacity and knowledge to effectively reduce crime and violence. Criminal justice practitioners, however, have made significant advancements in the last two decades toward evidence-based, comprehensive, and collaborative solutions to reduce violence. These promising approaches—including focused deterrence initiatives that partner law enforcement with academics, social service providers, medical professionals, and community members—should be our continued path forward.

References

Anderson, E. (1999). *Code of the Street: Decency, Violence, and the Moral Life of the Inner City*. New York: W. W. Norton and Company.

Andrews, D. A., and Bonta, J. (2006). *The Psychology of Criminal Conduct*. 5th ed. Newark: LexisNexis.

Andrews, D. A., Bonta, J., and Hoge, R. D. (1990). Classification for effective rehabilitation: rediscovering psychology. *Criminal Justice and Behavior, 17*, 19–52.

Arthur, J. A., and Marenin, O. (1995). Explaining crime in developing countries: the need for a case study approach. *Crime, Law, & Social Change, 23*, 191–214.

Braga, A. A. (2001). The effects of hot spots policing on crime. *Annals of the American Academy of Political and Social Science, 578*, 104–25.

Braga, A. A., and Weisburd, D. L. (2012). The effects of focused deterrence strategies on crime: a systematic review and meta-analysis of the empirical evidence. *Journal of Research in Crime and Delinquency, 49*, 323–58.

Dinh-Zarr, T. B., Sleet, D. A., and Shults, R. A. et al. (2001). Reviews of evidence regarding interventions to increase the use of safety belts. *American Journal of Preventative Medicine, 21*, 48–65.

Eck, J. E., Chainey, S, Cameron, J. G., Leitner, M., and Wilson, R. E. (2005). *Measuring Crime: Understanding Hot Spots*. Washington, D.C.: National Institute of Justice.

Engel, R. S., Tillyer, M. S., and Corsaro, N. (2013). Reducing gang violence using focused deterrence: evaluating the Cincinnati Initiative to Reduce Violence (CIRV). *Justice Quarterly, 30*, 403–39.

Engel, R. S., and Henderson, S. (2014). Beyond rhetoric: establishing academic-police partnerships that work. In: J. Brown (ed.), *The Future of Policing*. United Kingdom: Routledge, pp. 217–36.

Farrell, G., and Clark, K. (2004). *What Does the World Spend on Criminal Justice?* Helsinki: Helsinki European United Nations Institute for Crime Prevention and Control.

Farrell, G., and Pease, K. (1993). Once bitten, twice bitten: repeat victimization and its implications for crime prevention. Crime Prevention Unit Paper 46. London: Home Office.

Galtung, J. (1990). Cultural violence. *Journal of Peace Research, 27*, 291–305.

Gil-Garcia, J. R., Schneider, C. A., and Pardo, T. A. (2004). *Effective Strategies in Justice Information Integration: A Brief Current Practices Review*. Albany: Center for Technology in Government.

Grove, L., and Farrell, G. (2012). Once-bitten, twice shy: repeat victimization and its prevention. In: B. B. Welsh and D. P. Farrington (eds.), *The Oxford Handbook of Crime Prevention*. New York: Oxford Press, pp. 404–19.

Goldstein, H. (1990). *Problem-Oriented Policing*. New York: McGraw-Hill.

Harrendorf, S., Heiskanen, M., and Malby, S. (2010). *International Statistics on Crime and Justice*, Helsinki: Helsinki European United Nations Institute for Crime Prevention and Control.

Kennedy, D. M. (1997). Pulling levers: chronic offenders, high-crime settings, and a theory of prevention. *Valparaiso University Law Review, 31*, 449–84.

Mercy, J. A., Rosenberg, M. L., Powell, K. E., Broome, C. V., and Roper, W. L. (1993). Public health policy for preventing violence. *Health Affairs, 12*, 7–29.

Moore, M. H., Prothrow-Stith, D., Guyer, B., and Spivak, H. (1994). Violence and intentional injuries: criminal justice public health perspectives on an urgent national problem. In: A. J. Reiss, Jr. and J. A. Roth (eds.), *Understanding and Preventing Violence, Volume 4: Consequences and Control*. Washington, D.C.: National Academies Press, pp. 167–216.

Nagin, D. S. (1998). Criminal deterrence research at the outset of the twenty-first century. In: M. Tonry (ed.), *Crime and Justice: A Review of Research*. Chicago: University of Chicago Press, pp. 1–42.

National Research Council. (2004). *Fairness and Effectiveness in Policing: The Evidence*. Washington, D.C.: National Academies Press.

Rosenbaum, D. (2006). The limits of hot spots policing. In: D. Weisburd and A. Braga (eds.), *Police Innovation: Contrasting Perspectives*. New York: Cambridge University Press, pp. 245–66.

Sampson, R. J., and Lauritsen, J. L. (1994). Violent victimization and offending: individual-, situational-, and community-level risk factors'. In: A. J. Reiss, Jr. and J. A. Roth (eds), *Understanding and Preventing Violence, Volume 3, Social Influences*. Washington, D.C.: National Academies Press, pp. 1–114.

Shaw, M., van Dijk, J., and Rhomberg, W. (2000). Determining global trends in crime and justice: an overview of results from the United Nations surveys of crime trends and operations of criminal justice systems. *Forum on Crime and Society, 3*, 35–64.

Shults, R. A., Elder, R. W., and Sleet, D. A. et al. (2001). Reviews of evidence regarding interventions to reduce alcohol-impaired driving. *American Journal of Preventative Medicine, 21*, 66–88.

Transparency International. *Corruption Perceptions Index 2012*. Available at: http://cpi.transparency.org/cpi2012/ [Accessed 30 March 2013].

Tyler, T. R. (1990). *Why People Obey the Law*. New Haven: Yale University Press.

Weisburd, D., Bushway, S., Lum, C., and Yang, S. (2004). Trajectories of crime at places: a longitudinal study of street segments in the city of Seattle. *Criminology, 42*, 283–321.

Wilson, W. J. (1987). *The Truly Disadvantaged: The Inner City, the Underclass, and Public Policy*. Chicago: University of Chicago Press.

World Health Organization (2002). *World Report on Health and Violence*, Geneva: World Health Organization.

CHAPTER 15

The economic costs of violence

Phaedra Corso and Nathaniel H. Taylor

Introduction to the Economic Costs of Violence

As a leading cause of death and injury in many countries (Krug et al. 2002) violence has the potential to monetarily impact individuals, families, communities, and society as a whole (Patel and Taylor 2011). At the individual level, violence may result in treatment costs for medical and mental healthcare, losses in workplace productivity, and long-term decreases in educational and professional attainment. At the family level, violence may result in costs associated with the legal, judicial, and child welfare systems. Communities can be impacted by violence through decreases in social cohesion, economic development, and collective efficacy. Together, the economic impacts at the individual, family, and community levels are burdensome for the whole of society, particularly when considering the contribution of violence towards premature mortality and quality of life, both for the current and future generations of victims and perpetrators alike.

Estimating the Economic Costs of Violence

Estimates of the economic impact of violence have relevance for policymakers who want to highlight the burden of violence in a population, beyond impacts on morbidity and mortality, and to understand violence in the context of other health issues that may be impacting the population. Economic burden estimates also allow one to compare the costs of interventions, programmes, and policies targeting violence to the potential economic benefits of preventing the consequences of violence. An assessment of costs relative to potential benefits is referred to as benefit–cost analysis or return on investment (ROI) analysis (Haddix et al. 2003): a positive net benefit or ROI occurs when the benefits of a programme or policy outweigh the costs of a programme or policy. Thus a goal for estimating the economic costs of violence should be to determine the potential return on investment in prevention, for both the public and the private sectors.

As such, there are a number of studies that have systematically reviewed and summarized the economic costs of violence, either across or by typology. For example, the World Health Organization (WHO) published a report on the economic effects of interpersonal violence (defined as violence between family members and intimate partners, and violence between acquaintances and strangers), which included estimates of economic burden from 32 studies in 11 countries (Waters et al. 2004). In another publication, Waters et al. (2005) summarized the global economic costs of interpersonal violence, which ranged from US$67.9 million per year for homicides in New Zealand to US$84.1 billion per year for all forms of interpersonal violence in the United States (2003 USD). Other reviews of the costs of violence have been more narrowly defined. For example, Brown et al. (2011) summarized U.S. studies reporting both the short-term and long-term medical costs of child maltreatment and found that estimates ranged between $0 and $24,000 per episode with differences in research designs contributing to variability of estimates. In France, Nectoux et al. (2010) summarized the literature on the economic burden of intimate partner violence (IPV). The authors estimated the total cost of IPV in France at €2.5 billion.

In contrast to review papers, there are a number of studies that provide empirical evidence for the costs of violence, usually with a focus on a specific type of violence. For example, researchers in Ecuador used a number of primary data sources including a population-based survey on violence to estimate the medical and out-of-pocket health expenditures associated with intimate partner violence in the country (Roldos and Corso 2010). They found that the national costs were approximately US$182 million in 2004. In the United Kingdom, Dolan et al. (2005) estimated the total costs of non-partner sexual violence at £2.76 billion. Other researchers have focused on per person costs of violence, rather than national estimates. For example, Kruse et al. (2011) conducted a study in Denmark comparing total healthcare costs of women who were victims of violence to a reference population of non-victims. The authors used multivariate analyses to derive attributable costs from individually based register information for their estimates and found significantly higher costs in the affected population of approximately €1,800 per person annually. A similar study conducted in the United States also found significant increases in costs for a population of women experiencing physical intimate partner violence compared with those of never-abused women (Bonomi et al. 2009). The authors estimated annual healthcare costs, assembled over 7.4 years, associated with intimate partner violence by the timing of abuse (on-going, recent, and remote). They found increases in adjusted annual healthcare costs of 42 per cent for on-going violence versus no abuse, 24 per cent for recent violence (within the last 5 years), and 19 per cent for remote violence (more than 5 years past). Fishman et al. (2010) conducted a retrospective cohort analysis of a group of women exposed to intimate partner violence over a 10-year period following the end of exposure. They found that although the annual healthcare costs for the exposed group was higher than the non-exposed group, after 4 years the differences were no longer statistically significant.

For youth violence, several researchers in the United States (Cohen 1998; Cohen and Piquero 2009) have calculated lifetime costs of violence by estimating the costs saved by society for preventing juveniles from a life of crime, heavy drug use, and dropping out of high school. Recent research in the United Kingdom estimated the cost of crime perpetrated by males aged 10–50 years using longitudinal data from the Cambridge Study in Delinquent Development. The authors determined the annual cost of a male high-rate chronic offender to be an average of £18 per British citizen, with a lifetime cost of £742 per citizen (Piquero et al. 2013).

For child maltreatment, several authors have calculated the incremental increase in annual healthcare costs for adult survivors of abuse. Tang et al. (2006) conducted a study on the effects of child maltreatment on adult women's healthcare expenditures in Ontario, Canada. They found that the average annual healthcare cost for women with a history of childhood physical and sexual abuse was C$775 (1990 Canadian dollars), almost double that of women with no history of abuse. In the United States, Bonomi et al. (2008) reported that women who reported abuse as children had on average US$558 more in annual healthcare costs than women not reporting abuse as children. Other researchers have calculated the economic costs of child maltreatment by focusing less on the utilization of healthcare and more on the utilization of social services when the abuse of children occurs. For example, in the United States Conrad (2006) developed a model by which one could estimate actual costs of child maltreatment based on direct (associated costs of efforts to address child maltreatment and its negative outcomes), indirect (less tangible costs such as emotional suffering), and opportunity costs (costs of foregone choices) associated with each case. In Australia, the government reported spending $1.4 billion (2005 AUD) on child protection and out-of-home care services across the country in the 2005–2006 fiscal year (Productivity Commission 2007).

Comparison Difficulties in the Literature

Although these studies have contributed to our understanding of the economic impact of violence, it may not be possible to compare actual cost estimates from one study to the next, even if the violence typology and the underlying populations are the same. First, there are some basic study design elements that may be different, including how violence is defined. Lacking clear or consistent definitions of what constitutes violence and violent events makes determining both prevalence and incidence difficult, both of which are essential to assessing true costs. For example, in a study by Laing and Bobic (2002), the authors note that the definition of spousal abuse in the Australian literature ranged from physical and sexual abuse to emotional or psychological abuse. Additional definitional concerns occur when the underreporting of events obscures the true incidence and prevalence of violence in the community; and, second, when

cost estimations rely on medical records for accurate coding of causes of injury. Because universal screening for violence in medical settings is not widespread and there may be social stigmas associated with reporting violence, inaccuracies in reporting may occur.

Second, a common difference in economic burden estimates is whether costs are considered prevalence or incidence based. Costs that are incurred within a specified time period (typically a year), regardless of when the violent event occurred, are considered prevalence based. Costs that are considered over a longer period of time (typically lifetime) for violent events that occur within a defined time period (typically a year) are incidence-based estimates. Prevalence-based analyses are one approach for estimating economic burden and are often used by policymakers to determine how much of their total healthcare resources or per cent of gross domestic product are required (annually) to deal with the consequences of violence. For example, in the United States Finkelstein et al. (2004) estimated the costs of annual injury-attributable expenditures by analysing data on violence and injury prevalence and costs from the U.S. National Health Accounts. They determined that approximately 10 per cent of total U.S. medical expenditure in 2000 was attributable to intentional and unintentional injuries. In contrast, incidence-based analyses quantify the present value of current and future costs resulting from all consequences related to a violent episode that occurs during a particular time period. Incidence-based estimates are derived using another approach, and can provide cost per case data used to estimate the upper limit of potential resource savings due to prevention interventions. For example, Brand and Price (2000) conducted a study on the costs of crime in England and Wales in 1999. The authors used the British Crime Survey to create multipliers for each crime that tied the estimated total number of incidents to changes in the number of recorded offences from April 1999 to March 2000. The authors then applied these estimates to costs of individual crimes committed to determine average cost per incident. Finally, they were able to estimate the total cost of crime by multiplying the average cost by the estimated total number of crimes.

Next, studies that assess the economic costs of violence that are incidence based (present and future costs stemming from current violent events) may handle the valuation of future costs differently. For example, although studies may appropriately calculate the net present value of future costs of violence as recommended by published guidelines (Haddix et al. 2003), studies may differ in the discount rate used to make this calculation. Discounting is a technique used to adjust for differential timing in costs and benefits under the premise that immediate costs and benefits are valued higher than those that occur some time in the future. For example, while Corso et al. (2007) used a 3 per cent discount rate to convert future costs of injuries due to interpersonal and self-directed violence to present value, Palmer et al. (1995) used a 4 per cent discount rate to convert future costs of injuries due to self-directed violence—thus making these two studies incomparable.

Categories of Costs in Violence

But the main reason that most studies of the economic burden of violence are incomparable is because of the differences in the types of cost categories included. For violence defined as child maltreatment, youth violence (which includes bullying and gang violence), intimate partner violence, sexual violence, or elder abuse, the categories for which economic burden estimates could be generated are those delineated in Table 15.1, including the utilization of medical and mental healthcare; short-term work and household productivity losses; losses in educational or occupational attainment; legal and welfare system costs; costs to the non-profit sector; economic development and social cohesion costs; and costs associated with the impact that violence has on quality of life and premature mortality. These selected cost categories are representative of what one might

Table 15.1 Economic impacts of violence by type

	Child maltreatment (CM)	Youth violence (YV)[a]	Intimate partner violence (IPV)	Non-partner sexual violence (SV)	Elder abuse (EA)
Direct costs of violence					
Medical care utilization	X	X	X	X	
Mental healthcare utilization	X	X	X	X	X
Productivity losses in the workplace			X	X	
Productivity losses in school	X	X	X		
Household productivity losses			X	X	
Externalities of violence					
Losses in future educational/ occupational attainment	X	X			
Legal system costs	X	X	X	X	
Welfare system costs	X		X		
Costs to the non-profit sector			X	X	
Economic development/ tourism		X		X	
Social cohesion		X			
Effects on well-being					
Quality of life	X	X	X	X	X
mortality	X	X	X		
Pathways to violence					
Linkages to other forms of violence	IPV, YV, SV	CM, IPV, SV	CM	IPV	

[a]Includes bullying and gang violence.

find in the literature and are by no means definitive or exhaustive. For example, Chan and Cho (2010) conducted a review of studies presenting costs of domestic violence and they compare how costs are categorized, the cost components included in the analyses, and the ways to estimate costs in an integrated framework.

For each of these categories, costs can be considered both in terms of short-term (or immediate) and longer-term (or lifetime) or inter- or intra-generational impacts, depending on the type of analysis being conducted, prevalence or incidence-based, and the time frame over which costs are analysed for the latter approach. The inter- or intra-generational costs of violence occur when there is a trajectory of violence for the individual, within the family, or within the community, which is represented in Table 15.1 as the possible linkages of one cost of violence to another cost of violence. Further, who bears the burden of paying for each of these costs is also a relevant discussion when assessing economic burden. As framed at the beginning of this chapter, some costs are borne by the individual, and some are borne by the family. Some costs are borne by the victim and others by the perpetrator. The community bears many of these costs, and taken together, society as a whole is monetarily impacted by violence.

The first set of cost categories, utilization of medical care and productivity losses are standard types of costs included in the cost of illness (COI) approach for estimating economic burden (Cooper and Rice 1976; Rice 1994). COI analyses typically include some form of medical costs and productivity losses. Medical costs can include the costs of hospitalization, clinician visits, mental health counselling, diagnostic testing, prescription drugs, and other medical expenses. For some studies, a distinction is made between costs for medical care separately from costs for mental health services. Productivity losses include measuring the costs of resources forgone due to injury or illness, which are incurred while receiving or giving care. Productivity losses often include lost earnings due to missed work or the value of time spent performing non-wage activities such as caring for a victim of violence. Absenteeism, or absence from the workplace, has costs to both individuals and families (loss of income) as well as to community and society (loss of profit to businesses). Presenteeism, which is less easily defined or calculated for economic burden estimates, includes being present in the workplace but not working to full capacity. For example, Rothman and Corso (2008) found that a high propensity for abusiveness in a sample of men was positively associated with missing work and experiencing worse productivity on the job. Violence can impact other areas of productivity potential including schoolwork, housework, and leisure time. And finally, in the long term, violence has the potential to impact one's educational and occupational attainment. For example, Currie and Widom (2010) found that adults with documented histories of childhood abuse and/or neglect have lower levels of education, employment, earnings, and fewer assets as adults, compared to matched control children.

Additional Costs of Violence

Unlike the economic burden of other illnesses or injuries (like influenza, for example), violence may trigger the need for and cost of a whole host of other community-level resources as well. The legal system, in the form of law enforcement, legal representation, the courts, and incarceration services, is heavily impacted by violence and this represents a cost for the individuals involved and the taxpayers in the community. Likewise, when children are involved in violence, either as victims or witnesses of violence, there may be costs associated with child protective services and/ or the child welfare system. Victims of domestic violence may also be more likely to require other general welfare services, such as safe housing, relative to non-victims. The non-profit sector, at the local, national, and international levels, is also impacted and bears a cost of violence in the form of advocacy, education, training for providers, and delivery of services.

Finally, the effects of violence that are tangible in the community, like the destruction of property from gang violence or the fear of playing outside because of gunfire, have real impacts on social cohesion, community engagement, and ultimately on economic development and tourism. For example, Hilliard (2007) estimated that African countries lose an average of $18 billion (gross domestic product in constant year 2000 dollars) per year due to war and insurgencies, shrinking their economies by 15 per cent. Further, she found that between 1970 and 1997 countries in Africa lost a total of $25 billion in agricultural production due to armed violence. Violence in Africa has also had an impact on tourism. In the 5-year period leading up to 2005, South Africa lost 22 million visitors because of its reputation for violence (Cole 2005). A study of the cost of conflict in northern Uganda found that the country lost almost 14 per cent of its income from tourism due to armed conflicts (Dorsey and Opeitum 2002).

Impact of Violence on Quality of Life

Underlying all of these cost categories is the impact that violence has on quality of life, although this construct is difficult to measure and quantify. In economic burden assessments, quality of life is an important construct to measure because it can be used along with estimates of survival to calculate disability-adjusted life years, or DALYs (Murray and Lopez 1997). DALYs, developed in consultation with the World Health Organization, allow for international comparisons of the impact that illnesses and injuries have on population-level functional capacity and survival. In economic evaluations referred to as cost-effectiveness analyses or cost-utility analyses (Drummond et al. 2005; Gold et al. 1996), quality of life is also an important construct for developing a quality-adjusted life year, or QALY. The QALY is a health index, similar to that of the DALY, which combines health-related quality of life and life expectancy. When coupled with the costs of interventions/ policies/programs to prevent violence, less the costs of illness prevented, one can determine the cost per QALY (or DALY) saved comparing one intervention to another.

Another important component of the economic costs of violence is the impact of premature deaths on future productivity. Future productivity can be valued based on lifetime streams of potential future earnings, using the COI approach which uses wages as a proxy for productivity. For example, Fang et al. (2012) estimated that the future productivity loss for deaths resulting from child maltreatment in the United States was $2.19 billion in 2010 USD. Another approach is to calculate the value of a statistical life (VSL) lost from violence either through revealed or stated preferences of individuals in the community (Mitchell and Carson 1989). For example, when a sample of Ecuadorians were asked to state their willingness to pay for a mortality risk reduction associated with child maltreatment, their reported value for saving a child's life (or VSL) was ~$20 million (in 2012 USD) (Corso et al. 2013). Beyond future productivity losses for the victim experiencing premature mortality, it is also worthy to note that deaths resulting from violence may have impacts on family quality of life, and social cohesion and economic development as well, which are extremely important impacts of violence yet not easily quantified.

Challenges in Assessing the Costs of Violence

While the framework for elucidating the economic impact of violence laid out in Table 15.1 may be helpful, there are still many practical challenges in assessing the costs of violence. For incidence (or prevalence), there are challenges in consistent and accurate definitions of violence and reporting as mentioned previously. Establishing epidemiologic links to longer-term impacts of violence, such as sustained mental health problems for adult survivors of child maltreatment, is also a challenge. Further, to assess the full economic impact of violence across generations, these epidemiologic data are needed to model the developmental trajectory of violence within and across generations. For example, if it were possible to model the probability of future abuse by an intimate partner for those persons abused as children, then it would be possible to link these downstream costs of future violence to current episodes of violence. Finally, for incidence and prevalence, more information is needed on the attributable risk that violence has on other health outcomes, such as substance abuse, mental health disorders, and other chronic diseases. Once attributable risk is established, appropriate epidemiologic methods are needed to convert these risks to population-attributable fractions, as suggested by Brown et al. (2008) when discussing how to assess medical expenditures attributable to intimate partner violence.

There are also challenges in assessing the impact of violence on the unit cost side of the equation. For national estimation of the costs of violence, it is often the case that there are no available cost data for some of the cost categories outlined in Table 15.1, or the data are of poor quality. These challenges are particularly true for countries where national healthcare claims data or linkages between health and other social welfare systems are unavailable. And extrapolating unit costs from other countries may not be a viable alternative if it is the case that there are differences in healthcare systems, for assessing the medical costs of violence in particular. Further, it may not be appropriate to assume the same level of productivity losses from one setting to another, because productivity is based on the local economy (a farming economy versus an industrial economy, for example) and the local wage.

Recommendations for Future Research

Given these challenges in assessing the costs of violence, there is ample room for future research in this area to fill our gaps in knowledge to date. The following is a summary of four areas where future research on the costs of violence is needed: (i) determining the population attributable fraction of violence to other health conditions and assessing the economic impact of the attributed fraction; (ii) estimating the impact that violence has on the productivity of not just the victims of society, but on the perpetrators, family, and community; (iii) developing incidence-based models of the trajectory of violence outcomes and their costs, within and across generations; and (iv) quantifying the impact that violence has on quality of life. Until these challenges are met, our estimates of the costs of violence will only represent the tip of the iceberg in terms of the full economic impact on society.

References

Bonomi, A. E., Anderson, M. L., and Rivara, F. P. et al. (2008). Health care utilization and costs associated with childhood abuse. *Journal of General Internal Medicine*, 23, 294–9.

Bonomi, A. E., Anderson, M. L., Rivara, F. P., and Thompson, R. S. (2009). Health care utilization and costs associated with physical and nonphysical-only intimate partner violence. *Health Services Research*, 44, 1052–67.

Brand, S., and Price, R. (2000). *The Economic and Social Costs of Crime, Home Office Research Study, 217*. London: Home Office.

Brown, D. S., Fang, X. M., and Florence, C. S. (2011). Medical costs attributable to child maltreatment: a systematic review of short- and long-term effects. *American Journal of Preventive Medicine*, 41, 627–35.

Brown, D. S., Finkelstein, E. A., and Mercy, J. A. (2008). Methods for estimating medical expenditures attributable to intimate partner violence. *Journal of Interpersonal Violence*, 23, 1747–66.

Chan, K. L., and Cho, E. Y. N. (2010). A review of cost measures for the economic impact of domestic violence. *Trauma Violence & Abuse*, 11, 129–143.

Cohen, M. A. (1998). The monetary value of saving a high-risk youth. *Journal of Quantitative Criminology*, 14, 5–33.

Cohen, M. A., and Piquero, A. R. (2009). New evidence on the monetary value of saving a high risk youth. *Journal of Quantitative Criminology*, 25, 25–49.

Cole, B. (2005). *Crime Costs Tourism Millions*. Available at: http://www.iol.co.za/news/southafrica/crime-costs-tourism-millions-1.259784#.UZ2Ix5XstD8 [Accessed 22 February 2013].

Conrad, C. (2006). Measuring costs of child abuse and neglect: a mathematic model of specific cost estimations. *Journal of Health and Human Services Administration*, 29, 103–23.

Cooper, B. S., and Rice, D. P. (1976). Economic cost of illness revisited. *Social Security Bulletin*, 39, 21–36.

Corso, P. S., Ingels, J. B., and Roldos, M. I. (2013). A comparison of willingness to pay to prevent child maltreatment deaths in Ecuador and the United States. *International Journal of Environmental Research and Public Health*, 4, 1342–55.

Corso, P. S., Mercy, J. A., Simon, T. R., Finkelstein, E. A,. and Miller, T. R. (2007). Medical costs and productivity losses due to interpersonal and self-directed violence in the United States. *American Journal of Preventive Medicine*, 32, 474–82.

Currie, J., and Widom, C. S. (2010). Long-term consequences of child abuse and neglect on adult economic well-being. *Child Maltreatment*, 15, 111–20.

Dolan, P., Loomes, G., Peasgood, T., and Tsuchiya, A. (2005). Estimating the intangible victim costs of violent crime. *British Journal of Criminology*, 45, 958–76.

Dorsey, J., and Opeitum, S. (2002). The net economic cost of the conflict in the Acholiland sub region of Uganda. *Civil Society Organisations for Peace in Northern Uganda (CSOPNU) and Care USA*.

Drummond, M. R., Sculpher, M. J., Torrance, G. W., O'Brien, B. J., and Stoddart, G. L. (2005). *Methods for the Economic Evaluation of Health Care Programmes*. New York: Oxford University Press.

Fang, X. M., Brown, D. S., Florence, C. S., and Mercy, J. A. (2012). The economic burden of child maltreatment in the United States and implications for prevention. *Child Abuse & Neglect*, 36, 156–65.

Finkelstein, E. A., Fiebelkorn, I. A., Corso, P. S., and Binder, S. C. (2004). Medical expenditures attributable to injuries—United States, 2000. *Morbidity and Mortality Weekly Report*, 53, 1–4.

Fishman, P. A., Bonomi, A. E., Anderson, M. L., Reid, R. J., and Rivara, F. P. (2010). Changes in health care costs over time following the cessation of intimate partner violence. *Journal of General Internal Medicine*, 25, 920–5.

Gold, M. R., Siegel, J. E., Russell, L. B., and Weinstein, M. C. (1996). *Cost-effectiveness in Health and Medicine*. New York: Oxford University Press.

Haddix, A. C., Teutsch, S. M., and Corso, P. S. (2003). *Prevention Effectiveness: A Guide to Decision Analysis and Economic Evaluation*. New York: Oxford University Press.

Hilliard, D. (2007). *Africa's Missing Billions: International Arms Flows and the Cost of Conflict*. Oxford: The International Action Network on Small Arms and Oxfam International.

Krug, E. G., Mercy, J. A., Dahlberg, L. L., and Zwi, A. B. (2002). The world report on violence and health. *Lancet*, 360, 1083–8.

Kruse, M., Sorensen, J., Bronnum-Hansen, H., and Helweg-Larsen, K. (2011). The health care costs of violence against women. *Journal of Interpersonal Violence*, 26, 3494–508.

Laing, L., and Bobic, N. (2002). *Economic Costs of Domestic Violence*. Sydney: Partnerships Against Domestic Violence and the University of New South Wales.

Mitchell, R. C., and Carson, R. T. (1989). *Using Surveys to Value Public Goods: The Contingent Valuation Method*. Washington, D.C.: Hopkins University Press.

Murray, C. J. L., and Lopez, A. D. (1997). Global mortality, disability, and the contribution of risk factors: global burden of disease study. *Lancet*, 349, 1436–42.

Nectoux, M., Mugnier, C., Baffert, S., Albagly, M., and Thelot, B. (2010). An economic evaluation of intimate partner violence in France. *Sante Publique*, 22, 405–16.

Palmer, C. S., Revicki, D. A., Halpern, M. T., and Hatziandreu, E. J. (1995). The cost of suicide and suicide attempts in the United States. *Clinical Neuropharmacology*, 18, S25–S33.

Patel, D. M., and Taylor, R. M. (2011). *Social and Economic Costs of Violence: Workshop Summary*. Washington, D.C.: National Academies Press.

Piquero, A. R., Jennings, W. G., and Farrington, D. (2013). The monetary costs of crime to middle adulthood: findings from the Cambridge Study in Delinquent Development. *Journal of Research in Crime and Delinquency*, 50, 53–74.

Productivity Commission. (2007). *Report on Government Services* 2007. Melbourne: Steering Committee for the Review of Government Service Provision.

Rice, D. P. (1994). Cost-of-illness studies—fact or fiction. *Lancet*, 344, 1519–20.

Roldos, M. I., and Corso, P. S. (2010). The economic burden of intimate partner violence (IPV) in Ecuador: setting the agenda for future research and violence prevention policies.*Injury Prevention*, 16, A50.

Rothman, E. F., and Corso, P. S. (2008). Propensity for intimate partner abuse and workplace productivity—why employers should care. *Violence against Women*, 14, 1054–64.

Tang, B., Jamieson, E., Boyle, M., Libby, A., Gafni, A., and MacMillan, H. (2006). The influence of child abuse on the pattern of expenditures in women's adult health service utilization in Ontario, Canada. *Social Science & Medicine*, 63, 1711–9.

Waters, H. R., Hyder, A. A., Rajkotia, Y., Basu, S., and Buchart, A. (2005). The costs of interpersonal violence—an international review. *Health Policy*, 73, 303–15.

Waters, H. R., Hyder, A. A., Rajkotia, Y., Basu, S., Rehwinkel, J. A,. and Butchart, A. (2004). *The Economic Dimensions of Interpersonal Violence*. Geneva: World Health Organization Department of Injuries and Violence Prevention.

CHAPTER 16

Violence and the education system

Ross Deuchar and Denise Martin

Introduction to Violence and the Education System

Violence within the education system, and particularly in schools, has increasingly become regarded as a social problem around the world (Martin et al. 2011; Stephen 2011). Media reports allege that teachers are exposed to harassment and abuse on a daily basis and that extreme cases of violence are on the increase (Brown and Winterton 2010). Some suggest that teachers feel that they are facing growing difficulties in being able to exert their authority in class, and experience distress as a result (Blaya 2003; Martin et al. 2011). However, some research has reported that, while low-level disruption is increasing, serious incidents of physical violence in schools are actually rare (Brown and Winterton 2010; Munn et al. 2009).

Where violence does occur in the education system, the source of the problem is often viewed as being located with individual young people, families, and communities. However, in this chapter some of these views are challenged. By reviewing the existing literature and presenting the insights from empirical research in Scotland, this chapter seeks to present evidence-based illustrations of the way in which schools can inadvertently exacerbate the problems. It is argued that schools could do more to prevent the problem of youth violence from escalating, while also addressing the expectations associated with international legislation on children and young people's social rights.

International Perspectives on the Nature and Impact of School Violence

In many countries in the world, perceptions about violence in schools have been projected by the media (Osler and Starkey 2005). Indeed, it could be suggested that the wide interest in school violence over the past 20 years has emerged alongside a wider media-fuelled public concern about antisocial behaviour and juvenile delinquency (Brown and Munn 2008; Hayden and Martin 2011). However, there remains a high level of uncertainty about the extent to, and ways in, which violence impacts on the education system in a more general sense.

In the United States, it has been reported that administrative and senior management staff at 94 per cent of public middle and high schools have experienced one or more incidents of violent crime among students, while nearly one in ten students have been 'threatened or injured with a weapon on school property' (Hildenbrand et al. 2013, p. 408). In the 2009 national Youth Risk Behaviour Survey (YRBS) it was found that 32 per cent of high school students in the United States had engaged in a 'physical fight' during the last year, while 30 per cent admitted to having carried a weapon with them to school during the last 30 days prior to being surveyed (Maring and Koblinsky 2013). In the UK, there is no central register of violent incidents that occur in schools but a number of studies have attempted to explore the extent to which violence occurs (Martin et al. 2011). For instance, the National Association of Schoolmasters/Union of Women Teachers (NASUWT) surveyed a total of 1,007 teachers in England and Wales and identified that over a quarter viewed disruptive or violent pupils as a major concern in terms of the impact that they have on teaching and learning (cited in Martin et al. 2011). In Scotland, a survey by Munn and her colleagues (2009) identified some instances of serious violence in schools, but also that low-level incidents of indiscipline were more common. Indeed, in one survey of schools across the UK conducted by Brown and Winterton (2010, p. 8), it was found that 'extreme and serious incidents of violence, including violent assaults, are very rare in UK schools' but that teachers tend to report that low-level disruption, such as 'pupils being noisy in class' provide the biggest challenge to teaching and learning.

Concern about violence against teachers is not unique to the UK and countries such as the United States, Canada (Wilson et al. 2011) and Australia (Potts 2006) have also identified it as a growing concern. Research on violence against teachers has also been conducted across a number of other European countries (Smith 2003) including Luxembourg (Steffgen and Ewen 2007), Germany (Varbelow 2003 cited in Steffgen 2009) and France (Blaya 2003). In Luxembourg, a sizeable number of teachers have reported some form of verbal abuse and incidents of physical violence occurring in their classrooms, while similar levels of physical assault have been reported in Germany (Martin et al. 2011). Research conducted by Debarbieux (1996) in France has illustrated that the most common types of violent incidents are those involving student on student physical violence as opposed to violence against teachers.

Bullying can be defined as both physical and psychological act that can harm or injure an individual. According to a survey by the Youth Justice Board in 2009 in the UK (cited in Hayden 2009),

76% of children who had been victimized in school had experienced this form of abuse. Regardless of the extent and nature of violence, it is vital that researchers identify the causes of the behaviour where it does occur, as a first step towards preventing it from escalating further.

The Causes of Violence in Schools

In identifying the potential causes of violence within the education system, it has often been argued that disaffection from school can lead to active and aggressive resistance (Harber 2008). Further, Debarbieux (2003) has identified the impact of the 'school effect' on violence. He highlights the way in which schools in deprived communities are often the ones that experience the most violence, due to the wider issues of social exclusion and oppression that local families often experience. Indeed, Lindstrom (2001) presents evidence that schools in deprived urban areas are 'twice as likely to report violence than schools in privileged suburban areas' (cited in Martin et al. 2011, p. 135). Debarbieux (2003, p. 594) argues that 'any increase in inequality and social exclusion will lead to an increase in violence in schools and elsewhere'.

These findings are consistent with criminological theories that suggest that violence is a social product. According to Agnew (2006), social strains such as stressful life events, neighbourhood problems, goal blockage, challenging relationships with adults, or abusive peer relations can all conspire to bring about negative emotional reactions and attraction to violence and crime. In some cases, young people may experience a complex blend of social strains and, because of particular issues of emotional vulnerability, may interpret them as being so high in magnitude that they become compelled to cope with them through violence (Agnew 2006). Some studies have also shown that vulnerable young people may turn towards gang membership as a means of protection, social identity, and status (Deuchar 2009).

It has been argued, in both the literature and wider discourse on violence, that too much attention focuses on viewing the behaviour of young people as *the problem* (Brown and Munn 2008; Harber 2008; Stephen 2011). Indeed, in many parts of the world there is a growing tendency towards the criminalization of student misbehaviour (Harber 2008). Rather than stigmatizing young people further, it is important that we look towards identifying what it is that stimulates youth violence and ensuring that measures are put in place to prevent it. It has been argued that, where schools fail to provide a sense of social support and encouragement, violence may continue to dominate young lives (Twemlow and Sacco 2013). Harber (2008, p. 459) argues that schooling can be directly harmful to young people and can 'make society worse by perpetuating violence'. He draws attention to the prescriptive, rigid, and restrictive nature of many curricula, the competitive examination regimes and the authoritarian approaches to school discipline which often lead to disengagement among oppressed and marginalized young people and to increased violence (see also Osler and Starkey 2005). Indeed, evidence from England, Scotland, the United States, Greece, and Spain suggests that prescriptive national curricula restrict opportunities for active learning and democratic participation, demotivate pupils, and can ultimately lead to school exclusions (Harber 2008; Hayden 2011; Munn and Lloyd 2005; Osler 2010; Osler and Starkey 2010.

In drawing these perspectives together, it is useful to pay due regard to broader conceptualizations of 'school violence', beyond those commonly identified in the majority of research studies. Brown and Munn (2008, p. 227) refer to Bourdieu's concept of 'symbolic violence' in identifying the types of coercion that young people are often exposed to in schools without physical force. In particular, young people are often exposed to a curriculum that is 'culturally arbitrary and attuned to the social backgrounds of particular students', such as those from middle-class contexts, while disjunctive of the working class (Brown and Munn 2008, p. 227). The education system has an important moral obligation to ensure that the stimuli for violence are addressed and minimized, since failure to do so may lead disruptive young people to progress to wider forms of violence and crime beyond the immediate confines of schools.

Education's Role in Preventing Violence

Educational policy and practice must be underpinned by the principles within the UN Convention on the Rights of the Child (UNCRC). Articles 12 to 15 of the UNCRC affirm children's right to freedom of expression and to have their views and opinions given due weight within the learning context (Osler 2010). As a result, there has been an increased emphasis on the need for active, responsive learning and pupil consultation in education system of nation-states across the world (Deuchar and Ellis 2013). For instance, Denmark and other Scandinavian countries have a long history of encouraging pupils to have a voice in the planning of teaching and to have a direct influence on the running of schools (Scheerens 2011). In the Netherlands, Germany, Italy, Cyprus, and even emerging democratic states such as Guatamala, Nicaragua, and El Salvador, there has been an increased focus on pupil consultation and on informal approaches to learning (Baessa et al. 2002; Deuchar and Ellis 2013; McEvoy and Lundy 2007; Scheerens 2011).

However, in spite of the policy rhetoric on human rights and promoting the pupil voice, evidence suggests that many pupils are still subjected to education systems that are unresponsive to their opinions and values. Indeed, Osler and Starkey (2005, p. 211) argue that schools often remain as institutions that 'create failure, resentment and exclusion' and provide experiences that can reinforce violent attitudes. In light of these realities, Deuchar recently conducted a small qualitative study into the links between young people's experience of schooling, relationships with teachers, and their propensity towards violence.

Qualitative Research on Violence in Glasgow Schools

During 2011–2012, Deuchar implemented a small-scale study in three secondary schools in Glasgow, Scotland's largest city. Each of the schools was located within a community that all had a long history of social problems, including high levels of unemployment, widespread issues related to alcohol and drug abuse, and frequently reported issues of violence and crime.

Semi-structured interviews were conducted with 35 young people (aged 12–13 years and of mixed gender) who were selected because they had a history of engaging in disruptive behaviour within the schools and, in some cases, were known to be involved in, or on the periphery of, local territorial gang violence. Some also had a history of school exclusions (see also Deuchar and Ellis 2013). Interviews were also carried out with pastoral care and/or guidance teachers who worked closely with the young people.

The research sought to explore the relationship between the young people's perceptions of and experiences in their local communities and school, and their involvement in violence. On receipt of signed consent forms the pupil interviews were conducted in friendship pairs, wherever possible, as a means of putting young people at ease. Once transcribed, the interviews were analysed thematically to detect salient patterns (Strauss and Corbin 1990). In the sections that follow, the key insights from the small-scale research are outlined under specific themes, and key quotations emerging from interviews that were seen as being representative of participants' views highlighted.

Violence in the Community and Home

The majority of the young people who participated in interviews were regularly exposed to violence within their local communities:

> There's drug dealers where they're arguing about drugs and all that, and they they'll be all using knives and all that to fight. (Male pupil A)
>
> A boy goes to stab me and he's chased us a few times and he was waitin' for me after school a few times. (Male pupil B)
>
> The gangs, they have samurai swords, you see somebody run across wi' a samurai sword and you are like, 'what are you doin?' (Male pupil C)
>
> All the young team…everybody goes out and gets drunk and all that…people goin' out wi' hatchets and that, and samurai swords. (Male pupil D)

Teachers confirmed that the communities were characterized by territorial violence, and that several of the young people also experienced difficult home lives, which in some cases included exposure to domestic violence:

> In the summer months the motorway bridge is the big one—that's where you get a lot of fighting. (Teacher A)
>
> I think derelict spaces create the opportunity for young people to take part in the sort of 'toing and froing' of the gang fights…it's the sort of more dangerous level of chases and tag that goes on, there's a lot more threatening elements to it…from my own experience of them they are usually youngsters…with parents who have alcohol or drug issues of their own or stressful family situations that they're trying to deal with. (Teacher B)
>
> You look at the kind of issues in the family you can see they're dealing with, you know, quite a range of issues—there's a lot of domestic violence, there's quite a bit there, you know they've got that male who has in some cases subjected his partner to quite severe domestic violence. (Teacher C)

In many cases, the young people were either directly involved in territorial violence themselves, or were regularly on the periphery of violence out on the streets:

> I've been in hundreds of fights wi' like a couple of boys…'cos they say they're gonna stab me. (Male pupil E)

> I've got like a boyfriend that does gang fightin'…and if people call like my ma' a cow and that I just go up and smash them. (Female pupil A)
>
> It's sad that you've battered them but you are happy you did it. (Female pupil B)

Thus, it seemed that the young people experienced a complicated blend of social strains that stimulated their involvement in street violence (Agnew 2006). For instance, they all lived in economically deprived communities with low opportunities for accessing youth facilities or meaningful employment. They were clearly exposed to peer pressure that encouraged them to participate in recreational and territorial violence. And teachers indicated that they often suffered the traumatic experience of witnessing domestic violence, or experienced parental rejection due to alcohol or drug abuse. Many evidently learned about violence through a process of observation, behavioural rehearsal, and reinforcement (see also Deuchar 2013). They observed violence from a young age at home and out in the local neighbourhood, then rehearsed the use of violence out on the streets and subsequently were rewarded by achieving peer respect (Sprinkle 2006). In some cases, it seemed that they found the violence exhilarating and emotionally satisfying.

Experiences of Education, Relationships with Teachers, and Violence in Schools

Against this oppressive and violent local backdrop, one would hope that school might have provided the young people with a safe refuge and an opportunity for positive encouragement and support. However, in many cases it seemed that the very opposite was the case. The pupils often felt that the content of the curriculum was irrelevant to them, and preferred the limited opportunities that they had for active learning and pupil autonomy in subjects such as Physical Education and Technology. Many pupils felt that the ethos in school was too controlling and authoritarian in nature, that they were exposed to inflexible and inconsistent rules and felt frustrated about not having a voice (Deuchar and Ellis 2013; Harber 2008; Osler 2010):

> I talk sometimes in class—the slightest wee thing I get sent out. (Male pupil F)
>
> I don't like teachers who shout at you I don't like getting shouted at…when you try and reason wi' them, they try to bite the head off me. (Male pupil G)
>
> Sometimes the teachers, they give you a punishment exercise when you're just been turnin' around to ask somebody for a rubber and they think you've been talkin'. (Male pupil A)
>
> They don't let you go to the toilet…(and) if somebody else talks then they look at you and think you're talking…they don't give you a chance to say what you're sayin'. (Female pupil C)
>
> It's no' fair…like in maths, I was drinking a bottle of juice and then (the teacher) told me to put it away or else I'm going to get 'severely punished' and then I put it away and he started to drink his tea. (Female pupil D)
>
> If they just listened to us more and maybe considered some of the things we ask for. (Male pupil H)

Several of the young people in the sample described the way in which the authoritarian ethos they experienced in school, combined with the wider pressures on the young people's lives, led to intense feelings of anger and frustration:

> I asked for a rubber in class and the teacher didnae give me it so I hit my chair and…I was suspended…my ma' says I'm always angry. (Male pupil J)

I used to get angry n'that wi' the teachers...some of the teachers don't tell the truth n'all that and you're blamed for something you didnae dae. (Male pupil K)

Anger...normally I would call my teacher something. (Male pupil L)

In some cases, it seemed that the feelings of anger and frustration the young people felt led to them extending their violent activity out on the streets to inside the school buildings. While some attributed this directly to their negative relationships with teachers, it was also evident that some disturbing episodes of violence could occasionally emerge in classrooms:

Some of the teachers don't tell the truth and that and...you didnae do something but they think you done it and you get the blame...I get angry too easily and I take my anger out on the teachers...I hit (a teacher) with a chair...I was suspended for threatening behaviour. (Male pupil N)

I've tipped up a table and I've been violent to Miss X 'cos of what they say and stuff, and they blame me for something I never done. (Male pupil D)

I flung a chair and I got suspended. (Male pupil M)

I've been suspended because I battered (another pupil) in the changing rooms. (Female pupil A)

Accordingly, the young people interviewed mostly viewed school as an authoritarian, controlling institution with an ethos that undermined their sense of dignity and respect (reflecting earlier findings by Deuchar and Ellis 2013; Harber 2008; Osler 2010; Osler and Starkey 2010). Combined with the complex blend of social strains they were exposed to in their own homes and local communities, these young people's experiences of school led on to additional strains such as anger and frustration (Agnew 2006). Their feelings of angry frustration meant that they continued to experience alienated social bonds within school and became more vulnerable to participate in further violence within the school context (Agnew 2006). While this violence was sometimes directed at other pupils, it was also on occasions directed towards particular teachers whom the pupils resented. Some of the violent episodes that emerged clearly led to situations in class that could become potentially stressful for these teachers, as well as for other pupils.

Discussion

In a foreword to the study of the views of 15,000 pupils on schooling in the UK carried out in 2001, Becky Gardiner (2003, p. viiii) commented that young people in schools were often expected to 'fit into a structure and a curriculum that seemed to have been created without the first reference to what they might enjoy, or respond to...(and) were sick of not being listened to'. And in 2008, Clive Harber argued that the dominant model of schooling globally was 'authoritarian rather than democratic', focused on inculcating 'habits of obedience and conformity' which perpetuated violence, rather than preventing it (pp. 464–5). The evidence from the small-scale study in Glasgow reported previously corroborates some of these earlier findings.

This chapter began by making reference to the wide-ranging media reports that indicate that violence in schools is escalating, while also referring to the research reports that illustrate conflicting evidence about the nature and scale of violent incidents and how they impact on education. While some reports have suggested wide-ranging physical violence by pupils (Hildenbrand et al. 2013; Maring and Koblinsky 2013; Martin et al. 2011), others

have claimed that low-level disruptive behaviour is more common, while also drawing attention to symbolic violence (Brown and Munn 2008; Brown and Winterton 2010; Munn et al. 2009). It has been highlighted that, where violence occurs, some authors draw attention to the 'school effect' and the way in which social strains associated with neighbourhood problems, peer pressure, challenging adult and peer relationships, and social exclusion can lead to youth disorder (Agnew 2006; Debarbieux 2003). Most importantly, it is argued that schools can and must play a fundamental role in providing social support to those who are most vulnerable and oppressed, and ensure that the stimuli for violence are addressed and minimized.

One of the ways of achieving this could be the implementation of a democratic values model as promoted by the 'European Charter for the democratic citizenship'. This charter endorses the adoption of particular democratic rights, values and principles to reduce school violence. An evaluation of the charter's implementation in the UK (Holt et al 2011) found benefit when both staff and pupils invested in the principles of the charter and were positive about the change it could bring. However, issues in implementing such a programme remained including budget and staff training limitations.

In her evaluation of democratic initiatives in the United States, Bickmore (2008) found that the most effective programmes in reducing violence in schools were multi-faceted, sustained, educative and those that worked to facilitate both students' and teachers' social and cognitive competence. She also found that such programmes had the side-effect of contributing to students' academic engagement and learning (cited in Holt et al. 213).

There is an international focus on children's rights embedded within the UNCRC, and it is widely recognized that giving young people a voice and ensuring that they feel respected, supported, and included can minimize disaffection and violence. In spite of this, the data reported in this chapter indicates that some secondary schools in deprived communities may still create resentment, exclusion, and disaffection among youth (Osler and Starkey 2005).

It is unclear whether school teachers in the twenty-first century are exposed to more violence than they have been in the past. Where it occurs, every support needs to be given to teachers to deal with and manage these challenging situations. But, at the same time, a public health approach to violence suggests that treating young people with dignity and respect and avoiding humiliation may serve to prevent violence from emerging (Perry 2009). Accordingly, schools may need to change and become more flexible and responsive to the needs of young people in the modern world, thus ensuring that they are treated as full citizens with their rights upheld. In doing so, perhaps schools can move to a point where they avoid perpetuating violence and threatening the safety of those they are there to protect (Harber 2008). Previous research in Scotland has illustrated that educational programmes characterized by strong partnerships between teachers and local community youth workers can be highly effective in enabling young people to experience social support and empowerment, and can be conducive to helping them to manage the social pressures around them more effectively (Coburn and Wallace 2011; Deuchar and Ellis 2013). But these border-crossing partnerships need to become more commonplace in schools (Coburn and Wallace 2011).

The issue of violence in schools is one that will continue to stimulate discussion and debate among teachers, policy-makers and researchers over the years to come. We hope that this chapter may provide a valuable addition to that discussion and debate.

Acknowledgements

Special thanks go to the teachers and pupils from the three Glasgow schools for giving up their time to participate in the research study reported on within this chapter.

References

Agnew, R. (2006). *Pressurised into Crime: An Overview of General Strain Theory.* Los Angeles: Roxbury.

Baessa, Y., Chesterfiled, R., and Ramos, T. (2002). Active learning and democratic behavior in Guatemalan rural primary schools. *Compare: A Journal of Comparative and International Education,* 32, 205–18.

Blaya, C. (2003). School violence and the professional socialization of teachers: the lessons of comparatism. *Journal of Educational Administration,* 41, 650–68.

Brown, J., and Munn, P. (2008). 'School violence' as a social problem: charting the rise of the problem and the emerging specialist field. *International Studies in Sociology of Education,* 18, 219–30.

Brown, J., and Winterton, M. (2010). *Violence in UK Schools: What is Really Happening?* Cheshire: British Educational Research Association (BERA).

Coburn, A., and Wallace, D. (2011). *Youth Work in Communities and Schools.* Edinburgh: Dunedin.

Debarbieux, E. (1996). La Violence en Milieu Scolaire—1- Etat des Lieux. Paris: ESF.

Debarbieux, E. (2003). School violence and globalization. *Journal of Educational Administration,* 41, 582–602.

Deuchar, R. (2009). *Gangs, Marginalised Youth and Social Capital.* Stoke on Trent: Trentham Books.

Deuchar, R. (2013). *Policing Youth Violence: Transatlantic Connections.* London: Trentham/IOE Press.

Deuchar, R., and Ellis, J. (2013) 'It's helped me with my anger and I'm realising where I go in life': The impact of a Scottish youth work/schools intervention on young people's responses to social strain and engagement with anti-social behaviour and gang culture. *Research in Post-Compulsory Education—Special Issue: Reclaiming the Disengaged?,* 18, 98–114.

Gardiner, B. (2003). Foreword. In: C. Burke and I. Grosvenor (eds), *The School I'd Like: Children and Young People's Reflections on an Education for the 21st Century.* London: Routledge Falmer, pp. viiii–x.

Harber, C. (2008). Perpetuating disaffection: schooling as an international problem. *Educational Studies,* 34, 457–67.

Hayden, C. (2009). Deviance and violence in schools a review of the literature. *International Journal of School Violence,* 9, 8–35.

Hayden, C. (2011). Schools and social control. In: C. Hayden and D. Martin (eds), *Crime, Anti-Social Behaviour and Schools.* Hampshire: Palgrave MacMillan, pp. 35–55.

Hayden, C. and Martin, D. (eds) (2011). *Crime, Anti-Social Behaviour and Schools.* Hampshire: Palgrave MacMillan.

Hildenbrand, A. K., Daly, B. P., Nicholls, E., Brooks-Holliday, S., and Kloss, J. D. (2013). Increased risk for school violence-related behaviors among adolescents with insufficient sleep. *Journal of School Health,* 83, 408–14.

Holt, A. Martin, D., Hayden, C., and McNee, C. (2011) Schooled in Democracy? Promoting democratic values as a whole-school approach to violence prevention. *Crime Prevention and Community Safety* 13, 205–17.

Lindstrom, P. (2001). School violence: a multi-level perspective. *International Review of Victimology,* 82, 141–58.

Maring, E. F., and Koblinsky, S. A. (2013). Teachers' challenges, strategies, and support needs in schools affected by community violence: a qualitative study. *Journal of School Health,* 83, 379–88.

Martin, D., McKenzie, N., and Healy, J. (2011). Teachers' experience of violence in secondary schools. In: C. Hayden and D. Martin (eds), *Crime, Anti-Social Behaviour and Schools.* Hampshire: Palgrave MacMillan, pp. 119–40.

McEvoy, L., and Lundy, L. (2007). E-consultation with pupils: a rights-based approach to the integration of citizenship education and ICT. *Technology, Pedagogy and Education,* 16, 305–19.

Munn, P., and G. Lloyd. (2005). Exclusion and excluded pupils. *British Educational Research Journal,* 31, 205–21.

Munn, P., Sharp, S., and Lloyd, G. et al. (2009). *Behaviour in Scottish Schools 2009.* Edinburgh: Scottish Government Social Research. Available at: http://www.scotland.gov.uk/Publications/2009/11/20101438/0 [accessed 18 June 2013].

Osler, A., and Starkey, H. (2005). Violence in schools and representations of young people: a critique of government policies in France and England. *Oxford Review of Education,* 31, 195–215.

Osler, A (2010). *Students' Perspectives on Schooling.* Berkshire: Open University Press.

Osler, A., and Starkey, H. (2010). *Teachers, Human Rights and Education.* Stoke on Trent: Trentham.

Perry, I. (2009). Violence: a public health perspective. *Global Crime,* 10, 368–95.

Potts, A. (2006). Schools as dangerous places. *Educational Studies* 32(3): 319–30.

Scheerens, J. (2011). Indicators on informal learning for active citizenship at school. *Educational Assessment, Evaluation and Accountability,* 23, 201–22.

Smith, P. K. (2003). *Violence in Schools: The Responses in Europe.* London: Routledge.

Sprinkle, J. E. (2006) Domestic violence, gun ownership, and parental educational attainment: how do they affect the aggressive beliefs and behaviors of children? *Child and Adolescent Social Work Journal,* 24(2), 133–51.

Steffgen, G. (2009). Deviant behaviour and violence in Luxembourg Schools. *International Journal of Violence in Schools,* 10, 54–70.

Steffgen, G., and Ewen, N. (2007). Teachers as victims of school violence: The influence of strain and school culture. *International Journal on Violence and School* 3(April): 81–93.

Stephen, D. E. (2011) The problem with boys? Critical reflections on schools, inequalities and anti-social behavior. In: C. Hayden and D. Martin (eds), *Crime, Anti-Social Behaviour and Schools.* Hampshire: Palgrave MacMillan, pp. 56–72.

Strauss, A., and Corbin, J. M. (1990). *Basics of Qualitative Research: Grounded Theory Procedures and Techniques.* London: Sage Publications.

Twemlow, S. W,. and Sacco, F. C. (2013). Bullying is everywhere: ten universal truths about bullying as a social process in schools and communities. *Psychoanalytic Inquiry,* 33, 73–89.

Varbelow, D. (2003) Lehrer als Opfer von Schülergewalt. Eine quantitative Studie. Marburg: Tectum.

Wilson, C. M., Douglas, K. S., and Lyon, D.R. (2011). Violence against teachers: Prevalence and consequences. *Journal of Interpersonal Violence* 26(12): 2353–71.

SECTION 4

Evidence-informed programmes to reduce violence

CHAPTER 17

What is evidence in violence prevention?

Damien J. Williams, Anna J. Gavine, Catherine L. Ward, and Peter D. Donnelly

Introduction to Evidence in Violence Prevention

'Violence can be prevented. This is not an article of faith, but a statement based on evidence' (Dahlberg and Krug 2002, p. 3).

The assertion by Dahlberg and Krug is one of the key messages of the *World Report on Violence and Health*: that a public health approach can prevent violence. However, the evidence for violence prevention is limited and more evidence is needed to identify interventions that are both the most strategic *and* the most effective (Rutherford et al. 2007). This begs the question: *What is 'evidence' in violence prevention?*

Sources of Evidence in Violence Prevention

The definition of violence offered by the World Health Organization (WHO; see Dahlberg and Krug 2002) is considered one of the broadest in the field and includes actual *and* threatened actions, and a range of outcomes including physical and psychological harm, maldevelopment, and deprivation. Consistent with this broad definition, WHO recommended that different types of data be used to appreciate the full impact of violence and to evaluate interventions, including: mortality, morbidity, and other health data; self-report data; and community, crime, economic, and policy/legislative data (Dahlberg and Krug 2002). This list was not meant to be exhaustive (e.g. bullying data will be available from education; deprivation may come from social services) but clearly demonstrates that, in line with the multi-disciplinary nature of the public health approach, evidence in violence prevention will necessarily come from a wide range of sources in order to develop a detailed understanding.

What is Evidence?

The two main approaches to evidence generation are based in the quantitative and qualitative paradigms, each of which is associated with particular philosophical, ontological, and epistemological positions. Historically, the quantitative paradigm was underpinned by positivism which philosophically views all phenomena as being reducible to numerical indicators that represent 'the truth'; ontologically, it assumes only 'one truth, an objective reality that exists independent of human perception', and that

'[e]pistemologically the investigator and investigated are independent' (Sale et al. 2002, p. 44). Qualitative research, by contrast, is grounded in the constructivist paradigm, which views reality as being socially constructed; ontologically it assumes 'multiple realities or multiple truths'; and epistemologically that 'there is no external referent by which to compare claims of truth', viewing the creation of truth as the result of the interaction between investigator and investigated (Sale et al. 2002, p. 45).

In addition, one should recognize that a variety of research methods may be needed in the generation of evidence, requiring a more pragmatic approach (Johnson and Onwuegbuzie 2004). A mixed-methods approach, which is underpinned by pragmatism, values both quantitative and qualitative paradigms and considers the practical consequences of actions in terms of 'what works' (Sanderson 2009). The basic tenet of the mixed methods paradigm is to 'choose the combination or mixture of methods and procedures that works best for answering your research questions' (Johnson and Onwuegbuzie 2004, p. 17).

Evaluation in violence prevention

The best way to understand a problem is to attempt to solve it (Rittel and Weber 1973). Thus, intervention *and* evaluation are critical to understanding and preventing violence. The term 'evaluation' is often used as short-hand for 'outcome evaluation', which is typically associated with the quantitative paradigm and explores the effectiveness of an intervention through its impact on a pre-defined outcome measure (Stoto and Cosler 2008). However, Pawson and Tilley (1997) indicate that the preoccupation with 'what works' (associated with outcome) at the expense of 'how it works' (associated with process) is a significant limitation of much evaluation work. Process evaluation is typically associated with the qualitative paradigm and affords an understanding of the setting of the intervention, an exploration of the implementation, and can aid interpretation of results (Oakley et al. 2006). It can also offer important insights into why an intervention may have been found to be ineffective (Rychetnik et al. 2002). Thus, it is necessary to gather evidence regarding both outcome(s) and process(es) (Oakley et al. 2006) in order to fully evaluate a violence prevention intervention.

The quality of evidence in public health has typically been judged according to the hierarchy of evidence (Rychetnik et al. 2002), which considers the internal validity of the study design from which it was produced. Consequently, quantitative approaches, particularly experimental methods (i.e. randomized controlled trials, RCTs) are traditionally considered to constitute the strongest type of evidence, while qualitative methods are considered the weakest. However, systematic reviews of RCTs have now been placed at the top of the hierarchy as they further reduce the potential for bias (Rychetnik et al. 2002).

Because evaluation in public health generally, and violence prevention specifically, tends to draw on the quantitative paradigm, this approach will be discussed first, followed by a discussion of qualitative and mixed methods approaches, before moving on to consider evidence synthesis.

Quantitative Paradigm: Outcome Evaluation

A number of quantitative methods are used in outcome evaluation, the most rigorous of which is the RCT as it is associated with the greatest internal validity and lowest risk of bias (Oakley et al. 2006). In RCTs, participants are randomly allocated to either an intervention or comparator condition. Many violence prevention programmes are amenable to RCTs, such as parenting interventions (see Chapter 18 of this volume) or therapeutic interventions for high-risk youth (see Chapter 22 of this volume). However, RCTs are not always possible or appropriate due to feasibility and ethical issues around randomization (i.e. where there are too few people to make randomization meaningful, or where withholding a programme would cause harm). There are a number of viable quantitative alternatives to the RCT, some of which will be described.

Randomized Designs

* *Cluster-randomized trials* are appropriate when randomization at the individual level is not practical, but groups of individuals can be randomized to intervention or comparator conditions (Cochrane Effective Practice and Organisation of Care Group [CEPOCG] 2013). It is particularly useful to evaluate violence prevention interventions implemented in settings where individual randomization could result in contamination of the comparator group (e.g. schools and communities; see Chapter 21 of this volume).

* *Quasi-randomized trials* allocate individuals to either intervention or comparator groups but utilize methods that are not truly random (e.g. date of birth) thereby increasing the risk of selection bias (Reeves et al. 2011).

Quasi-Experimental Designs

Random assignment may not be feasible (or ethical) in all contexts, thus a variety of quasi-experimental approaches are considered appropriate to overcome this issue (Stoto and Cosler 2008).

* *Interrupted time series* (ITS) overcomes instances when it is not possible to include a comparator group. This design can be utilized if outcomes are measured at multiple time points before and after the intervention, with the effect being measured against the pre-intervention trend (CEPOCG 2013). This design is often used to study the effects of policy (i.e. firearm control policy; see Chapter 40 of this volume).

* *Controlled before-and-after studies* are used when allocation to intervention or control groups is not determined by the researchers. Observations are made pre- and post-intervention in both groups (CEPOCG 2013; see Chapter 20 of this volume for an example).

Economic Analysis

Evaluation of the impact of interventions tends to focus on effectiveness but as Maynard (2012, p. 12) notes: 'what is effective may not be cost-effective but what is cost-effective is always effective'. Economic evaluation is defined as a 'comparative analysis of alternative courses of action in terms of both their costs and consequences' (Drummond et al. 2005, p. 9). There are three methods of economic evaluation that can be undertaken alongside an experimental/quasi-experimental study or through decision analysis (see Drummond et al. 2005). Each will be briefly described in turn.

* *Cost–benefit analysis* (CBA) is rooted in welfare economics theory and considered the 'gold standard'. This method expresses both the inputs (costs) and outcomes (positive and negative) in monetary terms, and provides a measure of net benefit (the difference between inputs and outputs). A further benefit of CBA is that it allows comparison across studies also using CBA.

* *Cost-effectiveness analysis* (CEA) is perhaps the most widely used method, not least because of the difficulty in expressing outputs in monetary terms for CBA. This method expresses inputs in monetary terms, and outcomes in natural (non-monetary) values (e.g. number of injuries). This results in an incremental cost-effectiveness ratio that represents the change in cost for each unit change in outcome. The limitation of CEA is that it can only be compared with other evaluations that have used the same outcome measure.

* *Cost-utility analysis* (CUA) is a form of CEA except the outcomes are measured using a utility value (i.e. quality adjusted life years or QALYs) that is captured through measures of quality of life. Not only does this approach therefore account for the wider impact on health and well-being, it enables comparison with other evaluations that have used QALYs as the outcome. Moreover, it is the approach most commonly recommended in the health sector.

Owing to the potentially high costs of violence prevention interventions and the increasing requirement to consider economic implications in decision-making, economic evaluations are an important source of evidence in violence prevention (Dahlberg and Krug 2002).

The Quality of Quantitative Evidence

There are several sets of assessment criteria that draw on the hierarchy of evidence to judge the quality of evidence in violence prevention. For instance, the 'continuum of evidence' developed by the U.S. Centers for Disease Control and Prevention offers criteria which account for effect, programme and evaluation replication, external validity, and implementation guidance, and which rank interventions 'well supported' to 'unsupported/harmful' (Puddy and Wilkins 2011). Implicit in the use of the continuum is that only true experimental designs (i.e. RCTs) can ever be classified as 'well-supported'.

Using a similar approach, the Blueprints for Violence Prevention programme (Mihalic et al. 2001) outlines a rigorous review process and strict set of criteria by which to identify 'model programmes' and 'promising programmes'. The minimum criterion for certification as 'promising' is: "evidence of deterrent effect using a strong research design" (p. 2), particularly RCTs. Taxman and Belenko (2012) report that of the 900 programmes initially reviewed, only 11 were certified as model programmes, while 19 were certified as promising programmes.

Critique of the Quantitative Paradigm

As useful and important as this categorization of quantitative evidence is, it has several limitations relating both to the nature of many violence-related problems, and the paradigm on which the hierarchy of evidence is based.

First, violence is a multi-faceted problem that results from the complex interaction of factors at multiple levels of influence (individual, relationship, community, and societal), and interventions that operate at different levels simultaneously may not be amenable to relatively simple quantitative methods, such as the RCT (e.g. community-based interventions; see Chapter 34 of this volume). Smith and Petticrew (2010) describe the evaluation paradox whereby complex, 'macro-level' interventions are evaluated using techniques developed for 'micro-level' interventions. It has been suggested that one way to evaluate complex interventions is to operationalize them as a series of components (Rychetnik 2010). The main criticism of this kind of approach is that 'knowledge of the constituents is not knowledge of the whole or major parts' (Bettis and Prahalad 1995, pp. 10–1). This is particularly pertinent in the case of complex interventions where components often work synergistically (Schorr and Farrow 2011). Thus, the quality of any evaluation of a complex intervention depends on the careful synthesis of evidence across the various components (Rychetnik 2010). It is acknowledged that this is a developing area of evaluation science, and it is clear that as our understanding of how to evaluate complex interventions evolves, so will our understanding of the appropriate standards of evidence.

Secondly, the traditional hierarchy of evidence has received considerable criticism when applied to public health (Rychetnik et al. 2002) as it fails to account for external validity or generalizability and the different uses of evidence. Thirdly, many, even those who advocate the use of quantitative methods, disagree with the notion that such research is value- and theory-free, and adopt a post-positivist paradigm. This acknowledges that both the values of the investigator and the theory/hypotheses under investigation may influence the nature and outcomes of research (Teddlie and Tashakkori 2009), an issue that is inherently accepted within the qualitative paradigm.

One possible approach to overcome these limitations is to focus on the question being asked, rather than a preoccupation with the selection of the 'best' design (Johnson and Onwuegbuzie 2004). This implies that each design is suitable for certain questions under certain circumstances, and that the 'appropriateness of evidence' depends on the question being asked (Whitehead et al. 2004). Indeed, Gray (2009) recommends a typology of evidence

based on the relative contribution of different methods to evaluate different questions. The issue of importance here is that the evidence needs to be appropriately scrutinized (Rycroft-Malone et al. 2004) and judged on its own merits. Judging the quality of study designs requires transparent and detailed reporting, for which a number of guidelines exist (see www.equator-network.org).

Qualitative Paradigm: Process Evaluation

Quantitative methods are often also criticized for failing to capture the complexity of interventions (Oakley et al. 2006). Indeed, there is a call for the inclusion of qualitative components in evaluation strategies, to inform process evaluation. A number of traditional qualitative methods exist, and their selection depends on the perspective required in the evaluation.

◆ *Interviews* are typically undertaken one-to-one, and can be structured (specific questions to answer), semi-structured (following an 'agenda', but some degree of flexibility to pursue relevant topics) or unstructured/in-depth (driven by a theme, but no direct questioning). Participants generate an account in the context of the interview, which may lack naturalness.

◆ *Focus group discussions* are not simply group interviews but offer the additional benefit of concurrently exploring group dynamics as they are played out in the discussion. As focus group discussions capture real-world social processes, the output is believed to be more natural.

◆ *Observation* or ethnography is believed to generate the most natural account of behaviour. The observer can adopt a variety of roles ranging from covert to overt, which can have implications for the type of account generated.

While qualitative methods are typically a staple method for process evaluation (Oakley et al. 2006) both qualitative and quantitative data can be utilized in such evaluations. For example, the Blueprints for Violence Prevention programme employed a multi-method approach to identify strengths and weaknesses of interventions and the various sub-components (Mihalic and Irwin 2003). Thus, the depth of understanding achieved through the qualitative method(s) is complemented by the breadth of understanding achieved through the quantitative method(s).

Mixed Methods

In light of the limitations of quantitative and qualitative methods alone, the mixed methods approach seeks to integrate 'quantitative and qualitative research techniques, methods, approaches, concepts or language into a single study' (Johnson and Onwuegbuzie 2004, p. 7). Indeed, mixed methods approaches are commonly used in evaluations of complex interventions (e.g. Adamson 2005), for which a number of designs have been proposed. Creswell et al. (2003) describe a typology comprising six mixed methods designs:

◆ *Sequential explanatory designs:* quantitative data is prioritized and collected first with qualitative data being integrated to enhance interpretation.

◆ *Sequential exploratory designs:* qualitative data is prioritized and collected first with quantitative data being integrated to enhance interpretation. Particularly useful for testing emerging theories.

♦ *Sequential transformative designs:* quantitative or qualitative data is prioritized and collected first, but the perspective is made explicit. Enables an understanding of alternative perspectives.

♦ *Concurrent triangulation designs:* quantitative and qualitative data given equal priority and collected concurrently. Data are analysed separately and then integrated to corroborate results.

♦ *Concurrent nested designs:* priority given to either qualitative or quantitative data although data is collected concurrently and integrated during analysis. Enables the study of different groups within a single study.

♦ *Concurrent transformative designs:* priory given to the data that best answer the research question, but the perspective is made explicit. Data are collected concurrently and analysed separately before being integrated. Enables an understanding of alternative perspectives.

Realistic Evaluation

Pawson and Tilley (1997, p. 161) argue that it is necessary to go beyond the traditional concept of effectiveness and ask 'what works for whom in what circumstances?' Realistic evaluation is an example of the application of a mixed methods approach, which aims to evaluate programmes as theories through an exploration of the mechanism of the programme (i.e. how the programme results in any effects), context of the programme (i.e. social, biological, and economic conditions), and outcome patterns (i.e. intended and unintended consequences of the programme; Pawson and Tilley 1997). This information is then used to develop context–mechanism–outcome pattern configurations, which are models indicating how programmes activate mechanisms in certain populations, under certain circumstances, to result in behaviour change. The ability of realistic evaluations to consider context, mechanism, and outcome has been identified as a particular strength (van der Knaap et al. 2008).

The multiple approaches to, and applications of, mixed methods allow researchers to select approaches that address their research question(s) (Johnson and Onwuegbuzie 2004). Moreover, this approach is consistent with recommendations for the use of different 'perspectives, methodologies and outcomes' (Smith and Petticrew 2010, p. 6) in order to develop a greater understanding of violence prevention interventions.

Evidence Synthesis

It is increasingly difficult to identify, appraise, and interpret all available evidence to make informed decisions. As such, methods are needed to summarize the evidence in an accessible manner and uncover robust effects (Stoto and Cosler 2008). Evidence synthesis can take many forms including systematic reviews (with or without a meta-analysis) and realist reviews. Each of these will be discussed in turn.

Systematic reviews are considered the most versatile study design, and to provide the strongest type of evidence (Oxford Centre for Evidence-based Medicine 2009). While they traditionally focused on RCTs, Armstrong et al. (2011) identify the utility of other study designs in reviews of public health interventions. However, there is no firm consensus over which alternative study design should be included, although it has recently been recommended that randomized designs (i.e. cluster-randomized and

quasi-randomized trials) and quasi-experimental designs (i.e. ITS and controlled before-and-after studies) should be considered (CEPOCG 2013). Moreover, when there is homogeneity between interventions and study design, a meta-analysis can be undertaken, providing a quantitative summary.

The importance of qualitative data in further exploring participants' experiences of interventions has also been recognized within evidence synthesis. For instance, Noyes et al. (2011) indicate that for some reviews it may be appropriate to conduct a synthesis of qualitative studies to enhance the quantitative data. Indeed, a number of methods exist to enable the synthesis of qualitative studies (e.g. thematic synthesis, meta-ethnography) which involve analysing concepts from different studies to gain a better understanding of the feasibility and effectiveness of interventions (see Barnett-Page and Thomas 2009). The quantitative and qualitative data can be integrated using either multilevel (i.e. synthesized separately and then combined) or parallel synthesis (i.e. synthesized separately but the qualitative synthesis aids interpretation of the quantitative synthesis; see Noyes et al. 2011).

A more iterative and less prescriptive approach to evidence synthesis is the realist review, which seeks to understand why complex interventions succeed or not. It adopts a theory-driven approach by investigating programme theory integrity; adjudicating between rival programme theories; evaluating the same theory in comparative settings; and comparing intervention theory with actual practice (Pawson et al. 2005). Realist reviews are based upon the generative model of causality which argues that in order to establish a causal outcome between two events (e.g. pre- and post intervention) the underlying mechanism and the context in which it occurs need to be understood (Pawson et al. 2005). As such, mixed method approaches are favoured with less emphasis on RCTs.

In summary, realist reviews provide a depth of knowledge and understanding beyond the traditional forms of evidence synthesis; however, they do not provide firm conclusions or recommendations and, unlike systematic reviews, are not reproducible. Despite differences in methodology, approaches to evidence synthesis are increasingly acknowledging the importance of a variety of study designs, thus supporting the call to adopt a pragmatic approach to primary evaluation strategies.

From Evidence-Based to Evidence-Informed Practice

Traditionally, 'research evidence' has dominated evidence-based public health, which is defined as:

> 'a public health endeavour in which there is an informed, explicit, and judicious use of evidence that has been derived from any variety of science and social science research and evaluation methods' (Rychetnik et al. 2004, p. 538)

However, Culyer and Lomas (2006) indicate that research evidence is rarely complete, and can seldom be the sole source in the decision making process for practitioners and policymakers. For instance, Tilburt (2008) argues that implementing the 'most evidence-based' intervention may not be appropriate under certain societal conditions (including financial and logistic considerations), population norms or values, or the political culture of the target population (see also Chapter 43 of this volume for a discussion of policy transfer). In such circumstances, it may be necessary to adopt a more inclusive view of what constitutes evidence (Rycroft-Malone 2008).

Petticrew et al. (2004) recommend the use of a 'mixed economy' of evidence, in which diverse sources are synthesized to address different aspects of the issue in question. Indeed, Puddy and Wilkins (2011) suggest that 'experiential evidence' and 'contextual evidence' should be combined with research evidence. As a result of the need to account for a more inclusive evidence base—and greater context-sensitivity (Rycroft-Malone 2008) there has recently been a shift from the notion of *evidence-based practice* to *evidence-informed practice*. However, it is argued that the term 'evidence-informed' undermines the importance of rigorously generated evidence, and inflates the importance of biased experiential accounts (e.g. Sanderson 2009). Yet this does not mean that the quality of evidence should be disregarded: whatever the source of the evidence, it must be subject to scrutiny if it is to be used to inform policy and practice (Rycroft-Malone et al. 2004). Moreover, it is important that all forms of evidence be subjected to rigorous (research) enquiry (Sempik et al. 2007). In essence, it is imperative that all evidence is of high quality.

Conclusion

Violence is a multi-faceted public health problem and as such violence prevention often requires the use of various types of intervention design. Where interventions are considered relatively simple (i.e. programmes working with individuals), RCTs (or variants from the quantitative paradigm) can be used to examine effectiveness through outcome evaluation. However, even 'simpler' interventions could benefit from the inclusion of qualitative methods to undertake process evaluation (Oakley et al. 2006). Moreover, it is increasingly acknowledged that complex, multi-component interventions are necessary in preventing violence, which require that a myriad of 'perspectives, methodologies and outcomes' be utilized in the evaluation strategy (Smith and Petticrew 2010, p. 6). Evidence in violence prevention should, therefore, come from multiple sources, using multiple methods. Nonetheless the focus must be on the question, rather than the method.

Furthermore, the shift toward evidence-informed practice requires that contextual and experiential evidence be considered alongside research evidence. Moreover, as the acceptability of evidence varies between users (e.g. practitioners, policymakers, researchers) attention must also be paid to who will utilize the evidence. Nonetheless, regardless of the type, source, or user of the evidence it must be the subject of rigorous enquiry (Sempik et al. 2007) and scrutiny (Rycroft-Malone et al. 2004) to ensure it is of the highest quality.

Acknowledgements

Writing this chapter was supported in part by a grant from the University of Cape Town's Research Committee (URC) to the third author.

References

Adamson, J. (2005). Combined qualitative and quantiative design. In: A. Bowling, and S. Ebrahim (eds). *Handbook of Health Research Methods: Investigation, Measurement and Analysis.* Buckingham: Open University Press, pp. 230–45.

Armstrong, R., Waters, E., and Doyle, J. (eds.) (2011). Reviews in public health and health promotion. In: J. P. T. Higgins, and S. Green (eds).*Cochrane Handbook for Systematic Reviews of Interventions* [Online]. Cochrane Collaboration. Available at: http://handbook.cochrane.org/chapter_21/21_reviews_in_health_promotion_and_public_health.htm [Accessed 01 May 2013].

Barnett-Page, E., and Thomas, J. (2009). Methods for the synthesis of qualitative research: a critical review. *BMC Medical Research Methodology*, 9, 59.

Bettis, R., and Prahalad, C. K. (1995). The dominant logic: retrospective and extension. *Strategic Management Journal*, 16(1), 5–14.

CEPOCG (2013). *EPOC Resources for Review Authors* [Online]. Norwegian Knowledge Centre for the Health Services. Available at: http://epocoslo.cochrane.org/epoc-specific-resources-review-authors [Accessed 01 May 2013].

Creswell, J. W., Plano Clark, V. L., Gutmann, M., and Hanson, W. (2003). Advanced mixed methods research designs. In: A. Tashakkori and C. Teddlie (eds), *Handbook on Mixed Methods in the Behavioural and Social Sciences.* Thousand Oaks, CA: Sage, pp. 209–40.

Culyer, A. J., and Lomas, J. (2006). Deliberative processes and evidence-informed decision making in healthcare: do they work and how might we know? *Evidence and Policy*, 2(3), 357–71.

Dahlberg, L., and Krug, E. (2002). Violence: a global public health problem. In: E. Krug, L. Dahlberg, J. Mercy, A. B. Zwi, and R. Lozano (eds.).*World Report on Violence and Health.* Geneva: World Health Organization, pp. 1–21.

Drummond, M. F., Sculpher, M. J., Torrance, G. W., O'Brien, B. J., and Stoddart, G. L. (2005). *Methods for the Economic Evaluation of Health Care Programmes.* 3rd ed. Oxford: Oxford University Press.

Gray M. (2009). *Evidence Based Healthcare and Public Health: How to Make Decisions about Health Services and Public Health.* 3rd ed. Edinburgh: Churchill Livingston.

Johnson, R. B., and Onwuegbuzie, A. J. (2004). Mixed methods research: a research paradigm whose time has come. *Educational Researcher*, 33(7), 14–26.

Maynard, A. (2012). Public health and economics: a marriage of necessity. *Journal of Public Health Research*, 1(1), 11–3.

Mihalic, S. F., Irwin, K., Elliott, D., Fagan, A., and Hansen, D. (2001). *Blueprints for Violence Prevention* [Online]. US Department of Justice. Available at: https://www.ncjrs.gov/pdffiles1/ojjdp/187079.pdf [Accessed 15 April 2013]

Mihalic, S. F., and Irwin, K. (2003). Blueprints for violence prevention from research to real-world settings: factors influencing the successful replication of model programs. *Youth Violence and Juvenile Justice*, 1(4), 307–29.

Noyes, J., Popay, J., Pearson, A., Hannes, K., and Booth, A. (2011). Qualitative research and Cochrane reviews. In: J. P. T. Higgens, and S. Green (eds), *Cochrane Handbook for Systematic Reviews of Interventions* [Online]. Cochrane Collaboration. Available at: http://handbook.cochrane.org/chapter_20/20_qualitative_research_and_cochrane_reviews.htm [Accessed 01 May 2013].

Oakley, A., Strange, V., Bonell, C., Allen, E., Stephenson, J., and RIPPLE Study Team. (2006). Health services research: process evaluation in randomised controlled trials of complex interventions. *British Medical Journal*, 332(7538), 413–16.

Oxford Centre for Evidence-based Medicine. (2009). *Levels of Evidence* [Online]. University of Oxford. Available at: http://www.cebm.net/index.aspx?o=1025 [Accessed 11 Febuary 2013].

Pawson, R., and Tilley, N. (1997). *Realistic Evaluation.* London: Sage.

Pawson, R., Greenhalgh, T., and Harvey, G. (2005). Realist review: a new method of systematic review designed for complex policy interventions. *Journal of Health Services Research and Policy*, 10(Suppl 1), 21–34.

Petticrew, M., Whitehead, M., MacIntyre, S. J., Graham, H., and Egan, M. (2004). Evidence for public health policy on inequalities 1: the reality according to the policymakers. *Journal of Epidemiology and Community Health*, 58(10), 811–16.

Puddy, R. W., and Wilkins, N. (2011). *Understanding Evidence Part 1: Best Available Research Evidence. A Guide to the Continuum of Evidence of Effectiveness* [Online]. Centers for Disease Control and Prevention. Available at: http://www.cdc.gov/ViolencePrevention/pdf/Understanding_Evidence-a.pdf [Accessed 08 March 2013].

Reeves, B. C., Deeks, J. J., Higgins, J.P. T., and Wells, G. A. (2011). Including non-randomized studies. In: J. P. T. Higgins, and S. Green (eds). *Cochrane Handbook for Systematic Reviews of Interventions* [Online]. Cochrane Collaboration. Available at: http://handbook.cochrane.org/chapter_13/13_including_non_randomized_studies.htm [Accessed 01 May 2013]

Rittel, H. W. J., and Webber, M. M. (1973). Dilemmas in a general theory of planning, *Policy Sciences*, 4(2), 155-69.

Rutherford, A., Zwi, A. B., Grove, N. J., and Butchart, A. (2007). Violence: a priority for public health? (part 2). *Journal of Epidemiology and Community Health*, 61(9), 764–70.

Rychetnik, L. (2010). Is an 'evaluation jigsaw' a feasible way forward? *Journal of Public Health*, 32(1), 10–1.

Rychetnik, L., Frommer, M., Hawe, P., and Shiell, A. (2002). Criteria for evaluating evidence on public health interventions. *Journal of Epidemiology and Community Health*, 56(2), 119–27.

Rychetnik, L., Hawe, P., Waters, E., Barratt, A., and Frommer, M. (2004). A glossary for evidence based public health. *Journal of Epidemiology and Community Health*, 58(7), 538–45.

Rycroft-Malone, J., Seers, K., Titchen, A., Harvey, G., Kitson, A., and McCormack, B. (2004). What counts as evidence in evidence-based practice? *Journal of Advanced Nursing*, 47(1), 81–90.

Rycroft-Malone, J. O. (2008). Evidence-informed practice: from individual to context. *Journal of Nursing Management*, 16(4), 404–8.

Sale, J. M., Lohfeld, L. H., and Brazil, K. (2002). Revisiting the quantitative and qualitative debate: implications for mixed methods research. *Quality and Quantity*, 36(1), 43–53.

Sanderson, I. (2009). Intelligent policy making for a complex world: pragmatism, evidence and learning. *Political Studies*, 57(4), 699–719.

Schorr, L. B., and Farrow, F. (2011). *Expanding the Evidence Universe: Doing Better by Knowing More.* Washington, DC: Center for the Study of Social Policy.

Sempik, J., Becker, S., and Bryman, A. (2007). The quality of research evidence in social policy: consensus and dissension among researchers. *Evidence and Policy*, 3(3), 407–23.

Smith, R. D., and Petticrew, M. (2010). Public health evaluation in the twenty-first century: time to see the wood as well as the trees. *Journal of Public Health*, 32(1), 2–7.

Stoto, M. A., and Cosler, E. (2008). Evaluation of public health interventions. In: L. F. Novick, C. B. Morrow, and G. P. Mays (eds.), *Public Health Administration: Principles for Population-based Management.* 2nd ed. London: Jones and Bartlett Publishers, pp. 495–544.

Taxman, F. S., and Belenko, S. (2012). *Implementing Evidence-based Practice in Community Corrections and Addiction Treatment.* London: Springer.

Teddlie, C., and Tashakkori, A. (2009). *Foundations of Mixed Methods Research: Integrating Quantitative and Qualitative Approaches in the Social and Behavioral Sciences.* London: Sage.

Tilburt, J. C. (2008). Evidence-based medicine beyond the bedside: keeping an eye on context. *Journal of Evaluation in Clinical Practice*, 14(5), 721–5.

van der Knaap, L. M., Leeuw, F. L., Bogaerts, S., and Nijssen, L. T. J. (2008). Combining Campbell standards and the realist valuation approach: the best of two worlds? *American Journal of Evaluation*, 29(1), 48–57.

Whitehead, M., Petticrew, M., Graham, H., MacIntyre, S. J., Bambra, C., and Egan, M. (2004). Evidence for public health policy on inequalities 2: assembling the evidence jigsaw. *Journal of Epidemiology and Community Health*, 58(10), 817–21.

CHAPTER 18

Preventing child maltreatment and youth violence using parent training and home-visiting programmes

Jane Barlow

Theoretical Overview

Parent training and home-visiting programmes have a long history, especially in the prevention of child maltreatment.

Home-Visiting Programmes

Home-visiting programmes are typically underpinned by ecological theories about the importance of addressing diverse aspects of family functioning, many of which are related to poverty and social disadvantage (e.g. improving the educational and job prospects of the participating women). They have also been underpinned by other important theoretical approaches such as attachment theory. They have as such included components that are specifically targeted at promoting the type of parent–infant relationship that would promote later child resilience as a result of a secure infant attachment relationship with the primary caregiver. The Mother and Toddler programme, for example, focuses on improving parental reflective function, with the aim of impacting on parenting behaviours that promote attachment security (Suchman et al. 2010).

More recent home-visiting programmes such as Minding the Baby (Sadler et al. 2006) have continued core aspects of the model of delivery, but have incorporated methods of working that draw on recent research demonstrating the links between parental mentalization and reflective function, i.e. the ability to understand the behaviour of others in terms of mental states such as needs, feelings, and desires (Grienenberger et al. 2005).

Parent Training Programmes

Parent training programmes in contrast, have their theoretical origins in social learning theory, which provided an early empirical basis demonstrating a strong association between parenting practices and later child functioning, particularly

in terms of emotional and behavioural problems. For example, early research demonstrated a clear link between parenting practices characterized by harsh and inconsistent discipline, little positive parental involvement with the child, poor monitoring and supervision, and an increased risk of a range of poor outcomes including delinquency and substance abuse (Patterson et al. 1989).

Since then many parent training programmes have been developed that are underpinned by more diverse approaches to addressing such problems including family systems, Adlerian, and attachment theory. For example, insecure attachment in children has been shown to be related to a range of poor outcomes including behavioural problems (Sroufe et al. 2005) and delinquency (Garnier and Stein 1998), and a number of programmes explicitly targeting attachment have been developed (e.g. Circle of Security; Hoffman et al. 2006).

The success of parent training programmes in helping parents to manage children's behaviour has also resulted in their use to address more extreme forms of parenting behaviour, including physical and emotional abuse. Programmes such as Parent Child Interaction Therapy (PCIT), for example, involve additional work with parents focused on increasing parental motivation, and the use of clinic-based individual parent–child dyad sessions focused on enhancing skills and establishing daily positive parent–child interaction using guided play therapy. It also includes the teaching of positive methods of command-giving and discipline using live coached parent–child dyad sessions (Chaffin et al. 2004). Such programmes are underpinned by the recognition that maltreating parents may be driven in their use of emotional and physical abuse by their own dysregulated emotional states (e.g. extreme anger), often resulting from their own traumatic and abusive childhoods.

The most recent developments within the field of parent training have begun to build on what is described as the 'third wave of cognitive behavioural theory' with its emphasis on 'mindfulness', and the use of such techniques to help parents to regulate their own emotional states as a means of developing more measured approaches to children's behaviour (Dawe and Harnett 2012). Parents under Pressure is one such programme that targets substance dependent parents, and utilizes the teaching of mindfulness strategies alongside a range of other parenting techniques, with the aim of improving parental functioning and parenting practices (Dawe and Harnett 2007).

Intervention Procedures

Home-Visiting Programmes

Over the past 40 years more than 250 home-visiting programmes have been developed, ranging widely in their approach in terms of their content/curriculum, duration, and theory of change (Boller 2012). Despite this diversity, core features of early childhood home visitation programmes are the delivery of an intensive series of home visits beginning prenatally (in some models only), and continuing during at least the child's first 2 years of life by specially trained personnel who provide information, support, and training regarding child health, development, and care. The most comprehensive and effective (see 'Evidence about effectiveness' for further discussion) home-visiting programmes appear to be manualized interventions that have a clear underpinning theory in terms of the proposed mechanism for change, and a strong emphasis on staff training and supervision.

Although a majority of these programmes are delivered by professionals, a number of home-visiting programmes are delivered by paraprofessionals or volunteers. The limited research that has directly compared outcomes following delivery by professionals compared with paraprofessionals suggests that the former achieve significantly better outcomes (Olds et al. 2002; Peacock et al. 2013). In the UK, however, volunteer programmes such as HomeStart appear to be a good way of reaching disadvantaged families who may not be accessing other services, or who may be reluctant to trust a professional in the first instance (Crispin et al. 2005).

Parent Training Programmes

Standard parent training programmes are typically focused, short-term interventions, aimed at helping parents improve their functioning as a parent and their relationship with their child. The primary goal of most parent training programmes is preventing or treating a range of child emotional and behavioural problems by increasing the knowledge, skills, and understanding of the parents. Although most parent training programmes work directly with parents either on a one-to-one basis or in groups, a number of programmes have developed population level strategies that involve the delivery of a range of media-based strategies (e.g. radio programmes, advertising, etc.) aimed at raising awareness and changing population level practices (Prinz et al. 2009).

Parent training programmes typically involve the use of a manualized and standardized programme or curriculum, and are underpinned by a number of theoretical approaches including behavioural, cognitive behavioural, family systems, Adlerian, and mindfulness theories. They can involve the use of a range of techniques in their delivery including discussion, role-play, watching video vignettes, and homework. They are typically offered to parents over the course of eight to 12 weeks, for about one to two hours each week, in a range of settings including hospital/social work clinics and community-based settings such as general practitioner surgeries, schools, and churches. More recent approaches have involved the development of brief parent education programmes focused on issues such as reducing abusive head trauma, and are delivered to parents in hospital settings following the birth of a baby (Dias et al. 2005).

Evidence About Effectiveness

Home-Visiting Programmes

Home-visiting programmes have been evaluated to date in terms of their effectiveness in (i) preventing maltreatment in targeted (i.e. high risk) populations; (ii) improving outcomes related to youth violence and specifically, the emotional and behavioural functioning of children.

Child Maltreatment

A recent review of reviews (Mikton and Butchart 2009) identified 17 systematic reviews examining the effectiveness of around 149 studies of home-visiting programmes. The have produced somewhat diverse conclusions about the effectiveness of home-visiting programmes in preventing maltreatment—some reviews suggesting that they are effective (Daro and McKurdy 2007), some suggesting that that there is no evidence of effectiveness (Sweet and Appelbaum 2004), or highlighting problems in reaching any firm conclusion as a result of issues such a surveillance bias (Bull et al. 2004). Mikton and Butchart (2009) conclude that although there is evidence to suggest that home-visiting programmes are effective in improving risk factors associated with abusive parenting, there is very limited evidence of effectiveness in terms of objective measures, mostly confined to 15-year follow-up of the Nurse Family Partnership, which showed a 48 per cent reduction in actual child abuse (Olds et al. 1997).

Youth Violence

Although there is limited evidence concerning the impact of home-visiting programmes on youth violence, a review of reviews found that home-visiting programmes are effective in improving both early parenting practices and parent–infant interaction (Bull et al. 2004), both of which have been shown to be important precursors of later behavioural problems.

Evidence about the effectiveness of home visiting on children's social and emotional development (see Donelan-MacCall et al. 2012 for an overview) derives mostly from long-term follow-up studies of the Family Nurse Partnership Programme, which has demonstrated an impact in terms of reductions in arrests at 15 years of age (Olds et al. 1998), and reductions in both arrests and convictions for female participants at 19 years of age (Eckenrode et al. 2010); and in a separate study, use of substances and internalizing disorders in 12-year-old African-American children (Kitzman et al. 2010). This overview also cites evidence of an impact on child behavioural problems following the delivery of universal home visiting by Finnish nurses and in two further US-based home-visiting studies.

Parent Training Programmes

In contrast with home-visiting programmes, the bulk of the available evidence about parent training programmes is focused on their effectiveness in improving outcomes related to youth violence (e.g. behaviour and conduct problems). The more limited evidence about their effectiveness in preventing or treating maltreatment is summarized in the section below on child maltreatment.

Youth Violence

Parent training programmes have been shown in a number of recent reviews to be highly effective in improving a range of outcomes related to youth violence. In the UK, the National Institute for Health and Care Excellence (NICE) (2013) guidance recommends the use of parent training programmes for improving conduct-related problems in children aged 3–10 years of age. Similarly, a review of 47 randomized control trials (RCTs) of parent training programmes targeting children less than 5 years of age found a weighted effect size of around 0.35 corresponding to 50 per cent recidivism in the control group compared with 33 per cent recidivism in the experimental group (Piquero et al. 2008). The authors conclude that parent training is an effective intervention for reducing behaviour problems in young children.

Child Maltreatment

Although there have been numerous reviews of the effectiveness of parent training programmes in preventing or treating child maltreatment, many of these do not focus explicitly on the effectiveness of parent training and include diverse early prevention programmes, evidence taken from non-RCTs, or are comprehensive rather than systematic reviews. The evidence about 'what works' in the following section has been taken from reviews of RCTs of parent training programmes.

- *Targeted primary prevention*: A review of 23 studies found significant improvements in the region of 0.45–0.6 effect sizes for a range of outcomes including parents' attitudes toward abuse, emotional adjustment, child-rearing skills, and actual abuse (Lundahl and Nimer 2006).

- *Secondary prevention of recurrence*: Only one review has explicitly examined the effectiveness of parent training programmes in reducing the recurrence of physical maltreatment (i.e. treatment programmes; Barlow et al. 2006), and this found limited evidence to show that some parenting programmes may be effective in improving some outcomes that are associated with physically abusive parenting.

Since this review was conducted, however, there have been a number of further studies evaluating the effectiveness of parent training programmes in reducing maltreatment. Universal Triple P was evaluated in terms of its long-term impact on substantiated child abuse, following the implementation of a population-based approach including media and informational strategies. The study showed significantly reduced rates at 3 years of substantiated child maltreatment, hospitalizations, and emergency room visits due to suspected maltreatment-related injuries, and out of home placements (Prinz et al. 2009).

The Pathways Triple P parenting programme, which is explicitly designed for maltreating parents, has only been evaluated to date with families described as having 'borderline to clinically significant relationship disturbance'. The results of a study evaluating its effectiveness with this group, showed that following nine weeks of intervention consisting of parent skills training and cognitive behaviour therapy targeting negative attributions for child

behaviour, there were significant improvements in parent-child relationships and child behaviour problems, with gains maintained at three-month follow-up (Wiggins et al. 2009).

An RCT of the Parents under Pressure programme, which targeted substance dependent parents of children aged 2–8 years using a range of modules aimed at targeting parental affect regulation (e.g. 'mindfulness-based' techniques), alongside strategies to improve parent–infant interaction (i.e. video-guidance), found significant reductions in problems across multiple domains of family functioning, including child abuse potential, rigid parenting attitudes, and child behaviour problems (Dawe and Harnett 2007).

Implementation in Practice Settings and Transportability

Which Parenting Programmes are Effective in Practice?

A systematic review that examined the extent to which evidence-based parenting interventions could be transported across countries identified 17 studies (14 of which were RCTs) evaluating the effectiveness of four programmes originating in the United States or Australia in ten countries, mostly in Northern Europe, but also Asia, Latin America, and the Middle East (Gardner et al. 2013). The results show that while similar effect sizes were produced for other western countries, transportation to culturally different countries, including those with more traditional values in terms of family life and child-rearing showed higher effect sizes than countries with more secular, individualistic cultures. Effect sizes were also not influenced by local policy or resources (Gardner et al. 2013).

The two parent training programmes with the most evidence available are The Incredible Years and Triple P. One of the features of both of these programmes is that they offer different programme components for specific target audiences, and age groups of children, including both school-based interventions (The Dinosaur Social Skills and Problem Solving curriculum) and in the case of Triple P, programmes for children with disabilities (Stepping Stones), and for parents with a history of maltreatment (Pathways).

Recent additions now being made by many providers of parent training programmes explicitly target parents during pregnancy and the first year of life, with the aim of preventing the onset of problems. Although some of these programmes are targeted (e.g. First Steps), a number are being developed for population groups with the overall aim of preparing parents for the transition to parenthood (e.g. Parenting, Birth and Beyond).

Although there is currently very limited available evidence to support the use of standard parent training programmes in reducing the recurrence of child abuse, promising programmes are based on approaches such as cognitive behavioural therapy and child–parent interaction therapy. Other well-recognized interventions such as the Incredible Years Programme also appear to have a role in treating outcomes that are associated with abusive parenting. While behavioural child management programmes appear to have some benefit, the research suggests, however, the need for a wider focus to secure improvements in other aspects of parenting, and the most promising approaches currently would appear to include additional components that target parents affect regulation (e.g. stress and anger management modules) (Dawe and Harnett 2007).

Which Home-Visiting Programmes are Effective in Practice?

The evidence clearly indicates that not all home-visiting programmes are effective and in 2009 the U.S. Department of Health and Human Services (HHS) established the Home Visiting Evidence of Effectiveness (HomVEE) review, aimed at identifying home-visiting programmes that met evidence requirements to be provided as part of a 1.5 billion dollar federal initiative aimed at decreasing child maltreatment and improving parenting practices (Boller 2012). These programmes all target disadvantaged groups of mothers and children, some focusing explicitly on adolescent mothers with babies (Early Intervention Programme for Adolescent Mothers and Nurse Family Partnership), and others focusing more widely on disadvantaged parents of preschool children (e.g. Healthy Steps, Home Instruction for Parents of Preschool Youngers, and Parents as Teachers). They all involve the delivery of a series of home visits by a professional over an extended period of time, with the aim of breaking the cycle of disadvantage by promoting early parenting and educational outcomes (Boller 2012).

Transportability

The evidence suggests that both parent training and home-visiting programmes are highly transportable with parent training programmes such as the Webster–Stratton and Triple P both being delivered in over 40 countries internationally. Similarly, home-visiting programmes such as HIPPY (Home Instruction for Parents of Preschool Youngsters) and Nurse Family Partnership have been successfully transported to a range of international settings beyond the United States where they both originated.

The key factors associated with success in terms of the transportation of these programmes to new settings is their manualization, clear guidance and requirements in terms of the training and supervision of staff involved in their delivery, and a strong focus on integrity in terms of adherence to the original model. Some of these programmes also have licenses governing how and when they are delivered, and also target very specific groups (e.g. Nurse Family Partnership Programme, which only includes first-time, teenage mothers). Some of these programmes are, however, being delivered to groups who differ quite substantially from the original target group. For example, the HIPPY programme, which was first delivered to disadvantaged Israeli families, is now being successfully used with Canadian Aboriginal families.

Gaps in the Evidence

There is now extensive evidence to suggest that both parent training and home-visiting programmes are effective methods of working to prevent violence both in terms of reducing the incidence of maltreatment, and problems related to youth violence (i.e. conduct and behaviour problems). However, there is also extensive evidence to suggest that many home-visiting programmes are not effective, and that many parent training programmes are only effective with up to 50 per cent of participating parents (Webster-Stratton and Hammond 1990). Of relevance to both types of programme is the issue of 'readiness to change', and there is increasing recognition

that the type of psychological changes being sought using psychological interventions of this nature, require considerable commitment and readiness to change on the part of the parent. There are numerous ways in which such 'readiness to change' can be assessed prior to entering parents into treatment programmes of this type, and future research should identify the value of including this as part of an assessment of eligibility.

It has also been suggested that the skills training of parenting practitioners should include attachment theory, systems theory, cognitive factors, attribution theory, and motivational interviewing (Scott and Dadds 2009), and there is increasing recognition of the potential benefit of the concept of 'modularity' as an approach to therapeutic protocol design and application (Chorpita et al. 2005), and a need to evaluate the effectiveness of such an approach.

Home-Visiting Programmes

Two reviews of reviews both suggest that the evidence about the effectiveness of home-visiting programmes is highly variable (Bull et al. 2004; Mikton and Butchart 2009), with some programmes showing no benefits in terms of many of the outcomes measured, while others show wide-ranging benefits over extensive follow-up periods (e.g. Nurse Family Partnership). One of the biggest difficulties in evaluating the effectiveness of home-visiting programmes is the issue of surveillance bias, in which higher numbers of abuse are identified in the intervention group primarily as a result of the intensive nature and consequent additional surveillance involved. This issue is further compounded by the fact that most researchers regard a reduction in child abuse as being the desired outcome (i.e. lower numbers of recorded abuse in the intervention arm compared with the control arm), when in fact better detection might also represent a benefit of early intervention, particularly where the intervention is not bringing about change in some families. This requires long-term follow-up to identify whether home visiting is in fact resulting in an early identification of children, compared with the control arm, in which children are not identified until much later in their lives.

A second problem relating to the evaluation of the effectiveness of home-visiting programmes in preventing maltreatment is that many studies only use proxy, self-report measures of abusive parenting (e.g. parenting attitudes and behaviours) rather than objective measures of maltreatment (e.g. substantiated child abuse and neglect, or Emergency Room/Accident and Emergency visits). One of the consequences of this is that few home-visiting programmes have been demonstrated to be effective in reducing the incidence of actual abuse, and those that have been found to be effective, have involved limited groups of participants (i.e. the Nurse Family Partnership programme only recruits first-time, teenage parents). Further evaluation is needed of some of the innovative home-visiting programmes described above in terms of their use with wider populations of high-risk parents, and their impact on substantiated cases of abuse.

Recent research about the importance of parent–infant interaction, parental reflective function, and infant attachment security would suggest that future research should also assess the effectiveness of home visiting in producing sustainable change in these outcomes.

Parent Training Programmes

Although there is now extensive evidence about the effectiveness of parent training programmes, there is a paucity of evidence concerning their long-term effectiveness, and some evidence to suggest that the impact of such programmes is not sustained over time both in terms of their benefits directly for parents (Barlow et al. 2014), or for children's emotional and behavioural adjustment (e.g. Stewart-Brown et al. 2004). This suggests that there may be a need for 'top-up' programmes, and for research to assess whether such additional input improves their long-term impact.

There is also a need for further evaluation of the effectiveness of parent training programmes that have been explicitly designed for the purpose of preventing the recurrence of abuse in both physically and emotionally maltreating parents.

Other Means of Preventing Child Maltreatment

Two further methods of preventing child maltreatment—other than working with parents—have received attention in the literature. Enhanced paediatric care (training paediatricians to identify risk factors and refer parents as necessary) has been shown to reduce maltreatment, while school-based educational programmes teaching children to recognize the signs of potential abuse have been shown to increase knowledge but whether they prevent actual abuse is not known (MacMillan et al. 2009).

Programmes that address child maltreatment using other methods of this nature, should also be investigated further.

Conclusion

Both parent training and home-visiting programmes have a long developmental trajectory, and have evolved considerably over the past decade to reflect recent advances in theories about the causes of youth violence and maltreatment. They possibly represent two of the best-evidenced types of intervention explicitly targeting parents with the aim of improving outcomes in these domains. They are being delivered across diverse settings in over 40 countries internationally, providing strong testimony to their durability and transportability.

Although the evidence addressing their role in relation to youth violence is substantial, particularly in the case of parent training programmes, there is currently a paucity of evidence demonstrating the effectiveness of these programmes on actual abuse (i.e. as opposed to proxy measures of abuse), and limited evidence about what works in reducing the recurrence of abuse in maltreating parents. Future research should focus attention on some of the new models of both parent training and home-visiting programmes in terms of their benefits for more high-risk families.

References

Barlow, J., Simpkiss D., and Stewart-Brown, S. (2006). Interventions to prevent or ameliorate child physical abuse and neglect: findings from a systematic review. *Journal of Children's Services*, 1, 6–28.

Barlow, J., Smailagic, N., Huband, N., Roloff, V., and Bennett, C. (2014). Group-based parent training programmes for improving parental psychosocial health. *Cochrane Database of Systematic Reviews*, 5, CD002020.

Boller, K. (2012). Evidence for the role of home visiting in child maltreatment prevention. In: D. Spiker, and E. Gaylor (eds), *Encyclopaedia of Early Childhood Development*. Available at: http://www.child-encyclopedia.com/pages/PDF/BollerANGxp1.pdf [Accessed 13 November 2013].

Bull, J., McCormick, G., Swann, C., and Mulvihil, C. (2004). *Ante- and Post-natal Home-visiting Programmes: A Review of Reviews. [Evidence briefing]*. London: HAD. Available at: www.hda.nhs.uk/evidence [Accessed 13 November 2013].

Chaffin, M., Silovsky J. F., and Funderburk, B. et al. (2004). Parent-child interaction therapy with physically abusive parents: efficacy for reducing future abuse reports. *Journal of Consulting and Clinical Psychology*, 72, 500–10.

Chorpita, B. R., Daleiden, E. L., and Weisz, J. R. (2005). Modularity in the design and application of therapeutic interventions. *Applied and Preventive Psychology*, 11, 141–56.

Crispin, T., Milliken, D., and Bews, K. (2005). *Armbands in Deep Water: A Summary of Research into Home-Start's Home-visiting Volunteers*. Leicester: Home Start.

Daro, D., and McCurdy, K. (2007). Interventions to Prevent Maltreatment. In: L. Doll et al. (eds), *The Handbook of Injury and Violence Prevention*. New York: Springer, pp. 137–55.

Dawe, S., and Harnett, P. H. (2007). Improving family functioning in methadone maintained families: results from a randomised controlled trial. *Journal of Substance Abuse Treatment*, 32, 381–90.

Dias, M. S., Smith, K., deGuehery, K., Mazur, P., Li, V., and Shaffer, M. L. (2005). Preventing abusive head trauma among infants and young children: a hospital-based, parent education program. *Pediatrics*, 115, e470–77.

Donelan-McCall, N., Eckenrode, J., and Olds, D. L. (2009). Home visiting for the prevention of child maltreatment: lessons learned during the past 20 years. *Pediatric Clinics of North America*, 56(2), 389–403.

Eckenrode, J., Campa, M., and Luckey, D. W. et al. (2010). Long-term effects of prenatal and infancy nurse home visitation on the life course of youths: 19-year follow-up of a randomized trial. *Archives of Pediatric and Adolescent Medicine*, 164, 9–15.

Gardner, F., Knerr, W., and Montgomery P. (2013). *To What Extent Can Evidence-based Parenting Interventions for Child Problem Behaviour be Transported across Countries? Systematic Review and Meta-analysis*. Oxford: University of Oxford.

Garnier, H. E., and Stein, J. A. (1998). Values and the family: risk and protective factors for adolescent problem behaviours. *Youth and Society*, 30, 89–120.

Grienenberger, J., Kelly, K., and Slade, A. (2005). Maternal reflective functioning, mother-infant affective communication and infant attachment: exploring the link between mental states and observed caregiving. *Attachment and Human Development*, 7, 299–311.

Harnett, P. H., and Dawe, S. (2012). The contribution of mindfulness-based therapies for children and families and proposed conceptual integration. *Child and Adolescent Mental Health*, 17, 195–208.

Hoffman, K., Marvin, R., Cooper, G., and Powell, B. (2006). Changing toddlers' and preschoolers' attachment classifications: the Circle of Security intervention. *Journal of Consulting and Clinical Psychology*, 74, 1017–26.

Kitzman, H. J., Olds, D. L., and Cole, R. E. et al. (2010). Enduring effects of prenatal and infancy home visiting by nurses on children: follow-up of a randomized trial among children at age 12 years. *Archives of Pediatric and Adolescent Medicine*, 164, 412–8.

Lundahl, B. W., and Nimer, J. (2006). Preventing child abuse: a meta-analysis of parent training programmes. *Research on Social Work Practice*, 16, 251–62.

MacMillan, H. L., Wathen, C. N., Barlow, J., Fergusson, D. M., Leventhal, J. M., and Taussig, H. N. (2009). Interventions to prevent child maltreatment and associated impairment. *Lancet*, 373, 250–66.

Mikton, C., and Butchart, A. (2009). Child maltreatment prevention: a systematic review of reviews. *Bulletin of the World Health Organization*, 87, 325–404.

National Institute for Health and Care excellence (2013). *Antisocial Behaviour and Conduct Disorders in Children and Young People: Recognition, Intervention and Management*. Available at: http://publications. nice. org.uk/antisocial-behaviour-and-conduct-disorders-in-children-and-young-people-recognition-intervention-cg158 [Accessed 18 November 2013].

Olds, D. L., Eckenrode, J., and Henderson, C. R. Jr. et al. (1997). Long-term effects of home visitation on maternal life course and child abuse and neglect: fifteen-year follow-up of a randomized trial. *JAMA*, 278, 637–43.

Olds, D., Henderson, C. R. Jr., and Cole, R. et al. (1998). Long-term effects of nurse home visitation on children's criminal and antisocial behavior: 15-year follow-up of a randomized controlled trial. *JAMA*, 280, 1238–44.

Olds, D. L., Robinson, J., and O'Brien, R. et al. (2002). Home visiting by paraprofessionals and by nurses: a randomized, controlled trial. *Pediatrics*, 110, 486–96.

Patterson, G. R., DeBaryshe, D., and Ramsey, E. (1989). A developmental perspective on antisocial behavior. *American Psychologist*, 44, 329–35.

Peacock, S., Konrad, S., Watson, E., Nickel, D., and Muhajarine, N. (2013). Effectiveness of home visiting programmes on child outcomes: a systematic review. *BMC Public Health*, 13, 17.

Piquero, A. R., Farrington, D. P., Welsh, B. C., Tremblay, R., and Jennings, W. G. (2008). The effect of early family/parent training on antisocial behavior and delinquency. *Campbell Systematic Reviews*, 11.

Prinz, R. J., Sanders, M. R., Shapiro, C. J., Whitaker, D. J., and Lutzker, J. R. (2009). Population-based prevention of child maltreatment: the US Triple P system population trial. *Prevention Science*, 10, 1–12.

Sadler, L. S., Slade, A., and Mayes, L. (2006). Minding the Baby: a mentalization based- parenting programme. In: J. Allen, and P. Fonagy (eds), *Handbook of Mentalization Based Treatment*. Chichester, UK: Wiley, pp. 271–88.

Scott, S., and Dadds, M. (2009). Practitioner review: when parent training doesn't work: theory-driven clinical strategies. *The Journal of Child Psychology and Psychiatry*, 50, 1441–50.

Sroufe, L. A., Egeland, B., Carlson, E., and Colllins, A. W. (2005). *The Development of the Person: The Minnesota Study of Risk and Adaptation from Birth to Adulthood*. New York: The Guilford Press.

Stewart-Brown, S., Patterson, J., Mockford, C., Barlow, J., Klimes, I., and Pyper, C. (2004). Impact of a general practice based group parenting programme: quantitative and qualitative results from a controlled trial at 12 months. *Archives of Disease in Childhood*, 89, 519–25.

Suchman, N. E., DeCoste, C., Castiglioni, N., McMahon, T. J., Rounsaville, B., and Mayes, L. (2010). The Mothers and Toddlers programme, an attachment-based parenting intervention for substance using women: post-treatment results from a randomized clinical pilot. *Attachment and Human Development*, 12, 483–504.

Sweet, M. A., and Appelbaum, M. I. (2004). Is home visiting an effective strategy? A meta-analytic review of home visiting programmes for families with young children. *Child Development*, 75, 1435–56.

Webster-Stratton, C., and Hammond, M. (1990). Predictors of treatment outcome in parent training for families with conduct problem children. *Behavior Therapy*, 21, 319–37.

Wiggins, T. L., Sofronoff, K., and Sanders, M. R. (2009). Pathways Triple P-Positive Parenting programme: effects on parent-child relationships and child behavior problems. *Family Process*, 48, 517–30.

CHAPTER 19

Violence prevention through reduction of risks to child health and development in the years prior to school

Andrew Dawes

Theoretical Overview of Reduction of Risks to Child Health and Development in the Years prior to School

Early childhood is commonly regarded as extending from birth to 9 years. However, recent research has significantly extended our knowledge of the importance of the first 1,000 days (pregnancy plus the first 2 years) in the development of neurological processes and structures associated with higher mental functions and emotional regulation that lay the biological foundations for learning and socio-emotional functioning (Shonkoff 2012). These findings require that we include *foetal life* in our definition of early childhood and our approach to prevention. Interventions to reduce risks to development prior to birth are essential components of a strategy to promote child health and development and reduce early causes of violent behaviour (Tremblay 2006). The contribution of this chapter is twofold. First, risks to the health and intellectual development of young children that increase the risk of poor long-term developmental outcomes are outlined. Through complex interactions with other factors, these insults raise the risk of aggressive antisocial proclivities in the long term. The focus is on children in poverty environments, and more particularly in low- and middle-income countries (LMICs) where threats to sound development are more prevalent. Second, evidence for preventive and developmentally promotive interventions that can play a role in breaking the chain of influences associated with the development of antisocial behaviour is presented. The chapter does not consider development beyond the preschool period (around 6 years of age). As these are dealt with elsewhere in the volume, pathways to violent conduct (Chapter 5), interventions to prevent aggressive behaviour, child maltreatment (Chapter 4), and parenting interventions (Chapter 18) are not covered here.

Early interventions of the kind to be discussed in this chapter are likely to increase the probability that a significant proportion of children from poor backgrounds in both high-income countries (HICs) and LMICs will be ready to learn when they get to school and that a pathway towards school failure, dropout, antisocial behaviour, and inter-generational poverty is averted. As the majority of the world's children live in LMICs where finance for interventions is limited, the chapter pays particular attention to evidence for effective scalable interventions.

Threats to Early Development and their Implications for Preventive Interventions

Upstream structural and economic factors are primary determinants of disadvantaged childhoods and indeed of the violent pathways we seek to interrupt. Very significant numbers of children around the world are subject to what Johan Galtung (1969, p. 171) termed 'Structural Violence', which occurs when there is no actor and where:

> The violence is built into the (social) structure and shows up as unequal power and consequently as unequal life chances. Resources are unevenly distributed, as when income distributions are heavily skewed, literacy/education unevenly distributed, medical services existent in some districts and for some groups only, and so on.

Structural violence is associated with poverty but more importantly with societal inequality. While poverty has broad negative impacts on a range of developmental outcomes, inequality also structures well-being. More equal societies have lower poverty rates, better child outcomes, and greater equality in service provision (Schwebel and Christie 2001).

The majority of the world's young children live in environments in which the necessary affordances for a sound foundation in health, nutrition, and cognitive and language development are reduced. In such circumstances, a chain of developmental consequences ensues: individual potential is compromised, children are less likely to develop the capabilities required to benefit from schooling and ultimately to become productive adult members of society, and deviant developmental outcomes (including violent conduct) become more probable (Grantham-McGregor et al. 2007).

Reduction of poverty and inequality are therefore major public health imperatives if we are to reduce many of the sources of violent conduct that reside in families and communities burdened by poverty and inequitable access to the supports required for the sound health and development of the youngest members of our populations.

Early Child Health and Nutrition

The Status of the Evidence

Risks to child health both prenatally and in the first years of life are most common in the economically deprived areas of both HICs and LMICs. Antenatally, Mendes et al. (2009) identify insults to the child's developing neurological systems that have been linked to later aggression, including maternal tobacco, cocaine, and alcohol consumption and maternal malnutrition during the first two trimesters. Postnatally, they identify early malnutrition, maltreatment, and neglect. Liu's (2011) review points to factors that, while not directly associated with aggression, compromise early health and development: maternal stress and depression; birth complications (pre-eclampsia, preterm birth, and gestational diabetes); lead exposure; and head injury.

Paediatric HIV affects approximately 1 million LMIC children (Walker et al. 2007). Significant neurological impact and developmental delays are evident in these children. Although evidence of a link to later aggressive behaviour has not been systematically investigated, the neurological consequences of HIV infections suggest that an indirect link would be probable via lowered intellectual potential, school failure, and drop out.

Malnutrition is one of the most common preventable threats to normal neurological development and intellectual functioning. The impact depends on the period of life during which it is experienced and the duration of exposure. The first 1,000 days (pregnancy through the first 2 years) are particularly sensitive and the outcomes of early prolonged malnutrition are associated with long-term deficits. Victora and colleagues (2008, p. 23) report that stunting 'at 2 years was the best predictor of human capital and that under nutrition is associated with lower human capital'.

Limited attention has been paid to the role of malnutrition in the development of violent conduct until recently. Evidence of a link is emerging from longitudinal cohort and other studies in which early malnutrition has been shown to predict externalizing behaviour in middle childhood and adolescence. For example, a longitudinal study in Barbados has established links between malnutrition in the first year with executive functioning difficulties in middle childhood and adolescence that are associated with raised levels of aggression through to the mid-teens (Galler et al. 2011). The Mauritian birth cohort study (Liu 2011) provides supporting evidence: in that research, malnutrition by age 3 years predicted externalizing behaviour in middle childhood and adolescence. In addition, Walker et al. (2007) note that:

> prospective cohort studies consistently show significant associations between stunting (due to malnutrition) by age 2 or 3 years and later cognitive deficits school achievement, and dropout (p. 146).

They point to both foetal intrauterine growth restriction 'mainly due to poor maternal nutrition and infections' (p. 145), and malnutrition (mainly growth stunting) during the first three postnatal years as causing permanent neurological damage that leads to compromised cognitive development.

Further (though not conclusive) support for a link between maternal malnutrition and adult antisocial proclivities comes from studies of the adult offspring of women who experienced famine during early pregnancy. One example is the so-called *Hunger Winter Famine* in Nazi-occupied Holland during 1944–1945 (Neugebauer et al. 1999). The other is the Chinese famine of 1959–1961 that was associated with Mao's agricultural production policy during his *Great Leap Forward* (Huang et al. 2013). In both cases higher rates of antisocial personality disorder are evident. And in the Dutch study where records of mental status examinations of 18 year olds conceived during the famine were studied, a higher probability of violent antisocial personality disorder was found.

Finally, Liu (2011, p. 65) offers an interactive model in which early health risk factors are viewed as 'predictors of adverse outcomes, including childhood externalizing behaviour'. Brain dysfunction has direct effects (as in dysregulated behaviour), and also mediates the relationship between the early insult and the development of violent behaviour. For example, maternal nutrition during pregnancy (a biological process) interacts with psychosocial factors (the quality of antenatal care) to influence birth weight. Poor maternal nutrition is likely to be a function of food insecurity. In the absence of nutritional interventions, low birth weight children (<2,500g) are less likely to thrive and their neurological development is likely to be compromised. That in turn impacts intellectual capacity and ability to succeed in school increasing the risk of drop out and involvement with antisocial peers (should these be present in the child's environment).

These findings suggest that we should be paying more attention to pre- and postnatal nutrition as a probable source of aggressive behaviour in childhood and later, particularly in LMICs where the majority of affected children reside and who are most affected by malnutrition (United Nations Children's Fund, World Health Organization, and the World Bank 2012).

Interventions and Research Outcomes

Prevention of malnutrition, particularly in the first 1,000 days, is a simple low-cost intervention that can have a significant impact on school outcomes and human potential (e.g. Hoddinott et al. 2008). Prenatally, provision of iron, calcium, folate, and nutritional food reduce risks of maternal malnutrition. Postnatally, exclusive breast-feeding for at least the first 6 months, is the most effective way of preventing malnutrition and reducing the risk of childhood diseases common to children in poverty. Population level nutrition programmes including vitamin A, iodine, and iron supplementation play a key preventive role in children at risk for malnutrition through to and including the first years of school (Hendricks and Bourne 2010).

The risk of HIV infected children in resource-constrained environments progressing to advanced HIV infection (and associated neurological damage) is very high in the first 2 years of life (Ely 2010). Prevention of mother to child transmission treatment (PMTCT) is essential and affordable. In South Africa rates of infection have significantly decreased as access to free medication has improved (Ely 2010).

Prevention of alcohol and other drug use in pregnancy is also essential to prevent neurological damage. Findings indicate that messaging campaigns raise awareness of risk but do not change behaviour; screening of pregnant women plus brief counselling on risks has been shown to reduce alcohol intake; and relatively brief interventions for women who are at high risk can be effective (Hankin 2002).

In sum, interventions to prevent health risks during pregnancy will reduce the probability of neurological deficits that compromise children's capacity to succeed in school, and that are associated with dysregulated externalizing behaviour that in turn places the child at risk for the development of violent conduct in adolescence and adulthood.

Stimulation for Early Learning

The Status of the Evidence, Interventions, and Research Outcomes

There is clear evidence that children from economically disadvantaged homes who have quality early learning inputs do better in school and are less at risk for later drop out and associated troubles.

One of the key contributors to poor scholastic outcomes and the negative consequences that follow is inadequate preparation for the demands of schooling (Nores and Barnett 2010). Much of the evidence for effectiveness in improving school-related outcomes and reduction in antisocial behaviour has been produced in long-term follow-up studies of high-quality experimental preschool programmes for poor children in the United States such as the Perry Preschool and Abecedarian projects that commenced in the 1960s (Heckman et al. 2008, 2009; Sparling et al. 2007). While often heralded as examples of what is required to address the educational deficits of children from poor backgrounds, their cost makes them unscalable in HIC, let alone transportable to or affordable in LMICs.

Public programmes that have been taken to scale such as Early Head Start and Head Start in the United States have shown good child development outcomes at the end of kindergarten (Barnett 2011). And children who have participated in Early Head Start (which includes home visiting for particularly vulnerable children) have shown reduced aggressive behaviour at age 5 years when compared with controls (Administration for Children and Families, HHS 2006).

Early learning programmes are increasingly being implemented and evaluated in poor (frequently rural) communities in LMICs. They are delivered via several channels, including (i) preschools (e.g. Aboud 2006); (ii) home visiting (with a parent education focus or a two-generational approach involving both parent and child, e.g. Kagitcibasi et al. 2009); and (iii) parent education programmes (e.g. Evans, 2006). Home-visiting programmes often provide stimulation for early learning and parenting inputs delivered alongside nutrition, support for accessing social security, and health and welfare services (Aber et al 2012; Walker et al. 2011).

Engle et al. (2007) reviewed studies of LMIC early learning programmes and concluded that children who had the opportunity to attend a formal early childhood development programme (such as a preschool) had the edge over children who did not, showing higher levels of cognitive functioning; and gains in socio-emotional functioning were also evident. They were also more likely to enter school at the correct age, and to perform better. In the long term, they were less likely to fail a class. Nores and

Barnett's (2010) meta-analysis of the benefits of early education in both HIC and LMIC concurs. The findings are complex, but can be summarized as follows:

> Interventions that were either educational or mixed (e.g. stimulation and nutrition, care and nutrition, pre-K, pre-K and nutrition) evidenced the largest statistically significant effects on cognition. (p. 279)

Home visiting is commonly used as a delivery channel in LMIC for the promotion of early stimulation in the preschool years, primarily because access to formal preschools is very limited. Home visiting with early stimulation is delivered by paraprofessionals with the goal of improving cognitive and language outcomes prior to school has been shown to have positive outcomes. However, it is essential that visitors are carefully trained and supervised, quality is sound, and inputs are frequent (weekly) and of sufficient duration. Best outcomes are achieved when children are targeted from an early age (prior to 24 months). (Baker-Henningham and Boo 2010; Engel et al. 2007; Evans 2006; Kagitcibasi 2009).

Finally, the only study in a LMIC to permit scrutiny of the effects of home-based early stimulation on violent behaviour in adulthood is the Jamaican longitudinal study (Walker et al. 2011; Grantham-McGregor et al. 1991), which reports findings on participants at 22 years. Following weekly home visits for 24 months delivered by para-professional community health workers, participants reported fewer incidents of violent conduct and arrests when compared to controls.

Gaps in the Evidence

The material reviewed in this contribution is sourced from several disciplines each with their own literatures on research limitations and needs for further investigation. It is not possible to address the range of issues here. Some general points are made, in particular about interventions to promote early learning in disadvantaged LMIC.

There is a dearth of high-quality effectiveness studies outside the United States where high-quality preschool programmes have paid significant long-term dividends. For most countries, preschool interventions such as Perry Preschool or Abecedarian, or home-visiting programmes like the Nurse Family Partnership model (Olds et al. 2007), are simply not transportable.

If we are to take interventions to scale at population level, we need to extend the range of personnel available to provide developmental inputs to children to include non-professionals as in the Jamaican study referred to previously and a number of other examples (Cooper et al. 2009; Dawes et al. 2012; Kagitcibasi et al. 2009). There are many questions to be investigated regarding the selection, training, and mentoring of such workers so as to ensure effective programme implementation, and the quality of supervision and support in the field that are required to ensure sound implementation.

We have good evidence from several robust trials with high internal validity. However, when implemented in real-world conditions, we make the transition from science to service and it is here that the nature of the programme and all the things that influence the quality of delivery come into play. As Nores and Barnett (2010, p. 279) state:

> Overall, our findings indicate that program design matters, but that there is a lack of clarity about what dimensions matter how much and for what reasons.

We also need costing studies that compare different channels of delivery if we are to take interventions to scale, particularly in the majority world where resources are limited.

Finally, there is little consistency in the measures of cognitive, language, and emotional outcome in the evaluations that have been conducted. Are we measuring the same construct with different measures? And in non-Western countries there is a dearth of locally developed and standardized instruments.

Conclusion

The child's experience in the first 6 years has a critical bearing on later development. Recent evidence informs us that the *first 1,000 days* are especially important, and the call to prevent risks to child development during this period has gathered considerable momentum. There is a considerable body of evidence that social disadvantage prejudices the development of capabilities that children need to succeed in education and later life. Children in all countries are affected, but a far greater proportion resides in the majority world where risks are high, opportunities for support are limited, and the probability of long-term negative outcomes including perpetration of violence (by males) is significant.

Interventions to support young children's development should be tailored to the most pressing threats. As illustrated in this chapter, and on the basis of their prevalence, key health risks to early development that have been linked to violent conduct in later years include

- antenatally: poor maternal health care, inadequate nutrition, and alcohol or drug abuse;

- postnatally: child malnutrition (particularly in the first 2 years of life) and maltreatment (discussed elsewhere in the volume).

Threats to sound cognitive, language, and socio-emotional development in the years prior to school include

- limited stimulation of developmental capacities required for children to be ready to learn in school, and

- harsh and inconsistent parenting that compromises the development of self-regulation and in turn impacts executive functioning, the ability to learn, and also socio-emotional development.

We have clear evidence that interventions to promote maternal health and nutrition, and reduce intake of substances such as alcohol during pregnancy, will reduce the risk of neurological insults to the developing foetus. Promotion of maternal health is therefore a priority. We also know that maternal depression is highly prevalent in poor communities in both high- and low-income countries. While not directly associated with the development of externalizing behaviour and adult violence, the condition compromises the capacity to provide responsive affectionate care and is predictive of a broad range of risks to young children (Wachs and Rahman 2013). Provision of primary mental health interventions for vulnerable mothers and other primary caregivers therefore have the potential to substantially reduce risks to a large number of young children while promoting caregiver well-being.

In the majority world, early stimulation interventions have the potential to provide a good start for schooling, better school performance and attendance, lower risk of drop out, and ultimately reduced risk of engagement in antisocial conduct. But to make an impact, they need to be taken to scale in the most vulnerable populations. These services must be seen as a public good. Governments must come to the table. As Engle et al (2011, p. 1339) put it:

> Unless governments allocate more resources to quality early child development programmes for the poorest people in the population, economic disparities will continue and widen.

This contribution agrees whole-heartedly with Engle and her colleagues. However, we must also recognize that early intervention is not a panacea for the prevention of all later ills. As Loeber and Pardini (2008) demonstrate, developmental pathways to violence have complex determinants, and later periods in development bring their own risks as children enter new social spaces and encounter forces for positive and negative outcomes.

If we are to reduce the burden of disease attributable to violence—particularly those regions of the world most afflicted by poverty and structural inequality—it is crucial (and most cost-effective) to intervene early. But it is also necessary to continue to provide sustained support and protection for children growing up in challenging environments.

References

Aber, L., Biersteker, L., Dawes, A., and Rawlings, L. (2012). Social protection and welfare systems: implications for early childhood development. In: P. Rebello, P. Engle, and C. Super (eds), *Handbook of Early Childhood Development Research and Its Impact on Global Policy*. New York: Oxford University Press, pp. 260–74.

Aboud, F. E. (2006). Evaluation of an early childhood preschool program in rural Bangladesh. *Early Childhood Research Quarterly*, 21, 46–60.

Administration for Children and Families, HHS (2006). *Research to Practice: Preliminary Findings from the Early Head Start Prekindergarten Follow-Up, Early Head Start Research and Evaluation Project*. Washington, D.C.: HHS.

Alderman, H., Hoddinott, J., and Kinsey, B. (2008). Long-term consequences of early childhood malnutrition. *Oxford Economic Papers*, 58, 450–74.

Baker-Henningham, H., and Boo, F. L. (2010). Early childhood stimulation interventions in developing countries: a comprehensive literature review. *IZA Discussion Paper 5282*. Bonn: Institute for the Study of Labor (IZA). Available at: http://papers.ssrn.com/sol3/papers.cfm?abstract_id=1700451. [Accessed 25 April 2013].

Barnett, W. S. (2011). Effectiveness of early educational intervention. *Science*, 333, 975–8.

Cooper, P. J., Tomlinson, M., and Swartz, L. et al. (2009). Improving the quality of the mother-infant relationship and infant attachment in a socio-economically deprived community in a South African context: a randomised controlled trial. *British Medical Journal*, 338, b974.

Dawes, A., Biersteker, L., and Hendricks, L. (2012). *Towards Integrated Early Childhood Development. An evaluation of the Sobambisana Initiative*. Claremont, Cape Town: The D.G. Murray Trust. Available at: www.ilifalabantwana.co.za. [Accessed 29 August, 2013].

Ely, B. (2010). HIV, TB and child health. In: M. Kibel, L. Lake, S. Pendlebury, and C. Smith (eds), *South African Child Gauge 2009/2010*. Cape Town: Children's Institute, University of Cape Town, pp. 41–5.

Engle, P. L., Black, M. M., and Behrman, J. R., et al. (2007). Strategies to avoid the loss of developmental potential in more than 200 million children in the developing world. *The Lancet*, 369, 229–42.

Engle, P. L., Fernald, L. C. H., and Alderman, H., et al. (2011). Strategies for reducing inequalities and improving developmental outcomes for young children in low and middle-income countries. *Lancet*, 378, 1339–53.

Evans, J. L. (2006). *Parenting Programmes: An Important ECD Intervention Strategy*. Paris: UNESCO.

Galler, J. R., Bryce, C. P., and Waber, D. P., et al. (2011). Infant malnutrition predicts conduct problems in adolescents. *Nutritional Neuroscience*, 15, 186–92.

Galtung, J. (1969). Violence, peace, and peace research. *Journal of Peace Research*, 6, 167–91.

Grantham-McGregor, S., Bun Cheung, Y., and Cueto, S. (2007). Developmental potential in the first 5 years for children in developing countries. *Lancet*, 369, 60–70.

Grantham-McGregor, S. M., Powell, C. A., Walker, S. P., and Himes, J. H. (1991). Nutritional supplementation, psychosocial stimulation, and mental development of stunted children: the Jamaican Study. *Lancet*, 338, 1–5.

Hankin, J. R., (2002). Fetal alcohol syndrome prevention research. *Alcohol Health and Research*, 26, 58–65

Heckman, J. (2008). Schools, skills and synapses. *Economic Inquiry*, 46, 289–324.

Heckman, J. J., Moon, S. H., Pinto, R., Savelyev, P. A., and Yavitz, A., (2009). The rate of return to the High/Scope Perry Preschool program.*IZA Discussion Paper 4533*. Bonn: IZA.

Hendricks, M., and Bourne, L. (2010). An integrated approach to malnutrition in childhood. In: M. Kibel, L. Lake, S. Pendlebury, and C. Smith (eds), *South African Child Gauge 2009/2010*. Cape Town: Children's Institute, University of Cape Town, pp. 46–52.

Hoddinott, J., Maluccio, J. A., Behrman, J. R., Flores, R., and Martorell R. (2008). Effect of a nutrition intervention during early childhood on economic productivity in Guatemalan adults. *Lancet*. 371, 411–6.

Huang, C., Phillips, M. R., and Zhang, Y. et al (2013). Malnutrition in early life and adult mental health: Evidence from a natural experiment. *Social Science and Medicine*, 97, 259–66.

Kagitcibasi, C., Sunar, D., Baydar, N., and Cemalcilar, Z. (2009). Continuing effects of early enrichment in adult life: the Turkish early enrichment project 22 years later. *Journal of Applied Developmental Psychology*, 30, 764–99.

Liu, J. (2011). Early health risk factors for violence: conceptualisation, evidence, and implications. *Aggression and Violent Behaviour*. 16, 63–73.

Loeber, R., and Pardini, D. (2008). Neurobiology and the development of violence: common assumptions and controversies. *Philosophical Transactions of the Royal Society: Biological Sciences*, 363, 2491–503.

Mendes, D. D., Mari, J., Singer, M., Barros, G. M., and Mello, A. F. (2009). Study review of the biological, social and environmental factors associated with aggressive behaviour. *Review of Brazilian Psychiatry*, 31, 577–85.

Neugebauer R., Hoek, H. W., and Susser, E. (1999). Prenatal exposure to wartime famine and development of antisocial personality disorder in early adulthood. *Journal of the American Medical Association*, 4, 479–81.

Nores, M., and Barnett, S. W. (2010). Benefits of early childhood education interventions across the world. *Economics of Education Review*, 29, 271–82.

Olds, D. L., Sadler, L., and Kitzman, H. (2007). Programs for parents of infants and toddlers: recent evidence from randomized trials. *Journal of Child Psychology and Psychiatry*, 48, 355–91.

Schwebel, M., and Christie, D. 2001. Children and structural violence. In: D. J. Christie, R. V. Wagner, and D. D. Winter (eds), *Peace, Conflict, and Violence: Peace Psychology in the 21st Century*. New York: Prentice-Hall, pp. 120–30.

Shonkoff, J. (2012). Leveraging the biology of adversity to address the roots of disparities in health and development. *Proceedings of the National Academy of Sciences*, 109, 17302–7.

Sparling, J., Ramey, C. T., and Ramey, S. L. (2007). The Abecedarian experience. In: M. Eming Young and L. M. Richardson (eds), *Early Childhood Development. From Measurement to Action*. Washington D.C.: The World Bank, pp. 81–99.

Tremblay, R. E. (2006). Prevention of youth violence: why not start at the beginning? *Journal of Abnormal Psychology*, 34, 481–7.

United Nations Children's Fund, World Health Organization, and the World Bank (2012). *UNICEF WHO-World Bank Joint Child Malnutrition Estimates*. Geneva: World Health Organization.

Victora, C. G., Hallal, P. C., Araújo, C. L., Menezes, A. M., Wells, J. C., and Barros, F. C. (2008). Cohort profile: the 1993 Pelotas (Brazil) birth cohort study. *International Journal of Epidemiology*, 37, 704–9.

Wachs, T., and Rahman. A. (2013). The nature and impact of risk and protective influences on children's development in low and middle income countries. In: P. Rebello-Britto, P. Engle, and C. Super (eds.). *Handbook of Early childhood Development Research and its Impact on Global Policy*. New York: Oxford. pp. 85–160.

Walker, S. P., Wachs, T. D., and Meeks Gardner, J. et al. (2007). Child development: risk factors for adverse outcomes in developing countries. *Lancet*, 369, 145–57.

Walker, S. P., Chang, S. M., Vera-Hernández, M., and Grantham-McGregor, S. (2011). Early childhood stimulation benefits adult competence and reduces violent behaviour. *Pediatrics*, 127, 849–57.

CHAPTER 20

Preventing violence through positive youth development programmes

Abigail A. Fagan and Richard F. Catalano

Introduction to Preventing Violence through Positive Youth Development Programmes

Given the many short- and long-term negative consequences that involvement in violence poses for adolescents, and the fact that teenagers who engage in violence are at greater risk for offending during adulthood (Elliott 1994; Moffitt 1993), it is important to implement violence prevention programmes early in the life course, before violence has been initiated. This chapter reviews evidence regarding the ability of positive youth development programmes implemented in community settings to prevent youth aggression and violence by enhancing individual and social competencies of children and adolescents.

Theoretical Overview

There is evidence that interventions can effectively prevent problem behaviours like violence if they alter the known precursors of such behaviours (Catalano et al. 2012; Coie et al. 1993; O'Connell et al. 2009). Effective programmes seek to minimize risk factors, experiences which increase the likelihood that youth will engage in violent activities (in this case), and enhance protective factors, experiences which decrease the likelihood of violence or buffer the negative impact of risk factors. The positive youth development programmes described in this chapter focus on changing risk and protective factors to not only help youth avoid violence, but also to produce more competent individuals who will more positively contribute to society (Catalano et al. 2008; Weissberg and Greenberg 1998).

While they can take many forms, positive youth development programmes attempt to produce behavioural changes by promoting academic, emotional, social, and behavioural competencies such as self-management, effective communication, and responsible decision making (Durlak et al. 2011); emotional attachments between youth and positive adults and institutions; moral integrity; and caring, compassion, and/or spirituality (Catalano et al. 2004; Gavin et al. 2010; Roth and Brooks-Gunn 2003). Such programmes often occur in schools, but they can be implemented in other community settings. What is most important is that the intervention context is a supportive environment which provides opportunities and positive reinforcement for learning new skills (Roth and Brooks-Gunn 2003).

Given that Espelage has reviewed school-based interventions elsewhere in this volume, the current chapter focuses on interventions that occur at least partially outside the school setting and which involve more than classroom curricula or school-wide initiatives to build individual competencies. While school-based positive youth development programmes can successfully reduce violence (e.g. Hahn et al. 2007), their potential to enhance youth development will be limited if the broader environments in which youth spend time (e.g. peer groups, families, and communities) are not supportive of programme goals (Roth and Brooks-Gunn 2003; Wagenaar and Perry 1994). Social ecological theories emphasize that multiple contexts affect youth, and that factors may interact across settings to influence the development of violence and other problems (Bronfenbrenner 2005; Weissberg and Greenberg 1998). Such theories are supported by research indicating that risk and protective factors exist across multiple domains of influence (Catalano et al. 2011; Coie et al. 1993; Hawkins et al. 1992), and that the more risk factors and fewer protective factors encountered, the more likely one is to engage in violence (Herrenkohl et al. 2000). To have maximal impact, then, a youth development programme intent on preventing violence should ideally target multiple factors across multiple settings.

The Status of the Evidence regarding the Effectiveness of Positive Youth Development Programmes

Several reviews have previously assessed the effectiveness of positive youth development (Catalano et al. 2004; Gavin et al. 2010; Roth and Brooks-Gunn 2003; Weissberg and Greenberg 1998) and social and emotional learning programmes (Durlak et al. 2010, 2011). These studies have demonstrated that such interventions can enhance youth competencies, reduce risk factors, and positively affect diverse outcomes including academic success, conduct problems, delinquency, and violence. Interventions deemed effective have diverse content, settings, and targeted populations. They include universal interventions intended to reach the general population of youth, selective interventions targeting youth with elevated risk factors and/or depressed protective factors, and indicated programmes for those who have initiated but not yet reached elevated levels of problem behaviours (Coie et al. 1993; O'Connell et al. 2009).

While important in reviewing programme effectiveness, none of the cited reviews has focused on violence as an outcome or on interventions which take place at least partially outside the school setting. This chapter seeks to fill this gap by reviewing the degree to which positive youth development programmes implemented in community settings, with or without additional school-based programming, have reduced youth violence. We focus on services for children aged 5–18 years (in Grades 1–12). Programmes implemented earlier in childhood were not examined, as they are the focus of other chapters in this volume. Interventions deemed effective had to affect the perpetration of physical aggression and violence. Although broader behavioural problems (e.g. conduct disorder or general delinquency) may co-occur with violence and/ or have similar causes, we restricted our assessment to aggression and violence because these behaviours are of great concern to the public and are the most likely to lead to long-term, detrimental outcomes for youth. We largely excluded interventions that assessed aggression and violence using instruments which combined violent and nonviolent acts, to avoid the findings being driven by the less serious offenses.

We also limited the review to evaluations utilizing a well-conducted quasi-experimental or true experimental design with at least one experimental and one comparison group and at least two waves of data (i.e. pretests and post-tests). Evaluations were reviewed to ensure that threats to internal validity were minimal; for example, that there was appropriate assignment of participants to conditions, baseline comparability, minimal and non-differential attrition, an intent-to-treat analysis approach, valid and reliable instruments to assess outcomes, and appropriate statistical techniques. Only programmes demonstrating statistically significant effects using two-tailed tests and a significance level of at least $p<0.05$ were identified as effective.

The primary method for obtaining relevant literature was to examine the bibliographies of programmes cited in aforementioned reviews. We also consulted lists of evidence-based programmes from the Blueprints for Healthy Youth Development database (www.blueprintsprogrammes.com), the Campbell and Cochrane databases (www.campbellcollaboration.org and www.cochrane.org), the Communities That Care Prevention Strategies Guide (www.communitiesthatcare.net), the Office of Justice Programmes (www.crimesolutions.gov), and the National Registry of Evidence-based Programmes and Practices (http:// www.nrepp.samhsa.gov/).

Intervention Effects on Violence

Table 20.1 lists the 11 programmes considered effective according to these criteria: seven which included school- and family-focused components and four which took place in the school and/or community. For each intervention, Table 20.1 provides a brief programme description and information regarding the evaluation design, population participating in the study(ies), and statistically significant ($p<0.05$) programme effects on aggression and violence.

All of the effective interventions included child-focused programming, which was delivered by teachers, counsellors, or police officers as classroom curricula, or by adult facilitators of individual or small-group tutoring or mentoring sessions. The focus and content of services varied widely, but most programmes sought to promote cognitive, emotional, and social competencies including self-efficacy, decision making, problem solving, self-control, emotional regulation (including anger management), and effective communication. Many also promoted bonding and/or relationship building. Child-focused interventions often attempted to reduce individual and peer risk factors related to violence, such as having attitudes supportive of violent behaviour and interacting with deviant peers. Programmes all involved multiple sessions, with the duration ranging from one school semester (e.g. D.A.R.E. Plus and SAFE Children) to multiple years (e.g. Fast Track). Three interventions (Coping Power, the Seattle Social Development Programme, and the Multisite Violence Prevention Programme) included intensive training for teachers that emphasized the need for proactive classroom management and interactive teaching strategies to engage students.

Seven interventions included services for parents, typically delivered to small groups of families, and sometimes through home visits. A focus on strengthening families is important because parents who are more emotionally attached to children should be more likely to reinforce the competencies achieved during child-focused services (Tolan et al. 2004). Thus, most programmes try to improve parental warmth and parenting competencies such as monitoring, supervision, and discipline of children, as well as parental involvement in school and/or support for children's academic success. A few required that youth participate in home visits or group sessions in order to work more directly on parent/child communication, family bonding, and family conflict.

As shown in the last column of Table 20.1, interventions varied in the number, strength, and duration of effects. For five interventions, effects were assessed at post-test only; in the other six studies, follow-up periods ranged from 6 months to 9 years. Small to moderate reductions in aggression and violence were evidenced across all programmes. Four interventions had effects only for subgroups of participants. In the SAFE Children evaluation (Tolan et al. 2004), positive intervention effects on aggression were found only among first graders who were classified at baseline as being from high-risk families (those displaying poor parenting practices) or as high-risk individuals (rated by teachers and parents as having elevated aggression, hyperactivity, and concentration problems). In the Metropolitan Area Child Study (MACS) (2002), at post-test, reductions in aggression were found only for those receiving the full intervention (individual, school, and parent programmes) and who attended schools in low-income but high-resource neighbourhoods; aggression was increased among students who attended schools in inner-city neighbourhoods characterized by greater social and economic deprivation. The Reach for Health Community Service Programme was delivered to students in Grades 7 and 8, as both a stand-alone curriculum and a combined school- and community-based intervention, but violence was reduced only among 8th graders in the combined intervention (O'Donnell et al. 1999). Finally, the D.A.R.E. Plus intervention, which included content related to both substance use and violence prevention (e.g. decreasing intentions to be violent and increasing school and community norms opposed to violence) demonstrated positive effects on self-reported violence for boys but not girls (Komro et al. 2004).

Two interventions showed iatrogenic effects, increasing aggression or violence for intervention compared to control groups. In the MACS (2002), at post-test, high-risk students in schools receiving individually focused services were rated as more aggressive than those in the control group; iatrogenic effects were not found for the other two experimental conditions (excepting the outcome previously noted for students in inner-city neighbourhoods). In the Multisite Violence Prevention Project (2009), according to some but not all outcome measures, iatrogenic effects were found at post-test and 2-year follow-up for those in schools assigned to the universal curriculum and at post-test for those receiving school and family programming.

These iatrogenic effects are difficult to explain since both interventions addressed risk and protective factors associated with violence. However, given that both studies included a mix of high-risk and lower risk youth, 'deviancy training' (Dishion et al. 1999; Gottfredson 2010) may have occurred, such that the higher risk students may have modelled aggressive behaviours and attitudes, encouraged others to participate in such behaviours, and reinforced them for doing so (Metropolitan Area Child Study Research Group 2002). Similar interactions have been observed in other studies, particularly when adult facilitators fail to adequately monitor students or respond to inappropriate behaviour (Gottfredson 2010). It could also be that children in the high-risk, high-crime neighbourhoods in which the two programmes were delivered received messages from parents and adults endorsing the use of violence (e.g. to encourage youth to protect themselves in risky situations), which could have undermined programme effectiveness (Metropolitan Area Child Study Research Group 2002).

Transportability of Programmes Nationally and Internationally

In order to realize substantial reductions in youth violence, effective interventions must be widely disseminated. Yet, there are challenges to doing so. The interventions identified as effective in this review were nearly all tested with high-risk populations, and it is unclear if they would be effective for universal populations. Empirical research suggests that lower and higher risk youth tend to be influenced by similar risk and protective factors (Tolan et al. 2004), which offers hope that results can be broadly generalized, but this hypothesis needs further testing. Secondly, prevention science is generally more developed in higher income countries (especially the United States, although there is growing interest in Europe) than lower and middle-income nations, perhaps due to differences in funding opportunities, advances in research methods, and philosophical differences regarding the advantages and feasibility of preventive approaches (Catalano et al. 2012). In fact, all but one programme listed in Table 20.1 was designed and tested in the U.S., and further evaluation studies are needed to identify effective violence programmes in other nations. This can include programmes developed by other countries or replication of U.S.-based prevention models in other areas. For example, the Promoting Alternative Thinking Strategies (PATHS) programme, a school-based curriculum implemented as part of the Fast Track intervention shown in Table 20.1, reduced child reports

of aggressive behaviour in a replication in Switzerland, though no changes were demonstrated according to parent or teacher reports (Malti et al. 2011). Such results offer hope that the models reviewed here could be successfully transported to other nations, but such efforts need to be evaluated.

No matter the context, implementation challenges are likely to arise when communities replicate effective programmes (Gottfredson and Gottfredson 2002), and implementation is especially important for the multiple-component interventions reviewed in this chapter. These more complex programmes require the engagement, coordination, and monitoring of services across numerous service providers and agencies who may have different capacities, needs, resources, and ideas about what is needed to prevent violence (Wandersman and Florin 2003). There are no easy solutions to these challenges, but they are critical to address, as better implementation fidelity has been associated with more positive participant outcomes across diverse interventions (Durlak and DuPre 2008).

Gaps in the Evidence

Although the field of prevention science has been rapidly progressing (Catalano et al. 2012), youth continue to engage in violence at high rates and to suffer consequences from this behaviour, and more development and testing of violence prevention programmes is needed. There is a particular need for models created and evaluated in nations other than the United States, as well as studies that examine the transportability of programmes to different contexts and populations. Such research should include evaluation of effects on subgroups; for example, testing differences in outcomes according to gender, race/ethnicity, nationality, and so on. Doing so will not only help assess the generalizability of programmes, but also indicate if interventions have iatrogenic effects for certain types of individuals, which can occur even if programmes are well designed, implemented, and evaluated.

It is encouraging that all but one programme reviewed in this chapter involved both males and females, and that several evaluated whether or not programme effects differed by gender. Traditionally, violence-related research has focused exclusively on males because males are overrepresented as violent offenders. Although the gender gap in violent offending is indisputable, it is less clear if the same factors influence male and female offending. Experimental research testing differences in programme effects across genders can help answer this question.

Additional research is also needed to assess mediating effects; that is, whether or not the skills and competencies (or risk and protective factors) targeted by the programme are attained and if these improvements are associated with programme outcomes. These analyses can inform our understanding of how and why interventions work, and identify mechanisms that lead to unintended or iatrogenic effects. Finally, many of the interventions reviewed in this chapter included multiple components, but few evaluations compared the relative effectiveness of these elements. More information about which strategies contribute to positive change is important for programme development and for implementation; if some parts of the programme are not critical to success, they should be eliminated or enhanced to avoid wasting resources.

Table 20.1 Positive youth development programmes with significant effects on aggression and violence

Intervention evaluation citation	Programme components	Study design (QED or RCT[1])	Sample description	Significant effects (OR, ES) [2]
School- and family-focused				
Fast Track Study 1: CPPRG (1999) Study 2: CPPRG (2010)	*Universal School Programme*: multiyear programme *Selective Parent Programme*: small-group sessions and home visits *Selective Individual Programme*: small-group sessions	RCT: 55 elementary schools in four U.S. cities	*Study 1: Universal*: N=6,715 1st graders *Study 2: Selective*: N=891 1st graders already displaying aggressive and oppositional behaviours	*Study 1 (posttest, Grade 1):* Less aggression according to peer nominations; ES=0.22 *Study 2 (2yr f/u; Grade 12):* –Decreased the number (OR=0.71) and onset of juvenile arrests (OR=0.77) –Reduced the onset of adult (to age 19) arrests for severe, violent offenses; OR=0.82
Montreal Longitudinal and Experimental Study Study 1: Tremblay et al. (1992) Study 2: Barker et al. (2010)	*School Programme*: 2-year, 19-session programme *Parent Programme*: 2 years of home or clinic visits	RCT: individuals in Montreal	*Selective*: N=172 1st-grade boys from low-income neighbourhoods identified as disruptive by teachers	*Study 1 (4yr f/u, Grade 6):* Reduced teacher-reported fighting; ES=0.37 *Study 2 (9yr f/u, Grade 11):* Reduced self-reported violence from ages 13–17; ES=0.38
SAFE Children Tolan et al. (2004)	*Tutoring*: 22-week programme *Family Programme*: 22 small-group sessions	RCT: families in Chicago	*Universal/selective*: N=424 1st graders in low-income neighbourhoods	*6mo f/u (Grade 1):* Reduced teacher+parent-reported aggression for high-risk children (ES=0.16) and children in high-risk families (ES=0.12) *No effects for the full sample
Linking the Interests of Families and Teachers (LIFT) Eddy et al. (2000) Reid et al. (1999)	*School Programme*: 20-session programme *Parent Programme*: 6 small-group sessions and parent/teacher discussions	RCT: 12 schools in the northwest U.S.	*Universal/Selective*: N=671 1st and 5th graders in schools in high-crime areas	*Posttest (Grades 1 and 5):* Decreased observed physical aggression; ES=0.20 *Stronger effects (ES=0.36–0.57) for students aggressive at baseline
Metropolitan Area Child Study (MACS) Metropolitan Area Child Study Research Group (2002)	*Universal School Programme*: 2-year programme *Selective Individual Programme*: 2-year small-group sessions to improve peer relations *Selective Parent Programme*: 22 small-group sessions	QED: 16 middle schools randomly assigned to: 1) E1: School only 2) E2: Individual only 3) E3: All programmes 4) Control	*Selective*: N=2,181 2nd and 5th graders identified as aggressive by teachers and peers	*Posttest (Grades 3 and 6):* E2 vs. C: Iatrogenic effect: Increased teacher+peer-reported aggression (ES=0.18) *No effects for E1 vs. C or E3 vs. C *E3 vs. C: decreased aggression for students in neighbourhoods with more resources; increased aggression in neighbourhoods with fewer resources
Coping Power Lochman et al. (2009)	*School Programme*: 2-year programme *Parent Programme*: 2-year small-group programme *Teacher Enhanced Programme*: intensive training and technical assistance	RCT: counsellors in 57 elementary schools randomized to: 1) E1 (Coping Power) 2) E2 (CP + Teacher Enhanced) 3) Control	*Selective*: N=531 4th graders rated as aggressive by teachers	*Posttest (Grade 5):* E2 vs. C: decreased self-reported minor assault; ES=0.18 E1 vs. C: no effects

Table 20.1 continued

Intervention evaluation citation	Programme components	Study design (QED or RCT[1])	Sample description	Significant effects (OR, ES) [2]
Seattle Social Development Project (SSDP) Hawkins et al. (1999)	*School Programme*: 1-year programme *Teacher Programme*: 6-year programme with 5 annual sessions to increase proactive classroom management and interactive teaching skills *Parent Programme*: Small-group sessions	QED: 18 elementary schools in Seattle non-randomly assigned to: 1) E1 (Full: teacher programme in Gr 1-6; child+parent programmes in Gr 1 and 6) 2) E2 (Late, Gr 5-6 only) 3) Control	*Universal/Selective*: N=643 elementary students in schools in high-risk neighbourhoods	*6yr f/u (Age 18)*: E1 vs. C: decreased self-reported violence; OR=0.63 E2 vs. C: no effects
Multisite Violence Prevention Programme MVPP (2009)	*Universal School Programme*: 20-session programme *Universal Teacher Programme*: 10 small-group sessions to improve proactive classroom management *Selective Family Programme*: 15 small-group sessions for parents of aggressive children	RCT: 37 middle schools in four U.S. cities randomized within site to: 1) E1: Universal (school + teacher) 2) E2: Selective (family programme) 3) E3: All programmes 4) Control	*Universal/Selective*: N=5,625 6th graders in schools with high rates of low-income families	*Posttest (Grade 6)*: Iatrogenic effects –E1 vs. C, E3 vs. C: increased student-reported aggression; ES=0.09 for each –E1 vs. C: increased teacher+student-reported aggression for girls only; ES=0.16 *2yr f/u (Grade 8)*: –E2 vs. C: less growth in teacher+student-reported violence (ES=0.05) –E1 vs. C: iatrogenic effect: smaller decrease in teacher-reported aggression (ES=0.06)
Community-based				
Baltimore City Youth Bureaus Hanlon et al. (2002)	*Child programme*: 1 year of individual counselling, group mentoring, and educational and recreational field trips	QED: 2 clinics in Baltimore serving youth engaging in experimental drug use or delinquency or expelled from school	*Selective*: N=428 African American teens (aged 9–17, mean age 13) from high-risk neighbourhoods	*Posttest*: Decreased self-reported violence; ES=0.30
Big Brothers Big Sisters Tierney et al. (1995)	*Child programme*: One-on-one mentoring provided by volunteer adults for at least 1 year	RCT: 8 agencies in 8 cities across the U.S.	*Selective*: N=1,107 teens (aged 10-16, mean age 12) from single-parent homes	*6mo f/u*: Decreased self-reported minor assaults: ES=0.13
Drug Abuse Resistance Education (D.A.R.E.) Plus Komro et al. (2004)	*School Programme (D.A.R.E.)*: 10-session curriculum taught by police officers *Community Programme (D.A.R.E. Plus)*: Adds 4 peer-led classroom sessions, postcards mailed to parents, student-planned afterschool activities, and coalition-planned neighbourhood activities	RCT: 24 middle schools randomized to: 1) E1 (D.A.R.E. only) 2) E2 (D.A.R.E. Plus) 3) Control	*Universal*: N=4,976 7th graders	*Posttest (Grade 8)*: E2 vs. C: decreased self-reported violence for boys only; ES=0.10 E1 vs. C: no effects
Reach for Health Community Service Programme O'Donnell et al. (1999)	*School Programme*: 1-year, 35-session programme *Community Youth Service Programme*: 3 hours per week of community service activities	QED: 2 urban middle schools in New York City assigned: 1) E1: School only 2) E2: School+ community 3) E3: Control	*Selective*: N=914 7th–8th graders, 80% African American	*6mo f/u*: E2 vs. C: Decreased self-reported violence for 8th graders only: ES=0.46 E1 vs. C: no effects

[1] QED=Quasi-experimental research design; RCT=Randomized control trial.

[2] OR=Odds Ratio (reported for dichotomous outcomes); ES=Effect Size (reported for continuous outcomes).

Conclusion

It is encouraging that positive youth development programmes which impact youth aggression and violence are available for communities to implement. Because not all risk and protective factors for violence have been addressed, few programmes have been tested outside of schools, and few programmes have been tested outside the United States; more models are needed if youth violence is to be significantly reduced internationally. Our identification of these model programmes was based on a rigorous review of available evidence, and less stringent criteria might have identified an increased number of effective interventions. We advise caution, however, in promoting programmes that have not been evaluated using strong research designs, because design problems can lead to over- or underestimation of positive outcomes. Communities have limited resources, and efforts should be reserved for models that are most likely to lead to significant and meaningful reductions in violence. The programmes cited in this review have such evidence, but additional research is needed to expand this list.

References

Barker, E. D., Vitaro, F., and Lacourse, E., et al. (2010). Testing the developmental distinctiveness of male proactive and reactive aggression with a nested longitudinal experimental intervention. *Aggressive Behavior*, 36, 127–40.

Bronfenbrenner, U. (2005). *Making Human Beings Human: Bioecological Perspectives on Human Development*. Thousand Oaks, CA: Sage Publications.

Catalano, R. F., Berglund, L., Ryan, J. A. M., Lonczak, H. S., and Hawkins, J. D. (2004). Positive youth development in the United States: Research findings on evaluations of positive youth development programmes. *Annals of the American Academy of Political and Social Science*, 591, 98–124.

Catalano, R. F., Fagan, A. A., and Gavin, L. E., et al. (2012). Worldwide application of prevention science in adolescent health. *Lancet*, 379, 1653–64.

Catalano, R. F., Haggerty, K. P., Hawkins, J. D., and Elgin, J. (2011). Prevention of substance use and substance use disorders: the role of risk and protective factors. In: Y. Kaminer and K. C. Winters (eds), *Clinical Manual of Adolescent Substance Abuse Treatment*. Washington, D.C.: American Psychiatric Publishing, pp. 25–63.

Catalano, R. F., Hawkins, J. D., and Toumbourou, J. W. (2008). Positive youth development in the United States: History, efficacy, and links to moral and character education. In: L. P. Nucci, and D. Narvaez (eds), *Handbook of Moral and Character Education*. New York: Routledge, pp. 459–83.

Coie, J. D., Watt, N. F., and West, S. G., et al. (1993). The science of prevention: a conceptual framework and some directions for a national research programme. *American Psychologist*, 48, 1013–22.

Conduct Problems Prevention Research Group (1999). Initial impact of the Fast Track Prevention Trial for conduct problems: II. Classroom effects. *Journal of Consulting and Clinical Psychology*, 67, 648–57.

Conduct Problems Prevention Research Group (2010). Fast Track intervention effects on youth arrests and delinquency. *Journal of Experimental Criminology*, 6, 131–57.

Dishion, T. J., Mccord, J., and Poulin, F. (1999). When interventions do harm: peer groups and problem behavior. *American Psychologist*, 54, 755–64.

Durlak, J. A., and Dupre, E. P. (2008). Implementation matters: a review of the research on the influence of implementation on programme outcomes and the factors affecting implementation. *American Journal of Community Psychology*, 41, 327–50.

Durlak, J. A., Dymnicki, A. B., Taylor, R. D., Weissberg, R. P., and Schellinger, K. B. (2011). The impact of enhancing students' social and emotional learning: a meta-analysis of school-based universal interventions. *Child Development*, 82, 405–32.

Durlak, J., Weissberg, R. P., and Pachan, M. (2010). A meta-analysis of after-school programmes that seek to promote personal and social skills in children and adolescents. *American Journal of Community Psychology*, 45, 294–309.

Eddy, J. M., Reid, J. B., and Fetrow, R. A. (2000). An elementary school-based prevention programme targeting modifiable antecedents of youth violence and delinquency: Linking the Interests of Families and Teachers (LIFT). *Journal of Emotional and Behavioral Disorders*, 8, 165–76.

Elliott, D. S. (1994). Serious violent offenders: onset, developmental course, and termination. The American Society of Criminology 1993 Presidential Address. *Criminology*, 32, 1–21.

Gavin, L. E., Catalano, R. F., David-Ferdon, C., Gloppen, K. M., and Markham, C. M. (2010). A review of positive youth development programmes that promote adolescent sexual and reproductive health. *Journal of Adolescent Health*, 46, S75–S91.

Gottfredson, D. C. (2010). Deviancy training: understanding how preventive interventions harm: The Academy of Experimental Criminology 2009 Joan McCord Award Lecture. *Journal of Experimental Criminology*, 6, 229–43.

Gottfredson, D. C., and Gottfredson, G. D. (2002). Quality of school-based prevention programmes: results from a national survey. *Journal of Research in Crime and Delinquency*, 39, 3–35.

Hahn, R., Fuqua-Whitley, D., and Wethington, H., et al. (2007). Effectiveness of universal school-based programmes to prevent violence and aggressive behavior: a systematic review. *American Journal of Preventive Medicine*, 33, S114–S129.

Hanlon, T. E., Bateman, R. W., Simon, B. D., O'grady, K. E., and Carswell, S. B. (2002). An early community-based intervention for the prevention of substance abuse and other delinquent behavior. *Journal of Youth and Adolescence*, 31, 459–71.

Hawkins, J. D., Catalano, R. F., Kosterman, R., Abbott, R. D., and Hill, K. G. (1999). Preventing adolescent health-risk behaviors by strengthening protection during childhood. *Archives of Pediatric and Adolescent Medicine*, 153, 226–34.

Hawkins, J. D., Catalano, R. F., and Miller, J. Y. (1992). Risk and protective factors for alcohol and other drug problems in adolescence and early adulthood: implications for substance abuse prevention. *Psychological Bulletin*, 112, 64–105.

Herrenkohl, T. I., Maguin, E., and Hill, K. G. et al. (2000). Developmental risk factors for youth violence. *Journal of Adolescent Health*, 26, 176–86.

Komro, K., Perry, C. L., and Veblen-Mortenson, S. et al. (2004). Violence-related outcomes of the DARE Plus Project. *Health Education and Behavior*, 31, 335–54.

Lochman, J. E., Boxmeyer, C., and Powell, N. et al. (2009). Dissemination of the Coping Power programme: importance of intensity of counselor training. *Journal of Consulting and Clinical Psychology*, 77, 397–409.

Malti, T., Ribeaud, D., and Eisner, M. P. (2011). The effectiveness of two universal preventive interventions in reducing children's externalizing behavior: a cluster randomized controlled trial. *Journal of Clinical Child and Adolescent Psychology*, 40, 677–92.

Metropolitan Area Child Study Research Group (2002). A cognitive-ecological approach to preventing aggression in urban settings: initial outcomes for high-risk children. *Journal of Consulting and Clinical Psychology*, 70, 179–94.

Moffitt, T. E. (1993). Adolescence-limited and life-course persistent anti-social behavior: a developmental taxonomy. *Psychological Review*, 100, 674–701.

O'Connell, M. E., Boat, T., and Warner, K. E. (2009). *Preventing Mental, Emotional, and Behavioral Disorders among Young People: Progress and Possibilities*, Washington, D.C.: National Academies Press.

O'Donnell, L., Stueve, A., and San Doval, A. et al. (1999). Violence prevention and young adolescents' participation in community youth service. *Journal of Adolescent Health*, 24, 28–37.

Reid, J. B., Eddy, J. M., Fetrow, R. A., and Stoolmiller, M. (1999). Description and immediate impacts of a preventive intervention for conduct problems. *American Journal of Community Psychology*, 27, 483–517.

Roth, J. L., and Brooks-Gunn, J. (2003). Youth development programmes: risk, prevention and policy. *Journal of Adolescent Health*, 32, 170–82.

The Multisite Violence Prevention Project (2009). The ecological effects of universal and selective violence prevention programmes for middle school students: a randomized trial. *Journal of Consulting and Clinical Psychology*, 77, 526–42.

Tierney, J. P., Grossman, J. B., and Resch, N. L. (1995). *Making a Difference: An Impact Study of Big Brothers/Big Sisters*. Philadelphia: Public/Private Ventures.

Tolan, P. H., Gorman-Smith, D., and Henry, D. B. (2004). Supporting families in a high-risk setting: proximal effects of the SAFEChildren preventive intervention. *Journal of Consulting and Clinical Psychology*, 72, 855–69.

Tremblay, R., Vitaro, F., and Bertrand, L. et al. (1992). Parent and child training to prevent early onset of delinquency: The Montreal Longitudinal-Experimental Study. In: J. Mccord, and R. Tremblay (eds), *Preventing Antisocial Behavior: Interventions from Birth through Adolescence*. New York: Guilford, pp. 117–38.

Wagenaar, A. C., and Perry, C. L. (1994). Community strategies for the reduction of youth drinking: theory and application. *Journal of Research on Adolescence*, 4, 319–45.

Wandersman, A., and Florin, P. (2003). Community intervention and effective prevention. *American Psychologist*, 58, 441–8.

Weissberg, R. P., and Greenberg, M. T. (1998). School and community competence-enhancement and prevention programmes. In: I. E. Siegel, and K. A. Renninger (eds), *Handbook of Child Psychology. Vol 4: Child Psychology in Practice*. New York: Wiley, pp. 877–954.

CHAPTER 21

Preventing youth violence and bullying through social–emotional school-based prevention programmes and frameworks

Dorothy L. Espelage

Introduction to School-Based Prevention Programmes

School violence is a subset of youth violence and a broad public health problem (Centers for Disease Control 2010). Youth violence occurs between the ages of 10 and 24 years and is defined as the intentional use of physical force or power, against another person or group with the behaviour likely to cause physical or psychological harm (Centers for Disease Control 2010). Youth violence can include verbal and physical aggression, threatening, and intimidating behaviours that are associated with short- and long-term adverse academic and psychological outcomes for perpetrators and victims (Cook et al. 2010; Espelage et al. 2013; Low et al. 2013). Bullying is a subtype of aggressive behaviour among students that is repetitive and occurs among students of unequal power (Espelage 2012).

School-Based Social–Emotional Violence Prevention Approaches

Despite the personal and societal costs of youth aggression involvement and associated correlates, the efficacy of school violence and bullying prevention programmes have varied across countries and contexts (Espelage 2012; Ttofi and Farrington 2011). More recently, there has been an increase in bullying prevention/intervention programmes; however, their efficacy varies tremendously across contexts and programme effects are often modest (Ttofi and Farrington 2011) or have produced mixed results (Pearce et al. 2011). Two meta-analyses found that effects were non-existent or too small to be practically helpful (Merrell et al. 2008; Smith et al. 2004). A third found that programmes reduced bullying in non-U.S. countries but effects for U.S. studies were significantly lower (Ttofi and Farrington 2011). Programmes producing the greatest reductions in bullying consistently carve out class time to discuss bullying, improve disciplinary practices, but also include cooperative group work among students and opportunities for students to learn and practice social emotional learning

skills that would prevent aggression and manage conflicts (e.g. Ttofi and Farrington 2011).

In contrast, school-based violence prevention programmes that facilitate social and emotional learning skills, address interpersonal conflict, and teach emotion management have been very successful in reducing youth violence and disruptive behaviours in classrooms (Wilson and Lipsey 2007). Many of these social–emotional and social–cognitive intervention programmes target risk and promotive factors that have consistently been associated with aggression, bullying, and violence in cross-sectional and longitudinal studies (Basile et al. 2009; Espelage et al. 2003, 2011), including anger, empathy, perspective taking, respect for diversity, attitudes supportive of aggression, coping, intentions to intervene to help others, and communication and problem-solving skills.

In general, social emotional learning (SEL) involves the development of skills including self-awareness, social awareness, self-regulation, responsible decision-making, problem-solving, and relationship skills (Collaborative for Academic, Social, and Emotional Learning (CASEL) 2003). SEL programmes can provide schools, after-school programmes, and youth community centres with a research-based approach to building skills and promoting positive individual and peer attitudes that can contribute to the prevention of bullying. Although this chapter will focus on SEL programmes situated in schools, these programmes or frameworks are also being developed and implemented in settings outside of schools (see www.casel.org for a review).

A social emotional learning approach has emerged as a way to prevent many school-based problems. Social emotional learning as a framework emerged from influences across different movements that focused on resiliency and teaching social and emotional competencies to children and adolescents (Elias et al. 1997). SEL programmes use social skill instruction to address behaviour, discipline, safety, and academics to help youth become self-aware, manage their emotions, build social skills (empathy, perspective-taking, respect for diversity), friendship skill building, and make positive decisions (Zins et al. 2004). Recently, a study of more than 213 SEL-based programmes found that if a school implements a quality SEL curriculum, they can expect better student behaviour and an 11 percentile increase in academic test scores (Durlak et al. 2011). Schools elect to implement these programmes because of the gains that schools see in achievement and prosocial behaviour. Students exposed to SEL activities feel safer and more connected to school and academics, and SEL programmes build work habits in addition to social skills, and children and teachers build strong relationships (Zins et al. 2004).

It is not surprising that SEL approaches to prevention are yielding significant reductions in problematic behaviour given its rich developmental history. Social–emotional learning is a framework that was introduced at a 1994 convening of researchers, educators, and child advocates who were concerned that prevention and health promotion efforts were producing null results (Elias et al. 1997). These individuals explored efforts to enhance positive youth development, to promote social competence and emotional intelligence, to develop effective drug education, violence prevention, health promotion, character education, service learning, civic education, school reform, and school family–community partnerships. They believed that, unlike the many prevention programmes that targeted one specific problem, SEL programming addresses underlying causes of problem behaviour while supporting academic achievement. Thus, SEL approaches and programmes are based on many well-established theories including theories of emotional intelligence, social and emotional competence promotion, social developmental model, social information processing, and self-management. In addition, behaviour change and learning theories also informed the SEL framework, such as the health belief model, the theory of reasoned action, problem behaviour theory, and social–cognitive theory (e.g. Greenberg et al. 2003; Hawkins et al. 2004).

The Collaborative for Academic, Social, and Emotional Learning (CASEL) also emerged from this meeting with the goal of establishing high-quality, evidence-based SEL as an essential part of preschool through high school education (see www.casel.org). School-based SEL programmes developed to prevent school violence, including bullying, are predicated on the belief that academic skills are intrinsically linked to children's ability to manage emotions, regulate emotions, and to communicate and problem-solve challenges and interpersonal conflicts (Durlak et al. 2011). A SEL framework includes five interrelated skill areas: self-awareness, social awareness, self-management and organization, responsible problem-solving, and relationship management. Within each area, there are specific competencies supported by research and practice as essential for effective social–emotional functioning including emotion recognition, stress-management, empathy, problem-solving, or decision-making skills (Elias et al. 1997). Self-regulated learning is both directly and indirectly targeted in these programmes. As students are better able to control their feelings, thoughts, and actions, especially under emotional demands (i.e. cognitive complexity), academic learning is optimized. Further, exercises and opportunities to practice these skills and competences differ in their level of cognitive-emotional complexity across development in order to ensure SEL skills are sustainable.

In summary, social–emotional learning approaches to prevention are showing promise in reducing aggression and promoting prosocial behaviour (Brown et al. 2011; Espelage et al. 2013; Frey et al. 2005). This success is largely because SEL school-based programmes parallel the hallmarks of the prevention science framework. First, these programmes draw from the scientific literature on the etiological underpinnings of aggression, bullying, school violence, and other problematic behaviours among children and adolescents (Merrell 2010). Second, risk (e.g. anger, impulse control) and promotive (e.g. empathy, communication skills) factors are identified from the etiological literature and targeted through direct instruction of skills and opportunities to use skills in different contexts. Third, in relation to bystander intervention, these programmes include discussions and content about the barriers or challenges (e.g. fear of being targeted, losing friends) that youth face when they attempt to intervene on behalf of a victim of aggression. Several randomized clinical trials (RCTs) have attended to the rigorous evaluation of the intervention effects (Brown et al. 2011; Espelage et al. 2014), which is an additional hallmark of prevention science. RCTs of SEL programmes have identified implementation as critical components of producing reductions in aggression and increases in prosocial behaviour, but as the field moves forward a more deliberate focus on implementation, dissemination, and sustainability is needed in order to fully capture the prevention science impact of SEL programmes. As schools are increasingly pressed to find time in the day to address psychosocial issues, SEL programmes that prevent victimization and its correlates (e.g. social rejection) and also simultaneously improve academic engagement should be rigorously evaluated to make convincing arguments to teachers and school administrators that the use of these resources will produce noticeable benefits. Next, several school-based programmes with strong efficacy data are highlighted. These represent only a small sample of those programmes or approaches that are available to schools and communities (see www.casel.org for reviews of SEL programming).

Evidence Based School-Based Sel Programmes

Steps to Respect: A Bullying Prevention Programme

Steps to Respect: A Bullying Prevention Programme is designed to help students build supportive relationships with one another (Committee for Children 2001). The Steps to Respect programme promotes a whole-school primary- and secondary-level approach to bullying prevention by addressing factors at four levels: school staff, peer group, individual child, and family. Intervening at multiple levels, the programme developers believe, is the most effective way to reduce school bullying. Empirical support has shown reductions in playground bullying, acceptance of bullying behaviour, and argumentative behaviour. At the same time, it has demonstrated increases in agreeable interactions and perceived adult responsiveness in comparison with control schools (Frey et al. 2005) More recently, it has demonstrated reductions in observed aggression and destructive bystander behaviour, and higher teacher ratings of peer social skills (Brown et al. 2011; Hirschtein and Frey 2006). Steps to Respect relies heavily on adults to deliver scripted training from a curriculum and to continually emphasize those lessons throughout the school year. The Steps to Respect prevention programme is specifically respected for its well-established empirical support.

Primary bullying prevention strategies address risk factors from a systemic perspective that will influence the maximum number of students. Knowing that primary-level interventions have the potential to reach approximately 80 per cent of students in a school encourages school officials and stakeholders to invest time and effort into these systemic efforts (Walker and Shinn 2002). For example, the first component of the Steps to Respect programme is staff training for 'all adults' in the school building, emphasizing that the term includes janitors, bus drivers, mentors, receptionists, school nurses, volunteers, licensed staff, administrators, teachers, assistants, and other adults at school who are involved in the daily lives of students. Training meetings include a scripted training session that provides basic information on the Steps to Respect programme, information on bullying, and training on how to receive bullying reports from students. Administrators, teachers, or counsellors who will work directly with students who have been bullied or who are bullying others receive additional training.

The Steps to Respect curriculum includes lessons to increase students' social–emotional competence and positive social values. Specifically, the programme addresses three general skills: First, students learn skills of perspective-taking and empathy as well as how to manage their emotions. Second, academic skills are also encouraged by incorporating themes of friendship and bullying into literature unit activities such as oral expression, writing composition, and analytical reasoning. Third, the curriculum addresses students' social values by encouraging students' sense of fairness, and attempts to instil a desire for rewarding friendships. Frey and colleagues demonstrated (2005) a 25 per cent reduction in playground bullying incidents, compared with a control group, and a decrease in bystanders to bullying episodes who encouraged it. Furthermore, the effects of the Steps to Respect programme were most pronounced among students who were observed to do the most bullying before programme implementation. Another study's results included less observed victimization of all children who had previously been victimized and less destructive bystander behaviour among all children who had previously been observed contributing to bullying as bystanders (Hirschstein et al. 2007). In a more recent randomized clinical trial, evaluation of Steps to Respect in 33 California schools indicated that participation in a SEL bully prevention programme was associated with higher social skills, reductions in aggression, and reductions in bystanders assisting the bully among elementary school children (3rd–6th graders) (Brown et al. 2011).

Second Step: Student Success through Prevention

Second Step: Student Success through Prevention (Second Step—SSTP; Committee for Children 2008) is the middle school version of the K-8th grade Second Step Programme curriculum. Second Step is a social–emotional learning programme that also focuses on bullying prevention, sexual harassment, bullying in dating relationships, and substance abuse prevention. In 2008, the Second Step curriculum for grades 6–8 was revised to include a focus on sexual harassment, bullying in dating relationships, and substance abuse prevention. The only randomized controlled trial of this revised version is in its third and final year of evaluation across 36 multi-ethnic middle schools in Illinois and Kansas involving approximately 3,600 students. Participating students just recently completed the 8th grade curriculum (last year of 6th- 8th grade curriculum), and the last data collection is underway; the students

will transition to high school in the fall of 2013. Initial results indicated that students in the intervention group, as compared to controls, were 42 per cent less likely to report physical fights after 1 year of the 15-week 6th grade curriculum (Espelage et al. 2013).

Promoting Alternative Thinking Strategies

Promoting Alternative Thinking Strategies (PATHS; Kusche and Greenberg 1994). The PATHS programme, designed for children in kindergarten through 6th grade, was designated a Blueprints model programme by the Office of Juvenile Justice and Delinquency Prevention. Following the universal prevention model, PATHS was developed to integrate into existing curricula. Goals of the programme include enhancing social and emotional competence and reducing aggression. Some programme components are targeted at parents, but most are delivered by classroom teachers who are initially trained by PATHS project staff. Several randomized trials of PATHS have indicated positive outcomes including a reduction in aggressive solutions to problems and increases in prosocial behaviours (Greenberg et al. 1998, 2003).

KiVa National Anti-Bullying Programme in Finland

The KiVa programme, developed in Finland for elementary through high school students, is a universal school-based programme that addresses bullying at school by working with teachers, parents, families, community leaders, and students. Teacher training, student lessons, and virtual learning environments are all crucial aspects of this multi-component programme (Salmivalli et al. 2009a,b). Teachers use a manual for classroom instruction, which is supplemented by an anti-bullying computer game for primary school children and an internet forum—'KiVa Street'—for secondary school students. On KiVa Street students can access information pertaining to bullying or watch a short film about bullying. Both are designed to motivate students to apply learned skills. Early data show significant decreases in self-reported bullying and self- and peer-reported victimization in 4th–6th graders (Kärnä et al. 2011), and increases in empathy and anti-bullying attitudes.

Three-Tier Approach to School-Based Prevention

In terms of school-wide primary prevention efforts, SEL programmes are often implemented in tandem with a 'foundation' or 'behaviourally focused' school-wide comprehensive three-tiered model of prevention that encompasses academic, behavioural, and social components (Walker and Shinn 2002). In this three-tier approach, primary prevention strategies (those sometimes referred to as universal programmes, skills training, coping skills like SEL programmes) focus on 80 per cent of students of a school population that do not have serious behaviour problems. Secondary intervention strategies such as mentoring programmes target the 5–15 per cent of students in a school that are at risk for behaviour problems. Tertiary strategies (e.g. wraparound services) are directed at the 1–7 per cent of the student population that has intense and chronic problems.

Positive Behaviour Intervention and Supports

Positive Behaviour Intervention and Supports (PBIS) is a dominant paradigm in schools internationally and is currently being evaluated in over 9,000 U.S. schools and 40 U.S. states, and recently added several bully-related lessons to the curriculum. PBIS emerged as a result of the 1997 reauthorization of the Individuals with Disabilities Education Act (IDEA) and resulted in the National Centre on Positive Behavioural Interventions and Supports being formed at the University of Oregon. PBIS is used interchangeably with School-Wide Positive Behaviour Supports (SWPBS) and is based on principles of applied behaviour analysis and the prevention approach of positive behaviour support (Lewis and Sugai 1999; Sugai and Horner 2002; Sugai et al. 2000).

PBIS offers a primary, secondary, and tertiary level of intervention (Sugai and Horner 2002). A basic tenet of the PBIS approach includes identifying students in one of the three categories based on risk for behaviour problems. Interventions are specifically developed for each of these levels with the goal of reducing the risk for academic or social failure. Primary prevention strategies include effective teaching practices, evidence-based curricula, and explicit and direct instruction of appropriate behaviour within the school context. Other strategies focus on creating environmental contingencies that promote reinforcement of appropriate behaviour, where students are corrected at the first sign of inappropriate behaviour by all adults in the school in a consistent manner.

The primary prevention component of this approach involves faculty and staff establishing behavioural expectations (e.g. respect, responsibility, and best effort) and providing specific illustrations for all key settings in a school, e.g. classrooms, hallways, cafeterias, and playgrounds (Sugai and Horner, 2002). Ideally, these would be formulated with input from the parent community, with a goal of establishing culturally responsive expectations that are clearly understood by all parties. These expectations are then taught to all students and staff, providing students opportunities to practice and to be reinforced for meeting these expectations. When a student demonstrates that he or she has met a given expectation, an adult will intermittently reinforce the student by handing them a positive behaviour support (PBS) ticket paired with behaviour-specific praise. Students deposit the PBS tickets they receive into boxes strategically located throughout the school (e.g. in classrooms, the library, hallways) for access to prize drawings, assemblies, and other reinforcing activities (Sugai and Horner 2002).

In addition to these proactive components, schools also need to have a clearly articulated plan for responding to students who violate behavioural expectations. Specifically, faculty and staff need to establish and to implement consequences consistently for students who demonstrate major and minor rule infractions. The established consequences should be reasonable, feasible, and proportional. Teachers need to deliver the consequences—which need to be appropriate to the magnitude of the infraction—easily, without unnecessary interruption of instructional activities.

Minor and major infractions need to be delineated and operationally defined so that all parties are clear as to what constitutes each type of infraction. Then, the faculty and staff need to specify the procedures for responding to the various violations. The key is consistency—making sure consequences are allocated uniformly (Sugai and Horner 2002).

Several RCT evaluations of school-wide PBIS in elementary schools have shown that high-quality implementation of the model is associated with significant reductions in office discipline referrals and suspensions (Bradshaw et al. 2010; Horner et al. 2009) and teacher ratings of classroom behaviour problems and aggression, emotion regulation problems, bullying perpetration, and peer rejection (Bradshaw et al. 2010).

Conclusions

Youth violence continues to be a public health concern all over the world. Prevention of youth violence will require interventions at all levels of the social ecology, including working within families, communities, and schools. School-based interventions are becoming increasingly difficult to implement and to evaluate given the primary focus on academic test scores. Thus, it is critical to develop school-based programmes/frameworks that not only prevent and reduce youth violence, but also promote academic engagement and ultimately lead to better academic performance such as improved grades and scores on standardized tests. To this end, social–emotional learning approaches offer schools the ability to simultaneously minimize the risk factors associated with aggression, bullying, and other forms of violence and maximize the promotive factors that lead to greater prosocial, caring behaviours, and improved academic performance.

Of note, the majority of the programmes included in this review produced reductions in aggression, bullying, and victimization among elementary and middle school samples, but recent research indicates that the effect sizes among older adolescents are negligible (Yeager et al. in press). Yeager and colleagues caution against transporting programmes developed with children and young adolescents to older adolescents until more thought is given to the unique ways in which violence prevention messages are received by adolescents who are emerging adults. In addition to understanding transportability of programmes across age groups, much more attention needs to be paid to transporting of programmes across diverse contexts and cultures. Finally, programmes can only be effective if they are implemented with fidelity. Research needs to be conducted to determine how best to promote implementation integrity and sustainability over time.

References

Basile, K. C., Espelage, D. L., Rivers, I., McMahon, P. M., and Simon, T. R. (2009). The theoretical and empirical links between bullying behavior and male sexual violence perpetration. *Aggression and Violent Behavior*, 14, 336–47.

Bradshaw, C. P., Mitchell, M. M., and Leaf, P. J. (2010). Examining the effects of School-Wide Positive Behavioral Interventions and Supports on student outcomes: results from a randomized controlled effectiveness trial in elementary schools. *Journal of Positive Behavior Interventions*, 12, 133–48.

Brown, E. C., Low, S., Smith, B. H., and Haggerty, K. P. (2011). Outcomes from a school-randomized controlled trial of STEPS to RESPECT: a bullying prevention programme. *School Psychology Review*, 40, 423–43.

Centers for Disease Control and Prevention, National Center for Injury Prevention and Control. (2010). *Web-based Injury Statistics Query and Reporting System (WISQARS)*. Available at: www.cdc.gov/injury/wisqars/index.html [Accessed 14 June 2010].

Collaborative for Academic, Social, and Emotional Learning (CASEL). (2003). *Safe and Sound: An Educational Leader's Guide to Evidence Based Social and Emotional Learning (SEL) Programmes*. Chicago: CASEL.

Committee for Children. (2001). *Steps to Respect: A Bullying Prevention Programme*. Seattle: Committee for Children.

Committee for Children. (2008). *Second Step: Student Success through Prevention Programme*. Seattle: Committee for Children.

Cook, C. R., Williams, K. R., Guerra, N. G., Kim, T. E., and Sadek, S. (2010). Predictors of bullying and victimization in childhood and adolescence: a meta-analytic investigation. *School Psychology Quarterly*, 25, 65–83.

Durlak, J. A., Weissberg, R. P., Dymnicki, A. B., Taylor, R. D., and Schellinger, K. B. (2011). The impact of enhancing students' social and emotional learning: a meta-analysis of school-based universal interventions. *Child Development*, 82, 405–32.

Elias, M. J., Zins, J. E., and Weissberg, K. S. et al. (1997). *Promoting Social and Emotional Learning: Guidelines for Educators*. Alexandria, VA: Association for Supervision and Curriculum Development.

Espelage, D. L. (2012). Bullying prevention: a research dialogue with Dorothy Espelage. *Prevention Researcher*, 19, 17–9.

Espelage, D. L., Green, H., and Polanin, J. (2011). Willingness to intervene in bullying episodes among middle school students: individual and peer-group influences. *The Journal of Early Adolescence*, 32, 776–801.

Espelage, D. L., Holt, M. K., and Henkel, R. R. (2003). Examination of peer-group contextual effects on aggression during early adolescence. *Child Development*, 74, 205–20.

Espelage, D. L., Low, S., and De La Rue, L. (2012). Relations between peer victimization subtypes, family violence, and psychological outcomes during adolescence. *Psychology of Violence*, 2, 313–24.

Espelage, D. L., Low, S., Polanin, J., and Brown, E. (2013). The impact of a middle school programme to reduce aggression, victimization, and sexual violence. *Journal of Adolescent Health*, 53, 180–6.

Espelage, D. L., Low, S., Rao, M. A., Hong, J. S., and Little, T. D. (2014). Family violence, bullying, fighting, and substance use among adolescents: a longitudinal transactional model. *Journal of Research on Adolescence*, 24, 337–349. doi: 10.1111/jora.12060

Frey, K. S., Hirschstein, M. K., Snell, J. L., Edstrom, L. V., MacKenzie, E. P., and Broderick, C. J. (2005). Reducing playground bullying and supporting beliefs: an experimental trial of the *Steps to Respect* programme. *Developmental Psychology*, 41, 479–91.

Greenberg, M. T., Kusché, C., and Mihalic, S. F. (1998). *Blueprints for Violence Prevention, Book Ten: Promoting Alternative Thinking Strategies (PATHS)*. Boulder, CO: Center for the Study and Prevention of Violence.

Greenberg, M. T., Weissberg, R. P., and O'Brien, M. U. et al. (2003). Enhancing school-based prevention and youth development through coordinated social, emotional, and academic learning. American Psychologist, 58, 466–74.

Hawkins, J. D., Smith, B. H., and Catalano, R. F. (2004). Social development and social and emotional learning. In: J. E. Zins, R. P. Weissberg, M. C. Wang, and H. J. Walberg (eds), *Building Academic Success on Social and Emotional Learning: What Does the Research Say?* New York: Teachers College Press, pp. 135–50.

Hirschstein, M. K., Edstrom, L. V. S., Frey, K. S., Snell, J. L., and MacKenzie, E. P. (2007). Walking the talk in bullying prevention: teacher implementation variables related to initial impact of the Steps to Respect programme. *School Psychology Review*, 36, 3–21.

Hirschstein, M. K., and Frey, K. S. (2006). Promoting behavior and beliefs that reduce bullying: the Steps to Respect programme. In: S. Jimerson, and M. Furlong (eds), *The Handbook of School Violence and School Safety: From Research to Practice* Mahwah, NJ: Erlbaum, pp. 309–23.

Horner, R. H., Sugai, G., and Smolkowski, K. et al. (2009). A randomized, wait-list controlled effectiveness trial assessing school-wide positive behavior support in elementary schools. *Journal of Positive Behavior Interventions*, 11, 133–44.

Kärnä, Voeten, M., Little, T. D., Poskiparta, E., Kaljonen, A., and Salmivalli, A. (2011). A large-scale evaluation of the KiVa Antibullying Programme: grades 4-6. *Child Development*, 82, 311–30.

Kusche, C. A., and Greenberg, M. T. (1994). *The PATHS Curriculum*. South Deerfield, MA: Channing-Bete Co.

Lewis, T. J., and Sugai, G. (1999). Effective behavior support: a systems approach to proactive school-wide management. *Focus on Exceptional Children*, 31, 1–24.

Low, S., Polanin, J. R., and Espelage, D. L. (2013). The role of social networks in physical and relational aggression among young adolescents. *Journal of Youth and Adolescence* 42, 1078–89.

Merrell, K. W. (2010). Linking prevention science and social and emotional learning: the Oregon Resiliency project. *Psychology in the Schools*, 47, 55–70.

Merrell, K. W., Gueldner, B. A., Ross, S. W., and Isava, D. M. (2008). How effective are school bullying intervention programmes? A meta-analysis of intervention research. *School Psychology Quarterly*, 23, 26–42.

Pearce, N., Cross, D., Monks, H., Waters, S., Falconer, S. (2011). Current evidence of best practice in whole-school bullying intervention and its potential to inform cyberbullying interventions. *Australian Journal of Guidance Counselling*, 21, 1–21.

Salmivalli, C., Poskiparta, E., Tikka, A., and Pöyhönen, V. (2009a). KiVa: teacher's guide, unit 1. *Research into Practice Publication Series, No. 2*. Turku, Finland: University of Turka, Psychology Department.

Salmaivalli, C., Pöyhönen, V., and Kaukiainen, A. (2009b). KiVa: teacher's guide, unit 2. *Research into Practice Publication Series, No. 3*. Turku, Finland: University of Turka, Psychology Department.

Smith, J. D., Schneider, B. H., Smith, P. K., and Ananiadou, K. (2004). The effectiveness of whole-school antibullying programmes: a synthesis of evaluation research. *School Psychology Review*, 33, 548–61.

Sugai, G., and Horner, R. H. (2002). The evolution of discipline practices: school-wide positive behavior supports. *Child and Family Behavior Therapy*, 24, 23–50.

Sugai, G., Horner, R. H., and Dunlap, G. et al. (2000). Applying positive behavioral support and functional behavioral assessment in schools. *Journal of Positive Behavioral Interventions*, 2, 131–43.

Ttofi, M. M., and Farrington, D. P. (2011). Effectiveness of school based programmes to reduce bullying: a systematic and meta-analytic review. *Journal of Experimental Criminology*, 7, 27–56.

Walker, H. M., and Shinn, M. R. (2002). Structuring school-based interventions to achieve integrated primary, secondary, and tertiary prevention goals for safe and effective schools. In: M. R. Shinn, G. Stoner, and H. M. Walker (eds), *Interventions for Academic and Behavior Problems: Preventive and Remedial Approaches*. Silver Spring, MD: National Association of School Psychologists, pp. 1–21.

Wilson, S. J., and Lipsey, M. W. (2007). School-based interventions for aggressive and disruptive behavior: update of a meta-analysis. *American Journal of Preventive Medicine*, 33, S130–43.

Yeager, D. S., Fong, C. J., Lee, H. Y., and Espelage, D. L. (in press). Declines in efficacy of anti-bullying programmes among older adolescents: a developmental theory and a three-level meta-analysis. *Journal of Applied Developmental Psychology*.

Zins, J. E., Weissberg, R. P., Wang, M. C., and Walberg, H. J. (2004). *Building School Success through Social and Emotional Learning*. New York: Teachers College Press.

CHAPTER 22

Preventing youth violence through therapeutic interventions for high-risk youth

Scott W. Henggeler

Introduction to Preventing Youth Violence through Therapeutic Interventions for High-Risk Youth

This review is based on findings from the Blueprints for Violence Prevention project (Elliott 1998) that was launched in 1996 to identify and replicate violence prevention and intervention programmes that are effective. During the past 18 years, the highly respected and on-going Blueprints project (Elliott 2012) has reviewed more than 1,000 programmes that aim to reduce antisocial behaviour in youth. Based on selection criteria described subsequently, Blueprints identified eight prevention/interventions as model programmes—programmes that have strong evidence of effectiveness, favourable outcomes that were sustained for at least 12 months, and the capacity to be transported to community settings. An additional 36 prevention/interventions were identified as promising. Promising programmes also have the capacity to be transported to community settings, but have not demonstrated sustained intervention effects, and the body of supporting evidence is not as strong as that of their model programme counterparts.

Three of the eight model programmes provide therapeutic interventions in community settings for high-risk youth, and this chapter summarizes the theoretical rationales, clinical interventions, outcomes, and transportability of these programmes. The remaining model programmes are school-based (e.g. Project Toward No Drug Abuse; Sussman et al. 2012) or focus on early child development through the healthcare system (e.g. Nurse Family Partnership; Eckenrode et al. 2010), and these types of interventions are covered in preceding chapters. In addition, three of the 36 promising programmes provide therapeutic interventions for high-risk youth in community settings (the vast majority of the remaining programmes are school-based prevention programmes), and two of these programmes are briefly reviewed as well. The third, adolescent coping with depression (Clarke and DeBar 2010), is not discussed as it focuses on treatment of depression and has only modest support for attenuating co-occurring conduct problems.

Blueprints Criteria for Promising and Model Programmes

Blueprints programmes must meet a set of criteria that demonstrate their capacity to be adopted and implemented effectively (i.e. to achieve desired outcomes) in community settings (Blueprints 2013).

Intervention Specificity

The target population must be specified both clinically (e.g. juvenile offenders, youth with conduct disorder) and demographically (e.g. by age and gender). In addition, the programme's logic model should clearly identify the risk factors that are targeted by the intervention and how changes in these risk factors will impact the desired outcomes (i.e. reduced antisocial behaviour). Finally, the content of the intervention must be well specified in regard to clinical procedures, frequency, duration, mode of delivery, and setting of the interventions as well as the training of the providers.

Evaluation Quality

For model programmes, the effectiveness of the programme must be supported by at least two well-conducted randomized controlled trials (RCTs) or one RCT and one well-conducted quasi-experimental evaluation. The criteria for well-conducted outcome research include the use of valid measures, appropriate statistical analyses that include an intent-to-treat design, examination and control of baseline differences in intervention conditions, description of sample characteristics, and documentation of intervention intensity and fidelity. Promising programmes are supported by at least one high-quality RCT or two high-quality quasi-experimental evaluations.

Intervention Impact

For model programmes, the analyses must demonstrate a statistically significant treatment effect on ultimate outcomes (e.g. juvenile offending, violence, conduct problems) with at least one of these effects being sustained for a minimum of 12 months following the completion of the intervention. One-year sustainability of favourable post-treatment outcomes is not a criterion for promising programmes. Moreover, for both model and promising programmes, there must be no evidence of meaningful iatrogenic effects.

Dissemination Readiness

It is one thing for an intervention to achieve favourable outcomes in RCTs, but quite another to be transported effectively to community settings. Both model and promising programmes must have a demonstrated capacity for effective transport to community settings. Effective transport requires a purveyor organization to assure that adopters target a demographic and clinical sample appropriate to the intervention. In addition, protocols are needed for hiring appropriate providers, for training them in the intervention techniques, and to provide on-going quality assurance to support the fidelity of treatment implementation. Lastly, sustainable sources of funding must be identified and accessed if the programme is to endure.

Model Programmes

Multisystemic Therapy

Multisystemic therapy (MST) is a family- and home-based intervention that was first developed in the late 1970s and is currently one of the best-validated and most extensively transported evidence-based treatments of serious antisocial behaviour in adolescents.

Theoretical Overview of MST

Consistent with extensive longitudinal research on the determinants of antisocial behaviour in adolescents (Liberman 2008), MST follows a social–ecological conceptual framework. Behaviour is viewed as multi-determined through the reciprocal interplay of risk factors pertaining to the youth's cognitive functioning (e.g. problem-solving skills) and social networks (i.e. family, peer, school, and neighbourhood). Correspondingly, interventions are individualized to address pertinent risk factors while building protective factors.

Intervention Procedures of MST

MST clinical procedures are specified in Henggeler et al. (2009) and are implemented by master's-level therapists who work in MST programmes. Selection of interventions is guided by nine treatment principles, and intervention strategies typically incorporate evidence-based techniques from cognitive behavioural therapies, behavioural therapies, and pragmatic family therapies. Caregivers are viewed as critical change agents, and therapists work intensively to build parenting capacity of caregivers. For example, interventions often address barriers to effective parenting (e.g. caregiver drug abuse, family stress) and facilitate caregiver efforts to support, monitor, and discipline their children. Such efforts typically include strategies to increase youth responsibility at home, disengage youth from deviant peer relations, and improve school attendance and performance. Mediational research has supported the MST theory of change (e.g. Dekovic et al. 2012).

Fidelity of the MST treatment process is supported by an extensive quality assurance system. This system includes decision-making tools that guide the selection and sequence of interventions as well as extensive training and oversight by MST experts. For example, MST teams include two to four full-time therapists, with caseloads of four to six families each, and a supervisor who is at least half-time. Following specified and validated supervisory protocols, the supervisor provides targeted training, guidance, and support to help therapists sustain treatment fidelity and achieve desired outcomes. Similarly, via weekly conference call, an MST expert oversees the progress of each case. Additional procedures are put into place to assure the administrative and support and financial viability of the MST programme.

Research outcomes of MST

During the past 35 years, MST outcome research has transitioned from small efficacy trials conducted in university settings with graduate students as therapists to large-scale multi-site effectiveness studies conducted with community-based provider organizations and therapists. Currently, with 14 RCTs (six of which were independent of the developers) and one quasi-experimental study with juvenile offenders published, the model has been validated most extensively with this population. Across these studies, the median reduction in re-arrest was 39 per cent, and the median reduction in out-of-home placements was 53 per cent.

MST first became prominent as an effective community-based alternative to the incarceration of serious (i.e. chronic and/or violent) juvenile offenders with the publication of three RCTs in the 1990s. For example, in a community-based RCT with serious juvenile offenders at imminent risk of incarceration, Henggeler et al. (1992) showed that MST improved family relations and peer interactions while decreasing recidivism and incarceration for this challenging population. A subsequent RCT conducted by Borduin et al. (1995) included a 21.9-year follow-up (Sawyer and Borduin 2011), which showed that former MST participants, now in their mid-30s, had 36 per cent fewer felony arrests and 33 per cent fewer days in adult confinement than did counterparts who had received individual therapy. Favourable results from RCTs have also been observed by independent investigators in both the United States (e.g. Timmons-Mitchell et al. 2006) and Europe (Butler et al. 2011; Ogden and Hagen 2006).

MST has also been validated for challenging subgroups of juvenile offenders. For example, the effectiveness of MST with juvenile sex offenders has been supported in three RCTs, including a study (Borduin et al. 2009) that found large decreases in recidivism and incarceration across a 9-year follow-up as well as a broad array of other favourable outcomes (e.g. improved family relations, peer relations, and school performance; decreased youth mental health symptoms). Likewise, two further RCTs have focused on the use of MST with substance abusing or dependent delinquents and observed favourable outcomes. Please see Henggeler (2011) for a more extensive overview of MST outcome research.

Transportability of MST

In 1996 a purveyor organization, MST Services, was developed to meet an increasing demand for MST programmes. MST Services is licensed through the Medical University of South Carolina for the transport of MST technology and intellectual property. MST Services and its network partners (i.e. purveyor organizations trained by MST Services to carry out all aspects of programme development and implementation) currently provide the on-going training and quality assurance for the more than 500 MST programmes worldwide. These programmes, which are located in more than 30 states and 14 nations, have the capacity to serve up to 25,000 youths and their families annually. The effectiveness of MST has been supported in RCTs conducted in Norway, England, and the Netherlands; while an RCT in Sweden did not demonstrate significant treatment effects (see www.mstservices.com/outcomestudies.pdf).

Functional Family Therapy

The first Functional Family Therapy (FFT) outcome study with juvenile offenders was published 40 years ago (Alexander and Parsons 1973), and FFT has subsequently become one of the most widely transported family therapies worldwide.

Theoretical Overview of FFT

In FFT, the presenting problem is viewed as a symptom of dysfunctional family relationships. As such, rather than focusing on problem behaviours *per se*, interventions aim to change patterns of family behaviour in ways that lead to symptom change. A variety of cognitive and behavioural intervention techniques are used to facilitate such change.

Therapeutic Procedures of FFT

FFT clinical procedures are described most extensively by Alexander and colleagues (2013). This volume presents a five-phase process that aims to attenuate behavioural problems presented by adolescents and the family difficulties associated with these problems. FFT programmes typically include a team of three to eight master's-level therapists who carry caseloads of 12–15 families, and treatment duration averages about 12 sessions over 3–4 months. Services are delivered in home, clinic, and other community settings.

Engagement Phase

Therapists demonstrate their desire to resolve presenting problems through active listening, respect, and empathetic behaviours. To facilitate engagement, the therapist takes a strengths-based approach with the entire family and is highly available for communication and interactions (e.g. telephone outreach, home visits, arranging for transportation).

Motivation Phase

With the development of therapeutic engagement, the therapist is in a position to engender hope and positive expectations. Confrontation is avoided, and a non-blaming stance is taken by the therapist. The nature of family relations becomes the focus of treatment, with family strengths emphasized and negative interaction patterns interrupted. Reframing is often used to shift the family's focus from the problem behaviour to a more positive relationship emphasis.

Relational Assessment

The primary therapeutic task is to understand the association between the presenting problems and intra- and extra-family functioning. Through discussions with family members (e.g. to understand their values) and observations of their interactions (e.g. to understand the affective and instrumental nature of family relationships), the therapist analyses information and develops plans for the behaviour change and generalization phases of treatment.

Behaviour Change Phase

Based on the relational assessment, the primary aim of this phase is to change the problem behaviour by establishing new patterns of family interaction that replace the old patterns. Therapists use techniques such as communication training, modelling, teaching, assigning homework, and training in conflict resolution, to change family interactions in ways that decrease the identified problem behaviours.

Generalization Phase

The primary aims of this phase are to extend the favourable family changes to their social network (e.g. school, juvenile justice authorities) and to create relapse prevention plans. For example, the therapist helps the family develop positive relations with extra-familial systems (e.g. school, juvenile justice authorities)—relations that can be leveraged if behaviour problems recur.

Research Outcomes of FFT

Several efficacy (e.g. using graduate students as therapists) and effectiveness (e.g. using community-based therapists) outcome studies have been published. In one of the first successful RCTs conducted with juvenile offenders, Alexander and Parsons (1973) showed that FFT was more effective than three alternative interventions at improving family communication and decreasing status offending. Favourable effects on criminal behaviour were observed in two subsequent quasi-experimental efficacy studies (Barton et al. 1985; Gordon et al. 1988). More recently, in a complex four-condition efficacy RCT with substance-abusing adolescents, Waldron et al. (2001) demonstrated favourable outcomes for marijuana use post treatment. Thus, outcomes from efficacy research have been generally favourable.

The transition from successful efficacy research to effectiveness can be challenging. In an independent effectiveness RCT with substance-abusing adolescents, Friedman (1989) failed to find favourable FFT effects. Similarly, in a large multi-site independent effectiveness RCT, Sexton and Turner (2010) did not observe FFT treatment effects. Secondary analyses, however, showed a strong association between treatment fidelity and youth outcomes. Therapists with higher adherence to the FFT intervention protocols achieved lower rates of recidivism than did counterparts with poor FFT adherence. Indeed, implementation fidelity seems critical to the success of virtually all evidence-based interventions for youth violence (Mihalic 2004).

Transportability of FFT

FFT Inc. is the primary purveyor organization that provides training and certification of FFT programmes. Transport of FFT programmes includes three phases: clinical training, supervision training, and maintenance. The aim of clinical training is to build a local infrastructure that supports therapist adherence and competence in delivering FFT. During the supervision training phase the site is assisted in achieving greater self-sufficiency, especially the development of an effective on-site supervisor. The maintenance phase emphasizes the development of a partnering relationship with the provider agency, on-going monitoring and support to assure treatment fidelity, and problem solving regarding issues that impact programme functioning. Approximately 300 FFT programmes serving more than 20,000 families are currently operating worldwide. Two independent evaluations published in Swedish have supported the effectiveness of FFT transport (see Henggeler and Sheidow 2012).

Multidimensional Treatment Foster Care

Multidimensional Treatment Foster Care (MTFC; Chamberlain 2003) is a multi-faceted and well-conceived set of interventions that serves as an alternative to restrictive out-of-home placements for chronic juvenile offenders as well as a therapeutically oriented foster care intervention for children in the child welfare system (Leve et al. 2012). This review focuses on the use of MTFC with juvenile offenders.

Theoretical Overview of MTFC

MTFC interventions are implemented from a social ecological conceptual framework (i.e. explicitly considering the roles of cognitive, family, peer, and school factors) and are based on the principles of social learning theory. Thus, therapeutic techniques are primarily behavioural and cognitive behavioural in nature.

Therapeutic Procedures of MTFC

MTFC programmes surround highly trained foster parents, with one child per foster family, with extensive clinical support and resources. These resources include a programme supervisor who has daily contact with the foster parent and coordinates all interventions for the youth; an individual therapist who targets the youth's emotional and social skill development; a family therapist who prepares the biological or aftercare family for the youth's return home; and a skills trainer who coaches the youth in appropriate social behaviours in community settings such as school and the mall. Together, these individuals implement a detailed, individualized behavioural management plan that envelops the youth with adults and peers who reinforce prosocial behaviours and provides consistent consequences for negative behaviours. MTFC interventions are typically 6–9 months in duration, as youth are carefully transitioned back to their home environments.

Research Outcomes of MTFC

As detailed by Leve et al. (2012) and Henggeler and Sheidow (2012), MTFC has been evaluated in several clinical trials with chronic juvenile offenders directed by Chamberlain as well as independent research in Sweden (Westermark et al. 2011). Findings, including 2-year follow-ups, demonstrated favourable reductions in recidivism, incarceration, externalizing symptoms, and pregnancies. Moreover, key components of the MTFC theory of change have been supported, with reductions in antisocial behaviour mediated by improved foster parent supervision, decreased association with deviant peers, and increased completion of schoolwork (e.g. Eddy and Chamberlain 2000).

Transportability of MTFC

Training and technical assistance in developing and implementing MTFC programmes is provided by TFC Consultants Inc. Site visits are conducted to engage community stakeholders in the procedures necessary for implementing the model, and various protocols are used to support the fidelity of MTFC implementation among programme staff. MTFC programmes for adolescents have been transported to almost 100 sites across the United States and Europe, and the effectiveness of transport has been supported in the aforementioned Swedish RCT (Westermark et al. 2011).

Promising Programmes

As noted, three of the 36 programmes identified as promising by Blueprints provide therapeutic interventions to high-risk youth in clinic settings. Two of these programmes focus on children presenting disruptive behaviour disorders, and these are discussed.

Parent–Child Interaction Therapy

Parent–Child Interaction Therapy (PCIT) is a clinic-based therapeutic intervention that works with parent–child dyads to develop more nurturing attachment and parental limit setting for children presenting disruptive behaviour.

Theoretical Overview of PCIT

Based on extensive child development research, including attachment theory and social-learning theory, PCIT aims to teach authoritative parenting skills. Authoritative parenting is associated with a wide variety of favourable child outcomes and combines strong parent-child attachment with limit setting that is firm, consistent, and well reasoned.

Intervention procedures of PCIT

PCIT includes highly structured intervention protocols that comprise two phases (Zisser and Eyberg 2010). During the first phase, the parent is coached to engage in child-directed interaction. Here, for example, the parent is encouraged to show approval, express interest, and follow the child's appropriate behaviour during sessions. Commands, questions, and critical statements are avoided. Importantly, parental behaviour is carefully tracked, and mastery criteria must be met before moving to the second phase of treatment. During the second phase, the parent is coached in parent-directed interaction. Here, therapists teach the parent how to give commands in ways that maximize the probability of child compliance. For example, effective commands are direct, polite, and given one at a time and only when necessary. Special attention is devoted to the appropriate use of time out when the child is disruptive or disobeys. Significantly, PCIT is performance based rather than time limited. That is, standardized measures are used to track therapeutic progress, and treatment continues until outcome criteria are met and caregivers are confident in their ability to manage the child's behaviour. The average length of treatment is about 15 sessions.

Research Outcomes of PCIT

As described by Zisser and Eyberg (2010), the efficacy of PCIT has been examined in several RCTs (e.g. Bagner and Eyberg 2007; Nixon et al. 2003) with disruptive children. In addition, cross-cultural evaluations have supported the effectiveness of PCIT with Puerto Rican, Chinese, and Australian families, and its results with maltreating families have been examined (Chaffin et al. 2011). Mediational research (Bagner and Eyberg 2007) has supported the PCIT theory of change. Increases in positive parenting behaviour and decreases in negative parenting behaviour accounted for favourable changes in children's behaviour after treatment.

Transportability of PCIT

PCIT International certifies PCIT Master Trainers to provide on-site clinical training in PCIT. Master Trainers in several states and nations (e.g. Canada, Australia, Hong Kong) are currently certified to provide practitioner training.

The Incredible Years—Child Treatment

As described by Webster-Stratton (2011), The Incredible Years (IY) includes several variations and optional components including children, parents, and teachers that address the disruptive behaviour and social development of young children. The effectiveness of the array of IY interventions has been supported by numerous RCTs. Per the Blueprints designation, however, this summary focuses on the IY–Child Treatment programme.

Theoretical Overview of IY

Consistent with the evidence-based treatments discussed, IY is based largely on social learning theory and social ecological models of behaviour.

Intervention Procedures of IY

An overriding goal of the array of IY intervention protocols is to promote parent competencies—both positive parent–child bonding and improved parent control strategies. IY–Child Treatment, however, focuses on developing children's social skills and problem-solving skills in ways that promote academic and social development. The intervention is implemented by teams of two therapists, who work with groups of six or seven children during weekly 2-hour sessions for 18 weeks. Using video modelling, fantasy play, role play, and coaching, the therapists teach cognitive, affective, and behavioural skills that facilitate peer relations, academic performance, and positive classroom behaviour. Parents and teachers are kept informed about the programme.

Research Outcomes of IY

In its entirety, the IY programmes are among the most extensively validated of any evidence-based treatment. Numerous RCTs have been conducted by the developer (e.g. Webster-Stratton et al. 2011), independent investigators in the United States (e.g. Taylor et al. 1998) and internationally (e.g. Larsson et al. 2009). The most comprehensive overview of this research, including findings particular to the IY–Child Treatment programme, is provided by Webster-Stratton (2011).

Transportability of IY

IY has been transported to numerous states in the United States and internationally. Training and certification of group leaders is provided by The Incredible Years Inc. purveyor organization. Group leaders can be certified in any of four IY programmes, including IY–Child Treatment. Based on experience, performance, and additional training, these professionals can advance up the ranks to become IY mentors and trainers. Importantly, the effective transport of IY variations has been supported in studies conducted in the United Kingdom, Norway, and Jamaica (Webster-Stratton 2011).

Conclusions and Research Priorities

The Blueprints programmes share several pertinent commonalities in addition to those that define inclusion as a Blueprints programme (e.g. favourable outcomes from RCTs, intervention specification, existence of purveyor organization). First, they explicitly target risk and protective factors that have been identified in developmental research. Second, the models generally take a comprehensive approach to addressing these risk factors. Yet, third, their approaches are individualized to the specific circumstances of each child and family. Fourth, the techniques used in these interventions are primarily behavioural and cognitive behavioural in nature. Current and future efforts to develop and validate effective interventions for youth violence should be informed by these commonalities.

Finally, the interventions presented in this chapter have proven that they can effectively reduce antisocial behaviour in youth, and a subset of the interventions have proven effective in independent evaluations in the United States and internationally. In light of the international nature of this volume, two broad research priorities are suggested. First, additional RCTs are needed to clearly establish the effectiveness of those intervention models that have scant independent or international evaluations. Mediational studies that examine hypothesized mechanisms of change should be embedded within these trials. Second, extensive research is needed on the effective transport of evidence-based interventions. What are the most efficient and effective training strategies? How effective are purveyor organizations in developing programmes and supporting the therapists within these programmes? What are the key components of transport, and how do variations of these components influence youth outcomes? What are the best strategies for adapting evidence-based treatments to different cultures, while assuring that the effective components of the intervention remain intact? Again, it is one thing for an intervention to achieve favourable outcomes in RCTs, but quite another to be transported effectively and on a large scale to community settings.

Acknowledgement

This manuscript was supported by grants DA019892 and DA017487 from the National Institute on Drug Abuse.

References

Alexander, J. F., and Parsons, B. V. (1973). Short-term behavioral intervention with delinquent families: impact on family process and recidivism. *Journal of Abnormal Psychology*, 81, 219–25.

Alexander, J. F., Waldron, H. B., Robbins, M. S., and Neeb, A. A. (2013). *Functional Family Therapy for Adolescent Behavior Problems*. Washington, D.C.: American Psychological Association.

Bagner, D. M., and Eyberg, S. M. (2007). Parent-Child Interaction Therapy for disruptive behavior in children with mental retardation: a randomized controlled trial. *Journal of Clinical Child and Adolescent Psychology*, 36, 418–29.

Barton, C., Alexander, J. F., Waldron, H., Turner, C. W., and Warburton, J. (1985). Generalizing treatment effects of Functional Family Therapy: three replications. *The American Journal of Family Therapy*, 13, 16–26.

Blueprints (2013). *Blueprints Database Standards*. University of Colorado, Center for the Study and Prevention of Violence. Boulder, CO: Blueprints.

Borduin, C. M., Mann, B. J., and Cone, L. T. et al. (1995). Multisystemic treatment of serious juvenile offenders: long-term prevention of criminality and violence. *Journal of Consulting and Clinical Psychology*, 63, 569–78.

Borduin, C. M., Schaeffer, C. M., and Heiblum, N. (2009). A randomized clinical trial of Multisystemic Therapy with juvenile sexual offenders: effects on youth social ecology and criminal activity. *Journal of Consulting and Clinical Psychology*, 77, 26–37.

Butler, S., Baruch, G., Hickley, N., and Fonagy, P. (2011). A randomized controlled trial of MST and a statutory therapeutic intervention for young offenders. *Journal of the American Academy of Child & Adolescent Psychiatry*, 50, 1220–35.

Chaffin, M., Funderburk, B., Bard, D., Valle, L. A., and Gurwitch, R. (2011). A combined motivation and Parent-Child Interaction Therapy package reduces child welfare recidivism in a randomized dismantling field trial. *Journal of Consulting and Clinical Psychology*, 79, 84–95.

Chamberlain, P. (2003). *Treating Chronic Juvenile Offenders: Advances Made through the Oregon Multidimensional Treatment Foster Care Model*. Washington, D.C.: American Psychological Association.

Clarke, G. N., and DeBar, L. L. (2010). Group cognitive-behavioral treatment for adolescent depression. In: J. R. Weisz, and A. E. Kazdin (eds), *Evidence-Based Psychotherapies for Children and Adolescents. 2nd ed.* New York: Guilford, pp. 110–25.

Dekovic, M., Asscher, J. J., Manders, W. A., Prins, P., and van der Laan, P. (2012). Within-intervention change: mediators of intervention effects during Multisystemic Therapy. *Journal of Consulting and Clinical Psychology*, 80, 574–87.

Eckenrode, J., Campa, M., and Luckey, D. W. et al. (2010). Long-term effects of prenatal and infancy nurse home visitation on the life course of youths: 19-year follow-up of a randomized trial. *Archives of Pediatrics & Adolescent Medicine*, 164, 9–15.

Eddy, J. M., and Chamberlain, P. (2000). Family management and deviant peer association as mediators of the impact of treatment condition on youth antisocial behavior. *Journal of Consulting and Clinical Psychology*, 68, 857–63.

Elliott, D. S. (1998). *Blueprints for Violence Prevention*. University of Colorado, Center for the Study and Prevention of Violence. Boulder, CO: Blueprints.

Elliott, D. S. (2012, April). *Blueprints in 2012*. Keynote address at the Blueprints for Violence Prevention 2012 Conference. San Antonio, TX.

Friedman, A. S. (1989). Family therapy vs. parent groups: effects on adolescent drug abusers. *The American Journal of Family Therapy*, 17, 335–47.

Gordon, D. A., Arbuthnot, J., Gustafson, K. E., and McGreen, P. (1988). Home-based behavioral-systems family therapy with disadvantaged juvenile delinquents. *The American Journal of Family Therapy*, 16, 243–55.

Henggeler, S. W. (2011). Efficacy studies to large-scale transport: the development and validation of MST programs. *Annual Review of Clinical Psychology*, 7, 351–81.

Henggeler, S. W., Melton, G. B., and Smith, L. A. (1992). Family preservation using Multisystemic Therapy: an effective alternative to incarcerating serious juvenile offenders. *Journal of Consulting and Clinical Psychology*, 60, 953–61.

Henggeler, S. W., Schoenwald, S. K., Borduin, C. M., Rowland, M. D., and Cunningham, P. B. (2009). *Multisystemic Therapy for Antisocial Behavior in Children and Adolescents. 2nd ed.* New York: Guilford.

Henggeler, S. W., and Sheidow, A. J. (2012). Empirically supported family-based treatments for conduct disorder and delinquency. *Journal of Marital and Family Therapy*, 38, 30–58.

Larsson, B., Fossum, B., Clifford, G., Drugli, M., Handegard, B., and Morch, W. (2009). Treatment of oppositional defiant and conduct problems in young Norwegian children: results of a randomized trial. *European Child Adolescent Psychiatry*, 18, 42–52.

Leve, L. D., Harold, G. T., Chamberlain, P., Landsverk, J. A., Fisher, P. A., and Vostanis, P. (2012). Practitioner review: children in foster care—vulnerabilities and evidence-based interventions that promote resilience processes. *Journal of Child Psychology and Psychiatry*, 53, 1197–211.

Liberman, A. M. (2008). *The Long View of Crime: A Synthesis of Longitudinal Research*. New York, NY: Springer.

Mihalic, S. (2004). The importance of implementation fidelity. *Emotional & Behavioral Disorders in Youth*, 4, 81–109.

Nixon, R. D. V., Sweeny, L., Erickson, D. B., and Touyz, S. W. (2003). Parent-Child Interaction Therapy: a comparison of standard and abbreviated treatments for oppositional defiant preschoolers. *Journal of Consulting and Clinical Psychology*, 71, 251–60.

Ogden, T., and Hagen, K. A. (2006). Multisystemic Therapy of serious behavior problems in youth: sustainability of therapy effectiveness two years after intake. *Journal of Child and Adolescent Mental Health*, 11, 142–9.

Sawyer, A. M., and Borduin, C. M. (2011). Effects of MST through midlife: a 21.9-year follow up to a randomized clinical trial with serious and violent juvenile offenders. *Journal of Consulting and Clinical Psychology*, 79, 643–52.

Sexton, T., and Turner, C. W. (2010). The effectiveness of Functional Family Therapy for youth with behavioral problems in a community practice setting. *Journal of Family Psychology*, 24, 339–48.

Sussman, S., Sun, P., Rohrbach, L. A., and Spruijt-Metz, D. (2012). One-year outcomes of a drug abuse prevention program for older teens and emerging adults: evaluating a motivational interviewing booster component. *Health Psychology*, 31, 476–85.

Taylor, T. K., Schmidt, F., Pepler, D., and Hodgins, H. (1998). A comparison of eclectic treatment with Webster-Stratton's Parents and Children Series in a children's mental health center: a randomized controlled trial. *Behavior Therapy*, 29, 221–40.

Timmons-Mitchell, J., Bender, M. B., Kishna, M. A., and Mitchell, C. C. (2006). An independent effectiveness trial of Multisystemic Therapy with juvenile justice youth. *Journal of Clinical Child and Adolescent Psychology*, 35, 227–36.

Waldron, H. B., Slesnick, N., Turner, C. W., Brody, J. L., and Peterson, T. R. (2001). Treatment outcomes for adolescent substance abuse at 4- and

7-month assessments. *Journal of Consulting and Clinical Psychology*, 69, 802–13.

Webster-Stratton, C. (2011). *The Incredible Years Parents, Teachers, and Children's Training Series*. Seattle, WA: Incredible Years, Inc.

Webster-Stratton, C. H., Reid, M. J., and Beauchaine, T. (2011). Combining parent and child training for young children with ADHD. *Journal of Clinical Child and Adolescent Psychology*, 40, 1–13.

Westermark, P. K., Hansson, K., and Olsson, M. (2011). Multidimensional Treatment Foster Care (MTFC): results from an independent replication. *Journal of Family Therapy*, 33, 20–41.

Zisser, A., and Eyberg, S. M. (2010). Parent-Child Interaction Therapy and the treatment of disruptive behavior disorders. In: J. R. Weisz, and A. E. Kazdin (eds), *Evidence-based Psychotherapies for Children and Adolescents. 2nd ed.* New York: Guilford, pp. 179–93.

CHAPTER 23

Preventing violence through interventions in the health system

Christine Goodall

Theoretical Overview of Preventing Violence through Interventions in the Health System

Injury due to violence places a huge burden on healthcare systems worldwide. For every person who dies as a result of violence a further 20 to 40 require medical intervention; this amounts to 10–20 million patients annually, and many of these individuals may require lifelong healthcare as a result of their injuries (WHO 2005). The Global Burden of Disease Study 2010 measured the global burden of disease due to interpersonal violence using disability adjusted life years (DALYs) to represent an absolute measure of health loss due to disease (Murray et al. 2012). The total number of DALYs due to interpersonal violence in all age groups increased worldwide between 1990 and 2010 but the DALYs per 100,000 population showed only a small increase for interpersonal violence overall (+0.3 per cent) with the exception of assault with a sharp object where there was a bigger rise (+14.3 per cent). Gore et al. (2011) estimated DALYs for young people using data from the WHO 2004 Global Burden of Disease Study and found that violence was the second most common cause of DALYs in young men aged 20–24 years accounting for 8.1 per cent of DALYs, and the third most common cause for young men between 10 and 24 years, accounting for 5.8 per cent of DALYs. Patton et al. (2009) found that violence was the second most common cause of death in males aged 10–24 years, accounting for 9.2 per cent of deaths in this age bracket. Gore et al. (2011) and Patton et al. (2009) point out that a lack of investment in injury prevention has kept injury due to violence near the top of global burden of disease and mortality tables for young men and conclude that more needs to be done to improve this.

In addition to the interventions described in detail in this chapter, the clinical role of healthcare workers in the recognition and care of victims of violence should not be overlooked; nor should the potential for healthcare systems to develop better treatments for injured patients leading to improved survival rates and better long term outcomes.

Healthcare workers have an ideal opportunity to intervene with both current and historical victims of violence. Many interventions focus on the concept of the 'teachable moment'; this describes a period of time after an event (for instance, a violent attack) when patients may be more receptive to intervention and more ready to change. Williams et al. (2005) screened patients attending an emergency department for alcohol misuse and offered follow-up alcohol interventions. They concluded that the 'teachable moment' had a half-life of 2 days. Patients were much more likely to attend for a follow-up appointment soon after the incident which brought them to the emergency department. This would imply that patients have to perceive an association between their injury, the assault, and their drinking to be ready to make a change.

Advances in medicine and surgery result in continually improving outcomes from serious injury; however, healthcare professionals do not instinctively gravitate towards prevention despite being well placed to do so. There are a variety of reasons for this, not least lack of time and training. If these issues are addressed then they can effectively help patients with health behaviour change as has been shown with smoking, alcohol, and diet. It is fundamentally important that healthcare professionals do get involved as they may not only help prevent the individual and societal consequences of injury, but may influence an overall reduction in injury due to violence that would enable resources in often stretched healthcare systems to be more appropriately allocated.

The Status of the Evidence in Healthcare

As explained in Chapter 1 of this volume, the public health model of violence prevention developed by the World Health Organiziation (WHO) suggests that a problem should be defined, the protective and risk factors identified, and appropriate interventions developed, tested, and scaled up to reach the maximum number of individuals (WHO 2002). This model allows health professionals to frame violence as a disease and, although this perhaps oversimplifies the problem, it is a concept with which they are familiar.

Some areas of violence prevention in healthcare have been well evaluated and have resulted in the adoption of a particular approach. For example, with regard to injury surveillance, the sharing of data between Emergency Medicine Departments and police in Cardiff, UK, was robustly evaluated (Florence et al. 2011), and as a result has now been adopted as a standard approach by many other UK health boards. Similarly, in countries such as Jamaica it has also been well evaluated and firmly embedded in the healthcare system for many years (Ward et al. 2002).

In other areas there is background evidence on the willingness of healthcare workers and of patients to participate in violence prevention programmes, but also on the lack of training of healthcare professionals and the barriers to provision of violence prevention programmes in the healthcare arena. One example of this is the involvement of dentists in the recognition of domestic abuse. Dentists are well placed to identify the signs of domestic abuse in their patients, many of whom sustain injuries to the head and neck, yet few ask about abuse because they are not trained in how to respond and worry that they may offend the patient (Love et al. 2001). Conversely, victims of domestic abuse who attend the dentist with injuries would like to be asked how the injuries occurred and given the opportunity to disclose the abuse, but few are asked (Nelms et al. 2009), so there is a real missed opportunity. This background information led to the development of a training programme for dentists in the United States to give them the confidence to ask about abuse and signpost patients towards specialist services (Hsieh et al. 2006).

Medicine and other associated areas of healthcare provide treatment to patients using an evidence-based approach based on a hierarchy of evidence (Box 23.1). Generally speaking only the highest levels of evidence would result in a 'treatment' being widely adopted.

However, while double-blind placebo-controlled randomized controlled trials (RCTs) remain the gold standard in medicine, in terms of interventions for violence prevention, conducting a completely blinded RCT can sometimes be problematic as the shock of the injury itself and the screening tools that may be used can themselves act as forms of intervention so it can be difficult to identify what has caused any resultant effect (McCambridge and Day 2008). Nonetheless, the most robust evidence for the effectiveness of interventions will come from the use of this approach. Violence prevention in the health setting is a developing concept, so other lower forms of evidence will and do still lend valuable knowledge to the design of new interventions or their evaluations.

Box 23.1 The hierarchy of evidence in healthcare

- Ia: systematic review or meta-analysis of randomized control trials (RCTs).
- Ib: at least one RCT.
- IIa: at least one well designed controlled study without randomiziation.
- IIb: at least one well-designed quasi-experimental study, such as a cohort study.
- III: well-designed non-experimental descriptive studies, such as comparative studies, correlation studies, case-control studies and case series.
- IV: expert committee reports, opinions and/or clinical experience of respected authorities

---

RCT of interventions for violence have been carried out in the areas of domestic abuse (Feder et al. 2011), alcohol misuse associated with violence (Goodall et al. 2008; Smith et al. 2003), and youth violence prevention (Cunningham et al. 2012; Walton et al. 2010) (Table 23.1). These will be discussed in more detail in the following section. There is however a significant gap in this area and a lack of robust well-conducted RCTs of violence interventions.

Brief Description of Intervention Procedures

The majority of interventions for violence in healthcare fall under the umbrella of secondary or tertiary prevention; however, there are some examples of primary prevention.

Healthcare workers and their staff are very well placed to 'signpost' in relation to violence. Injury surveillance, a process whereby very basic and non-identifiable information about injured patients is shared with law enforcement agencies, can help to pinpoint locations where interpersonal violence resulting in injury occurs regularly. Healthcare workers may also identify individual patients as victims of particular sorts of violence or abuse (for example, domestic abuse, elder abuse, or child abuse). By encouraging them to disclose the abuse in the confidential surroundings of the healthcare setting they can help and encourage patients to access the appropriate help and support either through specialist agencies or the police. Disclosure in the healthcare setting, for example in the case of sexual assault, may also facilitate the collection of forensic evidence which can be stored for later use if the victim does not feel ready to report an assault to the police (Campbell et al. 2005).

Identification of victims is something that a broad range of healthcare professionals could be involved with; for example, community pharmacists are in a good position to identify victims of domestic abuse (Ford and Murphy 1996), but lack training. Identification of victims is not limited to healthcare professionals working with human victims as we know that the threat of harm or actual harm to animals is used to coerce or control human victims of domestic abuse so veterinary surgeons also have a role to play in identifying and helping victims (Gallagher et al. 2008).

There are several interventions designed to prevent re-injury or re-victimiziation aimed at individual patients or at groups of patients. These may directly target violent or aggressive behaviour, associated behaviours such as excess alcohol consumption (Chapters 32 and 42), or wider social issues.

There are interventions, or more accurately treatments, designed to help patients with the psychological aftermath of violence including acute stress disorder (ASD) and post-traumatic stress disorder (PTSD). PTSD affects a significant percentage of victims of violence (Hull et al. 2003) and is underreported, partly due to a lack of knowledge of how to identify victims. Healthcare workers need to be able to identify both ASD and PTSD, and either treat the patient psychologically or pharmacologically or refer them to specialist services for treatment.

There are also a few interventions falling under the umbrella of primary prevention that take healthcare workers out of the clinical environment to deliver interventions in schools, youth clubs,

Table 23.1 Examples of randomized controlled trials of interventions for violence and associated behaviours in healthcare settings

Intervention	Type of violence	Details of trial and outcomes	Country	Reference
IRIS (Identification and Referral to Improve Safety)	Domestic abuse	A cluster RCT of training to identify and refer female victims of domestic abuse in primary care. (n=48 GP practices)	UK	Feder et al. 2011
Weave	Domestic abuse	A cluster RCT to test an intervention for domestic abuse in primary care. (n=52 doctors and n=272 patients)	Australia	Hegarty et al. 2013
Alcohol Brief Intervention	Alcohol related violence and trauma	RCT compared a nurse-delivered alcohol brief intervention to a leaflet in maxillofacial clinics (n=151)	UK	Smith et al. 2003
Alcohol Brief Intervention	Alcohol related violence and trauma	RCT compared a nurse-delivered alcohol brief intervention to a leaflet in maxillofacial clinics (n=195)	UK	Goodall et al. 2008
SS-COVAID	Interpersonal violence/alcohol	RCT compared an alcohol brief intervention to a brief intervention designed to address both alcohol and violence (SS-COVAID) (n=187)	UK	Goodall et al. 2011
SafERteens	Youth violence	A three arm RCT of brief interventions to address violence and alcohol for patients aged 14-18 years delivered in the emergency department. This programme has a full year of follow up (n=726 individuals).	USA	Cunningham et al. 2012 Walton et al. 2010
Bridging the Gap	Youth violence	This RCT compared a hospital delivered brief violence intervention alone with a brief violence intervention plus community case management. (n=75)	USA	Aboutanos et al. 2011

or prisons with the aim of changing attitudes to violence (Goodall et al. 2010), and there is emerging evidence of their efficacy.

Lastly, there are those interventions aimed at reducing violence against healthcare workers themselves.

Injury Surveillance

The first step in the public health approach to violence is to define the problem. It is well known that violence is under-reported to the police. In the UK as many as 50–75 per cent of assaults presenting to hospitals are not reported (Shepherd et al. 2000); so it is incumbent on any other agency dealing with victims to try to bridge that gap in knowledge. Injury surveillance involves Emergency Medicine departments in the collection of anonymized demographic data on assaults when victims present to hospital. This information is shared with the police allowing them to build up a fuller picture of the extent of crime, the locations of assaults, the use of weapons, and the association with other behaviours such as drinking alcohol or drug taking. This, in turn, can lead to better deployment of police resources to areas and at times where violence is most prevalent, allows identification of trends in weapons use, may lead to the development of better and more effective interventions for violence, and could potentially improve the health and wellbeing of local communities. In the UK, the injury surveillance model was developed in Cardiff and is now being more widely deployed. Results of a three year evaluation in Cardiff showed that information sharing between Emergency Medicine and the police resulted in changes in policing which led to a significant and sustained reduction in violent injury, and an increase in police recording of minor injuries when compared to other cities with similar demographic profiles around the UK (Florence et al. 2011). It is still the case, however, that even if injury surveillance were widely deployed, violence would still be under-reported as many victims do not seek or need medical intervention.

Signposting of Victims of Domestic Abuse

Signposting is an area with particular relevance to victims of domestic abuse. Domestic abuse affects both genders but is much more prevalent in women, affecting one in four women in the UK in the course of their lifetime. These patients may not require urgent medical care but may present to a range of healthcare providers with more minor issues indicative of abuse or with chronic physical and mental health problems. There is a debate in the literature about whether all women should be asked about domestic abuse at each healthcare contact, and opinion is divided (Bacchu et al. 2002; MacMillan et al. 2009; Klevens et al. 2012). What is clear though is that in some countries, there is a real need to provide training in this area for healthcare professionals so that they are better placed to help victims. Healthcare workers in the United States have, for some years, received training on domestic abuse, and this has been shown to increase the identification of victims. Once identified victims can offered onward referral.

Interventions for Violence

There are several screening tools for aggression and alcohol-related aggression for use in the health care setting. There are, however, very few short programmes specifically designed to reduce violence that would be practical in a busy, clinical environment. There are even fewer with robustly tested outcomes (Table 23.1). Snider and Lee (2009) carried out a systematic review of secondary prevention initiatives in emergency departments and found only four suitable programmes, three case management programmes, two of which were RCTs, and another retrospective programme 'Caught in the Crossfire'; all had small sample sizes.

Most interventions for violence take the form of longer anger management courses, largely used in the criminal justice setting. One structured multi-session cognitive behavioural programme that deals specifically with alcohol-related aggression is Control of Violence for Angry Impulsive Drinkers (COVAID) (Bowes et al.

2012). It shows promising results but to date has only been tested on small numbers of offenders in the prison setting. This programme formed the basis for the development of a single session intervention (SS-COVAID) for use in healthcare. SS-COVAID produced a significant reduction in alcohol consumption over a year of follow-up, and that reduction was similar to that produced by an Alcohol Brief Intervention (ABI). However, it failed to show any change in alcohol-related aggression scores. This may be because the patients to whom the shorter intervention was provided were not inherently violent and had low baseline aggression scores (Goodall et al. 2012).

SafERteens was developed and tested on a group of male and female teenage attendees at an emergency department in the United States; not all were victims of violence. The programme was delivered using a combination of face-to-face contact with a therapist and use of a computer-based intervention to allow the exploration of more complex issues in a short time. The programme reduced peer victimiziation and aggression at 1 year but although changes alcohol consequences were seen at 3 and 6 months post intervention, this effect was not maintained at 1 year (Cunningham et al. 2012).

Interventions for Associated Health Behaviours

Some forms of violence, particularly interpersonal violence, are associated with alcohol or drug misuse. Many victims of interpersonal violence are assaulted while drinking alcohol and those patients who suffer repeated injury due to violence are more likely to have been drinking at the time of injury and to be chronic heavy drinkers (Gmel et al. 2007; Laski et al. 2004). A recent audit of patients presenting to Scottish Emergency Medicine departments with injuries due to interpersonal violence found 70 per cent to be alcohol related (Scottish Emergency Department Alcohol Audit (SEDAA) Group 2006). This is addressed in detail in a subsequent chapter (Chapter 31).

PTSD

Victims of violence may experience ASD or PTSD. PTSD is a psychiatric syndrome that may develop after either witnessing or experiencing an event that involves an actual or perceived threat to life resulting in a feeling of intense fear, horror, or helplessness (American Psychiatric Association 2000). PTSD may be preceded by ASD, which occurs within 4 weeks of a traumatic event and lasts for a maximum of 4 weeks. ASD may progress to PTSD and may in some cases be predictive of it, but PTSD can develop in patients who do not display ASD so the onset of symptoms in PTSD may be delayed (Bryant et al. 2012).

As many as 41 per cent of facial trauma patients display symptoms of PTSD 6 weeks post injury (Hull et al. 2003) so for some acute surgical specialties, practitioners need to be familiar with screening tools and with the signs and symptoms of PTSD. Whether patients present to primary or secondary care practitioners need to be able to direct them towards appropriate treatment services (NICE 2005). Interventions for PTSD take the form of psychotherapy or cognitive behavioural therapy, and pharmacological management with anti-depressants is also required in some cases.

Interventions for Violence against Healthcare Workers

Healthcare workers may be exposed to violence in the workplace. Pompeii and colleagues (2013) demonstrated a wide ranging prevalence from verbal abuse (22–90 per cent) to physical threats (12–64 per cent) and physical violence (2–32 per cent). A variety of measures have been put in place to protect staff including violence risk assessments, online courses designed to educate staff about prevention and aggression management, and the use of pharmacological and physical restraint (Kynoch et al. 2011).

Transportability of Programmes Nationally and Internationally

The WHO launched its first *World Report on Violence and Health* in 2002 (WHO 2002). Since then many countries have instituted national violence prevention programmes. Many interventions for violence have been developed in high-income countries and one of the biggest challenges faced by other countries trying to implement these programmes is financial. However, many countries have taken the view that an investment in effective preventive measures will show long-term benefits in terms of injury reduction.

Injury surveillance has been implemented in various countries, including South Africa, Colombia, a consortium of five African nations (Zavala et al. 2007), Jamaica (Ward et al. 2002), and England and Wales (Florence et al. 2011). All have faced significant challenges, not least financial and technical ones, but have achieved a reasonable degree of success. The projects have yielded a wealth of information that can be used to implement violence reduction programmes.

Programmes to signpost victims of child abuse, domestic abuse, elder abuse, and sexual violence are not costly to implement. Child protection procedures are accepted as standard practice in many countries. Healthcare workers need some training but this is not extensive. In low- and middle-income countries, however, signposting will inevitably lead to an increased demand for services to support victims and this may be challenging.

Short interventions for violence have yet to prove their true efficacy. Longer programmes exist but they are resource hungry and the result is that they cannot be provided to large numbers of individuals.

Gaps in the Evidence

There is good and high level evidence for the efficacy of some forms of intervention in healthcare, for injury surveillance, the treatment of PTSD, signposting of victims of domestic abuse, the use of interventions such as Alcohol Brief Interventions to address associated behaviours such as drinking, and emerging evidence for others such as the provision of interventions by healthcare workers in schools (Goodall et al. 2010). Many programmes directly targeting violent or aggressive behaviour and victimiziation have been used in healthcare settings; however, few have been robustly evaluated and there are significant gaps in the evidence in terms of what works in this area. Taking a more positive view it is clear that there is a will for healthcare workers to be involved in prevention and much of the evidence gathering to date has focused on their willingness to participate, their level of knowledge, and the acceptance of such a way forward for patients

Conclusions

Healthcare workers are in a good position to get involved in violence prevention at primary, secondary, and tertiary levels. However, violence prevention needs to be embedded as standard practice at grass roots level as part of undergraduate curricula and clinical training programmes. There is evidence from some countries that this has improved; however, much remains to be done to enable violence prevention to become a mainstream healthcare activity. This will inevitably also require a change to policy in many countries to allow clinicians to be less focused on targets and more on holistic clinical outcomes.

References

Aboutanos, M. B., Jordan, A., and Cohen, R. et al. (2011). Brief violence interventions with community case management services are effective for high-risk trauma patients. *Journal of Trauma, 71,* 228–36.

American Psychiatric Association. (2000). *Diagnostic and Statistical Manual of Mental Disorders (4th ed., text rev.).* Washington, D.C.: American Psychiatric Association.

Bacchu, L., Mezey, G., and Bewley, S. (2002). Women's perceptions and experiences of routine enquiry for domestic violence in a maternity service. *BJOG, 109,* 9–16.

Bowes, N., McMurran, M., Williams, B., Siriol, D., and Zammit, I. (2012). Treating alcohol-related violence: intermediate outcomes in a feasibility study for a randomized controlled trial in prisons. *Criminal Justice and Behavior, 39,* 333.

Bryant, R. A., Creamer, M., O'Donnell, M., Silove, D., and McFarlane, A. C. (2012). The capacity of acute stress disorder to predict post-traumatic psychiatric disorders. *Journal of Psychiatric Research, 46,*168–73.

Campbell, R., Patterson, D., and Lichty, L. F. (2005). The effectiveness of sexual assault nurse examiner (SANE) programs: a review of psychological, medical, legal, and community outcomes. *Trauma Violence Abuse, 6,* 313–29.

Cunningham, R. M., Chermack, S. T., and Zimmerman, M. A, et al. (2012). Brief motivational interviewing intervention for peer violence and alcohol use in teens: one-year follow-up. *Pediatrics, 129,* 1083–90.

Feder, G., Davies, R. A., and Baird, K., et al. (2011). Identification and Referral to Improve Safety (IRIS) of women experiencing domestic violence with a primary care training and support programme: a cluster randomised controlled trial. *Lancet, 378,* 1788–95.

Florence, C., Shepherd, J., Brennan, I., and Simon, T. (2011). Effectiveness of anonymised information sharing and use in health service, police, and local government partnership for preventing violence related injury: experimental study and time series analysis. *BMJ: British Medical Journal, 342;*d3313.

Ford, J., and Murphy, J. E. (1996). Chain pharmacists' attitudes on and awareness of domestic abuse. *Journal of the American Pharmaceutical Association, NS36,* 323–8.

Gallagher, B., Allen, M., and Jones, B. (2008). Animal abuse and intimate partner violence: researching the link and its significance in Ireland—a veterinary perspective. *Irish Veterinary Journal, 61,* 658–67.

Gmel, G., Givel, J. C., Yersin, B., and Daeppen, J. B. (2007). Injury and repeated injury—what is the link with acute consumption, binge drinking and chronic heavy alcohol use? *Swiss Medical Weekly, 13,* 642–8.

Goodall, C., A., Bowman, A., and Smith, I. et al (2012). A randomized trial of brief intervention strategies in patients with alcohol-related facial trauma as a result of interpersonal violence. *Addiction Science and Clinical Practice, 7,* A66.

Goodall, C. A., Devlin, M. F., and Koppel, D. A. (2010). Medics against violence—the development of a new violence prevention intervention for schools. *Dent Update, 37,* 532–4.

Goodall, C. A., Oakey, F., and Ayoub, A. F. et al. (2008). A prospective randomised controlled trial of nurse delivered brief interventions for alcohol misuse to hazardous drinkers with alcohol related facial trauma. *British Journal of Oral Maxillofacial Surgery, 46,* 96–101.

Gore, F. M., Bloem, P. J., and Patton, G. C. et al (2011). Global burden of disease in young people aged 10-24 years: a systematic analysis. *Lancet, 377,* 2093–102.

Hegarty, K., O'Doherty, L., and Taft, A. et al. (2013). Screening and counselling in the primary care setting for women who have experienced intimate partner violence (weave): a cluster randomised controlled trial. *Lancet, 382,* 249–58.

Hsieh, N. K., Herzig, K., Gansky, S. A., Danley, D., and Gerbert, B. (2006). Changing dentists' knowledge, attitudes and behavior regarding domestic violence through an interactive multimedia tutorial. *Journal of the American Dental Association, 137,* 596–603.

Hull, A. M., Lowe, T., Devlin, M., Finlay, P., Koppel, D., and Stewart, A. M. (2003). Psychological consequences of maxillofacial trauma: a preliminary study. *British Journal of Oral Maxillofacial Surgery, 41,* 317–22.

Kynoch, K., Wu, C. J., and Chang, A. M. (2011). Interventions for preventing and managing aggressive patients admitted to an acute hospital setting: a systematic review. *Worldviews Evidence Based Nursing, 8,* 76–86.

Klevens, J., Kee, R., Trick, W., et al. Effect of screening for partner violence on women's quality of life: a randomized controlled trial. *JAMA: Journal of the American Medical Association,* 2012;*308*(7):681–689.

Laski, R., Ziccardi, V., Broder, H. L., and Janal, M. (2004). Facial trauma: a recurrent disease? The potential role of disease prevention. *Journal of Oral Maxillofacial Surgery, 62,* 685–8.

Love. C., Gerbert, B., Caspers, N., Bronstone, A., Perry, D., and Bird, W. (2001). Dentists' attitudes and behaviors regarding domestic violence. The need for an effective response. *Journal of the American Dental Association, 132,* 85–93.

MacMillan, H. L., Wathen, C. N., and Jamieson, E. et al. (2009). Screening for intimate partner violence in health care settings: a randomized trial. *JAMA: Journal of the American Medical Association, 302,* 493–501.

McCambridge, J., and Day, M. (2008). Randomized controlled trial of the effects of completing the Alcohol Use Disorders Identification Test questionnaire on self-reported hazardous drinking. *Addiction. 103,* 241–8.

Murray. C. J. L., Vos, T., and Lozano, R. et al (2012). Disability-adjusted life years (DALYs) for 291 diseases and injuries in 21 regions, 1990–2010: a systematic analysis for the Global Burden of Disease Study 2010. *Lancet 380,* 2197–223.

National Institute for Health and Care Excellence (2005). *The management of PTSD in adults and children in primary care.* Clinical Guideline 26. London: National Institute for Clinical Excellence.

Nelms, A. P., Gutmann, M. E., Solomon, E. S., Dewald, J. P., and Campbell, P. R. (2009). What victims of domestic violence need from the dental profession. *Journal of Dental Education, 73,* 490–8.

Patton, G. C., Coffey, C., and Sawyer, S. M. et al. (2009) Global patterns of mortality in young people: a systematic analysis of population health data. *Lancet, 374,* 881–92.

Pompeii, L., Dement, J., and Schoenfisch, A. et al. (2013). Perpetrator, worker and workplace characteristics associated with patient and visitor perpetrated violence (Type II) on hospital workers: a review of the literature and existing occupational injury data. *Journal of Safety Research, 44,* 57–64.

Scottish Emergency Department Alcohol Audit (SEDAA) Group (2006). Understanding Alcohol Misuse in Scotland: Harmful Drinking. One: The size of the problem. Edinburgh: NHS Quality Improvement Scotland.

Shepherd, J. P., Sivarajasingam, V., and Rivara, F. P. (2000). Using injury data for violence prevention. Government proposal is an important step towards safer communities. *British Medical Journal, 321,* 1481–2.

Smith, A. J., Hodgson, R. J., Bridgeman, K., and Shepherd, J. P. (2003). A randomized controlled trial of a brief intervention after alcohol-related facial injury. *Addiction, 98,* 43–52.

Snider, C. E., and Lee, J. (2009). Youth violence secondary prevention initiatives in emergency departments: a systematic review. *Canadian Journal of Emergency Medicine*, 11, 161–8.

Walton, M. A., Chermack, S. T., and Shope, J. T. et al. (2010). Effects of a brief intervention for reducing violence and alcohol misuse among adolescents: a randomized controlled trial. *JAMA: Journal of the American Medical Association*, 304, 527–35.

Ward, E., Arscott-Mills, S., Gordon, G., Ashley, D., and McCartney, T. (2002). The establishment of a Jamaican all-injury surveillance system. *Injury Control and Safety Promotion*, 9, 219–25.

Williams, S., Brown, A., Patton, R., Crawford, M. J., AND Touquet, R. (2005). The half-life of the 'teachable moment' for alcohol misusing patients in the emergency department. *Drug Alcohol Dependence*, 77, 205–8.

World Health Organization (2002). *World Report on Violence and Health: Summary*. Geneva: WHO.

World Health Organiziation (2005). *Alcohol and Interpersonal Violence. Policy Briefing*. Geneva: WHO.

Zavala, D. E., Bokongo, S., and John, I. A. et al. (2007). A multinational injury surveillance system pilot project in Africa. *Journal of Public Health Policy*, 28, 432–41.

CHAPTER 24

Evidence-informed approaches to preventing sexual violence and abuse

Stephen Smallbone and Nadine McKillop

Introduction to Evidence-Informed Approaches to Preventing Sexual Violence and Abuse

Sexual violence and abuse (SVA) encompasses a very diverse set of problematic human behaviours, including sexual harassment; exploitation; trafficking; exposing others improperly to sexual acts or materials; the production, distribution, and viewing of child pornography; and 'hands-on' offences ranging from unwanted or age-inappropriate sexual touching through to violent sexual assaults causing physical injuries and on occasion death. Psychological effects vary widely, but often include serious short- and long-term harms. Offenders are generally adolescent and adult males; may be relatives, acquaintances, or (less often) strangers; and range from the ordinary to the dangerously psychopathic. Victims range in age from infancy to old age, and are usually women or (male or female) children. SVA occurs predominantly in domestic settings - usually offenders' and/or victims' homes, but also in organizational, public, and more recently 'virtual' settings.

Public health (e.g. World Health Organization (WHO)) definitions deal somewhat separately with sexual violence against women and the sexual abuse of children. These definitions describe the general features of the problem, but do not specify its dimensions or clarify its boundaries. Thus while there is little disagreement about prototypical cases, there may be significant legal and moral ambiguity about behaviours at the edges of the continuum.

Clinical definitions have their historical roots in psychiatry, and accordingly tend to focus on the offender's 'disordered' sexual preferences or preoccupations. Diagnostic classifications on one hand include unusual, but not generally illegal or abusive, sexual behaviours (e.g. fetishism, transvestic fetishism), and on the other hand exclude many behaviours that are illegal and clearly abusive (e.g. commercial sexual exploitation, rape). Clinical definitions focused on individual sexual psychopathology are therefore both over- and under-inclusive with respect to SVA.

Legal definitions are dynamic, changing across time and societies, reflecting the prevailing social and moral standards of the time. There is always disagreement and debate about whether legal boundaries are appropriate, and indeed these pressures are often the impetus to legal reforms. A key advantage of legal definitions is that they specify the boundaries of various kinds of SVA—in fact they are designed to rule individual cases in or out. In addition, consistent with public health concerns, they revolve around the key issues of consent and harm. Probably for these reasons, research, policy, and practice tend to rely predominantly on legal definitions.

Conceptualizing SVA as a primarily legal–criminal problem gives recognition to its conceptual and empirical connections to other kinds of crime—sexual offences, like other kinds of crime, fundamentally involve irresponsible social behaviour, rule-breaking, coercion or deception, exploitation of vulnerable others, unrestrained aggression or violence, and so on, and for many offenders SVA is part of a broader involvement in crime. Rather than seeing SVA as a unique problem requiring its own unique explanations and solutions, a legal–criminological perspective opens the door to a wealth of relevant knowledge about how and why crime (including sexual crime) occurs, and to the application of established and innovative crime prevention concepts and methods. Specific knowledge about SVA is of course also required to inform prevention efforts.

We adopt this legal–criminological perspective in the present chapter. Our task is to summarize evidence-informed approaches to preventing SVA. We begin by outlining key implications of an integrated theoretical perspective that we believe to be consistent with, and may further inform, a public health approach to the problem. We then comment on the status of evidence for SVA prevention efforts. The bulk of the chapter is devoted to summarizing prevention approaches and associated outcomes. We briefly address the question of transportability of interventions to different contexts, and finally outline the main gaps in knowledge, as we see them.

Theoretical Overview

One of the most readily recognized features of the public health model is the distinctions it makes between primary (or universal), secondary (or selected), and tertiary (or indicated) prevention. These distinctions have proved very useful in areas such as medicine and physical disease prevention, but have not always translated easily to the prevention of complex, multidimensional social and behavioural problems. There is no widely shared understanding of what these levels of prevention might mean when applied to crime, for example (see e.g. Tonry and Farrington 1995). Nuanced arguments about whether a particular intervention constitutes secondary or tertiary prevention, for instance, need not distract us here. The important point is that the public health model draws attention to the possibility that interventions may be directed to preventing SVA before it would otherwise first occur (primary or secondary prevention), as well as after the fact to prevent further offending and victimization (tertiary prevention).

Another feature of the public health model, particularly when applied to social and behavioural problems such as SVA, is its explicit adoption of a social ecological framework (see Krug et al. 2002). This situates individual offenders and victims within their natural ecological context, and locates risk and protective factors at various levels of the ecological systems in which the individual develops and lives. Thus the causes of SVA exist not just within individuals, but also within the family, peer, organizational, neighbourhood, and sociocultural systems within which they are embedded.

According to social ecology theory, the more proximal the system is to the individual concerned, the more direct and therefore more powerful its influence (Bronfenbrenner 2005). Thus the attitudes and behaviour of a child's family, a teenager's peers, or an adult's spouse or workmates, for example, are likely to be more influential than are neighbourhood or wider sociocultural factors. The most proximal elements of any behaviour, including SVA, are of course those present in the immediate setting in which the behaviour is enacted. Recognizing the role played by these immediate situational factors adds a crucial element to prevention efforts. Instead of conceptualizing the problem in terms of *individuals* within their social ecological context, we can conceptualize the problem in terms of *person–situation interactions* that occur within, and are shaped by, the wider ecological context. Situations include physical features of the setting, in-the-moment interactions between the offender and victim, as well as the presence/absence and behaviour of third parties such as guardians, co-offenders, and bystanders.

We accordingly conceptualize SVA in terms of individual, ecological, and situational factors. We have set out our integrated theory in detail elsewhere (see Smallbone et al. 2008; Smallbone and Cale in press). Here we briefly outline its key implications for designing and organizing public health-oriented SVA prevention strategies.

First, the theory assumes a universal biologically based potential among sexually mature males to engage in SVA. Unlike in clinical formulations, for example, the potential to behave in such ways is not confined to a deviant subset of individuals. The reason that comparatively few people actually do engage in SVA, at least at a legal threshold, is that human socialization and social control systems (e.g. social attachments, formal and informal social controls), as well as natural ecological and situational barriers (e.g. guardianship, risk of detection), are under most circumstances remarkably effective in constraining this potential. Indeed there is compelling evidence that social constraints have become progressively more effective over the course of human history such that human societies are now much less violent than ever before (Pinker 2011). Prevention strategies should therefore build on these effective personal and social constraints.

Second, and consistent with the public health approach, the theory points to risk and protective factors at various levels of

offenders' and victims' natural social ecologies. In accordance with the proximal–distal principle, interventions targeting individuals, peer and family systems, and specific organizations and places, are likely to be more effective than those targeting neighbourhood or sociocultural systems. Exceptions may include specific communities or whole societies where the usual restraints have not been adequately established or have broken down at a global level (e.g. tribal, war-torn, or marginalized communities).

Third, the theory recognizes immediate situations (or, more precisely, immediate person–situation interactions) as the most proximal cause of SVA. This opens the door to employing situational and place-based prevention strategies as part of the prevention armoury. Situational prevention strategies can be employed to reduce opportunities for already-motivated offenders, but should also include a focus on settings and circumstances that may precipitate SVA-related motivations that would otherwise not occur, at least not at that time or place.

Finally, SVA offending, like other operant behaviour, is shaped by its consequences. Prevention strategies that rely on stereotyped views of offenders based on the most serious and persistent cases (e.g. the prototypical 'paedophile' or serial rapist) miss the important point that SVA-related motivations may be very different for potential, novice, and persistent offenders. Preventing persistent offenders from continuing to engage in SVA, and preventing SVA from occurring in the first instance, may require very different prevention strategies.

Status of Evidence

Leading child abuse researcher David Finkelhor (2009) recently observed that 'as yet, no true evidence-based programs or policies exist in the area of preventing child sexual abuse' (p. 170). If we were to apply the same standards, we would have to similarly conclude that nor are there any 'true evidence-based programmes' in the area of preventing adult-victim sexual violence. This should not be taken to mean that there is no useful evidence, however. In fact there are a handful of relevant randomized controlled trials, a plethora of lesser-standard evaluation studies, a growing number of meta-analytic reviews, and a few recent innovative developments, that together indicate some promising directions. It is nevertheless the case that much of the existing SVA prevention research is at best equivocal.

While there have been major investments in SVA prevention over the last few decades, there is an overall lack of clarity and coherence concerning prevention targets and the logic linking various prevention activities with desired outcomes. In these respects we must agree with another of Finkelhor's (2009) observations that sexual abuse prevention is beset by 'evidentiary chaos...and philosophical disagreement' (p.170). Speaking of SVA more broadly, we would add that existing prevention approaches are theoretically muddled. Lack of coherent theory and logic underpinning prevention efforts raises fundamental questions about whether SVA intervention design and evaluation have been asking the right kinds of questions in the first place.

Interventions and Outcomes
Developmental Prevention

Developmental crime prevention is based on established developmental and ecological theories and an extensive evidence base linking developmental risk and protective factors to later involvement in delinquency and crime. Its aim is essentially to reduce individual criminal propensities by intervening early to forestall the negative effects of certain developmental circumstances and experiences (Homel 1999). In fact a broad range of individual (e.g. impulsivity), family (e.g. marital conflict), peer (e.g. association with antisocial peers), school (e.g. early school dropout), and neighbourhood risk factors (e.g. community disorganization) has been linked to a broad range of negative developmental outcomes, not just delinquency and crime (e.g. mental health problems, substance abuse, and educational problems; Loeber and Farrington 1998). For our present purposes it is of particular note that these same developmental risk factors are associated with problematic sexual outcomes, including early sexual activity, having multiple sex partners, early pregnancies, unstable relationships, and personal victimization. Developmental prevention may thus also be applied to reducing vulnerabilities for SVA victimization.

Developmental prevention projects have not reported outcomes specifically concerning SVA offending. Nevertheless, given the clear conceptual and empirical links between SVA and other kinds of serious crime, it is assumed that successful developmental prevention programmes would reduce SVA offending alongside other kinds of offending. Emerging evidence that sexual abuse in childhood may be a specific risk factor for later SVA offending (e.g. Ogloff et al. 2012) suggests this as an additional target for developmental prevention of SVA. Given the predominance of males as SVA offenders, reducing exposure particularly of young males to sexual abuse, and reducing harmful impacts of those who are exposed, may be important additions to the developmental prevention of SVA.

Child-Focused Protective Behaviours Programmes

School-based protective behaviours programmes are among the most widely implemented of all SVA prevention initiatives. These programmes generally aim to increase children's recognition of potentially abusive situations, teach resistance behaviours, and increase abuse disclosure. This approach is unique to the field of sexual abuse—there are no similar expectations that children could or should be taught to prevent adults from mistreating them in other ways, such as neglect or physical or emotional abuse. Evaluations of such programmes indicate that children can acquire and retain relevant concepts, can implement strategies in simulated conditions, and are usually not distressed by the programme content. There is much more limited evidence that such programmes increase disclosure when future abuse does occur; whether they reduce actual victimization is yet to be demonstrated (Finkelhor 2009, Zwi et al. 2007).

Apart from the philosophical objection that children should not be responsible for ensuring their own sexual safety, the main criticisms of protective behaviours programmes are that they are not aligned with evidence about how sexual abuse actually occurs. They do not, for example, generally cater separately to boys and girls of different ages even though the circumstances of sexual abuse vary across victim gender and age (e.g. girls are more likely to be abused at a younger age, repeatedly, within a family setting). Nor do they account for the fact that many abused children have complex dependent relationships with the abuser that make negotiating their own safety complicated, and nor do they account for

wide variations in SVA-related vulnerabilities. Some commentators have argued that this 'resistance training' model should be replaced with a 'resilience-building' model, whereby programmes would instead target evidence-based individual (e.g. low confidence, loneliness) and family vulnerability factors (e.g. insecure attachments, family violence; Smallbone et al. 2008). More rigorous evaluations of existing approaches are required to establish whether the concepts and skills acquired can be transferred to real life contexts, resulting in actual reductions in SVA.

Adult-Focused Sexual Assault Education

In response particularly to concerns about sexual assaults of college women, rape awareness and prevention programmes are now widely implemented across college campuses in the United States. These programmes aim to enhance resilience in women through education about risky situations and teaching rape avoidance concepts and skills, and to educate young men about responsible sexual attitudes and dating behaviour. Despite their popularity, meta-analytic reviews show their effectiveness to be limited (Anderson and Whiston 2005). Overall, evaluations suggest that multi-session programmes that are culturally relevant, interactive, skills-based, and implemented to single-gender audiences, are the most effective (Schewe 2007). However, while programmes seem to have immediate positive impacts on attitude change (e.g. reductions in rape supportive attitudes and rape myth acceptance), in many circumstances gains do not seem to be retained even over short follow-up periods. The evidence is even less compelling regarding behaviour change, and it remains unclear whether these approaches have any impact on reducing sexual victimization. Concerns have been raised that these approaches are unlikely to be effective for preventing SVA by intimate partners (Basile 2003).

Sexual Ethics Programmes

A relatively new direction in SVA prevention has been to engage with middle and early high-school children to prevent risky attitudes and behaviours concerning sexual and other relationship violence. The rationale is to educate children about appropriate and inappropriate relationship behaviour at the same time that their sexual identities are forming and their attitudes, beliefs, and behaviours toward romantic partners are beginning to develop (Schewe 2007). Programmes aim to enhance knowledge and skills for developing and maintaining healthy, respectful, and non-violent relationships, and to build awareness about the origins of, and effective responses to, sexual violence. The most rigorously evaluated programme to date, Safe Dates, has demonstrated reductions in sexual dating violence across several outcome studies (Foshee et al. 2005). Programmes targeting at-risk groups (e.g. male athletes), such as the Coaching Boys into Men Campaign, have also demonstrated some success in reducing problematic sexual norms and behaviour (Miller et al. 2012, Fellmeth et al. 2013).

Responsible Bystander Programmes

There has been a recent shift from engaging with children and young adults as potential victims or perpetrators of SVA to engaging with (especially male) youth and young adults as responsible peers and potential guardians. These approaches view males as partners and active agents-of-change in preventing of SVA, rather than as potential offenders, and aim to effect responsible bystander intervention before (e.g. by helping peers to avoid high-risk situations), during (e.g. by interrupting an offence), or after SVA has occurred (e.g. by providing timely and effective victim support). Programmes aim to increase recognition of risky situations, enhance perceived responsibility, overcome barriers to intervening with peers, and build skills to intervene safely. Emerging evidence supports the effectiveness of bystander interventions in producing attitudinal and behavioural change (Banyard et al. 2007), but follow-up studies are needed to determine their long-term impacts, including whether they result in actual reductions in SVA.

Preventing Re-Victimization

Services for identified SVA victims have proliferated over the last few decades. Interventions are generally focused on the immediate problem of ameliorating potential harms. Although it has long been known that SVA victims are at considerably increased risk of further victimization, surprisingly little attention has been given to testing the effectiveness of these services for preventing re-victimization.

For children and adolescents, the best-supported treatment approach for reducing psychological harms associated with SVA appears to be individual- or group-based trauma-focused cognitive behavioural therapy (TF-CBT), particularly when treatment includes parallel child and parent sessions (Trask et al. 2011). Adult survivors of childhood SVA have also benefited from TF-CBT, as well as present-focused CBT (PF-CBT; Classen et al. 2011). Structured individual CBT appears to be the most effective in reducing trauma-related symptoms in women who have experienced recent SVA (Taylor and Harvey 2009). PF-CBT is thought to be promising for reducing sexual re-victimization, but further evaluations are needed before this becomes clear (Classen et al. 2006). Specific rape risk-reduction programmes that target known personal and environmental risk factors have shown promise for increasing self-efficacy and enhancing risk perception, and possibly also for reducing re-victimization (Blackwell et al. 2003).

Preventing Re-Offending

Like victim services, treatment and risk management programmes for sexual offenders have proliferated over the last two decades. Meta-analytic reviews indicate that multisystemic therapy and CBT approaches are the most effective in reducing recidivism for youth offenders, and that pharmacological and CBT approaches are the most effective for adult offenders (Hanson et al. 2002; Lösel and Schmucker 2005), particularly for higher-risk offenders. There is some evidence that generic cognitive skills programmes may also be effective for adult sexual offenders (Robinson 1995).

Community-based programmes are more effective than are residential or prison-based programmes (MacKenzie 2002). For prisoners generally, post-release supervision and support is thought to be integral to maintaining rehabilitative gains and safely negotiating challenges associated with release and re-integration (Cullen and Gendreau 2000). Two studies have shown supervised release to be associated with lower recidivism specifically for adult sexual offenders (Boccaccini et al. 2009; Smallbone and Rallings 2013). One approach showing promise for socially isolated adult sexual offenders is Circles of Support and Accountability, with two recent evaluations showing significant reductions in sexual and violent recidivism up to 4.5 years post-release (Wilson et al. 2009).

In recent years many jurisdictions have introduced sexual offender registration and community notification schemes. Evaluations suggest that such schemes are ineffective in reducing re-offending (Sandler et al. 2008), and when applied to youth sexual offenders may be associated with increased arrests for minor offences and technical breaches (Letourneau et al. 2009).

Transportability

Much of the research on SVA prevention has been conducted in North America and other developed Western countries, and little is known about the transportability of prevention models and programmes developed in these settings to other social and cultural settings. The example of multisystemic treatment (MST), one of the most extensively evaluated interventions for antisocial youth, may be instructive. Originally developed in the United States, MST has been adopted in at least eight other countries, where significant adaptations were required to produce comparable client engagement and outcomes (Schoenwald et al. 2008). For prevention strategies more broadly, understanding how the local political, legal, and cultural context may affect the capacity and readiness for successful implementation may be a critical starting point (Mikton 2013). Evaluation models such as the 'realist' model (Pawson and Tilley 2004) offer nuanced approaches in which the specific context of the intervention becomes central to its design, implementation, and evaluation.

Gaps in Knowledge

The 'evidentiary chaos' in SVA prevention research makes it difficult to pinpoint specific gaps in the existing evidence base. The problem seems a much more fundamental one that the field has not yet established an agreed, coherent theoretical framework or overarching prevention model. The social ecological model that has long guided research and practice in related fields (e.g. public health, general child maltreatment, developmental criminology) has historically played only a marginal role in SVA prevention. The two dominant approaches seem to be a feminist model, which frames the problem at the broadest sociocultural level, and a clinical model, which typically frames the problem at the narrowest individual level. Feminist approaches have succeeded in drawing widespread attention to the problem, but have contributed comparatively little to the empirical evidence base. Clinical approaches have by contrast produced a large body of empirical literature, but this has focused narrowly on the psychological characteristics of convicted offenders and individual-level risk factors for recidivism. Even here there is a lack of theoretical guidance—much is now known about individual characteristics associated with recidivism, for example, but very little is known about why these associations exist, or about ecological and situational risk and protective factors associated with either the original offending or with recidivism. The biggest gap is arguably the lack of knowledge about how and why sexual offences first occur, and how this knowledge might be developed to inform primary and secondary prevention efforts.

There is also a large empirical literature on adult-focused and especially child-focused protective behaviours programmes, the results of which remain equivocal with respect to preventing actual SVA. Arguably it is more appropriate, and theoretically and empirically more defensible, to focus prevention efforts on reducing vulnerabilities in at-risk children and young adults, and on intervening to reduce exposure to risky situations and to make risky places safer. Among other things, creating safer environments requires improving the capacity for adult guardianship. Responsible bystander training is one recent type of intervention that aligns with this approach. Wortley and Smallbone (2006; 2012) have outlined how situational crime prevention principles might be applied to make physical, social, and online environments safer to reduce various forms of SVA, although as yet there is little evidence demonstrating the effectiveness of this approach.

Conclusions

A fundamental challenge for SVA prevention is to come to grips with the multifaceted nature of the problem itself. What might be done to prevent, say, the sexual abuse of 10–12-year-old girls in family settings, is likely to be very different from what is needed to prevent the abuse of 12–14-year-old boys in educational, recreational, or pastoral care settings, the sexual trafficking of adolescents or young adults, the proliferation of internet child pornography, sexual assaults of young women in and around bars, sexual harassment or assault in sporting or military settings, or rape in combat zones. Indeed these problems highlight the stark limitations of the mainstays of current prevention efforts—teaching children and young adults to resist offenders, and treating offenders once they are caught and convicted. Getting serious about prevention will require a much more sophisticated approach that enables the most serious problems to be identified and prioritized, the dimensions, scope, and dynamics of these specific problems to be established, and prevention strategies designed to fit the problem at hand. As we have argued elsewhere (Smallbone et al. 2008), a comprehensive prevention framework is needed that focuses on key targets—(potential) offenders, (potential) victims, specific situations, and relevant ecological (peer, family, organizational, and neighbourhood) systems—across all prevention levels (primary, secondary and tertiary).

References

Anderson, A. A., and Whiston, S. C. (2005). Sexual assault education programs: a meta-analytic examination of their effectiveness. *Psychology of Women Quarterly*, 29, 374–88.

Banyard, V. L., Moynihan, M. M., and Plante, E. G. (2007). Sexual violence prevention through bystander education: an experimental evaluation. *Journal of Community Psychology*, 35, 463–81.

Basile, K. C. (2003). Implications of public health for policy on sexual violence. *Annals New York Academy of Sciences*, 989, 446–63.

Blackwell L. M., Lynn, S. J., Vanderhoff, H., and Gidycz, C. (2003). Sexual assault revictimization: toward effective risk-reduction programs. In: L. J. Koenog, L. S. Doll, A. O'Leary, and W. Pequegnat (eds), *From Child Sexual Abuse to Adult Sexual Risk: Trauma, Revictimization and Intervention*. Washington, D.C.: American Psychological Association, pp. 269–95.

Boccaccini, M. T., Murrie, D. C., Caperton, J. D., and Hawes, S. W. (2009). Field validity of the Static-99 and MnSOST-R among sex offenders evaluated for civil commitment as sexually violent predators. *Psychology, Public Policy, and Law*, 15, 278–314.

Bronfenbrenner, U. (2005). The bioecological theory of human development. In: U. Bronfenbrenner (ed.), *Making Human Beings Human: Bioecological Perspectives on Human Development*. Thousand Oaks, CA: Sage, pp. 3–15.

Classen, C. C., Cavanaugh, C. E., and Kaupp, J. W. et al. (2011). A comparison of trauma-focused and present-focused group therapy for survivors of childhood sexual abuse: a randomized control trial. *Psychological Trauma: Theory, Research, Practice and Policy*, 3, 84–93.

Classen, C. C., Palesh, O. G., and Aggarwal, R. (2006). Sexual revictimization: a review of the empirical literature. *Trauma, Violence and Abuse*, 6, 103–29.

Cullen, F. T., and Gendreau, P. (2000). Assessing correctional rehabilitation: policy, practice, and prospects. In: J. Horney (ed.), *Criminal Justice 2000: Volume 3—Policies, Processes, and Decisions of the Criminal Justice System*. Washington, D.C.: National Institute of Justice, pp. 109–75.

Fellmeth GL, Heffernan C, Nurse J, Habibula S, Sethi D. (2013) Educational and skills-based interventions for preventing relationship and dating violence in adolescents and young adults. *Cochrane Database Syst Rev*, 6:CD004534. doi:10.1002/14651858.CD004534. pub3

Finkelhor, D. (2009). The prevention of childhood sexual abuse. *The Future of Children*, 19, 169–94.

Foshee, V. A., Bauman, K. E., Ennett, S. E., Suchindran, C., Benefield, T., and Linder, G. F. (2005). Assessing the effects of the dating violence prevention program 'safe dates' using random coefficient regression modelling. *Prevention Science*, 6, 245–58.

Hanson, R. K., Gordon, A., and Harris, A. J. R. et al. (2002). First report of the collaborative outcome data project on the effectiveness of psychological treatment of sex offenders. *Sexual Abuse: A Journal of Research and Treatment*, 14, 169–95.

Homel, R. (1999). *Pathways to Prevention: Developmental and Early Intervention Approaches to Crime in Australia*. Canberra: Commonwealth of Australia.

Krug, E. G., Dahlberg L. L., Mercy, J. A., Zwi, A. B., and Lozano, R. (2002). *World Report on Violence and Health*. Geneva: World Health Organization.

Letourneau, E. J., Bandyopadhyay, D., Sinha, D., and Armstrong, K. S. (2009). The influence of sex offender registration on juvenile sexual recidivism. *Criminal Justice Policy Review,* 20, 136–53.

Loeber, R., and Farrington, D. P. (1998). *Serious and Violent Juvenile Offenders: Risk Factors and Successful Intervention*. Thousand Oaks, CA: Sage.

Lösel, F., and Schmucker, M. (2005). The effectiveness of treatment for sexual offenders: a comprehensive meta-analysis. *Journal of Experimental Criminology*, 1, 117–46.

MacKenzie, D. L. (2002). Reducing the criminal activities of known offenders and delinquents: crime prevention in the courts and corrections. In: L. W. Sherman, D. P. Farrington, B. C. Welsh, and D. L. Mackenzie (eds), *Evidence-based Crime Prevention*. New York: Routledge, pp. 330–404.

Mikton, C. (2013). Review of the evidence for effectiveness of programmes to prevent child maltreatment. Presented at the Unicef East Asia and Pacific Regional Meeting, *Research on Violence against Children: Building Evidence for Action*, 23-27 June 2013, Bangkok, Thailand.

Miller, E., Tancredi, D. J., and McCauley, H. L. et al. (2012). Coaching Boys into Men: a cluster-randomized controlled trial of a dating violence prevention program. *Journal of Adolescent Health*, 51, 431–8.

Ogloff, J., Cutajar, M., Mann, E., and Mullen, P. (2012). *Child sexual abuse and subsequent offending and victimization: a 45 year follow-up study.* (Trends & Issues in Crime & Criminal Justice No. 440). Canberra: Australian Institute of Criminology, pp. 1–6.

Pawson, R., and Tilley, N. (2004). Realist evaluation. In: S. Matthieson (ed.). *Encyclopaedia of Evaluation*. Thousand Oaks, CA: Sage Publications, pp. 359–67.

Pinker, S. (2011). *The Better Angels of our Nature: Why Violence has Declined*. New York, N.Y.: Penguin Books.

Robinson, D. (1995). *The Impact of Cognitive Skills Training on Post-release Recidivism among Canadian Federal Offenders*. Ottawa: Correctional Services of Canada.

Sandler, J. C., Freeman, N. J., and Scocia, K. M. (2008). Does a watched pot boil? A time-series analysis of New York State's sex offender registration and notification law. *Psychology, Public Policy and Law,* 14, 284–302.

Schewe, P. A. (2007). Interventions to prevent sexual violence. In: L. S. Doll, S. E. Bonzo, J. A. Mercy, D. A. Sleet, and E. N. Haas (eds), *Handbook of Injury and Violence Prevention*. New York: Springer, pp. 223–40.

Schoenwald, S. K., Heiblum, N., Saldana, L., and Henggeler, S. W. (2008). The international implementation of multisystemic therapy. *Evaluation and the Health Professions*, 31, 211–25.

Smallbone, S., and Cale, J. (in press). An integrated life-course developmental theory of sexual offending. In: A. Blokland and P. Lussier (eds), *Sexual Offenders: A Criminal Careers Approach*. New York: Wiley, pp. 1–44.

Smallbone, S., Marshall, W. L., and Wortley, R. (2008). *Preventing Child Sexual Abuse: Evidence, Policy and Practice*. Cullompton: Willan.

Smallbone, S., and Rallings, M. (2013). Short-term predictive validity of the Static-99 and Static-99-R for Australian indigenous and non-indigenous sexual offenders. *Sexual Abuse: A Journal of Research and Treatment*, 25, 302–16.

Taylor, J. E., and Harvey, S. T. (2009). Effects of psychotherapy with people who have been sexually assaulted: a meta-analysis. *Aggression and Violent Behaviour*, 14, 273–85.

Tonry, M., and Farrington, D. P. (1995). Strategic approaches to crime prevention. In: M. Tonry, and D. Farrington (eds), *Building a Safer Society: Strategic Approaches to Crime Prevention*. Chicago: University of Chicago Press, pp. 1–20.

Trask, E. V., Walsh, K, and DiLillo, D. (2011) Treatment effects for common outcomes of child sexual abuse: a current meta-analysis. *Aggression and Violent Behavior*, 16, 6–19.

Wilson, R. J., Cortoni, F., and McWhinnie, A. J. (2009). Circles of Support and Accountability: a Canadian national replication of outcome findings. *Sexual Abuse: A Journal of Research and Treatment*, 21, 412–30.

Wortley, R., and Smallbone, S. (2006). Applying situational principles to sexual offenses against children. In: R. Wortley and S. Smallbone (eds), *Situational Prevention of Child Sexual Abuse*. Monsey, NY: Criminal Justice Press, pp. 7–35.

Wortley, R., and Smallbone, S. (2012). *Internet Child Pornography: Causes, Investigation and Prevention*. Santa Barbara: Praeger.

Zwi, K., Woolfenden, S., Wheeler, D., O'Brien, T., Tait, P., and Williams, K. (2007). School-based education programmes for the prevention of child sexual abuse. *Cochrane Database of Systematic Reviews*, 3, 1–39. DOI:10.1002/14651858.CD004380.pub2.

CHAPTER 25

Preventing intimate partner violence

Lori Heise

Overview of Preventing Intimate Partner Violence

Intimate partner violence arguably represents the most significant 'violence burden' on women's health and well-being, especially in low- and middle-income countries. At the population level, it greatly exceeds the prevalence of all other forms of physical and sexual abuse (Heise 2012b).

The chapter reviews programmes and evidence related to five areas of interest: shifting gender-related roles, norms, and beliefs, including notions of male authority and female obedience; reducing exposure to violence during childhood; the contributing role of problematic alcohol abuse; women's economic status and empowerment; and increasing the 'cost' of violence through legal and justice system interventions.

The first three topics are highlighted because there is relatively strong evidence that these factors contribute to the overall likelihood that partner violence will occur, or in the case of alcohol, that incidents of violence will be more frequent and their consequences more severe (Heise 2012b). The practical implication is that interventions that successfully reduce these factors among individuals or in communities will also reduce the prevalence and severity of women's experience with partner violence.

The second two topics—women's economic empowerment and legal and justice systems—are reviewed here because donors and advocates have long considered such interventions critical to violence reduction and have invested considerable resources accordingly.

Significantly, the factors that increase an individual woman's risk of violence are not necessarily the same as those that account for the distribution of partner violence across settings. One of the key contributions that public health has to offer violence prevention is its focus on population-level drivers of risk. Interventions that shift the distribution curve of key determinants of partner violence (such as norms of female obedience or acceptability of violence), hold promise to greatly reduce overall levels of abuse.

The State of Evidence

The field of partner-violence prevention is still in its infancy, especially in low- and middle-income countries. While it benefits from several decades of practice-based learning (World Health Organization (WHO) and London School of Hygiene and Tropical Medicine (LSHTM) 2010), rigorous evaluations are largely lacking on how effective programmes have been in reducing violence. Moreover, existing evaluation research has concentrated on assessing the effectiveness of interventions designed to identify and assist victims through formal institutions, such as the health and justice system, or to reduce repeat violence by male partners or repeat victimization among women. Programmes geared toward primary prevention of partner violence have been few and far between.

In a field as complex and 'new' as violence prevention it is vital that innovation be encouraged; many worthy strategies may lack evidence not because they don't work, but because they have not been evaluated. Some of the most 'effective' strategies may remain to be discovered.

Changing Social Norms and Gender-Related Beliefs

Both qualitative and quantitative data suggest that social norms and beliefs related to gender and family privacy contribute to physical and sexual violence (Boudet et al. 2013). Social norms are shared expectations of specific individuals or groups regarding how people should behave (Paluck and Bell 2010). Norms act as powerful motivators either for or against change in individual attitudes and behaviours, largely because individuals who deviate from group expectations are subject to shaming, sanctions, or disapproval by others who are important to them. If it is considered socially unacceptable for a woman to get a divorce or live alone, for example, this can serve as a powerful deterrent to her leaving an abusive relationship, even if she has the legal right to do so.

Box 25.1 points to the kinds of social and cultural norms that support violence against women in low- and middle-income settings, especially within the family. Particularly salient are norms related to gender.

In many countries wife beating is normative, with women as well as men expressing support for partner violence under certain circumstances (WHO 2005). Implicit support for violence is frequently couched in terms of men's need to 'discipline' women for various infractions, generally related to gendered expectations regarding female behaviour or deference to male authority.

The acceptability of violence appears strongly linked to both the nature of the perceived transgression and the severity of abuse. Violence that is viewed as 'without just cause' or is perceived as excessive is more likely to be condemned by women themselves

---

Box 25.1 Examples of social and cultural norms that promote violence against women

- A man has a right to assert power over a woman and is considered socially superior

- A man has a right to physically discipline a woman for 'incorrect' behaviour

- Physical violence is an acceptable way to resolve conflict in a relationship

- Intimate partner violence is a 'taboo' subject

- Divorce is shameful

- Marriage grants men un-restricted sexual access to his wife

- Sexual activity (including rape) is a marker of masculinity

- Girls are responsible for controlling a man's sexual urges

Adapted with permission from World Health Organization/ London School of Hygiene and Tropical Medicine, *Preventing Intimate Partner and Sexual Violence against Women*, World Health Organization, Geneva, Switzerland, Copyright © 2010, available from http://whqlibdoc.who.int/publications/2010/9789241564007_eng.pdf.

---

and by others. This opens the possibility of intervening at multiple levels—to challenge the underlying beliefs that define the range of acceptable male and female behaviour; to build a new social consensus that all violence, regardless of severity, is unacceptable in families; and to foster informal sanctions against men who abuse their wives.

Among strategies to shift norms, attitudes, and beliefs related to gender, the three that have been most rigorously evaluated are (i) small group, participatory workshops designed to challenge existing beliefs, build pro-social skills, promote reflection and debate, and encourage collective action; (ii) larger-scale 'edutainment' or campaign efforts coupled with efforts to reinforce media messages through street theatre, discussion groups, cultivation of 'change agents', and print materials; and (iii) theory-informed community mobilization strategies. Each of these strategies has demonstrated modest changes in reported attitudes and beliefs—and in some cases, reductions in reported rates of partner violence (Heise 2012b).

Participatory Group Workshops

Two programmes in South Africa (Stepping Stones and IMAGE) and one programme in Burundi (Iyengar and Ferrari 2011) have been rigorously evaluated using community randomized trials. The IMAGE programme—a participatory gender and HIV training grafted onto an existing microfinance programme—reduced partner violence by 55 per cent over 2 years, improved a range of household economic measures, and increased women's self efficacy (Pronyk et al. 2006). A follow up study suggests that the positive impacts on empowerment, violence, and HIV-related behaviours derived largely from the gender and HIV component, rather than the underlying microfinance intervention (Kim et al. 2009).

By contrast, a second randomized experiment in Burundi increased decision-making for women but did not decrease domestic violence (Iyengar and Ferrari 2011). The project in

Burundi combined a village savings scheme with discussion groups that encouraged couples to discuss how household decisions are made and promoted greater respect for women's contributions and opinions.

Stepping Stones, a stand-alone group intervention that has been adapted and used in 40 countries, is designed to build knowledge, risk awareness, and communication skills around gender, HIV, violence, and relationships. Most versions involve at least 50 hours of critical reflection and training over 10–12 weeks, delivered in 15 sessions.

The Stepping Stones Curriculum has been evaluated using a community-randomized trial in South Africa and a large quasi-experimental study in India. Generally, these evaluations demonstrate that Stepping Stones, when properly implemented, can increase knowledge and have a positive impact on male behaviour, including decreasing the likelihood that they will abuse their partner, engage in transactional sex, or drink excessively (Jewkes et al. 2008). Stepping Stones, however, did not have similarly positive effects on women's behaviour or outcomes (e.g. transactional sex, abuse by a partner, unwanted pregnancy), suggesting that as a stand-alone intervention, it may be inadequate to overcome the social and economic factors that condition women's risk. Moreover, neither Stepping Stones nor IMAGE has demonstrated a clear ability to diffuse novel beliefs or behaviours beyond workshop participants into the wider community. This is key if strategies for transforming norms are to be taken to scale.

Edutainment and other Social Media Strategies

An increasingly popular approach to changing norms and behaviours is the creative use of media and/or entertainment culture together with strategies to encourage dialogue and reinforce social change messages at a community level (Lacayo and Singhal 2008).

Among the most innovative groups doing this work are the Soul City Institute for Health and Development in South Africa (now working regionally); Breakthrough, a non-governmental organization in India; and Puntos de Encuentro in Nicaragua. All include a mass media component, with Puntos and Soul City running pro-social television dramas that have achieved remarkable popularity and viewership within their setting. Evaluations of all three programmes are cautiously optimistic, demonstrating reductions in violence-supportive beliefs, attitudes, and norms (CMS Communication 2011; Solorzano et al. 2008; Usdin et al. 2005).

A typical 1-year Soul City series, for example, includes 13 1-hour episodes of a prime-time television series, 45 15-minute radio drama episodes, three booklets distributed at the community level, and an 'advertising/publicity' campaign on a series-related topic. Series 4 specifically focused on partner violence featuring a story line about Matlakala, who is the wife of an abusive husband, Thabang. The show promoted a new injunctive norm against abuse by depicting neighbours banging on pots and pans to communicate their disapproval and disrupt partner violence.

An evaluation of Series 4 found a consistent association between exposure to the Soul City programmes and both support-seeking (e.g. calling the helpline or writing down the number) and support-giving (e.g. did something concrete to stop domestic violence during the evaluation period). Eight months after being established, 41 per cent of respondents nationally had heard of the helpline. Some communities had adopted the pot-banging strategy modelled in the series (WHO and LSHTM 2010).

Reducing Childhood Exposure to Violence

Hundreds of multivariate studies from both high and low-income countries have found that children who witness violence between their parents or who are physically abused themselves are more likely to use violence in their relationships as adults (Ellsberg et al. 2000; Vung and Krantz 2008; Whitfield et al. 2003). The pattern is not inevitable, however, and a key question for future research is what genetic, situational, socio-cultural, and life course factors distinguish those who later become violent from those who go on to form healthy relationships.

Longitudinal research from high-income countries likewise demonstrates that early exposure to violence can leave emotional and developmental scars that predispose a child to later behavioural problems, including poor school performance, bullying, and antisocial behaviour in adolescence (Anda et al. 2006). Left unchecked, this developmental pathway is highly predictive of later engagement in partner violence (Ireland and Smith 2009). There is evidence that early trauma can affect the developing brain, interfering with a child's ability to develop trust and empathy, and heightening the tendency to perceive benign overtures as threats (Neigh et al. 2009). There is an urgent need to establish whether the developmental pathway between early violence, antisocial behaviour in adolescence, and partner violence in adulthood is similarly operative in low-income countries, and whether and how it interacts with norm-driven violence.

Reducing partner violence therefore requires reducing exposure to violence in early childhood. Strong evidence is available from high-income countries that parenting programmes can improve parent-child interactions. (Eshel and et.al. 2006; Gilbert et al. 2009). Likewise, a systematic 'review of reviews' in the *Bulletin of the World Health Organization* ranked parenting education among four interventions showing promise for the prevention of child maltreatment (Mikton and Butchart 2009). It is not clear the extent to which these findings from North America, Australia, and Europe will generalize to realities elsewhere. A recent review of studies evaluating parenting interventions in low- and middle-income countries found parenting training and support programmes promising (Knerr et al. 2013). The authors noted, however, an almost stunning lack of content in parenting curricula on the benefits of promoting less rigid and more equitable roles between boys and girls.

Less data are available on the effectiveness of programmes in low-income countries. In many settings, the same logic that justifies the beating of children is applied to the beating of adult women. Both are framed as physical 'correction' for transgression against authority—men's authority in the case of women and parent's authority in the case of children. Much progress has been made globally toward outlawing corporal punishment in schools, with 43 per cent of states in Africa and 52 per cent in East Asia and the Pacific now outlawing violent discipline in schools (Global Initiative to End all Corporal Punishment of Children 2011). However, attitudes are much more ambivalent about interfering with 'parents' rights' to discipline their children.

A comparative study of the effects of banning corporal punishment in five European countries suggests that prohibiting corporal punishment *does* facilitate reductions in the use of violence, but only where reforms are accompanied by intensive on-going efforts to publicise the law and to introduce and reinforce positive forms of discipline (Bussmann et al. 2011).

Addressing Problematic Alcohol Use

A wide range of evidence establishes excessive alcohol use, especially binge drinking by men, as a key factor that increases the frequency and severity of partner violence. One systematic review found that harmful use of alcohol by men was associated with a 4.6-fold increased risk of exposure to intimate partner violence compared to mild or no alcohol use (Gil-Gonzalez et al. 2006). While alcohol use is neither necessary nor sufficient for abuse to occur, data suggest that lowering the rates of binge drinking could reduce the overall level and severity of partner violence.

Various strategies have been demonstrated effective in reducing the harmful consequences of drinking (See Chapter 41, this volume). Studies have demonstrated a reduction in domestic violence after the implementation of strategies to reduce alcohol availability in the United States, Greenland, and Australia (Room 2003), as well as reduction of violence after abusers have been treated for alcohol abuse (Murphy and Ting 2010). Replication of WHO's 'brief counselling' intervention by health workers has shown promise in South Africa and India (Peltzer et al. 2008); however, evaluated programmes, especially those that specify partner violence as an outcome, are rare in the developing world.

Women's Economic Empowerment

Compared to alcohol abuse (where the association with partner violence is consistent), the role of economic factors on women's risk of violence appears to be complex, context-specific, and contingent on other factors (such as partner's employment or education). Current research suggests that economic empowerment of women in some situations can perversely increase the incidence of partner violence, at least in the short term (Vyas and Watts 2008). This seems especially common in situations where a man is unable to fulfil his gender-ascribed role as 'bread-winner' and a woman is beginning to contribute relatively more to family maintenance, or where a woman takes a job that defies prevailing social convention (Atkinson et al. 2005).

To date, evaluations of economic empowerment strategies have focused on two short-term strategies—micro-finance programmes and conditional cash transfers. The premise of micro-finance programmes is that access to small amounts of affordable credit can help families cope with events such as illness without going into debt and can help to unleash entrepreneurial talent and initiative among the poor (Sanyal 2009). Findings suggest that such schemes can have either a positive or negative effect on a woman's risk of partner violence, depending on other aspects of her situation. However, most currently available studies come from one country, Bangladesh, so the broader relevance to other settings is not clear.

Only a handful of evaluations have examined the impact of conditional cash transfers on women's risk of partner violence.

These evaluations have focused almost exclusively on Mexico's *Oportunidades* programme, which targets poor households and dispenses cash to women provided that they attend health and nutrition classes, send their children to school, and receive periodic health checkups. One study that looked back 5–9 years post-enrolment demonstrated no effects on partner violence from the programme (Bobonis and Castro 2010). A second study found that the cash transfers decreased alcohol-related violence by 37 per cent across all *Oportunidades* households. However, violence increased in households where men had low levels of education (and presumably more traditional gender expectations) and the wife was entitled to large transfers (Angelucci 2008). In this situation it appears that the loss that men experience over status and control exceeds the benefits they perceive from increased income. Thus, the risk of violence increases.

Indeed, the effect that any one economic variable may have on women's risk of violence—women's entry into employment, her ownership of property, access to income through transfers of microfinance schemes—all appear to be defined by variables extending beyond the economic implications of the shift: To what extent do women's resources improve the household's economic security, and does the husband see this as an asset or a threat? Do community and family norms support a woman taking on new economic roles? How does the change affect the existing gendered division of labour?

Future research on the short-term impacts of economic empowerment must explore this wider field of questions. Programmes must also recognize that the short and long-term effects of economic empowerment strategies may differ. Economic and feminist theory strongly suggests that increasing a woman's access to and control over resources over the long term will reduce her risk of partner violence. Moreover, historical studies and ecological studies confirm that gender roles tend to become more equitable as more women enter the formal wage economy and attain higher status jobs (Heise 2012a).

Implementing Legal and Justice System Reforms

Coalitions of women's organizations and human rights groups have been remarkably successful in reforming criminal and civil laws related to domestic violence and rape. As of April 2011, 125 countries had passed legislation on domestic violence (United Nations Women 2011). These laws have often broadened the legal definition of partner violence to include psychological and financial abuse by a partner, as well as physical and sexual violence. The effectiveness of legal reform as a mechanism to redefine the boundaries of acceptable behaviour is theoretically strong, but studies documenting its impact in this regard are largely absent.

By contrast, a substantial body of research exists on the effectiveness of justice system interventions, largely from the United States, United Kingdom, and Australia. The United States in particular—which adopted a 'criminal justice system' approach to domestic violence—has generated little convincing evidence that pro-arrest policies, pro-prosecution policies, domestic violence courts, and court-referred perpetrator treatment programmes (whether considered individually or taken together) have worked to substantially reduce rates of recidivism or make women feel safer (Maxwell and Garner 2012). Many of these interventions are now being implemented in various developing countries.

By contrast, research from the United States suggests that protective orders do reduce repeat violence for some victims some of the time. A review of 32 studies (Spitzberg, 2002) estimates that about 40 per cent of protective orders are violated on average. A more recent study that followed 698 women found that 60 per cent experienced violations within 12 months of the order, although the majority of these women—even those who experienced a violation—reported feeling 'safer' with the order, with three-quarters saying that the order was either 'extremely' (51 per cent) or 'fairly' (27 per cent) effective at addressing the abuse (Logan and Walker 2009).

Women-only police stations are the justice system reform that has been most widely evaluated in developing countries. Designed to facilitate reporting of rape and domestic violence, women's police stations have received mixed reviews in terms of effectiveness. Women frequently arrive at these stations seeking emergency shelter, guidance, support, and legal advice; and most stations are not set up to meet these needs. Often, women must initiate a legal case in order to obtain protection orders, even though most do not want to pursue prosecution or send their partners to jail. An evaluation of women's police stations in Brazil, Ecuador, Nicaragua, and Peru concludes that although they may contribute to changing norms about violence against women, there is no evidence that they reduce violence or give women better access to justice (Jubb et al. 2010).

A wide range of other innovative strategies are underway in developing countries that have yet to be evaluated, including experiments with 'restorative justice', use of protection orders, and non-formal approaches to public shaming and community sanctioning. Priority should be given to evaluating the impact of these strategies on repeat offending and on changing community norms. Especially needed are studies that focus on community-led responses to violence. In the WHO multi-country study on domestic violence and women's health, 55–95 per cent of physically abused women had never sought help from formal services or from individuals in authority (e.g. village or religious leaders). Only in the capitals of Brazil, Namibia, and Peru did more than 15 per cent of abused women report seeking help from the police (WHO 2005). Programmes must move beyond formal services if they are to reach the bulk of female victims, especially in the developing world.

Conclusion

For decades small women's groups have attempted to put the issue of violence in intimate partnerships squarely on the global agenda. They have succeeded. But now the challenge is even greater: How to design and implement effective strategies to dramatically reduce levels of partner violence.

Based on our current state of knowledge, a comprehensive programme of violence reduction would include the following elements:

i. A focus on reducing the population prevalence of known risk factors for partner violence in developing countries, including:

  a. norms, attitudes, and beliefs that encourage partner violence and harsh discipline of children;

  b. binge drinking;

  c. childhood exposure to violence.

ii. An effort to change how family and friends—the 'first responders' to abuse—react to both victims and perpetrators. The goal would be to encourage more supportive attitudes towards victims and a more critical stance toward perpetrators, as well as to model how to respond constructively. This strategy could help lay a foundation for a more community-led approach to sheltering and supporting victims and sanctioning perpetrators that does not rely on formal services and systems.

iii. Safe spaces for facilitated discussion, reflection, and debate around key norms and beliefs that support violence against women and children. Frequently, this will include discussions about power, norms around gender and authority, and the long-term impact of violence on children. Such groups become a vehicle for empowerment and leadership development and a launch pad for collective action.

iv. A theory-informed communications effort designed around specific, staged goals linked to the objectives (i) and (ii). Such an effort might variously employ street theatre, roving vans, leaflets, and other small-scale media, or radio and television programming aimed at modeling new behaviours and

sparking community reflection and debate. These communication efforts can also be used to publicize changes in relevant laws such as those related to domestic violence, family law or divorce.

v. A parallel effort to enact or reform laws and policies to strengthen women's bargaining power in marriage and other sexual partnerships. This might include reforming formal and customary laws on age at marriage, divorce, maintenance, and child custody; increasing women's access to income through formal employment; and keeping girls in school. Each of these factors have been linked to overall levels of partner violence at a country level (Heise 2012a).

Together these strategies could begin to build a world where children are not beaten, women and men enjoy equal and satisfying relationships, and violence is no longer tolerated. Average levels of abuse vary 10–15-fold across countries and settings, confirming that societies, families, and relationships *can* be structured to reduce abuse. The challenge now is to refine our knowledge of 'what works' to prevent partner violence and to mobilize the political will to do so.

References

Anda, R. E., Felitti, V. J., and Bremner, J. D. et al. (2006). The enduring effects of abuse and related adverse experiences in childhood: a convergence of evidence from neurobiology and epidemiology. *European Archives of Psychiatry and Clinical Neuroscience*, 256, 174–86.

Angelucci, M. (2008). Love on the rocks: domestic violence and alcohol abuse in rural Mexico. *The B.E. Journal of Economic Analysis & Policy*, 8, 1682–766.

Atkinson, M. P., Greenstein, T. N., and Lang, M. M. (2005). For women, breadwinning can be dangerous: gendered resource theory and wife abuse. *Journal of Marriage and Family*, 67, 1137–48.

Bobonis, G., and Castro, R. (2010). The role of conditional cash transfers in reducing spousal abuse in Mexico: short-term vs. long-term effects. Available at: http://homes.chass.utoronto.ca/~bobonis/BC_dviolence2_mar10.pdf%3E [Accessed 15 April 2011].

Boudet, A. M. M., Petesch, P., and Turk, C. (2013). *On Norms and Agency: Conversations about Gender Equality with Women and Men in 20 Countries*. Washington D.C.: The World Bank.

Bussmann, Kai-D, Erthal, C., and Schroth, A. (2011). Effects of banning corporal punishment in Europe: a five-nation comparison. In: J. Durrant, and A. B Smith (eds.). *Global Pathways to Abolishing Physical Punishment: Realizing Children's Rights*. New York: Routledge, pp. 299–322.

CMS Communication (2011). *Endline Survey on Domestic Violence and HIV/AIDS, 2010*. New Dehli: Breakthrough.

Ellsberg, M., Peña, R., Herrera, A., Liljestrand, J., and Winkvist, A. (2000). Candies in hell: women's experiences of violence in Nicaragua. *Social Science and Medicine*, 51, 1595–610.

Eshel, N., Daelmans, B., Mello, M. C. D., and Martines, J. (2006). Responsive parenting: interventions and outcomes. *Bulletin of the World Health Organization*, 84, 991–8.

Gil-Gonzalez, D., Vives-Cases, C., Alvarez-Dardet, C., and Latour-Pérez, J. (2006). Alcohol and intimate partner violence: do we have enough information to act? *European Journal of Public Health*, 16, 278–84.

Gilbert, R., Kemp, A., and Thoburn, J. et al. (2009). Recognising and responding to child maltreatment. *Lancet*, 373, 167–80.

Global Initiative to End all Corporal Punishment of Children (2011). *Prohibiting all Corporal Punishment in Schools: Global Report 2011*. London: Global Initiative to End all Corporal Punishment of Children.

Heise, L. L. (2012a). Determinants of partner violence in low and middle-income countries: exploring variation in individual and population-level risk. *PhD Dissertation*. United Kingdom: London School of Hygiene and Tropical Medicine.

Heise, L. L. (2012b). What works to prevent partner violence: an evidence overview (Version 3.0 edn.). *STRIVE Briefing Papers*. London: London School of Hygiene and Tropical Medicine.

Ireland, T., and Smith, C. (2009). Living in partner-violent families: developmental links to antisocial behavior and relationship violence. *Journal of Youth and Adolescence*, 38, 323–39.

Iyengar, R., and Ferrari, G. (2011). Discussion sessions coupled with microfinance may enhance the role of women in household decision-making in Burundi. *NBER Working Paper Series*. Washington, D.C.: National Bureau of Economic Research.

Jewkes, R., Nduna, M., and Levin, J. et al. (2008). Impact of Stepping Stones on incidence of HIV and HSV-2 and sexual behaviour in rural South Africa: cluster randomised controlled trial. *British Medical Journal*, 337, a506–16.

Jubb, N., Camacho, G., and D'Angelo, A. et al. (2010), *Women's Police Stations in Latin America: An Entry Point for Stopping Violence and Gaining Access to Justice*. Quito, Ecuador: Centre for Planning and Social Studies.

Kim, J. C., Ferrari, G., and Abramsky, T. et al. (2009). Assessing the incremental effects of combining economic and health interventions: the IMAGE study in South Africa. *Bulletin of the World Health Organization* 87, 824–32.

Knerr, W., Gardner, F., and Cluver, L. (2013). Improving positive parenting skills and reducing harsh and abusive parenting in low and middle income countries: a systematic review. *Prevention Science*, 14, 352–63.

Lacayo, V., and Singhal, A. (2008). *Pop Culture with a Purpose! Using Edutainment Media for Social Change*. The Hague: Oxfam/Novib.

Logan, T. K., and Walker, R. (2009). Civil protective order outcomes: violations and perceptions of effectiveness. *Journal of Interpersonal Violence*, 24, 675–92.

Maxwell, C. D., and Garner, J. H. (2012). The crime control effects of criminal sanctions for intimate partner violence. *Partner Abuse*, 3, 469–500.

Mikton, C., and Butchart, A. (2009). Child maltreatment prevention: a systematic review of reviews. *Bulletin of the World Health Organization*, 87, 353–73.

Murphy, C. M., and Ting, L. A. (2010). The effects of treatment for substance use problems on intimate partner violence: a review of empirical data. *Aggression and Violent Behavior*, 15, 325–33.

Neigh, G., Gillespie, C. F., and Nemeroff, C. B. (2009). The neurobiological toll of child abuse and neglect. *Trauma, Violence and Abuse*, 10, 389–410.

Paluck, E. L., and Bell, L. (2010). *Social Norms Marketing Aimed at Gender Based Violence: A Literature Review and Critical Assessment*. New York: International Rescue Committee.

Peltzer, K., Matskeke, G., and Azwihangwisi, M. (2008). Evaluation of alcohol screening and brief intervention in routine practice of primary care nurses in Vhembe district, South Africa. *Croatian Medical Journal*, 49, 392–401.

Pronyk, P., Hargreaves, J. R., and Kim, J. C. et al. (2006). Effect of a structural intervention for the prevention of intimate-partner violence and HIV in rural South Africa: a cluster randomised trial. *Lancet*, 368, 1973–83.

Room, R (2003), *Alcohol in Developing Societies: A Public Health Approach*. Geneva: World Health Organization.

Sanyal, P. (2009). From credit to collective action: the role of microfinance in promoting women's social capital and normative influence. *American Sociological Review*, 74, 529–50.

Solorzano, I., Bank, A., Peña, R., Espinoza, H., Ellsberg, M., and Pulerwitz, J. (2008). Catalyzing personal and social change around gender, sexuality and HIV: Impact evaluation of puntos de encuentro's communication strategy in Nicaragua. *Horizons Final Report*. Washington, D.C.: Population Council.

Spitzberg, B. (2002). The tactical topography of stalking victimization and management. *Trauma, Violence and Abuse*, 3, 261–88.

United Nations Women (2011). *In Pursuit of Justice: Progress of the World's Women 2011-2012*. New York: UN Women.

Usdin, S., Scheepers, E., Goldstein, S., and Japhet, G. (2005). Achieving social change on gender-based violence: a report on the impact evaluation of Soul City's fourth series. *Social Science & Medicine*, 61, 2434–45.

Vung, N. D., and Krantz, G. (2008). Childhood experiences of interparental violence as a risk factor for intimate partner violence: a population based study from northern Vietnam. *Journal of Epidemiology and Community Health*, 63, 708–14.

Vyas, S., and Watts, C. (2008). How does economic empowerment affect women's risk of intimate partner violence in low and middle income country settings?: a systematic review of published evidence. *Journal of International Development*, 21, 577–602.

Whitfield, C. L., Anda, R. F., Dube, S. R., and Felitti, V. J. (2003). Violent childhood experiences and the risk of intimate partner violence in adults: assessment in a large health maintenance organization. *Journal of Interpersonal Violence*, 18, 166–185.

World Health Organization (2005). *WHO Multi-Country Study on Women's Health and Domestic Violence Against Women: Report on the First Results*. Geneva, Switzerland: WHO.

World Health Organization and London School of Hygiene and Tropical Medicine. (2010). *Preventing Intimate Partner and Sexual Violence against Women*. Geneva, Switzerland: WHO.

CHAPTER 26

Preventing intimate partner violence through advocacy and support programmes

Gene Feder and Lynnmarie Sardinha

Introduction to Preventing Intimate Partner Violence through Advocacy and Support Programmes

Intimate partner violence (IPV) rates are high globally (see Chapter 6, this volume), and it leads to a wide range of short- and long-term physical, mental, and sexual health problems (Howarth and Feder 2013; Trevillion et al. 2012). Over and above support that should be offered by professionals when women disclose abuse (Feder et al. 2006a), there is growing evidence that specialist advocacy can improve outcomes for survivors of IPV. In this chapter we review this evidence, treating IPV advocacy interventions as a type of secondary and tertiary prevention of IPV. We have included evidence from interventions initiated in any setting, including healthcare, social care, and the voluntary sector, focusing on those interventions that report abuse, quality of life, or health outcomes. We have not reported outcomes for children from those studies that reported them.

Theoretical Overview Of IPV

While interventions for IPV are often not based on an explicit conceptual framework or model, most of the advocacy interventions that we describe in this chapter are based around the concept of empowerment—talking through potential solutions with the woman (rather than being prescriptive and telling her what she ought to do), helping the woman to achieve the goals she has set (rather than being directive and setting the goals for her), and helping her to understand and make sense of the situation and her responses to it (Campbell and Humphreys 1993). As articulated by Dutton, empowerment is about helping women feel more in control of their lives and take decisions about their future (Dutton 1992). In situations when the harm to oneself is inflicted through a relationship, it is often necessary for the rebuilding to take place through other safe, mutual, and empowering relationships where the woman's experiences are validated. The quality of those relationships is central to the healing process.

What is Advocacy?

In the context of IPV services, advocacy is a term that varies widely, depending on institutional settings and historical developments of the role of advocates (Feder et al. 2006b). Advocates typically engage with individual clients who are being abused, aiming to empower them and linking them to community services. In some settings they may also have a role in bringing about system change and catalysing increased recognition of women experiencing abuse by healthcare and other professionals. Despite variations, the core role of advocacy can be characterized as provision of legal, housing, and financial advice, facilitating access to and use of community resources such as refuges or shelters, emergency housing, provision of safety planning advice, and provision of on-going support. Depending on the specific advocacy model, advocates can also be involved in psychological interventions and counselling.

Thus, the aims of advocacy programmes are multifaceted and may include helping abused women to access services, the reduction or cessation of abuse, and the improvement of abused women's physical or psychological health. Advocacy may be offered as a stand-alone service, but may also be part of a multi-component (and possibly multi-agency) intervention. In multi-component interventions where advocacy is included, it is theorized that offering advocacy addresses an abused woman's immediate needs which, in turn, allows her then to be receptive to other interventions (such as psychotherapy or parenting support).

The duration and intensity of advocacy varies. Crisis or short-term advocacy involves the advocate working with the abused woman for a limited period of time (although the woman may then be referred on to other more specialized agencies). The duration of such advocacy depends on the needs of the abused woman but generally can range from a single meeting up to about 12 hours (Metters 2009). Longer-term advocacy entails weekly sessions of up to 12 months' duration.

How Advocacy Interventions Might Work

The needs of abused women—for information, advice, legal protection, emergency refuge, permanent accommodation, financial support, and safe arrangements for children—cross the boundaries of agency roles and services. A common understanding of the continuum of services or a multi-agency approach required to provide comprehensive assistance to victims of violence and prevent further harm, has emerged (Council of Europe, http://www.coe.int/t/dg2/equality/domesticviolencecampaign/fact_sheet_en.asp). The range of services includes helplines and shelters, which offer immediate services with 24-hour access to counselling and safe accommodation for women and children; early proactive services; short-term counselling and advocacy; trauma care and long-term support; as well as outreach work and mobile services (Council of Europe 2008). All these health and social services need to be combined with legal aid and advocacy, children's services, other health and social services such as mental health services, measures to guarantee rights, affordable housing, perpetrator programmes, and coordinated community responses.

This chapter is largely based on a systematic review commissioned by the United Kingdom Health Technology Assessment programme and a Cochrane review of advocacy interventions for partner violence (Feder et al. 2009), updated by the World Health Organization (WHO) guidelines on the healthcare response to IPV and the evidence review underpinning the UK National Institute for Health and Care Excellence (NICE) guidelines on domestic violence and abuse, including studies published up until May 2012 (NICE 2014; WHO 2013). Electronic databases searched for these reviews included Medline, Embase, Cinahl, British Nursing Index, and PsycInfo. Searches included relevant websites, reference lists, and forward citation tracking of eligible studies. Principal investigators and experts in the field were contacted. Eligible research designs included randomized control trials, parallel group, and before and after studies.

Advocacy in Healthcare Settings

IPV against pregnant women affects not only the health and well-being of the pregnant mother but also that of the infant (Cokkinides et al. 1999; Parker et al. 1994). Therefore, identification of violence against pregnant women and providing specific intervention efforts targeted at them (Jasinski 2004) should be a priority. In addition, pregnancy is an opportune time to offer interventions as it may be the only time a healthy woman has regular scheduled contact with healthcare professionals (McFarlane et al. 2000).

Tiwari and colleagues (2005) evaluated the effectiveness of an empowerment intervention in reducing IPV and improving health status among Chinese pregnant women. The intervention group received empowerment training including advice on safety, choice-making, and problem-solving, while the control group received a referral card listing community services. The intervention sessions lasted about 30 minutes, and women were given a brochure reinforcing the information provided. At 6-weeks follow-up women in the experimental group had significantly improved physical functioning and role limitation due to physical problems and emotional problems, and reduced psychological (but not sexual) abuse, minor (but not severe) physical violence, and postnatal depression scores. However, they reported more bodily pain.

Findings of a parallel group intervention study conducted by McFarlane and colleagues (1997, 1998) and Parker and colleagues (1999) also showed that advocacy and associated services were beneficial to pregnant abused women who were still in a relationship with the abuser. The women, attending an antenatal clinic, were offered an intervention of three brief sessions of individual advocacy—education, referral, and safety planning—spread over their pregnancies. The women receiving the intervention significantly increased their use of safety behaviours. At the 12-month follow-up, women in the intervention group reported significantly improved resource use but not use of the police, and there were also significant reductions in violence, threats of violence, and nonphysical abuse, as compared with the control group.

A pilot study by Cripe and colleagues (2010) in Peru examined the effectiveness of an empowerment-based intervention for abused pregnant women. The study found that, compared with women in the control group, women in the empowerment group adopted more safety behaviours, although this difference was not statistically significant. Also, there was no statistically significant difference in health-related quality of life, and use of community resources between the two groups.

In another study by McFarlane and colleagues (2000), Hispanic pregnant women were allocated to one of three intervention groups: (i) 'brief', where women were offered a card with information on community resources and a brochure; (ii) 'counselling', where for the duration of the pregnancy women were offered unlimited access to an IPV advocate who was able to provide support, education, referral, and assistance in accessing resources; and (iii) 'outreach', which included all aspects of the 'counselling' intervention, plus the additional services of a non-professional mentor mother who offered support, education, referral, and assistance in accessing resources. Findings showed a statistically significant decrease in severity of abuse across time for all intervention groups, and no statistically significant differences between the intervention groups. Use of resources was low for each of the groups and did not differ significantly by type of intervention.

Kiely and colleagues (2010) evaluated the efficacy of a psycho-behavioural intervention for reducing IPV recurrence and improving birth outcomes for pregnant and postpartum African-American women. The integrated cognitive-behaviour intervention was aimed at reducing smoking, second-hand smoke exposure, depression, and IPV during pregnancy. The intervention focused on safety and safety planning, information on types of abuse and the cycle of violence, risk assessment, the provision of preventive options, and a list of community resources. Intervention components were delivered over four to eight sessions, for 20 to 50 minutes per session. In addition, two 'booster sessions' were provided. Findings from this study suggest that the intervention was associated with reductions in some adverse pregnancy outcomes and recurrent risk of IPV at the second and third trimesters, and the 8- to 10-week postpartum follow-up.

An Australian cluster-randomized controlled trial by Taft and colleagues (2011) examined the effectiveness of an intervention for reducing IPV and depression among pregnant women and postpartum women. Intervention involved mentorship from non-professionals providing befriending, advocacy, parenting support, referrals, and legal and self-care support. Findings at the 12-month follow-up suggest that non-professional mentor support is associated with modest improvements in pregnant women or mother's safety and physical and mental well-being following IPV or risk of IPV.

An individually randomized controlled trial conducted by McFarlane and colleagues (2006) in two urban primary care health clinics compared a nurse case management intervention with a referral card that listed a safety plan and sources of partner violence services. Advocacy sought to empower the women through encouraging the use of a safety-promoting behaviour checklist, supplemented with supportive care, anticipatory guidance by a nurse, and guided referrals tailored to the women's individual needs, such as job training. There were five 20-minute nurse case management sessions. The control group received standard refuge services. No effect for the intervention was found at the 24-month follow-up: all outcomes (use of safety behaviours and community resources, threats, assault, homicide risk, and work harassment) improved over time, regardless of group allocation.

Feighny and Muelleman (1999) conducted a before-and-after study in a hospital's accident and emergency department where the woman met with the advocate 30 minutes after disclosure. The advocate discussed the incident with her, addressed safety issues, provided education about the cycle of violence, and informed her of community resources. Women receiving advocacy significantly increased their use of refuges and refuge-based counselling services in comparison with pre-intervention controls. However, there was no effect on subsequent experience of abuse as measured by the number of repeat visits to the department, nor was there any significant difference in access to police services.

Community and Shelter/ Refuge-Based Interventions

In two separate evaluations conducted by Sullivan and colleagues (1999, 2002), undergraduate psychology students were trained to provide 10 weeks of community-based advocacy to severely abused women exiting from refuges. Advocacy was tailored to the individual women's needs to help them to access community resources (such as housing, employment, legal assistance, and childcare), as well as empowering the women themselves. At 10 weeks post intervention, the women who received advocacy reported improvement in their quality of life, and this was maintained at 6 months after the cessation of the programme. Initial improvements in perceived effectiveness in obtaining resources and perceived social support were no longer statistically significant at 6 months. However, when followed up 2 years after the cessation of advocacy, women in the advocacy group reported significantly less physical abuse and still had a significantly higher quality of life than women in the control arm.

Another study by Sullivan and colleagues (2002) tested the effect of an advocacy intervention aimed at abused women and their children. Advocacy was based on the individual needs of the mother and child, but all sessions actively assisted mothers in accessing community resources. A multi-component intervention consisted of a highly trained paraprofessional who advocated for 16 weeks for mothers and children, and a 10-week support and education group attended by the children. At a 4-month follow-up, women in the intervention group had significantly reduced depression and improved self-esteem. Mothers who received advocacy also reported better quality of life than mothers in the control group, although this was not statistically significant. However, the intervention did not have an effect on the incidence of abuse or on social support.

A study by Price and colleagues (2008) examined the outcomes of the first 18 months of the Domestic Violence Intervention Programme (DVIP) in three London boroughs. The interventions offered included one-to-one group programmes, telephone support, and outreach meetings at the children's centre of social work offices. The main aims were to improve women's safety, emotional and mental health, to improve knowledge about IPV, to provide realistic expectations of the perpetrator programme, to improve empowerment of women, and to connect women to other available local services. Self-report surveys at 3-, 6- and 18-month follow-up revealed that the majority of women reported improvements in their safety and quality of life and their children's safety; case workers also supported improvements in the majority of women's and children's safety.

A third advocacy study by the same group (McFarlane et al. 2002, 2004) was based in a family violence unit of a large urban district attorney's office. All women received the usual services of the unit, which included processing of civil protection orders and optional advocacy referral, the phone number of a caseworker for further assistance, and a 15-item safety-promoting behaviour checklist. In addition the intervention group received six follow-on phone calls over 8 weeks to reinforce the advice on adopting safety behaviours. The number of safety promoting behaviours increased significantly in the intervention group, and this was sustained up to 18 months later.

Tiwari and colleagues (2010) conducted a study in Hong Kong to determine whether an advocacy intervention would improve the depressive symptoms of Chinese women survivors of IPV. The intervention group received a 12-week advocacy intervention comprising empowerment and telephone social support. The women in the control group received usual community services including child care, healthcare, and recreational programmes. The evaluation concluded that the intervention did not result in a clinically meaningful improvement in depressive symptoms.

A United States based study by Constantino and colleagues (2005) tested the feasibility and effectiveness of a social support intervention with a therapeutic component with women living in a shelter. The intervention comprised eight weekly sessions (each lasting 90 minutes) and sought to empower abused women through the provision of four dimensions of social support: belonging, evaluation, self-esteem, and tangible support (BEST). It provided resources to the women as well as information on further resources; it allowed them time to access resources when these were available; and provided an environment where they could talk with a counsellor and friends. At the end of the programme the experimental group had significant improvements on the 'belonging' function of social support, and had significant reductions in psychological distress and healthcare utilization. Non-significant improvements in 'tangible' social support and total social support were reported.

Advocacy Interventions in Other Contexts

Advocacy interventions have been conducted in settings other than healthcare and community or shelters/refuges. Two examples are programmes evaluated by Howarth and colleagues (2009) and Bair-Merritt and colleagues (2010).

A study by Howarth and colleagues (2009) examined the effectiveness of Independent Domestic Violence Advisor (IDVA) services for increasing safety and well-being of female victims of IPV who were deemed to be at high risk of harm or homicide. The main components of the IDVA services included: a focus on safety as the primary goal, the targeting of victims at high risk of harm or homicide due to IPV, the provision of intervention from the point of crisis, and the proactive provision of help to reduce immediate risks to safety and improve long-term safety. Overall, findings revealed that although there were no statistically significant differences in participants' frequency of physical abuse, sexual abuse, or jealous behaviour, following IDVA services, over half the women/victims experienced a cessation in the abuse; the majority of victims (76 per cent) reported feelings of safety; IDVAs also reported reduced risk in 79 per cent of the cases. At 6 months after case closure, the majority of women surveyed (82 per cent) reported no further abuse.

A U.S.-based trial by Bair-Merritt and colleagues (2010) examined the impact of a home visitation programme after childbirth on mothers. The study included new mothers engaged in the 'Hawaiian Healthy Start' home visitation programme who had an infant at high risk of maltreatment, and who were not involved in child protective services. The intervention included home visits by paraprofessionals aimed at improving family functioning and child health and decreasing maltreatment. Families were connected to community services, and taught about child development, role modelling, problem-solving, and providing emotional support. Results indicated that in the home visiting group, as compared to the control group, rates of IPV victimization and perpetration decreased significantly during the 3 years of programme implementation. When the children were 7–9 years of age, rates of IPV victimization and perpetration had decreased for both intervention and control mothers and there were no longer statistically significant differences between the two groups (Bair-Merritt et al. 2010).

Overview of Findings

Studies of IPV advocacy intervention show that such interventions, particularly for women who have actively sought help from professional services (particularly those leaving a refuge), can reduce abuse, increase social support and quality of life, and lead to increased safety behaviours and accessing of community resources. Evidence regarding the effectiveness of advocacy interventions is weakest for women who are still in an abusive relationship. The evidence for the effectiveness of advocacy with a less intensive intervention or for women identified in healthcare settings is less robust, either because study designs were more prone to bias or because the conduct or analysis of the studies was flawed. Yet the majority of studies show some benefit from advocacy for some outcomes and therefore this is a legitimate option for intervention. Continued severe abuse or re-victimization was the outcome most resistant to advocacy, although this may partly be a function of short follow-up, as one of Sullivan's trials showed no decrease in abuse at four months follow-up but did find it at 2 years after the advocacy intervention (Sullivan et al. 2002). Moreover, abuse is the outcome over which the survivor has least direct control.

The duration of the interventions varied considerably and, to a large extent, this was related to the settings in which the women were recruited. In general, where women were recruited outside of healthcare settings interventions were of longer duration both in terms of the length of sessions and the duration over which the sessions were offered. Typically, these types of interventions took place over a period of months and provided advocacy totalling approximately 12 hours (Constantino et al. 2005) and 60–80 hours (Sullivan and Davidson 1991, 1992). The one exception is where the women were recruited within a community centre setting (Tiwari 2010): an initial face-to-face session (lasting about 30 minutes) was followed by 3.5–4.5 hours of telephone advocacy (about 15–20 minutes per call).

While all of the interventions were administered by trained advocates there was some variability in their professional status. Three interventions were administered by research nurses (Constantino 2005; McFarlane et al. 2006; Tiwari et al. 2005), three by social workers or psychologists (Cripe et al. 2010; Kiely 2010; Tiwari 2010), and three of the trials were led by trained para-professional students (Sullivan et al. 1994, 1999, 2002). Two studies were somewhat different in that they evaluated the effectiveness of advocacy provided by 'lay people'. In the first of these (McFarlane et al. 2000), advocacy was provided by a professional advocate supplemented by the services of a trained non-professional 'mentor mother', while in the second (Taft et al. 2011) the intervention was provided wholly by non-professional 'mentor mothers'.

These studies of advocacy/empowerment interventions have both their methodological strengths and limitations. While most studies were randomized controlled trials, the limitations included a lack of description of the randomization process or outcome assessment, and high attrition rates resulting in very underpowered studies and a high risk of bias. One of the main challenges in interpreting the studies was the sparse information about the interventions and the overlap between psychological and advocacy/empowerment interventions, in so far as the former often have components of non-psychological support and the latter may include psychological support such as counselling. In addition, in many studies the interventions were not described in enough detail to distinguish between formal psychological interventions and psychological support.

There is thus moderate evidence that advocacy services may improve safety and women's access to community resources, and reduce rates of IPV, with weaker evidence of improvements in mental health or quality of life. Interventions included community-based mentorship, home visitation advocacy services, Independent Domestic Violence Advisory services (IDVA), emergency department advocacy services, advocacy services for rural women, shelter/refuge, and post-shelter advocacy services. The strongest evidence comes from shelter/refuge settings.

Transferability

All but one of the studies was conducted in high-income countries, making problematic the extrapolation of findings to the majority of the world's population. The generalizability of some findings may also be limited to the specific sub-populations targeted, including women using shelter/refuge services, rural African-American women, and pregnant and post-partum women. Some studies included women abusing substances, and their findings may be applicable to women with this co-occurring problem.

There is evidence that structural interventions from outside healthcare settings, such as microfinance (Pronyk et al. 2006), can reduce IPV, but despite the existence of promising projects, there is no evidence from controlled studies of system level interventions to improve responses to IPV (Ulbrich and Stockdale 2002) amongst women experiencing IPV.

Until there is further evidence, there is no certainty about which models of IPV advocacy are appropriate for which countries or care settings and different models can legitimately be implemented, but what works best and is the most cost-effective in different contexts should be determined through careful evaluation.

Whatever model is used, it should aim to reduce the number of services and providers that a woman has to contact and facilitate access to services she may need.

Conclusion

In this chapter we have shown that there is some evidence for effectiveness of IPV advocacy in some settings. Further development of advocacy models is needed to improve outcomes and they need to be tested in different care and country settings. Within the study reports we have examined, most authors recommend more rigorous research designs for evaluating effectiveness, longer follow up of IPV survivors exposed to the intervention, and cost-effectiveness analysis.

References

Bair-Merritt, M. H., Jennings, J. M., and Chen, R. et al. (2010). Reducing maternal intimate partner violence after the birth of a child: a randomized controlled trial of the Hawaii Healthy Start Home Visitation Program *Archives Paediatric Adolescent Medicine* 164, 16–23.

Campbell, J. C., and Humphreys, J. C. (1993). *Nursing Care of Survivors of Family Violence.* St Louis: Mosby.

Cokkinides, V. E., Coker, A. L., Sanderson, M., Addy, C., and Bethea, L. (1999). Physical violence during pregnancy: maternal complications and birth outcomes. *Obstetrics and Gynaecology*, 93, 661–6.

Constantino R. K. Y., and Crane P. A. (2005). Effects of a social support intervention on health outcomes in residents of a domestic violence shelter: a pilot study. *Issues in Mental Health Nursing*, 26, 575–90.

Cripe, S. W., Sanchez, S. E., and Sanchez, E. et al. (2010). Intimate partner violence during pregnancy: a pilot intervention program in Lima, Peru. *Journal of Interpersonal Violence*, 25, 2054–76.

Dutton, M. A. (1992). *Empowering and Healing Battered Women: A Model for Assessment and Intervention.* New York: Springer Publishing Co.

Feder, G., Ramsay, J., and Dunne, D. et al. (2009). How far does screening women for domestic (partner) violence in different health-care settings meet criteria for a screening programme? Systematic reviews of nine UK National Screening Committee criteria. *Health Technology Assessment*, 13, iii–xiii.

Feder, G. S., Hutson, M., Ramsay, J., and Taket, A. R. (2006a). Women exposed to intimate partner violence: expectations and experiences when they encounter health care professionals: a meta-analysis of qualitative studies. *Archives of Internal Medicine*, 166, 22–37.

Feder, G., Ramsay, J., and Zachary, M. (2006b). Clinical response to women experiencing intimate partner abuse: what is the evidence for good practice and policy? In: G. Roberts, K. Hegarty, and G. Feder (eds), *Intimate Partner Abuse and Health Professionals: New Approaches to Domestic Violence.* London: Elsevier, pp. 93–110.

Feighny, K. M., and Muelleman, R. L. (1999). The effect of a community-based intimate-partner violence advocacy program in the emergency department on identification rate of intimate-partner violence. *Missouri Medicine*, 96, 242–4.

Howarth E., and Feder G. (2013). Prevalence and physical health impacts of domestic violence. In: L. M. Howard, G. Feder, and R. Agnew-Davies (eds), *Domestic Violence and Mental Health.* London: RCPsych Publications, pp. 1–17.

Howarth, E., Stimpson, L., Barran, D., and Robinson, A. (2009). *Safety in Numbers: A Multi-site Evaluation of Independent Domestic Violence Advisor Services.* London: Henry Smith Charity.

Jasinski, J. (2004). Pregnancy and domestic violence: a review of literature. *Trauma, Violence and Abuse*, 5, 47–64.

Kiely, M., El-Mohandes, A. A. E., El-Khorazaty, M. N., and Gantz, M. G. (2010). An integrated intervention to reduce intimate partner violence in pregnancy. *Obstetrics and Gynaecology*, 115, 273–83.

McFarlane, J., Groff, J. Y., O'Brien, J. A., and Watson, K. (2006). Secondary prevention of intimate partner violence: a randomized controlled trial. *Nursing Research*, 551, 52–61.

McFarlane, J., Parker, B., Soeken, K., Silva, C., and Reel, S. (1998). Safety behaviours of abused women after an intervention during pregnancy. *Journal of Obstetrics, Gynaecology and Neonatal Nursing*, 27, 64–9.

McFarlane, J., Soeken, K., Reel, S., Parker, B., and Silva, C. (1997). Resource use by abused women following an intervention programme: associated severity of abuse and reports of abuse ending. *Public Health Nursing*, 22, 59–66.

McFarlane, J., Soeken, K., and Wiist, W. (2000). An evaluation of interventions to decrease intimate partner violence in pregnant women. *Public Health Nursing*, 17, 443–51.

McFarlane, J., Malecha, A., Gist, J., Watson, K., Batten, E., Hall, A., and Smith, S. (2002). An intervention to increase safety behaviors of abused women: Results of a randomized clinical trial. *Nursing Research*, 51, 347–54.

McFarlane, J., Malecha, A., Gist, J., Watson, K., Batten, E., Hall, A., and Smith, S. (2004). Protection orders and intimate partner violence: An 18-month study of 150 Black, Hispanic and White women. *American Journal of Public Health*, 94, 613–18.

Metters, C. (2009). (Director of a domestic abuse service for abused women). *Personal Communication.*

National Institute for Health and Care Excellence. *Public Health Draft Guidance. Domestic Violence and Abuse: How Health Services, Social Care and The Organisations They Work with Can Respond Effectively.* Available at: http://www.nice.org.uk/nicemedia/live/14384/66668/66668.pdf [Accessed 2 June 2014].

Parker, B., McFarlane, J., and Soeken, K. (1994). Abuse during pregnancy: effects in maternal complications and birth outcomes in adult and teenage women. *Obstetrics and Gynaecology*, 84, 323–8.

Parker, B., McFarlane, J., Soeken, K., Silva, C., and Reel, S. (1999). Testing an intervention to prevent further abuse to pregnant women. *Research in Nursing and Health*, 22, 59–66.

Price, P., Rajagopalan, V., Langeland, G., and Donaghy, P. (2008). *Domestic Violence Intervention Project Improving Women and Children's Safety: Report and Evaluation of the East London Domestic Violence Service January 2007—September 2008* London: DViP.

Pronyk, P. M., Hargreaves, J. R., and Kim, J. C. et al. (2006). Effect of a structural intervention for the prevention of intimate-partner violence and HIV in rural South Africa: a cluster randomised trial. *Lancet*, 368, 1973–83.

Sullivan, C. M., and Bybee, D. I. (1999). Reducing violence using community based advocacy for women with abusive partners. *Journal of Consulting and Clinical Psychology*, 67, 43–53.

Sullivan, C. M., Bybee, D. I., and Allen, N. (2002). Findings from a community based program for battered women and their children. *Journal of Interpersonal Violence*, 17, 915–36.

Sullivan, C. M., Campbell, R., Angelique, H., Eby, K. K., and Davidson, W. S. (1994). An advocacy intervention program for women with abusive partners: six-month follow-up. *American Journal of Community Psychology*, 22, 101–22.

Sullivan, C. M., and Davidson, W. S. (1991). The provision of advocacy services to women leaving abusive partners: an examination of short-term effects. *American Journal of Community Psychology*, 19, 953–60.

Taft A, Small, R., Hegarty, K. L., Watson, L. F., Gold, L., and Lumley, J. A. (2011). Mothers Advocates in the Community (MOSAIC)—non-professional mentor support to reduce intimate partner violence and depression in mothers: a cluster randomised trial in primary care. *BMC Public Health*, 11, 178–87.

Tiwari, A., Leung, W. C., Leung, T. W., Humphreys, J., Parker, B., and Ho, P. C. (2005). A randomised controlled trial of empowerment training for Chinese abused pregnant women in Hong Kong. *BJOG*, 112, 1249–56.

Tiwari, A., Salili, F., Chan, R. Y. P., Chan, E. K. L., and Tang, D. (2010). Effectiveness of an empowerment intervention in abused Chinese women. *Hong Kong Medical Journal* 16, 33–7.

Trevillion, K., Oram, S., Feder, G., and Howard, L. M., (2012). Experiences of domestic violence and mental disorders: a systematic review and meta-analysis. *PLoS ONE*, 7, e51740.

Ulbrich, P. M., and Stockdale, J. (2002). Making family planning clinics an empowerment zone for rural battered women.. *Women Health* 35, 83–100.

World Health Organization (2013). *Responding to Intimate Partner Violence and Sexual Violence against Women: WHO Clinical and Policy Guidelines*. Geneva: World Health Organization. Available at: http://apps.who.int/iris/bitstream/10665/85240/1/9789241548595_eng.pdf [Accessed 18 November 2013].

CHAPTER 27

Preventing male violence

Michael Flood

Introduction to Preventing Male Violence

Most violence is men's violence. While most men do not use violence, when violence occurs it is perpetrated largely by men. This is true particularly of violence against women, but also true of violence against men. Reflecting the influence of feminist advocacy and scholarship, there has for several decades been substantial attention to the gendered character and dynamics particularly of men's violence against women, and increasingly of men's violence against other men. In efforts to prevent men's violence, there is an increasing focus on engaging men and boys in prevention.

This chapter provides an outline and assessment of efforts to engage men and boys in the prevention of men's violence. It focuses on *primary* prevention efforts in particular—activities which take place before violence has occurred to prevent initial perpetration or victimization. Because most violence prevention activities aimed self-consciously at men and boys concern forms of violence against women, much of the chapter addresses these, but it also addresses prevention efforts regarding other forms of interpersonal violence perpetrated by men.

Involving Men in Prevention

While many forms of prevention activity involve men or boys among their target audiences, only some do so in *gender-conscious* ways. That is, only some violence prevention efforts addressing men or boys attend to the gendered identities, practices, and relations of men and boys. Where violence prevention efforts which self-consciously address men or boys have been most developed is in relation to the prevention of men's violence against women—of the forms of violence highlighted by such terms as 'domestic violence', 'family violence', 'intimate partner violence', and 'sexual violence', perpetrated largely by men and often against women.

There are growing efforts to involve boys and men in various capacities in the primary prevention of men's violence against women: as participants in education programmes, as targets of social marketing campaigns, as policymakers and gatekeepers, and as activists and advocates (Flood 2005–2006, 2011). There is a groundswell of community-based prevention activity directed at men and boys, exemplified by the White Ribbon Campaign, with, for example, over 400 events and 250,000 ribbons distributed in the 2012 Australian campaign. There is significant policy support for male involvement in violence prevention, evident in recent plans of action by governments at both Federal and state levels in Australia, and affirmed by overseas governments and international agencies (Flood et al. 2010).

There is an obvious rationale for addressing men in ending violence against women. First and most importantly, efforts to prevent violence against women must address men because largely it is men who perpetrate this violence. Second, constructions of masculinity—the social norms associated with manhood and the social organization of men's lives and relations—play a crucial role in shaping violence against women. Third, and more hopefully, men and boys have a positive role to play in helping to stop violence against women, and they will benefit personally and relationally from this (Expert Group 2003). None of this is to say that efforts to prevent violence against women now should focus primarily on men and boys. There remains a powerful rationale for women-focused and women-only initiatives, and efforts focused on boys and men should complement these.

Much the same rationale can be applied to many other forms of violence. Interpersonal violence in public locations such as streets or pubs is perpetrated largely by men and often against other men and structured in part by dynamics of masculinity and gender (Flood 2007). Male–male violence is shaped by, and itself helps to constitute, social codes and relations of masculinity, across such diverse contexts as wars and civil conflicts, in crime and among gangs, and in prisons, schools, and workplaces (Messerschmidt 1997; Polk 1994).

However, efforts to prevent forms of violence other than those involving men's violence against women have paid far less attention to dynamics of masculinity. In comparison to violence prevention initiatives engaging men and boys in the prevention of violence against women, there are only a small number engaging men and boys in gender-conscious ways in preventing other forms of violence. In a 2007 review by the World Health Organization (2007), only one of 15 programmes addressing gender-based violence included substantial attention to male–male violence, 'Building a Culture of Peace' among marginal men and women in Nicaragua. A later review documents other programmes including an educational programme among young men in Northern Ireland (International Planned Parenthood Federation 2010). Two other initiatives are worth noting. In the Western Balkans, CARE Northwest Balkans has worked with young men aged 13–19 to challenge their attitudes and behaviours regarding both male–female and male–male violence, addressing the culture of violence which is a legacy in part of the Yugoslavian Wars of 1991–2001. In South Africa, Sonke Gender Justice has had a lengthy involvement in advocacy, education, and policy work in prisons, focused on the prevention of male–male sexual violence and HIV transmission. Both the Western Balkans project and the South African prisons work embody the recognition that gender inequalities and narrow constructions of masculinity fuel both male–male and male–female violence and that tackling them is central to prevention.

Trends in Men's Violence Prevention

Efforts to engage men in the prevention of men's violence against women are marked by several trends: increased regional and global networking, increasing diversity in prevention strategies, an orientation towards 'scaling up', increased engagement in policy, and an increasing emphasis on evaluation.

Increased regional and global networking is visible both in relation to particular campaigns focused on men and in the emergence of regional and international networks and organizations. The White Ribbon Campaign, in which men wear a white ribbon on and around the International Day for the Elimination of Violence Against Women (25 November) to show their commitment never to condone nor commit violence against women, is one of the most prominent violence prevention efforts aimed at men.

Regional and international networks focused on men's roles in building gender equality and non-violence has emerged in the last decade. In 2004, a global alliance of non-governmental agencies and United Nations agencies seeking to engage boys and men to achieve gender equality formed, called MenEngage. MenEngage members at the national level include more than 400 non-governmental organizations from sub-Saharan Africa, Latin America and the Caribbean, North America, Asia, and Europe. Another significant regional network is Partners for Prevention (P4P), a UN regional joint programme for gender-based violence prevention in the Asia-Pacific which began in 2008. These multi-country programmes and projects are complemented by substantial websites such as EngagingMen.net and XYonline.net.

There is growing diversity in the strategies used to engage or address men in violence prevention. One can conceptualize prevention strategies in terms of a spectrum organized by scale, with the smallest and most localized strategies at one end and the most large-scale at the other (Davis et al. 2006). Much prevention activity has taken place at the level of community education, involving face-to-face education programmes in schools and universities and communications and social marketing strategies. These are now increasingly complemented by activities at other points on the spectrum, including efforts to engage and mobilize communities, change organizational practices, and influence policies and legislation. In addition, within each level of the spectrum, there is increasing diversity in the strategies used. For example, at the level of community education, there is growing specialization in the adoption of particular approaches such as bystander intervention, social norms approaches, and so on.

Another dimension of this diversity is an expansion in the domains of social life or social practice through which men are engaged in violence prevention. Internationally, men's anti-violence work often is part of wider initiatives regarding men and gender inequalities. Thus one sees efforts in various countries which engage men across such domains as sexual and reproductive health, HIV/AIDS, and economic inequalities. However, there has been an increase, for example, in efforts to engage men in violence prevention through particular domains such as parenting. The MenCare project is the preeminent example of this.

MenCare is a global campaign to promote men's involvement as equitable, responsive, and non-violent fathers and caregivers. The campaign is coordinated by Promundo and Sonke Gender Justice (Sonke) in collaboration with the MenEngage Alliance. Using media, programme development, and advocacy, the campaign works at multiple levels to engage men as caregivers and as fathers: engaging men as participants in fathers' groups, advocating for progressive family legislation, and encouraging institutions to see engaging men as caregivers as a key dimension of gender equality. The campaign is described as having a preventative effect on men's violence against women by encouraging fathers to treat mothers with respect and care, diminishing the corporal punishment which feeds into cycles of family violence, involving fathers in preventing sexual violence against children, and contributing to boys' adoption of peaceful and progressive masculinities and girls' empowerment (MenCare 2010).

There is growing attention to violence prevention work with men and boys in conflict and post-conflict settings in particular. Recognition of the need for this was exemplified in the 'Advocacy Brief' released by the global network MenEngage and the United Nations Population Fund at the 57th UN Commission on the Status of Women in New York in March 2013 (MenEngage and UNFPA 2013b). There are fledgling efforts at gender-conscious violence prevention among men and boys in conflict and post-conflict settings. These include the Young Men Initiative in the Western Balkans, educational programmes engaging men in the prevention of rape as a weapon of war in the Democratic Republic of Congo (International Planned Parenthood Federation 2010), and training programmes in Timor-Leste, Sudan, Liberia, and Chad with UN peacekeepers concerning sexual violence. On the other hand, there is only limited recognition of men's potential roles in the prevention of violence in these settings by bodies such as the Security Council (MenEngage and United Nations Population Fund (UNFPA) 2013b).

Echoing wider trends in violence prevention, there is some evidence of an increasing orientation towards change efforts addressed to systemic and structural supports for men's violence. As a recent World Health Organization (WHO) report notes:

> Most work with men has tended to be local in scale and limited in scope. To be more widely effective—that is, to transform the pervasive gender inequalities that characterize many societies globally—efforts to transform men's behaviour need to be significantly scaled up. (Flood et al. 2010, p. 9)

'Scaling up' here includes the need to address the social and structural determinants of gender inequalities, contribute to the development or consolidation of policies and programmes promoting gender equality and non-violence, scale up existing initiatives already being run by NGOs and other actors, and strengthen policy implementation (Flood et al. 2010).

The Mobilising Men programme, developed by the Institute for Development Studies since 2009, is a strong example of the shift from a focus on changing individual men's attitudes and behaviours to an emphasis on the need to change systemic and structural gender inequalities (Greig and Edström 2012). In India, Kenya, and Uganda, activists in the programme have, for example, lobbied local governments to enforce domestic violence laws, addressed the failure of authorities on college campuses to adopt adequate institutional processes for addressing sexual harassment, worked to improve the coordination of services for victims and survivors of violence, and conducted human rights work with refugees, asylum seekers, and marginalized communities (Greig & Edström 2012).

One aspect of this increasing focus on shifting institutional relations is an increased engagement with public policy. The WHO report urges that we 'mainstream' men into policies addressing gender, health, and violence. To strengthen the use of government policies to engage men in preventing men's violence and building gender equalities, the report calls for involving affected communities, building institutional capacity and expertise, and strengthening civil society capacity to monitor policy compliance and implementation (Flood et al. 2010).

Two significant examples of such approaches include the work of Sonke Gender Justice and Partners for Prevention (P4P). Sonke Gender Justice (Sonke) is a South African NGO working across Africa to strengthen government, civil society, and citizen capacity to support men and boys to take action to promote gender equality, prevent domestic and sexual violence, and reduce the spread and impact of HIV and AIDS. Among other efforts, Sonke works to hold the South African government accountable for the adoption and implementation of appropriate policies regarding gender-based violence (Sonke 2009). Similarly, P4P, based in the Asia-Pacific, supports research on men, gender-based violence, and policy; engages in awareness-building and advocacy with decision makers; and builds capacity for policy research and advocacy. This emphasis on engagement in public policy was visible most recently at the 57th UN Commission on the Status of Women in New York, in March 2013. The global network MenEngage launched a '10 Point Call for Action', emphasizing ten concrete steps that the UN and national governments should take immediately to engage men and boys in preventing violence against women.

Finally, there is an increasing emphasis on evaluation. As is the case in the violence prevention field and associated fields more generally, there is an increasingly pervasive expectation that prevention efforts will be complemented by examination of their effectiveness.

It is possible that similar trends are under way in relation to prevention efforts addressing other forms of men's violence, although this field is far less well developed.

The Effectiveness of Violence Prevention Efforts among Men

Evidence is emerging that violence prevention efforts among men and boys can make a difference, and that if done well they can shift the attitudes among boys and men that lead to physical and sexual violence. They may even shift behaviours, reducing males' actual perpetration of violence.

However, it has to be conceded that evaluations of violence prevention are often either absent or lacking. Most primary prevention efforts have not been evaluated, including those engaging men in prevention (Flood 2005–2006). Where impact evaluations *have* been done, often they are limited in methodological terms (Flood 2011). Nevertheless, there is a growing evidence base for the effectiveness of violence prevention strategies among men and boys. There is an increasing body of evidence that well-designed interventions can make a difference to males' violence-related attitudes and behaviours. With regard to the range of forms of violence by men, this evidence is most well established for interventions addressing men's violence against women.

An international review by the World Health Organization (2007), titled *Engaging Men and Boys in Changing Gender-Based Inequity in Health*, documents 58 interventions with evaluations. It reports that well-designed programmes *do* show evidence of leading to change in behaviour and attitudes (WHO 2007). Programmes which are gender-transformative—which seek to transform gender roles and promote more gender-equitable relationships between men and women—had a higher level of effectiveness, as did programmes which were integrated within community outreach, mobilization and mass-media campaigns and thus reached beyond individuals to their social contexts (WHO 2007). A follow-up review documents 12 further programmes or interventions promoting gender equality and positive masculinities: most were effective, with gender-transformative programmes more effective than others (International Planned Parenthood Federation 2010), although the standards used for 'effectiveness' were relatively low.

In engaging men and boys in violence prevention, the largest body of evidence for effectiveness concerns education programmes addressing domestic and sexual violence and delivered in schools and universities. This partly reflects the fact that such programmes are a common form of violence prevention. Another strategy, social marketing or media campaigning, also has a sizeable body of evidence. What are some examples of violence prevention efforts among men and boys that have been shown to make a positive difference?

Community Education

Violence prevention education programmes can have positive effects on participants' attitudes towards and participation in violence. For example, male school and university students who have attended rape education sessions show less adherence to rape myths, express less rape-supportive attitudes, and/or report greater victim empathy than those in control groups. Some programmes have reduced men's reported likelihood to rape, while some have reduced men's actual perpetration of sexual aggression. To give some examples:

- In Brazil and Mexico, young men exposed to weekly educational workshops and a social marketing campaign showed improved attitudes towards violence against women and other issues (Pulerwitz et al. 2006).

- In India, young men in the intervention sites showed declines in their support for gender-inequitable norms and in self-reported violence against a partner relative to a comparison group (Verma et al. 2008).

- In South Africa, men who participated in workshops run by the Men As Partners project were less likely than non-participants to believe that it is acceptable to beat their wives or rape sex workers (White et al. 2003).

- In the United States, among adult men in a multi-module education programme, five months after the programme, while some men had 'rebounded', others continued to show improvement on attitudinal and behavioural measures (Heppner et al. 1999).

Not all evaluation results are positive. Existing evaluations show that not all educational interventions are effective, the magnitude of change in attitudes often is small, changes often 'rebound' to pre-intervention levels 1 or 2 months after the intervention and some even become worse, and improvements in men's violence-supportive attitudes do not necessarily lead to reductions in their perpetration of violence.

Nevertheless, it is possible to produce lasting change in attitudes and behaviours. For example, evaluations of the Safe Dates programme among American adolescents found that 4 years after the programme, adolescents who had received the programme continued to report less physical and sexual dating violence perpetration and victimization than those who had not (Foshee et al. 2004).

Communication and Social Marketing

There is evidence that social marketing campaigns can produce positive change in the attitudes and behaviours associated with men's perpetration of violence against women (Donovan and Vlais 2005). For example,

♦ Men Can Stop Rape's 'My strength is not for hurting' campaign uses media materials, in tandem with schools-based Men of Strength (MOST) Clubs for young men and other strategies, to build norms of sexual consent, respect, and non-violence. An evaluation of the Californian campaign documents that students exposed to the campaign had slightly more respectful and equitable attitudes, while schools with MOST Clubs had more favourable social climates (Kim and White 2008).

♦ In Nicaragua, a mass media campaign among heterosexual men aged 20–39 generated increased support for the ideas that men can prevent gender-based violence and that men's violence affects community development (Solórzano et al. 2000).

Two further communication-based strategies include 'social norms' and 'bystander intervention' approaches. 'Social norms' campaigns seek to close the gap between men's perceptions of other men's agreement with violence-supportive and sexist norms and the actual extent of this agreement. Bystander approaches focus on the ways in which individuals who are neither the perpetrators nor victims of violence can intervene, in order to prevent and reduce harm to others. Again, such strategies can be effective among men:

♦ After a recent social norms initiative on a U.S. university campus, college males reduced their overestimation of other males' sexist beliefs and comfort with sexism (Kilmartin et al. 2008).

♦ Experimental evaluations among U.S. undergraduates show that approaching men (and women) as potential bystanders or witnesses to behaviours related to sexual violence can improve attitudes, knowledge, and behaviour (Banyard et al. 2007).

There are other strategies which have strong rationales for use in violence prevention among men and boys, such as community development and community mobilization. While they have been implemented only rarely and evaluated even less often, their powerful rationale makes them critical elements in future violence prevention efforts. Community mobilization strategies can catalyse broader social change by shifting social norms and power relations (Flood 2011). There are only a handful of studies globally of men's involvements in community-based violence prevention, all but one from North America, and none involve impact evaluation (Casey and Smith 2010).

Gender-conscious programmes focused on or addressing men's violence against other men have been evaluated even less often. In the Young Men's Initiative in the Western Balkans discussed earlier, there are tentative findings of positive shifts in gender attitudes, reductions in bullying behaviour, and reductions in ethnic-based prejudices among the boys and young men who took part (MenEngage and UNFPA 2013b). Various other programmes do address male–male violence and other forms of interpersonal violence, as already noted, but robust evidence of their effectiveness is limited.

Challenges

Violence prevention efforts aimed at men and boys have a powerful rationale, are on the public agenda, and are being adopted and funded increasingly widely. There is growing experience regarding gender-conscious prevention work among men and boys, and a growing body of evidence testifying to its effectiveness if done well. At the same time, there are important limitations and challenges. I briefly highlight four.

First, much of the work engaging men and boys in violence prevention is conceptually simplistic. Much is not informed by contemporary scholarship either on interpersonal violence and its prevention or on men and masculinities. This causes a number of problems. Many interventions fall short of the elements identified as 'best practice' in prevention (Flood et al. 2009). Many lack a theory of change—of how the strategies they use will lead to intended effects. They do not necessarily address relevant predictors or causal factors for violence or its antecedents. Their actual activities may not generate the intended change, because they are too short, one-dimensional, or limited in other ways.

The violence prevention field's lack of engagement with scholarship on men, masculinities, and gender also causes problems. In many projects boys and men are addressed as a homogeneous group, all sharing the same relationships to violence against women. There has been little attention to how men's lives (like women's) are shaped by multiple forms of social difference including ethnicity, class, age, and sexuality (Heppner et al. 1999). The field has been marked by a focus on individual attitudes, whereas the evidence is that violence *and* non-violence are shaped at least as much by collective relations (among peers for example) and by contextual and institutional factors (local cultures and contexts and their features) (Flood and Pease 2009).

Second, the growing focus on engaging men and boys in prevention is politically delicate and, in some instances, dangerous. Mobilizing men to end violence against women and gender inequalities involves mobilizing members of a privileged group to dismantle that same privilege (Flood 2004). In practice, a number of problems have been visible in violence prevention efforts focused on or led by men. In some instances, funding or resources for these have been at the expense of, or in competition with, women-only and women-focused programmes. Not all 'work with men' shares a feminist-informed commitment to gender justice, and some is motivated instead by problematic understandings of men or boys as victims (Pease 2008). 'Work with men' sometimes has ceased to be the strategy and has become the goal, perceived as an end in itself rather than as one means of pursuing violence prevention and gender equality. More widely, a focus on 'working with men' or 'male involvement' can omit or marginalize the pressing need to address unequal *relations* of gender between men and women.

Third, there is much which is unknown about the effectiveness of violence prevention efforts among men and boys. First, few programmes have been evaluated, so that the evidence base as a whole is weak. Then there are other questions. Are some strategies more effective among some groups of men or boys than others, and why? For example, there is evidence that rape prevention efforts among men are less effective among those men at higher risk of perpetrating sexual coercion (Stephens and George 2009). What are the mediators of change, those factors which influence whether and how change occurs? What factors sustain men's and boys' involvement in and commitment to prevention activities? How do the contextual features and dynamics of organizations, communities, and cultures influence efforts to engage men and boys in violence prevention? How is men's and boys' participation in the prevention of violence against women shaped by the wider dynamics of gender and sexuality and other forms of social difference? Given the evidence that culturally relevant interventions are more effective than 'colour-blind' ones (Heppner et al. 1999), to what extent are programmes or interventions transferable across cultural and national boundaries?

Finally, among efforts to address men, masculinities, and gender in preventing men's violence, there has been a profound neglect of men's violence against other men. There are two sides to this. On the one hand, activities aimed at the prevention or reduction of violent and criminal behaviour which largely involve male–male violence—gun violence, public assaults, and so on—are usually gender-blind. On the other, gender-sensitive programmes focused on men's violence against women often have neglected the links or similarities between this and men's violence against men. Still, there are small signs of dialogue or rapprochement across these.

In preventing men's violence, there is both good news and bad news. Men's violence-supportive and gender-inequitable attitudes are declining around the globe, albeit unevenly, and there are signs of positive shifts in men's familial, social, and economic relations with women (MenEngage and UNFPA 2013a). There are signs of increased momentum and mobilization in men's violence prevention: increased public advocacy, a growing range of male-focused interventions, and increased policy support (Flood 2010). There is a growing evidence base for violence prevention among men and boys. There is bad news too. Men's violence against women is rooted in entrenched gender inequalities which are hard to change. Many men are resistant to violence prevention campaigns and educational interventions. Some efforts among men or boys produce neutral or negative impacts. Few men actually take up the cause of preventing violence against women, and those who do sometimes are complicit with gender inequalities. Nevertheless, men have a vital and positive role to play in ending men's violence.

References

Banyard, V., Moynihan, M., and Plante, E. (2007). Sexual violence prevention through bystander education. *Journal of Community Psychology*, 35, 463–81.

Casey, E., and Smith, T. (2010). 'How Can I Not?': men's pathways to involvement in anti-violence against women work. *Violence against Women*, 16, 953–73.

Davis, R., Parks, L., and Cohen, C. (2006). *Sexual Violence and the Spectrum of Prevention*. Enola, PA: National Sexual Violence Resource Center.

Donovan, R. J., and Vlais, R. (2005). *VicHealth Review of Communication Components of Social Marketing/Public Education Campaigns Focused on Violence Against Women*. Melbourne: Victorian Health Promotion Foundation.

Expert Group. (2003). *The Role of Men and Boys in Achieving Gender Equality*. DAW in collaboration with ILO and UNAIDS, 21-24 October 2003, Brasilia, Brazil.

Flood, M. (2004). Men's collective struggles for gender justice. In: M. Kimmel, R. W. Kimmel, and J. Hearn (eds), *Handbook for Studies of Masculinities*. Thousand Oaks, CA Sage, pp. 458–66.

Flood, M. (2005-2006). Changing men. *Women against Violence: A Feminist Journal*, 18, 26–36.

Flood, M. (2007). Violence, men as victims of. In: M. Flood, J. K. Gardiner, B. Pease, and K. Pringle (eds), *The International Encyclopedia of Men and Masculinities*. London & New York: Taylor & Francis, pp. 616–7.

Flood, M. (2010). *Where Men Stand*. Sydney: White Ribbon Prevention Research Series, No. 2, Sydney: White Ribbon Australia.

Flood, M. (2011). Involving men in efforts to end violence against women. *Men and Masculinities*, 14, 358–77.

Flood, M., Fergus, L., and Heenan, M. (2009). *Respectful Relationships Education*. Melbourne: Department of Education and Early Childhood Development, State of Victoria.

Flood, M., Peacock, D., Stern, O., Barker, G., and Greig, A. (2010). *World Health Organisation Men and Gender Policy Brief*. Johannesburg: Sonke Gender Justice Network.

Flood, M., and Pease, B. (2009). Factors influencing attitudes to violence against women. *Trauma, Violence and Abuse*, 10, 124–42.

Foshee, V., Bauman, K. E., Ennett, S. T., Linder, G. F., Benefield, T., and Suchindran, C. (2004). Assessing the long-term effects of the safe dates program and a booster in preventing and reducing adolescent dating violence victimization and perpetration. *American Journal of Public Health*, 94, 619–24.

Greig, A., and Edström, J. (2012) *Mobilising Men in Practice*. Brighton: Institute of Development Studies

Heppner, M. J., Neville, H. A., Smith, K., Kivlighan, D. M., and Gershuny, B. S. (1999). Examining immediate and long-term efficacy of rape prevention programming with racially diverse college men. *Journal of Counseling Psychology*, 46, 16–26.

International Planned Parenthood Federation. (2010). *Men are Changing*. London: IPPF.

Kilmartin, C., Smith, T., Green, A., Heinzen, H., Kuchler, M., and Kolar, D. (2008). A real time social norms intervention to reduce male sexism. *Sex Roles*, 59, 264–73.

Kim, A. N., and White, M. L. (2008). *Evaluation of California's MyStrength Campaign and MOST Clubs*. United States: California Department of Public Health, Epidemiology and Prevention for Injury Control Branch.

MenCare (2010). *MenCare—A Global Fatherhood Campaign: Prospectus*. Washington, D.C. and Cape Town: Sonke Gender Justice and Promundo.

MenEngage and UNFPA. (2013a). *Engaging Men, Changing Gender Norms*. Washington, D.C.: MenEngage and UNFPA.

MenEngage and UNFPA. (2013b). *Sexual Violence in Conflict and Post-Conflict*. Washington, D.C.: MenEngage and UNFPA.

Messerschmidt, J. W. (1997). *Crime as Structured Action*. Thousand Oaks, CA: Sage.

Pease, B. (2008). Engaging men in men's violence prevention. *Australian Domestic & Family Violence Clearinghouse Issues Paper*, 17.

Polk, K. (1994). *When Men Kill*. Cambridge & New York: Cambridge University Press.

Pulerwitz, J., Barker, G., Segundo, M., and Nascimento, M. (2006). Promoting more gender-equitable norms and behaviors among young men as an HIV/AIDS prevention strategy. *Horizons Final Report*. Washington, D.C.: Population Council.

Solórzano I., Abaunza, H., and Molina, C. (2000). *Impact Evaluation of the Campaign 'Violence against Women: A Disaster We Can Prevent as Men'*. Managua: CANTERA.

Sonke Gender Justice Network (2009). *South Africa Report for the 54th Session of the United Nations Commission on the Status of Women, 2010*. Johannesburg & Cape Town: Sonke Gender Justice.

Stephens, K. A., and George, W. H. (2009). Rape prevention with college men. *Journal of Interpersonal Violence*, 24, 996–1013.

Verma, R., Pulerwitz, J., and Mahendra, V. S. et al. (2008). Promoting gender equity as a strategy to reduce HIV risk and gender-based violence among young men in India. *Horizons Final Report*. Washington, D.C.: Population Council.

White, V., Greene, M., and Murphy, E. (2003). *Men and Reproductive Health Programs*. Washington, D. C.: Synergy Project.

World Health Organisation. (2007). *Engaging Men and Boys in Changing Gender-Based Inequity in Health*. Geneva: WHO.

CHAPTER 28

Evidence-informed programmes to reduce violence: preventing elder abuse

Liesbeth De Donder

Theoretical Overview of Preventing Elder Abuse

Elder abuse has been associated with a number of negative consequences such as reduced quality of life (Luoma et al. 2011), negative health outcomes, suicidality (Olofsson et al. 2012), and a threefold greater likelihood of mortality (Lachs et al. 1998). This becomes an urgent issue given the rapidly increasing number of older adults worldwide: In the more developed regions, the population aged 60 and over is expected to increase by 45 per cent by 2050, in less developed regions the numbers are expected to triple (from 554 million in 2013 to 1.6 billion in 2050; United Nations 2013). Given the negative implications of elder abuse and the demographic evolution, it is particularly important to develop and implement effective prevention programmes. Although numerous prevention programmes have been put in place to address elder abuse (Sethi et al. 2010), a recent systematic review demonstrates that evidence-based interventions to prevent elder abuse are few and far between (Ploeg et al. 2009).

This chapter will provide an understanding of the potential for prevention of each of these programmes, while addressing a number of shortcomings. Since interventions must be evidence based before being taken to scale, the chapter starts with an overview of the status of the evidence in preventing elder abuse. Next, a brief description of existing prevention programmes is provided, followed by a discussion on the transportability of programmes (inter)nationally. Finally, the most important gaps are highlighted and future paths for research and practice are discussed.

In doing so, the chapter adopts a systematic multi-dimensional approach. First, four stages of prevention can be distinguished (Reay and Browne 2002). Primary prevention is the earliest intervention, and involves all programmes aimed at avoiding the occurrence of elder abuse. Secondary prevention aims at identifying and detecting elder abuse early, before it causes significant problems and to prevent it from getting worse. The goal of tertiary prevention is to stop abuse and provide tools to preventing revictimization. Finally, quaternary prevention is not often incorporated in classical categories of prevention, but refers to actions to mitigate or avoid unnecessary, adverse, or excessive interventions in the life of the older person, such as the relocation of victims (e.g. to nursing homes).

Second, the ecological framework is often used as structure for understanding the risk factors of elder abuse but could be used as well to classify programmes to reduce and prevent elder abuse. Micro-level elder abuse prevention looks at both individual victims as well as individual perpetrators. Meso-level prevention targets small groups such as families and households. Exo-level prevention involves larger groups such as communities, neighbourhood, local organizations, and institutions. Finally, macro-level prevention targets the general public.

A combination of both frameworks will be used to categorize the different types of prevention programmes (Table 28.1). Primary, secondary, tertiary, and quaternary preventions apply to each ecological level. The categorization used in this chapter is not intended to suggest a rigid framework of prevention programmes that should be used at certain stages, but rather to identify what prevention programmes are available.

The Status of the Evidence in Preventing Elder Abuse

High-quality evaluation studies use rigorous research designs to investigate the effectiveness of prevention programmes. In terms of strength of evidence it has been argued that the best data on whether an intervention does more good than harm comes from experimental designs (i.e. randomized controlled trials), followed by strong quasi-experimental designs (i.e. non-randomized controlled trials) (Deeks et al. 2003). However, such research designs are often lacking in the field of elder abuse prevention. The most recent systematic review conducted by Ploeg and colleagues (2009), for instance, discovered only eight such high-quality studies in the review. Meta-analysis at this stage was not possible due to the heterogeneity of samples, interventions, and outcomes across studies.

Table 28.1 Elder abuse prevention programmes: a multi-dimensional framework

	Macro	Exo	Meso	Micro
Primary	Public information campaigns on elder abuse[a]	Awareness and education among professional carers[d]	Social network strengthening[a]	
	Public anti-ageist campaigns[a]	Anti-ageist campaigns: intergenerational programmes[b]	Informal caregiver support programme[a]	
	Enhancement of care services[b]	Restraint reduction programmes[b]		
Secondary		Screening and detection[a]	Mandatory reporting[a]	Helplines[a]
				Awareness and education among (potential) victims[a]
Tertiary			Peer social support and self-help groups[a]	Home visits by police officer or volunteers[c]
			Safe houses and emergency shelters[a]	Adult protective services[c]
				Psychological programmes for perpetrators[d]
Quaternary				

[a] Lacks any scientific, high-quality evaluation.

[b] Has impact on the targeted risk factors.

[c] Has negative or adverse effects on elder abuse.

[d] Shows promising effects on elder abuse.

Source: data from Nahmiash, D., and Reis, M., Most successful intervention strategies for abused older adults, *Journal of Elder Abuse and Neglect*, Volume 12, Issue 3–4, pp. 53–70, Copyright © 2000; Pillemer, K. et al., Interventions to prevent elder mistreatment in L. Doll, S et al., (eds.), *Handbook of Injury and Violence Prevention*, pp. 241–56, Springer, New York, USA, Copyright © 2007; and Ploeg, J. et al., A systematic review of interventions for elder abuse, *Journal of Elder Abuse and Neglect*, Volume 21, Issue 3, pp. 187–210, Copyright © 2009.

Since evidence-based studies on the effectiveness of programmes preventing elder abuse are rare, we will give a broad overview of existing evidence-informed intervention procedures, allowing for the inclusion of programmes that build on other forms of evidence, such as demonstrated risk factors or effective programmes from other violence disciplines.

Brief Description of Intervention Procedures

Interventions for elder abuse have been reviewed a number of times, and these reviews suggest a variety of approaches for the prevention, detection, assessment, and management of elder abuse (Nahmiash and Reis 2000; Pillemer et al. 2007; Ploeg et al. 2009). Table 28.1 summarizes the prevention programmes and categorizes them in a multi-dimensional framework.

Primary Prevention

Primary prevention involves the developments of a range of *macro-strategies*. First, public information campaigns on elder abuse are used to raise awareness and knowledge of elder abuse in the general population and stimulate people to seek information and support services (Sethi et al. 2011). A second type of campaign, targeting the general public, concerns public anti-ageist campaigns. Stereotyping, prejudices, and discriminating against people based on their old age may make elder abuse more tolerable in society (Krug et al. 2002). Consequently, such public campaigns challenge stereotypes and focus on human rights and respect for older people. A third primary prevention programme

on the macro-level can be described as 'enhancement of care services'. Developing care services to provide nursing, day care, and residential care for older adults, while providing caregivers respite care to relieve the care burden temporarily (e.g. adult day programmes, residential respite care, night-sitting) are named as beneficial in order to increase quality of care, and reduce derailed care (Reay and Browne 2002). Although programmes to enhance the organizational, social, and physical environment of care services and facilities seems an important area to intervene to prevent elder abuse, this is practiced only in 38 per cent of (European) countries (Sethi et al. 2010). No worldwide information on this topic is currently available.

At the *exo-level*, three types of primary prevention programmes are found. A first type concerns anti-ageist campaigns such as intergenerational programmes. In line with the anti-ageist programmes at the national level, these programmes aim to encourage positive attitudes and behaviour towards older people. However, instead of developing large-scale campaigns, stereotypes and prejudices are challenged through offering opportunities for meaningful interaction between different generations (Sethi et al. 2011). Examples are direct interactions between students and older people in discussions and cultural projects (Meshel and McGlynn 2004). Second, at the organizational level of professional care several primary prevention actions are undertaken. Professional training and education programmes aim to increase professional awareness and knowledge of elder maltreatment among health professionals (Bond 2004) or social workers (Richardson et al. 2002). Such education programmes often include identifying signs and symptoms of elder abuse, how to manage suspected cases, and the role of the professional in protecting potential victims and ethical issues. Within professional training and education programmes 'restraint reduction programmes' play a specific role. Restraining older people with bedrails, belts, and chairs in residential facilities and hospitals is a much-debated policy as restraining is abusive (Dixon et al. 2010). It should only be used in life-threatening situations after being approved by a medical doctor (European Social Network 2010). Subsequently several education-based restraint reduction programmes have been established (Möhler et al. 2012).

The first primary prevention programme at the *meso-level* builds on the social network model. Since studies demonstrate that social isolation and loneliness are risk factors for elder abuse and neglect (Dong and Simon 2009; Garre-Olmo et al. 2009), the social network model aims at strengthening the social surroundings of the person at high risk. One type of prevention programme, for instance, aims to train older people to serve as visitors to potential victims (Sethi et al. 2010). Next, the stress model suggests that overburdened caregivers can be potential perpetrators, since caring for an older person can be a serious source of stress (Iborra 2008). Consequently, an informal caregiver support programme could have potential to prevent elder abuse. At a primary prevention level, this focuses on supporting informal caregivers from the start, promoting their mental health, and enabling social interaction (Sethi et al. 2011).

Secondary Prevention

The main goal of secondary prevention at the *exo-level* is screening for factors that put older people at risk for abuse, to identify and detect elder abuse at an early stage. The premise of screening and detection interventions is clear: elder abuse remains unknown until the problem is brought to light (Pillemer et al. 2007). There are a number of programmes where a systematic screening of elder abuse is put in place. In hospitals this approach could in theory be especially beneficial as hospitals are venues where older victims interact in a profound way with professionals (Cohen et al. 2006) however clear evidence of effectiveness is currently lacking.

Mandatory reporting is a secondary prevention programme at the *meso-level*. In countries with laws on mandatory reporting, professionals have an obligation to report elder abuse as soon as suspicion arises. Cases of elder abuse should be brought to the attention of an agency in order that services can be initiated to prevent revictimization (Pillemer et al. 2007).

Aside from mandatory reporting by professionals, victims themselves can report their abuse (*micro-level*). Helplines (free of charge) can provide emotional support as well as information and follow-up services for callers. However, only a small proportion of victims presently call for help. One of the main reasons could be the reluctance of older people to report abuse due to feelings of powerlessness, shame, or guilt (Luoma et al. 2011). Consequently, an important secondary prevention programme at the micro-level concerns awareness and education programmes for older people. Such programmes aim to empower and encourage victims to report elder abuse as early as possible and to seek help.

Tertiary Prevention

Tertiary prevention involves case-specific actions aimed at reducing harmful consequences of elder abuse and preventing revictimization in the future. At the *meso-level*, some programmes include peer social support for the older victim, often through the use of self-help groups. Such self-help groups recognize that practical and emotional support is needed both for victims who left the abusive situations and for victims who were still living in them. These programmes provide opportunities to talk about the abuse, and may include long-term supportive or therapeutic work (Pritchard 2003). Next, in terms of immediate action when the abuse has been detected, some countries have safe houses and emergency shelters offering victims temporary, safe accommodation (Pillemer et al. 2007). Typically these shelters have no age restrictions, they are often used by younger women and children escaping situations of intimate partner violence, and are not always adapted for older people (Sethi et al. 2011). Consequently, older victims are often admitted to a hospital or nursing home because of the lack of alternative accommodation (Reay and Browne 2002).

The first tertiary prevention programme at the *micro-level* concerns home visits. The aim is to reduce revictimization by providing regular follow-up home visits. While some programmes focus on home visits by volunteers, others focus on law enforcement involvement and organize home visits by a team of a police officer and a domestic violence counsellor. Second, some social services organizations may have departments targeting elder abuse. Such adult protective services are mainly active in the United States (though also in a few other countries). They are responsible for investigating reports of suspected elder abuse. Based on the investigation they can decide if, and which, protective services need to be put in place, such as medical care, legal services, fiscal service, housing-related services, or social services. Third, specific psychological programmes for perpetrators have been developed. Aspects of these promising psychological programmes include a one-to-one intervention with a clinical psychologist, anger management and education about the nature of the older person's illness, the area services available, and the nature of caring for an older person (Reay and Browne 2002).

Quaternary Prevention

Finally, quaternary prevention programmes are the actions to prevent unnecessary, adverse, or excessive interventions in the life of the older person. Quaternary prevention completes the different prevention levels by keeping guard over the process and collecting information on the outcome of the prevention actions on the lives of older people. It focuses on quality assurance and improvement processes (Gofrit et al. 2000). Although the World Organization of National Colleges, Academies, and Academic Associations of General Practitioners/Family Physicians (WONCA) has adopted the concept of quaternary prevention in healthcare since 2003, to date to our knowledge no study on elder abuse has taken into account quaternary prevention actions, protocols, or strategies.

Research Outcomes

In general, it is demonstrated that a large number of diverse preventive actions are designed to address elder abuse. However, these programmes almost always lack any scientific, high-quality evaluation. To our knowledge, no high-quality evaluations exist for the effectiveness of public information campaigns on elder abuse, public anti-ageist campaigns, social network strengthening, screening and detection, mandatory reporting, helplines, awareness and education among (potential) victims, peer social support and self-help groups, safe houses, and emergency shelters.

Moreover, when prevention programmes are examined, studies often examine the impact of the prevention programme on the targeted risk factors and not its impact on the occurrence of elder abuse. In terms of quality of care, for example, Mason et al. (2007) concluded in their systematic review of respite care that some (weak) positive effects were found on burden and depressions amongst caregivers. Participation in intergenerational programmes has been found to have a decrease in ageist attitudes, and an increase of positive attitudes towards older people (e.g. Belgrave 2011), at least in the short term. As for restraint reduction programmes, the empirical evidence is relatively weak and mixed, with some studies reporting a decline in restraining use, but one reporting an increase (Möhler et al. 2012). Whether such campaigns have positive effects on elder abuse have yet to be established.

Despite the general paucity of evidence, a number of high-quality evaluations of elder abuse prevention programmes do exist, although with mixed findings. Some studies unexpectedly revealed that prevention programmes had negative or adverse effects. Those programmes are all situated in tertiary prevention at the micro-level. The two studies that evaluated the impact of adult protective services found negative effects, such as a higher likelihood of being placed in nursing homes or greater mortality than non-clients (Pillemer et al. 2007). Furthermore, older people receiving home visits, both by volunteers and by police officers, report more abuse following the intervention than did the control group (Pillemer et al. 2007; Sethi et al. 2011). Although a number of methodological questions arise which could have affected the outcomes, these are troubling findings which require further clarification in future studies.

Finally, some high-quality evaluations of prevention programmes on elder abuse show promising results. Evaluations of education among professional carers showed an increased knowledge of elder abuse (e.g. Richardson et al. 2002), and increased care-giving knowledge, but even more so, also showed a decrease in psychologically abusive behaviour from staff to the elderly in their care (Hsieh et al. 2009). Additionally, evidence is emerging for interventions that target perpetrators and abusive caregivers. Psychological programmes, education, and anger management training may help prevent revictimization (Nahmiash and Reis 2000; Reay and Browne 2002).

Transportability of Programmes

Interventions need to be evidence-based before being taken to scale. However, since there have been very few high-quality evidence-based prevention programmes, there is even more limited research on transportability of programmes nationally and internationally. Studies have so far failed to consider how prevention programmes need to be implemented in order to be successful.

Likewise, there is a paucity of translation of effective prevention strategies from other forms of (family) violence to elder abuse, although this could be a promising avenue to advance knowledge

and expertise (Pillemer et al. 2007). Nevertheless, this is not a straightforward appeal to adopt prevention strategies from other areas. As Davis and Medina-Ariza (2001) demonstrate, one programme that was found effective in a partner violence sample produced negative effects in the elder abuse sample. New incidents of elder abuse were more frequent among households that both received home visits and public education in housing projects.

Gaps in the Evidence

As demonstrated, there has been very limited attention for evaluating prevention programmes targeting elder abuse. This comes especially to the fore in comparison with other types of violence. In a systematic review of prevention programmes for family violence in 1998, Chalk and King found 78 high-quality studies of child abuse interventions, 34 high-quality studies of domestic violence interventions, and only two high-quality studies of elder abuse interventions. Although the authors emphasized even then the need for more rigorous evaluations of elder abuse preventive programmes, Ploeg and colleagues (2009) found very little progress more than 10 years later.

A second important gap in evidences derives from several methodological problems. On the one hand, most literature reviews do not involve a systematic assessment of the methods of the studies, including design, procedures, and outcomes of intervention studies for elder abuse (Pillemer et al. 2007). On the other, most studies of elder abuse prevention strategies are descriptive in nature and high-quality evaluation studies are lacking (Pillemer et al. 2007). A number of interventions may have the potential to have a positive impact on preventing or reducing elder abuse but if they are not evaluated more rigorously, no conclusions can be drawn. The reviewed studies are often of low methodological quality, creating difficulty in quantifying and interpreting the reported outcomes (Ploeg et al. 2009). Some of the most important methodological shortcomings include:

- An unclear delineation of the object of study. Most studies are weakened by their undifferentiated treatment of various types of elder abuse (Pillemer et al. 2007). Since risk factors differ according to type of abuse (Jackson and Hafemeister 2011), it is also important to differentiate by type of abuse when identifying effective prevention strategies. Measurement of these different types in future intervention studies is necessary to determine which interventions offer the best chance for reducing which type of elder abuse.

- Different determination of the population at risk of elder abuse (Pillemer et al. 2007). As in current prevalence studies, the specific age group being researched differs from study to study. Some take the age of 55 as the lower limit, whereas others only start from the age of 75 (De Donder et al. 2011).

- Lack of valid and reliable measurement instruments. In a recent overview of European prevalence studies, De Donder and colleagues (2011) conclude that studies hardly ever use a substantiated operationalization. Hardly any of the publications discussed objectivity, reliability, and validity of the measurement instrument(s), and statistical information is scarce. A poor measurement tool may lead to an inaccurate estimation of the extent of elder abuse, which in case of effectiveness studies is crucial. Consequently, measures should always provide information on the psychometric properties of the instruments used (Ploeg et al. 2009).

- Lack of randomized controlled trials. Using an experimental group that follows the prevention programme, and a control group that receives nothing throughout the study, are necessary conditions to determine effectiveness of a prevention strategy (Ploeg et al. 2009). If a study employs a non-randomized controlled design, it risks that baseline differences between both groups may confound the results of the study. Because the two groups are non-randomly composed, group characteristics may not be balanced. For example, typical confounding variables—age, gender, and health, for instance—are also risk factors for elder abuse. One possibility to address this problem is first to collect data from the experimental group, and afterwards to match the control group as equivalently as possible to the test group (Deeks et al. 2003).

- Lack of rigorousness in experimental studies. Studies sometimes use small sample sizes, lack power analyses, or have inadequate follow-up rates of less than 80 per cent (Ploeg et al. 2009).

Conclusions

The literature review in this chapter shows that the elder abuse literature does not yet provide consistent guidelines for prevention programmes. A large number of preventive actions have been specifically designed to address elder abuse, but there have been very few high-quality evaluations of such programmes so far. Not only is more prevention research seriously needed, studies should be methodologically rigorous, addressing each of the aforementioned methodological limitations. Where possible randomized controlled trials, or non-randomized controlled trials with carefully matched groups, should be conducted in the field of elder abuse interventions. This will provide information on 'what works and what does not work', and will aid to determine the cost effectiveness of elder abuse prevention strategies.

In addition to rigorous quantitative study designs, qualitative studies could generate insights into the mechanisms of why some prevention strategies are successful or not (Creswell and Clark 2007). Intervention studies fail to provide reasons why some prevention programmes work and others do not. Examining the processes of the interventions could provide insights into this matter.

Consequently, in order to gain a better understanding why some projects are successful or not, studies should include a process evaluation: monitoring and mapping of strategic, tactical, and operational processes from which decisions and impacts become more comprehensive and interchangeable to other projects (WHO 1998). One aspect of the process, for example, is enabling older participants to have some control over and input into the intervention. Involving the target population at the different levels throughout the process (gathering their expectations, designing, executing, and evaluating the intervention, in co-creation with the target population) can increase the quality and effectiveness of the programmes (WHO 2007).

Although prevention classifications often distinguish between primary, secondary, and tertiary prevention, in testing prevention programmes specific attention needs to be given to quaternary prevention. Programmes put in place to prevent or reduce elder abuse should ensure they do not have negative effects on those persons they are designed to help (Pillemer et al. 2007), such as the relatively high rates of relocation of abused older adults (e.g. to nursing homes). Although relocation may generate a safe environment for the abused person, it does so at the cost of placement in unfamiliar surroundings and likely reduction in independence and disruption of social networks (Ploeg et al. 2009). Additionally, some studies demonstrate that intervention groups obtained higher rates of recurrence of elder abuse than the control groups (Davis and Medina-Ariza 2001). Future research should not only measure the benefits, but also clarify any potentially harmful effects of prevention programmes on older victims of abuse.

In addition to measuring the outcomes of existing preventions programmes, the development of new prevention programmes also merits attention (Pillemer et al. 2007). Prevention programmes require an understanding of factors that lead to elder abuse. There has been a substantial literature on the risk factors for elder abuse (see Chapter 9, this volume) pointing towards a number of risk factors, which could be framed in the ecological framework. Notwithstanding this knowledge, several risk factors remain unaddressed in elder abuse prevention. New, innovative prevention programmes could benefit from knowledge of risk factors and directly targeting them, producing evidence-informed programmes. Richard and colleagues (2008), for instance, suggest investing more in the creation of supportive environments. In addition, Lachs and Pillemer (2004) propose that interventions should be context-specific. Elder abuse in community-dwelling older people occurs in a different context from elder abuse in nursing home. Consequently, prevention programmes should lead to different actions in different contexts.

Other authors emphasize the need for recognizing diversity among older (potential) victims. In terms of tertiary prevention, this would require thorough assessment of each person's needs, followed by a case-specific intervention package (Reay and Browne 2002). For example, most research suggests that elder abuse differs across gender. Notwithstanding that older men also experience abuse, evidence suggests that women are more often victims of abuse than men (Iborra 2008). Consequently, preventing elder abuse could possibly benefit from a gender-specific approach.

References

Belgrave, M. (2011). The effect of a music therapy intergenerational program on children and older adults' intergenerational interactions, cross-age attitudes, and older adult's psychosocial well-being. *Journal of Music Therapy*, 48, 486–508.

Bond, C. (2004). Education and a multi-agency approach are key to addressing elder abuse. *Professional Nurse*, 20, 39–41.

Chalk, R., and King, P. A. (1998). *Violence in Families: Assessing Prevention and Treatment programs*. Washington: National Academy Press.

Cohen, M., Halevi-Levin, S., Gagin, R., and Friedman, G. (2006). Development of a screening tool for identifying elderly people at risk of abuse by their caregivers. *Journal of Aging and Health*, 18, 660–85.

Creswell, J. W., and Clark, V. L. P. (2007). *Designing and Conducting Mixed Methods Research*. Thousand Oaks: Sage.

Davis, R. C., and Medina-Ariza, J. (2001). Results from an elder abuse prevention experiment in New York City. *National Institute of Justice Research in Brief*, pp. 1–7. Available at http://www.ncjrs.gov/pdffiles1/nij/188675.pdf [Accessed 17 November 2013].

De Donder, L., Luoma, M.-L., and Penhale, B. et al. (2011). European map of prevalence rates of elder abuse and its impact for future research. *European Journal of Ageing*, 8, 129–43.

Deeks, J. J., Dinnes, J., and D'Amico, R. et al. (2003). Evaluating non-randomised intervention studies. *Health Technology Assessment*, 7, 1–179. Available at http://www.hta.ac.uk/fullmono/mon727.pdf [Accessed 17 November 2013].

Dixon, J., Manthorpe, J., and Biggs, S. et al. (2010). Defining elder mistreatment: reflections on the United Kingdom study of abuse and neglect of older people. *Ageing & Society*, 30, 403–20.

Dong, X., and Simon, M. A. (2009). Loneliness and mistreatment of older women: does social support matter? *Journal of Women & Aging*, 21, 293–302.

European Social Network (2010). *Contracting for Quality. An ESN Research Study on the Relationships between Financer, Regulator, Planner, Case-manager, Provider and User in Long-term Care in Europe*. Brighton: ESN.

Garre-Olmo, J., Planas-Pujol, X., Lopez-Pousa, S., Juvinya, D., Vila, A., and Vilalta-Franch, J. (2009). Prevalence and risk factors of suspected elder abuse subtypes in people aged 75 and older. *Journal of the American Geriatrics Society*, 57, 815–22.

Gofrit, O. N., Shemer, J., Leibovici, D., Modan, B., and Shapira, S. C. (2000). Quaternary prevention: a new look at an old challenge. *Israel Medical Association Journal*, 2, 498–500.

Hsieh, H. F., Wang, J. J., Yen, M., and Liu, T. T. (2009). Educational support group in changing caregivers' psychological elder abuse behavior toward caring for institutionalized elders. *Advances in Health Sciences Education: Theory and Practice*, 14, 377–86.

Iborra, M. I. (2008). *Elder Abuse in the Family in Spain*. Valencia: Queen Sofia Center.

Jackson, S. L., and Hafemeister, T. L. (2011). Risk factors associated with elder abuse: the importance of differentiating by type of elder maltreatment. *Violence and Victims*, 26, 738–57.

Krug, E., Dahlberg, L. L., Mercy, J. A., Zwi, A. B., and Lozano, R. (2002). *World Report on Violence and Health*. Geneva: World Health Organization. Available at http://www.who.int/violence_injury_prevention/violence/world_report/en/ [Accessed 17 November 2013].

Lachs, M. S., and Pillemer, K. (2004). Elder abuse. *Lancet*, 364, 1263–72.

Lachs, M. S., Williams, C. S., O'Brien, S., Pillemer, K. A., and Charlson, M. E. (1998). The mortality of elder mistreatment. *Journal of the American Medical Association*, 280, 428–32.

Luoma, M.-L., Koivusilta, M., and Lang, G. et al. (2011). *Prevalence Study of Abuse and Violence Against Older Women*. Available at: www.thl.fi/AVOW [Accessed 17 November 2013].

Mason, A., Weatherly, H., and Spilsbury, K. et al. (2007). The effectiveness and cost-effectiveness of respite for caregivers of frail older people. *Journal of the American Geriatrics Society*, 55, 290–9.

Meshel, D. S., and McGlynn, R. P. (2004). Intergeneration contact, attitudes, and stereotypes of adolescents and older people. *Educational Gerontology*, 30, 457–79.

Möhler, R., Richter, T., Köpke, S., and Meyer, G. (2012). Interventions for preventing and reducing the use of physical restraints in long-term geriatric care—a Cochrane review. *Journal of Clinical Nursing*, 21, 3070–81.

Nahmiash, D., and Reis, M. (2000). Most successful intervention strategies for abused older adults. *Journal of Elder Abuse & Neglect*, 12, 53–70.

Olofsson, N. K., Lindqvist, K., and Danielsson, I. (2012). Fear of crime and psychological and physical abuse associated with ill health in a Swedish population aged 65-84 years. *Public Health*, 126, 358–64.

Pillemer, K. A., Mueller-Johnson, K. U., Mock, S. E., Suitor, J. J., and Lachs, M. S. (2007). Interventions to prevent elder mistreatment. In: L. Doll, S. Bonzo, D. Sleet, J. Mercy, and E. Hass (eds), *Handbook of Injury and Violence Prevention*. New York: Springer, pp. 241–56.

Ploeg, J., Fear, J., Hutchison, B., MacMillan, H., and Bolan, G. (2009). A systematic review of interventions for elder abuse. *Journal of Elder Abuse & Neglect*, 21, 187–210.

Pritchard, J. (2003). *Support Groups for Older People Who Have Been Abused: Beyond Existing*. New York: Jessica Kingsley Publishers.

Reay Campbell, A. M., and Browne, K. D. (2002). The effectiveness of psychological interventions with individuals who physically abuse or neglect their elderly dependents. *Journal of Interpersonal Violence*, 17, 416–31.

Richard, L., Gauvin, L., Gosselin, C., Sapinski, J.-P., and Trudel, M. (2008). Integrating the ecological approach in health promotion for older adults: a survey of programs aimed at elder abuse prevention, falls prevention and appropriate medication use. *International Journal of Public Health*, 53, 46–56.

Richardson, B., Kitchen, G., and Livingston, G. (2002). The effect of education on knowledge and management of elder abuse: a randomized controlled trial. *Age and Ageing*, 31, 335–41.

Sethi, D., Mitis, F., and Racioppi, F. (2010). *Preventing Injuries in Europe: From International Collaboration to Local Implementation*. Copenhagen: WHO Regional Office for Europe.

Sethi, D., Wood, S., and Mitis, F., et al. (2011). *European Report on Preventing Elder Maltreatment*. Rome: World Health Organization.

United Nations, Department of Economic and Social Affairs, Population Division (2013). *World Population Prospects: The 2012 Revision, Key Findings and Advance Tables*. Working Paper No. ESA/P/WP.227. New York: United Nations.

World Health Organization (2007). *Global Age-Friendly Cities: A Guide*. Geneva: World Health Organization.

WHO European Working Group on Health Promotion Evaluation (1998). *Health Promotion Evaluation: Recommendations to Policy Makers*. Copenhagen: World Health Organization.

CHAPTER 29

Preventing gang violence

Erika Gebo, Ellen E. Foley, and Laurie Ross

Gang Distinction and the Public Health Model

Gang violence is generally seen as a distinct youth violence category because gang membership has a violence enhancing effect. Gang members commit more violence, more serious violence, and use weapons more often as part of a gang than they would have otherwise, even if they were part of a non-gang delinquent peer group (Krohn and Thornberry 2008). The prevalence of gang membership in the youth population of cities with gangs is low. Studies have found that between 14 and 30 per cent of youthful community members ever become gang members (Thornberry et al. 2003). The incidence of serious violence attributed to gangs, in contrast, is high. Approximately 50–60 per cent of all serious violence can be attributed to gangs (Thornberry et al. 2004). Thus, preventing gang violence can significantly impact the overall violence levels in communities.

Definitions of a gang and a gang member are contested. Gangs and gang members have been defined in a variety of ways, each with its own definitional problems that could misidentify gangs and gang youth. Howell (2012) identifies five components to defining a gang: (i) five or more members; (ii) members share identity (i.e. name and/or symbols); (iii) members view themselves as a gang and are recognized by others as a gang; (iv) the group has some permanence and organization; and (v) the group is engaged in criminal activity. This definition offers a broad framework that can be modified by researchers, policymakers, and programme staff, as they identify the components that are relevant for addressing the violence in their communities and affected populations.

Gang member definition systems include self-nomination, where a youth identifies him or herself as part of a gang, and survey item–response indicators, such as the Eurogang Programme definition, wherein a series of questions provides identification of gang members, as well as a series of outside familial, peer, and authoritative validation (Matsuda et al. 2012). Overall, however, the self-nomination definition has been shown to be a robust indicator of gang membership (Matsuda et al. 2012). Defining and identifying gang members is complicated by two realities. Gang membership is typically transitory, with most youth spending less than 2 years in gangs, and commitment to the gang varies between and within individuals over time (Thornberry et al. 2003). Even though gang membership may be fleeting from a life course perspective, it is now clear that gang membership itself can have lasting negative effects on many areas of an individual's life, including physical and mental health and family well-being (i.e. Melde and Esbensen 2011). The community consequences of gangs, including the further erosion of social cohesion and community institutions, the loss of economic vitality, and the increase in fear of crime, are described elsewhere in this volume.

Gangs are typically found in large urban cities with populations over 100,000 people, but they are becoming more common in smaller cities and city suburbs (Esbensen and Weerman 2005; Miller 2001). Gang membership is typically made up of young, ethnic minority males (Howell 2012). Females generally constitute less than a quarter of gang members; yet, female gang members commit more violence than delinquent, non-gang member males (Peterson and Carson 2012).

Much of the research on gangs is from the United States, where the gang problem is believed to be more entrenched than in many other regions of the world (Klein et al. 2001). Preventing the formation of gangs and the violence they cause is an important public health issue. Addressing the socio-economic processes that facilitate the proliferation of gangs and minimizing the impact that gang violence has on public safety, morbidity, and mortality has tremendous potential to improve quality of life. Reducing the risk factors for gangs and gang membership and increasing protective factors, provides a positive foundation on which to support the overall potential for future generations. Preventing gang violence is analysed in this on three core levels: preventing the formation of gangs, preventing gang membership, and preventing gang violence.

Preventing Gang Formation

From the earliest days of gang research, social scientists have questioned how particular environments and social processes offer a context within which gangs develop. Macro-level forces, from government instability to poverty and the accompanying social disorganization of communities, create the context in which gangs form and in which gang membership offers individuals (typically minority males) a space of belonging and protection (Short and Hughes 2006). The macro-structural forces at work include patterns of immigration and migration and the segregated urbanization of cities in the United States (and elsewhere). Historical and institutionalized racism, social and cultural repression, and fragmented institutions shape the ecological context in which many urban, minority youth face the challenges of childhood, adolescence, and young adulthood (Vigil 2002).

These broad socioeconomic and racial inequalities result in fractured or failing community-level social structures. Schools, families, neighbourhoods, law enforcement, and other social institutions in marginal communities regularly lack the resources needed to properly socialize young people, to offer them opportunities for success, or to operate as an effective mode of social control. For youth growing up in these fragile communities, the 'street' can become a primary locus of socialization and gangs become a means of coping with street realities. As Vigil (2003) argues, some young people who have spent most of their early lives in the street gravitate to gangs as teens to resolve their 'age/gender identity crisis'. He suggests that in adolescence, 'the more group-oriented preteen activities coalesce and merge into that of the street gang, and in most instances it is a continuous process' (2003, p. 230).

Gangs therefore operate in the absence of supportive social institutions and provide a means for young people to navigate the dangers and unpredictability of street life. Gang members are typically youth who experience 'multiple marginalities' (neighbourhood effects, poverty, culture conflict, and sociocultural marginalization) (Vigil 2002).

At present, most approaches to youth and gang violence focus on reducing the effects of the previously mentioned multiple marginalities on young people rather than addressing the sources of these marginalities. The increase in gangs in the United States in the last 40 years has been attributed in large part to these macro-structural effects. These include basic poverty, misguided government policies, the illicit drug trade, immigration, the expansion of national gangs with a federated structure (e.g. Crips and Bloods), the rise of single-parent households among minorities, and the mainstreaming of gang sub-culture, such as gangsta rap and gang fashions (Miller 2001).

Since both the formation of gangs and their attractiveness to vulnerable adolescents stem from the cumulative effects of social and economic distress, preventing the formation of gangs requires intervention at multiple levels. These interventions require an approach that considers both proximate and distal factors in gang formation. In addition to the long-term objective of eradicating poverty, investment in schools and educational resources, the creation of adequate and accessible housing, economic development and employment opportunities for distressed urban zones, and combating racial and cultural discrimination could operate as pillars of gang prevention (see generally Decker and Weerman 2005; Miller 2001).

Preventing Gang Membership

Preventing a young person from joining a gang requires a good understanding of which individuals are most likely to join gangs. Research suggests that young people who join gangs have an accumulation of risk factors across multiple developmental domains (e.g. individual, family, peer, school, community), including a high prevalence and incidence of trauma. Common risk factors for gang involvement include growing up in low-income neighbourhoods, single-headed households, association with gang-involved peers, school failure, and early use of drugs and alcohol (Hill et al. 2001). Yet, not all youth exposed to these risk factors join a gang, nor is it understood which specific risk factors with what intensity at what points in a young person's life are likely to cause him or her to join a gang (Decker et al. 2013; Howell and Egley 2005). Little is known about the risk factors associated with female gang membership, although there are strong correlations between gang membership and female victimization and low school commitment (Peterson

and Carson 2012; Thornberry et al. 2003). Further, surprisingly little is known about how protective factors (Howell 2012), buffering factors (Lösel and Farrington 2012), or maintaining factors mediate or moderate the effects of risk factors in young people's lives.

Even if young people most likely to join gangs were identified accurately, the knowledge of programmes and approaches that prevent them from joining is in its infancy. Few programmes have undergone rigorous evaluation (Howell 2010); notable exceptions include two school-based programmes that have shown gang prevention effects. Schools may be an ideal location for such prevention programming where education is compulsory. The Montreal Preventive Treatment programme, a longitudinal study addressing anti-social behaviour among white, low-income boys ages 7–9 years who had shown behavioural problems in kindergarten, demonstrated reduced delinquency and gang membership (Gatti et al. 2005). Social skills training, parent training, and school collaboration are core features of this programme. The revised Gang Resistance Education and Training Programme (G.R.E.A.T.) resulted in reductions in the likelihood of gang membership in middle school students (approximately aged 10–14) in ethnically diverse urban areas in North America (Esbensen et al. 2011). This is a school-based skills curriculum wherein students are taught to resist gang membership and learn about the negative consequences of gang membership through interactive modules facilitated by trained police officers.

One reason relatively few gang prevention programmes have undergone rigorous evaluation is that most lack theoretically grounded conceptual frameworks (Klein and Maxson 2006; Miller 1990). Resiliency theory provides a foundation on which to build a conceptual framework for preventing young people from joining gangs. Resiliency theory posits that resilient young people may be exposed to significant threats or severe adversity but are able to adapt positively and move through developmental stages in spite of the exposure to serious risks (Jain and Cohen 2013). Resilient youth not only present an absence of antisocial behaviour and psychopathology, but in the face of significant adversity they still display positive behaviours and competency in a variety of developmental domains (Luthar et al. 1993).

Consistent with resiliency theory, Positive Youth Development (PYD) principles can inform thinking about individual and community level approaches that enhance positive features and protective factors for young people to develop resilience and avoid gang membership (Butts and Roman 2010; Catalano et al. 2004). PYD emphasizes a strengths based approach (as opposed to a deficit approach) to defining youth development. PYD identifies the features of settings that have been shown through programme evaluations to promote positive development, such as promotion of positive social norms, opportunities for skill building, physical and psychological safety, and opportunities to belong (Eccles and Gootman 2002). PYD outcomes, such as enhanced self-control, increased problem-solving abilities, and improved perception of family support can be used to evaluate whether individual development is occurring in various developmental domains, including family, schools, and communities (Eccles and Gootman 2002; McDonald et al. 2011). Multisystemic Therapy (MST), described in depth elsewhere in this volume, is an example of a rigorously evaluated resilience-building programme that is based on PYD principles and has been shown to be effective in addressing violent behaviour. Using a family ecological systems approach to work with serious violent or substance abusing juvenile offenders, MST has been found to reduce recidivism, enhance family functioning, and improve peer relations (Ogden and Hagen 2006). This intensive home-based programme is driven by the family's goals and strengths, and teams of therapists are available to the family 24 hours a day, 7 days a week. Programmatic interventions, such as MST, informed by resiliency theory and infused with principles of Positive Youth Development that enhance protective factors, hold promise to prevent young people with multiple risk factors from joining gangs (McDonald et al. 2011).

Preventing Violence from Gang Members

Suppression is generally the first strategy communities turn to in addressing gang activity; yet the use of suppression tactics in isolation, such as police and prosecution, has been shown to be limited in effectiveness (Howell 2010). These tactics may reduce the social capital of communities, or a community's ability to effectively address youth and violence, by relying on formal social control mechanisms. The Pulling Levers approach, a focused deterrence strategy in which suppression is part of a multi-pronged initiative that includes the provision of services, has been shown to be successful in reducing violent crime, a large portion of which is committed by gang members (Braga and Weisburd 2012). The programme was developed in Boston (otherwise known as Boston Ceasefire) and has spread to other parts of the U.S. and Europe. Under this programme, the most active gangs are identified by law enforcement and are brought into face-to-face meetings with law enforcement and key community leaders, such as clergy, to be collectively put on notice that their gangs are being watched closely. They are informed that if their gangs commit violence, the individuals responsible will be prosecuted to the fullest extent of the law. The objective of these meetings is to address the group behaviour of gangs in order to encourage the informal social controls of the gang to police its members. When violence occurs and individuals are prosecuted, these are held as examples to others of what can happen when the warning is not heeded (Kennedy 2011).

An important part of this approach is addressing group dynamics, not just individual level factors. Tackling group cohesion is an essential element of effective gang violence reduction (Decker et al. 2013); though outcomes may vary depending on how tightly connected gang members are to each other and to the gang (Papachristos 2013). Often, with the Pulling Levers strategy, law enforcement collaborates with a variety of community agencies and stakeholders to provide alternatives to the gang lifestyle. This typically includes a cadre of employment and educational programmes, clergy and community leader counselling and mentoring, as well as mental health and social service programmes. At the time of this writing, there is a lack of evaluation of the effectiveness of these social service provisions (Engel et al. 2013), though research shows that gangs must be addressed at the individual, group, and community levels across the life course (Decker et al. 2013).

Interventions thought to address gangs at multiple levels are street worker programmes. These programmes have been shown to be a promising approach to entice gang members in alternatives to gang life (Skogan et al. 2009). Improper implementation,

however, could increase gang cohesion and crime (Papachristos 2013). Street workers are usually people from the same community as the gang members, and often are former gang members. They typically have more street credibility to reach gang youth than other individuals who may have dissimilar life experiences. Street workers attempt to steer gang members towards prosocial activities and institutions, provide mentorship, and mediate gang disputes. From a public health perspective, street workers explicitly or implicitly attempt to change the normative culture of violence among gangs and gang members (Skogan et al. 2009). Services for gang members are then provided by other entities.

The Comprehensive Gang Model (CGM) usually incorporates streetworker programmes into their strategies and is considered by the United States Office of Juvenile Justice and Delinquency Prevention to be an 'effective' comprehensive programme to address gang violence (Howell 2010; Spergel 1997). The CGM aims to build new community collaborative systems and structures and function across ecological domains. CGM strategies segment a community's youth population according to levels of risk and then direct supports and interventions based on their particular risk factors and delinquency history (i.e. youth 'at-risk' requiring prevention activities to 'proven-risk' requiring intervention or suppression activities). These could include the Pulling Levers and street worker programmes already described. In addition to multiple levels of prevention, intervention, treatment, and suppression, the CGM also requires organizational change within and across community institutions, such as police, social service agencies, and schools to alter the way they do business in order to more effectively address gang violence. Community mobilization also is an essential element for persistent violence reduction and community change (Howell 2010). Utilization of research partners to assist in problem definition, data management, process evaluation, and outcome evaluation is also important in the process of implementing and sustaining the CGM.

The initial pilot programme of the CGM in the Little Village neighbourhood of Chicago showed significant reductions in gang members' serious violent and property crimes as well as in the frequency of other types of crimes (Spergel 2007). The CGM implementation in other cities in the United States, however, has shown mixed results. Formative evaluations of the CGM point out two key reasons for mixed results (Klein and Maxson 2006). The first has to do with myriad implementation problems that accompany such a complex initiative. The second reason is that communities may not be using evidence-based prevention and intervention programming. Gebo and Bond's (2012) overview of the Commonwealth of Massachusetts' implementation of the CGM at the state level demonstrates the challenges in comprehensive approaches to gang prevention. To address these problems, communities are encouraged to undergo more rigorous community assessments of the youth and gang violence problem before assembling strategies and partners within the CGM framework (Howell 2010). A comprehensive approach, however, is commensurate with a public health perspective to reduce risk factors for gang involvement as well as the criminal activities of gang members.

Intervention programming for gang members is in its early stages. To date, there are no rigorously evaluated programmes that have been shown consistently to work to reduce gang member violence and to facilitate exodus from the gang;

yet, there is a plethora of programmes, particularly employ-ment and educational programmes, while mental health and other services may serve gang members as part of their total caseloads. Programmes are widely varied as is the dosage of services provided. Few programmes working with gang mem-bers appear to be utilizing evidence based programming or a validated risk assessment tool, which takes into account risk factors, needs, and responsiveness to treatment, to match individual needs and risks with appropriate programming (Andrews et al. 2006). Although more research needs to be conducted on how well validated instruments work on a gang population, research consistently shows that only medium to high risk violent individuals should be placed in intensive ser-vices (Lowenkamp et al. 2006). Placing low-risk individuals in such programmes is likely to have iatrogenic effects. Currently, there is a Functional Family Therapy (FFT) pilot programme being conducted through the University of Maryland on gang youth which utilizes the evidence-based FFT programme com-bined with what is known about working with gang youth and their families. No evaluative results of FFT on the gang popula-tion are available at the time of this writing.

The Challenges of Gang Violence Prevention Work

There is no programme blueprint for what works best to reduce the likelihood of gang formation, gang membership, or violence among gang members. Sound theoretical underpinnings (Miller 1990) and incorporation of knowledge about gangs, adolescent development, gender, and culturally competent programming is critical for gang prevention and intervention programming to succeed. Further, rigorous evaluations of programmes that address gangs and those most at-risk for gang membership are needed, but lacking (Klein and Maxson 2006). The fact that few youth in the community ever become gang members can be problematic for such evaluations as the statistical power to assess programme effects is low; there may not be enough

individuals engaged in programming to determine whether or not the programme is successful. Effective programming may also vary across race, ethnicity, gender, and in different urban contexts.

Addressing individual needs of those who are at-risk for gang membership or who are already gang members is one key to reducing gang violence (Spergel 1997); yet gang members are more difficult to engage and keep engaged than most youth. This must be taken into account in any approach that takes on the issue of gang members. They also are likely to present with a host of risk factors, and while not exclusive to gangs, addressing individuals with those risk factors is likely to be more involved than tackling the risk factors of youth with general delinquency (Gebo and Sullivan 2014). Unfortunately, we know little about the protective factors and maintaining factors of gang mem-bers that may further our knowledge of what works. The group behaviour of those who are in gangs must also be addressed. Violence escalates as part of the group process, and that cannot be ignored.

There are five main points about gang violence prevention worth repeating. First, preventing gangs from developing and perpetuating involves investing in structural changes. Second, evidence-based early intervention programmes that target risk factors do seem to show residual gang suppression effects. Third, programming for gang members must address the host of risk fac-tors of gang members, not just the behaviour that is manifested. Fourth, targeted suppression may be somewhat effective as a short-term strategy, but without a comprehensive approach that cross-cuts the socio-ecological landscape, it is unlikely to be sus-tainable and may reduce social capital of community that would organically suppress gang behaviour. Finally, implementation of evidence-based programming with gang members based on results from validated Risk–Need–Responsivity assessment tools would be an important advance to what is currently being done. Smart programming is to utilize what we know about youth vio-lence prevention generally and apply those programmes to what we know about gangs.

References

Andrews, D. A., Bonta, J., and Wormith, J. S. (2006). The recent past and near future of risk and/or need assessment. *Crime & Delinquency*, 52, 7–27.

Braga, A. A., and Weisburd, D. (2012). The effects of 'Pulling Levers' focused deterrence strategies on crime. *Campbell Systematic Reviews*, 6, 1–90.

Butts, J. A., and Roman, C. G. (2010). A community youth development approach to gang control programs. In: R. J. Chaskin (ed.), *Youth Gangs and Community Intervention*. New York: Columbia, pp. 175–205.

Catalano, R., Berglund, M. L., Ryan, J. A. M., Lonczak, H. S., and Hawkins, J. D. (2004). Positive Youth Development in the United States: research findings on evaluations of positive youth development programs. *The ANNALS of the American Academy of Political and Social Science*, 591, 98–124.

Decker, S. H., Melde, C., and Pyrooz, D. C. (2013). What do we know about gangs and gang members and where do we go from here? *Justice Quarterly*, 30, 369–402.

Decker, S. H., and Weerman, F. M. (2005). *European Street Gangs and Troublesome Youth Groups*. Lanham, MD: AltaMira Press.

Eccles, J., and Gootman, J. (2002). *Community Programs to Promote Youth Development*. Washington, D.C.: National Academy Press.

Engel, R. S., Tillyer, M. S., and Corsaro, N. (2013). Reducing gang violence using focused deterrence: evaluating the Cincinnati Initiative to Reduce Violence (CIRV). *Justice Quarterly*, 30, 403–39.

Esbensen, F., Peterson, D., and Taylor, T. J. et al. (2011). Evaluation and evolution of the Gang Resistance Education and Training (G.R.E.A.T.) program. *Journal of School Violence*, 10, 53–70.

Esbensen, F. and Weerman, F. M. (2005). A cross-national comparison of youth gangs and troublesome youth groups in the United States and the Netherlands. *European Journal of Criminology*, 2, 5–37.

Gatti, U., Tremblay, R. E., Vitaro, F., and McDuff, P. (2005). Youth gangs, delinquency and drug use: a test of selection, facilitation, and enhancement hypotheses. *Journal of Child Psychology and Psychiatry*, 46, 1178–90.

Gebo, E., and Bond., B. J. (2012). *Looking Beyond Suppression: Community Strategies to Reduce Gang Violence*. Lanham, MD: Lexington.

Gebo, E., and Sullivan. C. J. (2014). A statewide comparison of gang and non-gang youth in schools. *Youth Violence & Juvenile Justice*, 12, 191–208.

Hill, K. G., Lui, C. J., and Hawkins, J. D. (2001). *Early Precursors of Gang Membership: A Study of Seattle Youth*. Bulletin. Washington, D.C.: U.S. Department of Justice, Office of Justice Programs, Office of Juvenile Justice and Delinquency Prevention.

Howell, J. C. (2010). *Gang Prevention: An Overview of Research and Programs*. Washington, D.C.: Office of Juvenile Justice and Delinquency Prevention.

Howell, J. C. (2012). *Gangs in America's Communities*. Thousand Oaks, CA: Sage.

Howell, J. C., and Egley, A., Jr. (2005). Moving risk factors into developmental theories of gang membership. *Youth Violence & Juvenile Justice*, 3, 334–54.

Jain, S., and Cohen, A. (2013). Fostering resilience among urban youth exposed to violence: a promising area for interdisciplinary research and practice. *Health Education and Behavior*, 40, 651–62.

Kennedy, D. M. (2011). *Don't Shoot*. New York: Bloomsbury.

Klein, M. W., Kerner, H., Maxson, C. L., and Weitekamp, E. G. M. (2001). *The Eurogang Paradox: Street Gangs and Youth Groups in the U.S. and Europe*. New York: Springer.

Klein, M. W., and Maxson, C. L. (2006). *Street Gang Patterns and Policies*. New York: Oxford.

Krohn, M. D., and Thornberry, T. (2008). Longitudinal perspectives on adolescent street gangs. In: A. Liberman (ed.), *The Long View of Crime: A Synthesis of Longitudinal Research*, New York: Springer, pp. 138–60.

Lösel, F., and Farrington, D. (2012). Direct protective and buffering protective factors in the development of youth violence. *American Journal of Preventive Medicine*, 43, S8–S23.

Lowenkamp, C. T., Latessa, E. J., and Holsinger, A. M. (2006). The risk principle in action: what have we learned from 13,676 offender and 97 correctional programs? *Crime & Delinquency*, 52, 77–93.

Luthar, S. S., Doernberger, C., and Zigler, E. (1993). Resilience is not a unidimensional construct: insights from a prospective study of inner-city adolescents. *Development and Psychopathology*, 5, 703–17.

Matsuda, K. M., Esbensen, F., and Carson, D. (2012). Putting the 'gang' in 'Eurogang': characteristics of delinquent youth groups by different definitional approaches. In: F. Esbensen, and C. Maxson (eds), *Youth Gangs in International Perspective: Results from the Eurogang Program of Research*. New York: Springer, pp. 17–33.

McDonald, C. C., Deatrick, J. A., Kassam-Adams, N., and Richmond, T. S. (2011). Community violence exposure and positive youth development in urban youth. *Journal of Community Health*, 36, 925–32.

Melde, C., and Esbensen, F. (2011). Gang membership as a turning point in the life course. *Criminology*, 49, 513–52.

Miller, W. B. (1990). Why the United States has failed to solve its youth gang problem. In: R. C. Huff (ed.), *Gangs in America*. Newbury Park, CA: Sage, pp. 263–87.

Miller, W. B. (2001). *The Growth of Youth Gang Problems in the United States: 1970-1998*. Washington, D.C.: Office of Juvenile Justice and Delinquency Prevention. Available at: https://www.ncjrs.gov/pdffiles1/ojjdp/181868-1.pdf [Accessed 27 August 2013].

Ogden, T., and Hagen, K. A. (2006). Multisystemic Therapy of serious behaviour problems in youth: sustainability of therapy effectiveness 2 years after intake. *Child and Adolescent Mental Health*, 11, 142–49.

Papachristos, A. V. (2013). The importance of cohesion for gang research, policy, and practice. *Criminology & Public Policy*, 12, 49–58.

Peterson, D., and Carson, D. (2012). The sex composition of groups and youths' delinquency: a comparison of gang and non-gang peer groups. In: F. Esbensen, and C. Maxson (eds), *Youth Gangs in International Perspective: Results from the Eurogang Program of Research*. New York: Springer, pp. 189–210.

Short, J. F., Jr., and Hughes, L. A. (2006). *Studying Youth Gangs*. Lanham, MD: AltaMira Press.

Skogan, W., Hartnett, S. M., Bump, N., and Dubois, J. (2009). *Evaluation of Ceasefire Chicago*. Available at: https://www.ncjrs.gov/pdffiles1/nij/grants/227181.pdf [Accessed 8 August 2013]

Spergel, I. A. (2007). *Reducing Youth Gang Violence: The Little Village Project in Chicago*. Lanham, MD: AltaMira Press.

Thornberry, T. P., Huizinga, D., and Loeber, R. (2004). The Causes and Correlates Studies: findings and policy implications. *Juvenile Justice*, 10, 3–19.

Thornberry, T. P., Krohn, M. D., Lizotte, A. J., Smith, C. A., and Tobin, K. (2003). *Gangs and Delinquency in Developmental Perspective*. New York: Cambridge.

Vigil, J. D. (2002). *A Rainbow of Gangs: Street Cultures in the Mega-City*. Austin, TX: University of Texas Press.

Vigil, J. D. (2003). Urban violence and street gangs. *Annual Review of Anthropology*, 32, 225–42.

CHAPTER 30

Chicago, I do mind dying

John M. Hagedorn

Introduction to Chicago, I Do Mind Dying

Chicago in 2012 was constantly in the United States news over a reported 'spike' in homicides. Both the Chicago Police Department (CPD), and the highly publicized CeaseFire programme were unable to reduce the death toll. This chapter addresses three questions:

i. Did murders actually 'soar' in Chicago in 2012 and how do we understand homicide trends in that city?

ii. From an international comparative perspective, what factors influence the overall level of homicide and major fluctuations?

iii. Why did the all-out efforts of the Chicago Police Department and others fail to reduce the number of murders in 2012?

The main argument of this chapter reduces to the truism that violence reduction strategies must be based on analysis of the actual nature of violence at a given time and place. This chapter begins by looking at variations in murder around the world through the lens of the 2011 United Nations Global Study on Homicide (GSH). Internationally, homicide is most strongly related to level of development, inequality, and the desperation of the socially excluded. The highest levels of homicide are related to wars between gangs, cartels, or other similar social actors.

Second, using Uniform Crime Report (UCR) data and social science findings on the rise and fall of homicide, I compare trends of homicide in Chicago with other U.S. cities and look at some international comparisons. I note that by 2000 organized gang wars in Chicago had ended and homicide rates by 2008 had already fallen by half. The data show that 2012 did not represent a 'spike' in Chicago homicides whose murder rate had stabilized for the past decade.

I conclude that targeted interventions can be effective in incrementally reducing homicides, but operate within certain parameters. The findings of the GSH imply that absent major environmental changes addressing social exclusion, city homicide rates are unlikely to appreciably change.

The 2011 United Nations Global Study of Homicide

This important study establishes three significant facts: (i) homicide in most of the world in the past decade has been on a gradual decline; (ii) high levels of homicide generally are correlated with lack of development, inequality, and the desperation of unemployed young men; (iii) countries with the highest homicide rates are plagued by gang or organized crime warfare and it is in these countries where we see the most substantial fluctuations over

time. A review of this report (Me et al. 2011) sets the stage for understanding variations in the United States by city and gives a clearer picture of what is happening now in Chicago.

Of the factors that influence homicide, the GSH finds the strongest correlation with lack of development and inequality (GSH 2011; see also Fajnzylber et al. 2003). The report summarizes:

> lethal violence is often rooted in contexts of paucity and deprivation, inequality and injustice, social marginalization, low levels of education and a weak rule of law. (Me et al. 2011, p. 29)

But these are not the only factors correlated with high levels of homicide.

In fact, the only exception to the pattern of the general correlation of high rates of homicide with lack of development are in some developed countries in the Americas, 'where other factors such as organized crime and inequality play a more important role than average human development levels' (GSH 2011, p. 30). The GSH excludes deaths due to civil wars and ethnic conflicts, but it finds the highest rate of homicide and most extreme fluctuations are associated with gang wars and organized crime.

In the Americas, fully 25 per cent of all homicides are linked to gangs, cartels, and organized crime, as compared to only 5 per cent of homicides in Asia and Europe. While homicide has dropped in most of the world over the past decade, Central America and Mexico have seen sharp increases during the same time—sometimes as much as 100 per cent—linked to drug trafficking wars. This is consistent with historical trends: for example, sharp increases in homicide in Italy in the 1990s were due to mafia wars (see Dickie 2004); the Cali versus Medellín cartel wars in Colombia in the 1980s (Guitierrez and Jaramillo 2004); the U.S. 'beer wars' during Prohibition and 'crack wars' of the 1990s. The GSH concludes 'the presence of organized criminal groups can provoke a surge in violence and homicides' (GSH 2011 p. 49).

In countries characterized by gang and organized crime warfare, the lifetime risk of a 20-year-old male's being murdered can be as high as 2 per cent—which means in those countries one in every 50 young men will be murdered before the age of 31. The GSH finds this risk for young males is 400 times larger than in countries without gang warfare. The international context of the GSH sheds light on homicide in the United States and Chicago.

Trends in Homicide In the United States

Every death is wrenching for loved ones and touches anyone possessing a trace of empathy. On the other hand, homicide in the U.S. is at its lowest levels in over a century. This is not quite a trend:

the U.S. murder rate in 2010 was at about the same rate as it was in both 1950 and 1910:4.6 per 100,000. Lower rates of homicide since the 1800s are consistent with Elias's (1939/1994) notion of a 'civilising effect' while murders in the U.S. have always been somewhat higher than in Europe (see Pinker 2011). There is considerable variation by city, and these variations are tied to both extreme poverty of the U.S. African-American population and periods of gang warfare. Compare Chicago's higher rates with overall U.S. trends (Table 30.1).

Prior to the 1960s, the highest rates of homicide in the United States were during the period of alcohol Prohibition in the 1920s, where organized crime groups fought a series of 'beer wars' against one another and the government. In both Chicago and Detroit, researchers have estimated that about one-third of all homicides during prohibition years were gang related (Zahn 1989). After repeal of Prohibition most U.S. homicides were domestic disputes or bar room quarrels between men. Over that time homicide rates dropped and stabilized until the 1960s when African-Americans faced oppressive conditions as they migrated to large cities. A mass social movement broke out alongside numerous urban riots. Black gangs grew in numbers and crime rates, including homicide, rose sharply.

A look at the trends in homicide in Chicago, New York City, Los Angeles, and Detroit (Figure 30.1) supports the GSH's contention of the correlation of homicide rates with lack of development, as well as indicating that large fluctuations in homicide may be gang related.

Note the sharper slope, higher rates, and larger increases in Detroit starting in the mid-1960s than in other major U.S. cities. There is surely a common sense, if not demonstrably causal, relationship between the 50 per cent loss of jobs in Detroit since the 1970s and truly 'soaring' murder rates (Loftin et al. 1989). Georgakas and Surkin's (1975) poignant *Detroit, I Do Mind Dying* (from which this chapter borrows its name) is among the works that bring to life the desperation of African-Americans in the former auto capital of the world (see also Sugrue 1996).

Table 30.1 Homicide rates in Chicago and United States 1900–2010

	Chicago	**United States**
1900	6.0	1.2
1910	9.2	4.6
1920	10.5	6.8
1930	14.6	8.8
1940	7.1	6.3
1950	7.9	4.6
1960	10.3	5.1
1970	24.0	7.9
1980	28.7	10.2
1990	32.9	9.4
2000	22.1	5.5
2010	15.4	4.8*

Source: data from United States Federal Bureau of Investigation, *Uniform Crime Report*, 2014, available from http://www.fbi.gov/about-us/cjis/ucr/ucr.

The higher rate of homicide in Detroit is also consistent with the general analysis of the GSH. Detroit remains home to a disproportionate number of desperate, angry, unemployed African-American men with one of the highest urban homicide rates in the country. As Lane argues in his seminal study on homicide, 'the historical evidence' convincingly shows murder is related to 'changes in the structure of employment' as it particularly affects African-Americans (Lane 1997, p. 342). The battle for control of Detroit's heroin and later crack markets by the Chambers Brothers and other gangs in the 1970s and 1980s contributed to even higher homicide rates in that city (Taylor 1989).

Homicide rose across the United States in the 1970s and reached its all time high in 1980, for the first and only year exceeding ten per 100,000 nationally, the UN threshold for a homicide 'epidemic' (see http://www.disastercenter.com/crime/uscrime.htm for a year by year report of homicide numbers and rate over the past century). The higher U.S. rates were driven by sizeable increases in homicide in larger cities, as Figure 30.1 has shown.

U.S. Studies on the History of Homicide

A review of the scholarship on the history of violence in the United States strongly supports the twin contentions of the GSH that homicide is generally related to lack of development, inequality of minority groups, and the resulting desperation of young men, and that large fluctuations are typically related to gang wars and youth gun violence. I particularly focus on three remarkable edited volumes: Ted Gurr's *History of Crime* (1979), Michael Tonry and Mark Moore's *Youth Violence* (1998), and Alfred Blumstein and Joel Wallman's *The Crime Drop* (2000).

The selections in Gurr's volume provide a broader perspective on the post 1960s sharp rise in violence in the United States Gurr pointed out at the onset that any abrupt changes in homicide need to be placed in historical perspective.

> Since homicide is a relatively rare event it is highly variable over the short run.....homicide rates are best used as an indicator of middle and long-run trends in interpersonal violence. (1979, p. 26)

The volume argues that the United States appeared to be in the midst of a long-term decline in homicide rates that have been interrupted only by small spikes in the aftermath of world war and internal gang wars.

Eric Monkkonen, in the same volume, compared homicide rates in the United States and United Kingdom and saw both in a state of decline. Since 1870, Monkonnen concluded, homicide has declined rapidly in the United Kingdom but more modestly in the United States, which he found continues to be more violence-prone than its European cousin.

Roger Lane (1989), in his essay *On the Social Meaning of Homicide Rates in America* (also in the same volume), looks inside the U.S. decline and finds homicide to be concentrated largely among unemployed African-American males. He concludes in words consistent with the GSH: '...in the real world, homicide in modern societies is overwhelmingly done by and to marginal people, often members of minority groups' (1989, p. 75).

After the drug wars of the 1990s, two more major edited volumes collected the nation's top scholars to weigh in and again

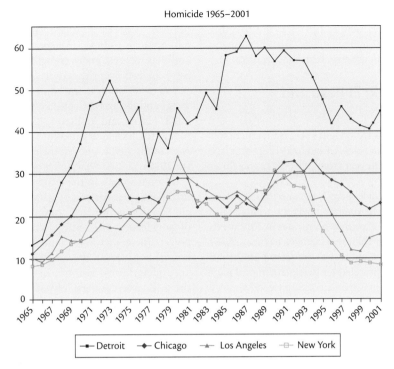

Fig. 30.1 Homicide in four cities: 1965 and 2001.

Source: data from United States Federal Bureau of Investigation,*Uniform Crime Report*, 2014, available from http://www.fbi.gov/about-us/cjis/ucr/ucr.

their findings foretold the substance of the GSH 20 years later. In the University of Chicago's Annual Review of Research, Tonry and Moore (1998) debunk the notion that the increase in violence was a mechanical product of an increase in the youth population and 'super-predators' (Dilulio 1995). Rather, they argue in public health terms that there was in fact an 'epidemic' of youth violence in the 1990s, though they caution that the contagious aspect of the term epidemic is 'a matter to be investigated, not assumed' (Tonry and Moore 1998, p. 6).

Phil Cook and John Laub analyse the epidemic and discover that while property crimes by youth remained constant, in the late 1980s and early 1990s, youth violence, particularly among black males, exploded to 'levels with no precedent in this century' (1998, p. 28). In fact, homicide rates for all males 25 and over actually declined during the epidemic. But by 1993 homicide rates for black male offenders 13–17 years had skyrocketed to 120 per 100,000 and for those 18–24 years, to an astounding 280 per 100,000! Explaining how this could occur in a country where overall homicide rates were less than ten per 100,000 was a major task of the volume.

Cook and Laub firmly reject Dilulio's assertion that the increase in violence was related to the character of a specific set of youth, a 'cohort effect'. Rather Cook and Laub argue that what was occurring was a 'period effect', since violence did not follow the career of the cohort but rather was concentrated on a period of time. One characteristic of the period was increased use of firearms, particularly in gang-related killings. They pointed out, 'all of the epidemic of increase in killing by adolescents and young adults in the late 1980s was accomplished with firearms' (1998, p. 54).

In two other essays, one by Fagan and Wilkinson (1998) and a second by this author (Hagedorn 1998), the relationship between

gang wars and homicide is explored using multiple literatures. What Cook and Laub call a 'period effect' was translated by these researchers as a period of gang wars over crack and cocaine distribution.

Why the 'epidemic' suddenly came to an end was the question explored by Blumstein (2000). He pointed out that the change in violent offending was sudden and related to changes in crack markets. Johnson et al. (2000) give a detailed ethnographic picture of how changes in crack markets in the 1990s led to decreases in violence. As competition for markets declined among gangs of drug sellers, violence dropped. Johnson et al.'s chapter suggested that police tactics were effective in suppressing drug gangs. Ric Curtis (1998), in an important essay (unfortunately not in that volume) expands on Johnson's argument by pointing out that since New York City did not have institutionalized gangs who controlled drug sales as in Chicago, police suppression was particularly effective. Once the newly formed New York City drug posses were arrested, there simply were no organized gangs to take their place and violence sharply declined. In Chicago, police arrests simply added opportunities for a new and willing cohort of younger gang members to step up and take their place. Violent gang rivalries over drug markets in Chicago continued long after their decline in New York.

Eck and Maguire (2000) provide a fitting transition between what is now classic homicide research and why nothing seemed to work in Chicago. They begin by pointing out that there are no studies that find a significant correlation between numbers of police officers in a city and the crime drop of the 1990s. While there is a mixed bag of studies that find a police effect on crime, it is unclear whether increased numbers of police were the cause or the effect of the 1990s crime drop. In fact, crime began dropping in major

U.S. cities, including New York City, *before* increases in policing and the introduction of various new tactics. Eck and Maguire also look at 'hot spots' and other policing tactics that they suggest might have a localized effect, but draw no firm conclusions.

Chicago and New York; El Paso and Juarez

The first conclusion we can draw from Figure 30.2 is that there was no significant 'spike' in homicides in Chicago in 2012. In fact, the homicide rate in Chicago in each year from 2004–2012 was *lower* than at any time since 1967.

This does not mean that homicide today is not a serious problem, particularly in very poor African-American neighbourhoods. But the 'soaring' media attention to Chicago's homicides in 2012 needs to be explained by factors other than real changes in the number of homicides which even in raw numbers were *less* in 2012 than 2008. It is beyond the scope of this chapter to explain 'moral panics' and media 'crime waves' (e.g. Cohen 1972; Surette 1998).

What *was* going on? It is here that the GSH proves valuable. Chicago, like other large cities, saw large increases in violence in the 1970s as the U.S. economy restructured and poverty vastly increased in black neighbourhoods. William Julius Wilson's (1987) studies of Chicago's 'underclass' starkly demonstrated this shift. The increases in poverty, unemployment, and other measures of 'social isolation' are what the GSH means by underdevelopment, inequality, and desperation. This is also consistent with Lane's (1997) analysis of the reasons for higher rates of homicide for African-Americans.

In Chicago, however, desperate conditions coincided with the institutionalization of its city's gangs who in turn became key in how we understand homicide in that city. In the 1970s and 1980s gang wars produced the highest rates of violence in Chicago's history, reaching a horrific 970 murders in 1974, nearly twice as many as the 507 in 2012. The killing fields of those years were one reason for the formation of the well-known 'People' and 'Folks' gang coalitions. These groupings of 'nations' were put together to organize crime, but also to reduce violence, both in the prisons as well as the streets.

Gang efforts produced some reductions in violence in the 1980s, but in the 1990s, two sets of gang wars erupted; one between the Gangster Disciples and Black Disciples, and a second a 'war of the families' between the allied gangs of the Maniac Latin Disciples and Spanish Cobras (Hagedorn forthcoming). These sustained conflicts were examples of *organized gang warfare*, and cost thousands of lives over the decade.

The result of these wars was the fracturing of Chicago's major gangs and the loss of 'legitimacy' of their leaders (Hagedorn 2006, 2008; Moore and Williams 2010). The gang violence occurring today in Chicago is different in nature and severity than in the wars of the 1990s, or even the pre-People and Folks battlefields of the 1970s.

In other words, in the 1970s and 1990s the jumps in homicide in Chicago were driven by gang wars which reflected the desperate conditions in black communities but also the self interests of gang leaders attempting to control drug markets and exercise power. The gang wars wound down by the end of the 1990s and homicide dropped, but only gradually, not precipitously. While an undetermined amount of violence is still gang connected, the killings are indeed 'out of control' of both police and gang leaders. Violence in Chicago today is basically a reflection of the desperation in Chicago's black community, not organized gang warfare.

Gang Wars and Truces

Both CeaseFire and the Chicago Police Department prior to 2012 were claiming credit for relatively lower rates of homicide. A popular movie, *The Interrupters*, celebrated what CeaseFire leaders claimed were 'statistically significant' reductions in all neighbourhoods (Papachristos 2011; Skogan et al. 2007). But a rise in homicides could not be stemmed as both CeaseFire and the CPD tried a variety of tactics. The practices of CeaseFire and the CPD were based in part on negotiating with or intimidating gang leaders and getting them to call a halt to the violence. That didn't work—not because the idea of gangs calling off violence was flawed, but mainly because the notion that Chicago gang leaders had the power to call off retaliation was inaccurate.

Gangs with strong leaders and control over their members can call violence on and off and there are many international examples of gangs' capacity to end the wars they start. For example, in El

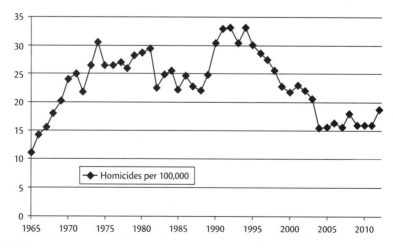

Fig. 30.2 Chicago homicides 1965–2012.

Source: data from United States Federal Bureau of Investigation, *Uniform Crime Report*, 2014, available from http://www.fbi.gov/about-us/cjis/ucr/ucr.

Table 30.2 A tale of two cities

City	Population	Number of homicides	Homicide rate per 100,000
El Paso	800,647	5	< 1
Juarez	1,300,000	3075	229

Source: data from United States Federal Bureau of Investigation, *Uniform Crime Report*, 2014, available from http://www.fbi.gov/about-us/cjis/ucr/ucr.

Salvador, a truce called by incarcerated gang leaders has reportedly dropped killings by a third (e.g. Archibold 2012).

The capacity of gangs to control violence is even better seen in two sets of cities on the U.S.–Mexican border. El Paso, consistently cited as the nation's safest city, is located across a river from Juarez, where a gang war rages (Table 30.2).

Similarly, in 2010, Tijuana saw 818 homicides but San Diego had just 29. The cities have a comparable population but a drug war is going on in Tijuana that has not spilled over a few miles north in San Diego. Cartel leaders are making conscious decisions on *where* to kill. In other words, some gangs can control violence to a substantial degree and their decisions can have a major effect on rates of violence in any place. Clearly, as in El Salvador, gang truces can have immediate effects on homicide rates on the streets when gang leaders have 'legitimate' authority and can command allegiance from their soldiers.

This is *not* the situation in Chicago. My own research and other studies of homicide (Papachristos 2013) report that much of Chicago's gang violence of the last decade was intra-gang, confirming the fracturing of gangs and the loss of control by gang leaders. While 'interrupting' the angry retaliation of loose groups of renegade gang members is valuable, an overall strategy of pressuring, bribing, or intimidating gang leaders is simply misplaced in today's Chicago.

Housing and Homicide

Chicago and other cities are trying frantically to replicate the crime drop in New York City. While police tactics are popularly cited as the principle reason for New York City's drastic reductions in crime, I can only note that the list of New York Police Department tactics (Zimring 2012) claimed to have had an effect are all being implemented in other cities, including Chicago, with only limited success. This suggests the New York Police Department tactics probably interacted with other environmental factors to cause such major reductions.

Frank Zimring concludes that major changes in crime rates 'are possible without major structural changes in the city' (2012, p. 199). But he fails to note that there *were* major structural changes

in New York City over the same period as the crime drop, specifically Mayor Koch's multi-billion dollar 180,000 unit investment in housing (Petro 2013; Association of Neighborhood Housing Development 2013). This bold and transformative development policy stands in stark contrast to Chicago's destruction of public housing and dispersal of its black population in the same period. At least one study (Hagedorn and Rauch 2007) suggested that housing policy had a significant effect on the different trends in homicide of those two cities.

Massive investments in infrastructure and development in poor communities internationally have been demonstrated as having significant impacts on violence, consistent with the GSH thesis. For example, in Medellín, Colombia, a determined urban plan of investments in housing played a major role in reductions in homicide between 2003 and 2007 that were even more drastic than in those in New York City (Escobar 2010). In Medellín, however, self-interested decisions by gang leaders to call off wars and start them again also played key roles in the zig-zag fluctuations in homicide over the past decades (Felbab-Brown 2011).

The example of Medellín supports both aspects of the GSH analysis and helps explain why programmes such as CeaseFire and those of the CPD were unable to reduce violence in 2012. Medellín embarked on a New York City-style urban rebuilding that weakened the hold of the drug lords on their soldiers by increasing a stake in their homes and in a city that was investing in their future. The favelas on the hills surrounding Medellín, where most of the violence occurred, were the locus of massive redevelopment. At the same time, city leaders also embarked on an urban peace strategy that encouraged gang leaders themselves to curtail violence.

In Chicago in 2012, there were no gang wars nor gang leaders with significant clout. Chicago was a city with a major budget crisis and lacked the resources—and mayoral resolve—to make serious investments in stabilizing the poorest African American communities and its education policy of closing schools contributed to uncertainty. It is not 'easy' to drop a city's homicide rate, and short of massive investments in poor black communities of the scale of New York and Medellín significant reductions in homicide are not likely in Chicago.

It is beyond the scope of this chapter to examine the effectiveness of specific intervention tactics. But programmes like CeaseFire or the CPD's Violence Reduction Strategy can be effective only within given parameters, particularly when there are no gang wars to be stopped. Applying the GSH to Chicago, we can conclude that it is underdevelopment, inequality, and unstable black communities that need to be at the centre of Chicago's violence reduction policy, not gangs.

Chicago, I do mind dying. But please, address the real reasons why so many of our young black men are desperate enough to kill.

References

Archibold, R. C. (2012). *Gangs' Truce Buys El Salvador a Tenuous Peace.* New York Times, 27 August 2012.

Association of Neighborhood Housing Development, Inc. (2013). *The Visionary Koch Housing Plan.* Available at: http://www.anhd.org/2775[Accessed 08 March 2013].

Blumstein, A. (2000). Disaggregating the violence trends. In: A. Blumstein, and J. Wallman (eds), *The Crime Drop in America.* Cambridge: University of Cambridge Press, pp. 13–44.

Blumstein, A., and Wallman, J. (2000). *The Crime Drop in America.* Cambridge: University of Cambridge Press.

Cohen, S. (1972). *Moral Panics and Folk Devils,* London: MacGibbon & Kee.

Cook, P. J., and Laub, J. H. (1998). The unprecedented epidemic in youth violence. In: M. Tonry, and M. H. Moore (eds), *Crime and Justice: An Annual Review of Research, Vol. 24. Youth Violence* Chicago: University of Chicago, 1998, pp. 27–64.

Curtis, R. (1998). The improbable transformation of inner-city neighborhoods: crime, violence, drugs, and youth in the 1990s. *The Journal of Criminal Law and Criminology,* 88, 1233–76.

Dickie, J. (2004).*Cosa Nostra: A History the Sicilian Mafia.* New York City: Palgrave.

Dilulio, J. (1995).*How to Stop the Coming Crime Wave.* New York: Manhattan Institute.

Escobar, J. (2010). *Reducing Urban Violence: Lessons from Medellín, Colombia.* Master's Thesis, Boston: Urban Studies and Planning, Massachusetts Institute of Technology.

Fagan, J., and Wilkinson, D.(1998). Guns, youth violence, and social identity in inner cities. In: M. Tonry, and M. Moore (eds),*Crime and Justice: An Annual Review of Research, Vol. 24. Youth Violence.* Chicago: University of Chicago, pp. 105–88.

Fajnzylber, P, Lederman, D., and Loayza, N. (2003). *Determinants of Crime Rates in Latin America and the World: An Empirical Assessment.* Washington D.C.: World Bank.

Felbab-Brown, V. (2011). *Reducing Urban Violence: Lessons from Medellín, Colombia.* Brookings Institute. Available at: http://www.brookings.edu/research/opinions/2011/02/14-colombia-crime-felbabbrown. [Accessed 21 November 2013].

Eck, J., and Maguire, E.(2000). Have changes in policing reduced violent crime? In: A. Blumstein, and J. Wallman (eds),*The Crime Drop in America.* Cambridge, U.K.: Cambridge University Press, pp. 207–65.

Elias, N. (1939/1994). *The Civilizing Process: The History of Manners.* Oxford: Blackwell.

Georgakas, D., and Surkin, M. (1975). *Detroit: I Do Mind Dying.* New York: St. Martin's Press.

Guitierrez S, F., and Jaramillo, A.M. (2004). Crime, [counter]insurgency, and the Privatization of Security: the case of Medellín, Colombia. *Environment and Urbanization,* 16, 1–14.

Gurr, T. R. (1989). Historical Trends in Violent Crime: Europe and the United States. In: T. R. Gurr (ed.), *Violence in America: The History of Crime.* Vol. 1. Newbury Park, CA: Sage, pp. 21–54.

Hagedorn, J. M. (1998). Post-industrial gang violence. In: M. Tonry, and M. H. Moore (eds), *Crime and Justice: An Annual Review of Research, Vol. 24. Youth Violence.* Chicago: University of Chicago, pp. 457–511.

Hagedorn, J. M. (2006). Race not space: a revisionist history of gangs in Chicago. *Journal African America History,* 91, 194–208.

Hagedorn, J. M., and Rauch, B. (2007). Housing, gangs, and homicide: what we can learn from Chicago. *Urban Affairs Review,* 42, 435–56.

Hagedorn, J. M. (2008). *A World of Gangs: Armed Young Men and Gangsta Culture.* Minneapolis: University of Minnesota Press.

Hagedorn, J. M. (forthcoming). *The In$ane Chicago Way. The Daring Plan by Chicago Gangs to Create a Spanish Mafia.* Chicago. University of Chicago Press.

Johnson, B. D., Golub, A., and Dunlap, E. (2000). The rise and decline of hard drugs, drug markets, and violence in inner-city New York. In: A. Blumstein, and J. Wallman (eds.). *The Crime Drop in America.* Cambridge, UK: Cambridge University Press, pp. 164–206.

Lane, R. (1989). On the social meaning of homicide rates in America. In: T. R. Gurr (ed.), *Violence in America: The History of Crime.* Vol. 1. Newbury Park, CA: Sage, pp. 55–79.

Lane, R. (1997). *Murder in America: A History.* Columbus: Ohio State University Press.

Loftin, C., Mcdowall, D., and Boudouris, J. (1989). Economic change and homicide in Detroit, 1926-1979. In: T. R. Gurr (ed.), *Violence in America: The History of Crime.* Vol. 1. Newbury Park, CA: Sage, pp. 163–77.

Me, A., Bisogno, E., Malby. S. (2011). *Global Study of Homicide.* Vienna: United Nations Office on Drugs and Crime.

Moore, N, and Williams, L. (2010). *The Almighty Black P. Stone Nation.* Chicago: Lawrence Hill Books.

Papachristos, A. V. (2011). Too big to fail: the science and politics of violence prevention. *Criminology and Public Policy,* 10, 1053–61.

Papachristos, A. V. (2013). *Personal Correspondence* (13 March 2013).

Petro, J. (2013). A closer look at Ed Koch's affordable housing legacy. *Next City.* Available at: http://nextcity.org/daily/entry/a-closer-look-at-ed-kochs-affordable-housing-legacy. [Accessed 21 November 2013].

Pinker, S. (2011). *The Better Angels of our Nature: Why Violence has Declined.* New York: Viking.

Sugrue, T.J. (1996). *The Origins of the Urban Crisis: Race and Inequality in Postwar Detroit.* Princeton, NJ: Princeton Press.

Surette, R. (1998). *Media, Crime, and Criminal Justice: Images and Realities.* Belmont, CA: West/Wadsworth.

Taylor, C. (1989). *Dangerous Society.* East Lansing, MI: Michigan State University Press.

Tonry, M., and Moore, M. H. (1998). Youth Violence. In: M. Tonry, and M. H. Moore (ed.), *Crime and Justice: An Annual Review of Research, Vol. 24. Youth Violence.* Chicago: University of Chicago, pp. 1–26.

United States Federal Bureau of Investigation. *Uniform Crime Reports.* Available at: http://www.fbi.gov/about-us/cjis/ucr/ucr. [Accessed 21 November 2013].

Wilson, W. J. (1987). *The Truly Disadvantaged.* Chicago: University of Chicago.

Zahn, M. A. (1989). Homicide in the twentieth century: trends, types, and causes. In: T. R. Gurr (ed.). *Violence in America: The History of Crime.* Vol. 1. Newbury Park, CA: Sage, pp. 216–34.

Zimring, F. E. (2012). *The City that Became Safe.* Oxford: Oxford University Press.

CHAPTER 31

Preventing violence through interventions for substance abuse

Christine Goodall

Substance Misuse and Violence

Alcohol is undoubtedly our preferred and most abused legal drug; it is also a major risk factor for violence. The World Health Organization (WHO) lists the harmful use of alcohol as the third global cause of premature death, disability, and incapacity (WHO 2010). Worldwide, alcohol accounts for the deaths of 2.5 million people annually (3.8 per cent of all deaths) and for 4.5 per cent of the global burden of disease and injury. Males, particularly those in the 15–59 year age group, are at much greater risk of alcohol-related mortality than women across all world regions. Alcohol also contributes to widening the health inequalities gap across a number of disease entities and so the relative risk of death and disability from those diseases associated with alcohol, including injuries resulting from violence, is greater for those of low socioeconomic status than those of higher socioeconomic status (Anakwe et al. 2011; Conway et al 2010). The impact of alcohol on health is felt most in middle-income countries largely because they do not seem to benefit from the modest protective effects of low levels of alcohol consumption seen in high-income countries (Hansel et al. 2010).

Death and disability due to alcohol misuse far outweigh those due to the misuse of illicit substances, which result in 99,000–253,000 deaths annually (0.5–1.3 per cent of deaths in the 15–64 year age group) and 0.9 per cent of the global burden of disease (UNODC 2012). Much of the mortality is due either to unintentional overdose or to suicide rather than to interpersonal violence (Degenhardt and Hall 2012). It is often the case, however, that drug-related deaths attract more public and political attention than alcohol-related death and disability, possibly due to the illicit and unregulated nature of the drug market.

Substance misuse behaviours can and do co-exist, and many psychoactive substances will act either synergistically to potentiate the effects of one or both substances, or will interact to produce a new psychoactive substance. For example, cocaine and alcohol are often taken in combination because the resulting substance—cocaethylene—results in a prolonged and more intense feeling of euphoria than cocaine alone. However, using alcohol and cocaine in combination is also associated with a variety of adverse health effects, not least drug-related death. Another effect resulting from this combination of substances is an increase in violent thoughts and behaviour (Pennings et al. 2002). Studies have shown that while both alcohol and cocaine will individually increase the likelihood of violent behaviour, the combination of the two may increase the severity of violence (Chermack and Blow 2002). It is therefore important when thinking about interventions to consider a coordinated approach to both substance misuse behaviours.

Twelve per cent of alcohol-attributable deaths globally are due to intentional injuries, including violence and suicide. There is a recognized link, albeit a complex one, between alcohol and violence perpetration and victimization (WHO 2006). Offenders report high levels of alcohol problems both using validated screening tools and by discursive self-report. Coulton and colleagues (2012), using the Alcohol Use Disorders Identification Test (AUDIT), found that 73 per cent of participants in prisons, custody suites, or probation offices in England had scores over 8 (indicating a hazardous drinking habit), and those individuals were more likely to have been involved violent offending than those with scores below 8; this finding was almost exactly mirrored in a Scottish prison study (MacAskill et al. 2011). In addition, 36 per cent of offenders in the Scottish prison had AUDIT scores in excess of 20, consistent with possible alcohol dependence. Many offenders associate their criminality with alcohol misuse, particularly young offenders and those who have committed a violent offence. Self-report data suggest that 50 per cent of all male offenders in Scotland were under the influence of alcohol at the time of their offence, rising to 77 per cent among young offenders aged 16–21 (McKinlay et al. 2009). Additionally, 63 per cent of victims of violent crime perceived the perpetrator to be drunk at the time of the offence (Scottish Government 2011). Offenders also associated drug taking with their criminality, usually in combination with alcohol (MacAskill et al. 2011; McKinlay et al. 2009). There is clearly a high level of unmet need within the offending population in relation to both alcohol and drug issues and, while it is possible that addressing these may help reduce recidivism, there is a wider public health and social need to tackle these issues.

Alcohol excess and misuse is also associated with victimization. Studies in healthcare settings demonstrate a clear association between injuries due to violence and alcohol consumption on the part of both perpetrator and victim (Scottish Emergency Department Alcohol Audit (SEDAA) Group 2006).

While it is understood those who misuse alcohol either chronically or by binge drinking have a higher risk of becoming both victims and perpetrators of violence, confounding factors often make it difficult to prove a direct causal link. Boden et al. (2012) tried to dissociate the link between alcohol and violence from other factors using a birth cohort studied to age 30, and concluded tentatively that, in their study carried out in New Zealand, persons aged 17–30 displaying five or more symptoms consistent with alcohol misuse or dependence were 1.91–3.58 times more likely to be involved in violent offending, to be victims of violence, or to be perpetrators of domestic violence. Indeed they suggest that alcohol misuse accounted for 5–10 per cent of violent offending in this group.

Alcohol misuse acts to increases the likelihood of violence in several ways. Intoxicated individuals have both reduced self-control and reduced awareness of risk, making them more likely to become both a victim and a perpetrator (Welte and Wieczorek 1998). Alcohol also leads to changes in impulse control and in some individuals will also increase aggressiveness (Gmel et al. 2006). Some other substances of abuse also have these effects. It would seem appropriate, therefore, that any individualized alcohol intervention seeking to reduce violence should attempt to address or raise awareness of these issues.

The Status of the Evidence

There is a need to tackle both alcohol misuse and substance misuse at population, community, and individual levels. Only by taking this public health approach will there be a change in how individuals and communities view their relationship with alcohol and drugs. Part of this is about changing social norms, and this is discussed in Chapter 33 of this volume.

There is a robust body of evidence on the efficacy of both individual interventions for alcohol in health settings and a wealth of research on 'community interventions' in drinking environments perhaps due to the very wide-reaching and burgeoning health consequences of alcohol misuse, and the resulting imperative to find effective ways to tackle the issue. We know that the majority of perpetrators and victims of violence are deprived young men (Houchin 2005; Leyland and Dundas 2010) and that for most drinking alcohol and the drinking environment is associated with their crime or injury (Goodall et al. 2008)—so it makes sense to try to regulate that environment. Some young men, for example in gangs, also use drinking as a way to prepare for violence because it lowers inhibitions.

The majority of individuals who misuse alcohol do so at a hazardous as opposed to a dependent level and brief advice and brief interventions are an effective and cost-effective way of addressing this level of drinking. Similarly, replacing glassware in bars with plastic or shatterproof glass will not reduce levels of drinking, but this measure effectively removes access to weapons and has been shown to reduce injury (Warburton and Shepherd 2000).

There is less evidence, although evidence is now emerging, for the efficacy of interventions for alcohol in the offender management sector (Newbury-Birch et al. 2009). Programmes for drug misuse including brief interventions are also well evaluated in the health sector but not in the criminal justice system. Longer, more intensive programmes for alcohol, alcohol and violence, and substance misuse that address more serious issues around dependence are effective in certain settings. What is less clear is whether interventions for alcohol and substance abuse can or will bring about a real reduction in levels of violence.

Brief Description of Intervention Procedures

Interventions in Drinking Environments

The alcohol industry in the United Kingdom has in recent years made improvements to the safety of drinking environments a priority. These improvements include measures such as training for bar staff in the identification of underage drinkers and intoxicated customers, use of closed-circuit television, and substitution of glass with plastic and shatterproof glassware. However, a recent Cochrane review (Ker and Chinnock 2008) found little good-quality evidence for the effectiveness of such interventions in drinking environments in reducing injury; few good randomized controlled trials exist, and, furthermore, compliance with interventions by bar staff was a significant issue.

It has also been argued that even if effective, these interventions would simply displace the problems associated with alcohol misuse, such as violence, to areas remote from the bars and clubs because they do nothing to address the fundamental issue of drinking to excess (Bellis and Hughes 2011). This may result in a more difficult issue for the police and emergency services in dealing with violence and its aftermath.

Individual Level Interventions

Alcohol misuse is a factor in many health issues and brief interventions (BIs) also known as Brief Motivational Interventions (BMIs) and, when directed towards drinking behaviour as Alcohol Brief Interventions (ABIs), have been commonplace in health settings for many years with a wealth of good-quality evidence on their efficacy and cost-effectiveness in different cultural settings (Babor and Higgins-Biddle 2001; Bien et al. 1993; WHO Brief Intervention Study Group 1996).

To be properly targeted BI should be delivered after screening and a variety of screening tools have been developed for use in different settings. The gold standard screening tool is the AUDIT, developed as part of the WHO brief intervention project. It consists of ten questions that categorize drinkers as non-hazardous, hazardous, harmful or possibly dependent. Individuals can then be allocated to a suitable intervention or treatment (Babor et al. 2001).

BI is a behaviour change style of counselling, developed to help change substance abuse behaviours but now used across a range of health behaviours. The intervention makes use of the Prochaska and DiClemente's Transtheoretical Model or Cycle of Change (Prochaska and DiClemente 1998). The Cycle of Change describes the five stages that individuals go through when making a change in their behaviour: pre-contemplation, contemplation, preparation, action, and maintenance. This model includes lapse and relapse both of which can occur during behaviour change. BI uses the results of screening to help give feedback to patients allowing them to understand the gap between their actual and ideal behaviour and aims to narrow that gap.

A BI can take several forms but one commonly used template is FRAMES (Miller and Sanchez 1993). Using the FRAMES approach, the counsellor gives feedback on the patient's level of drinking (Feedback); gives the patient the responsibility for making a change (Responsibility); gives advice (Advice); provides a range of options for change (Menu); expresses understanding of the patient's situation (Empathy); and encourages the patients to be optimistic about the possibility of change (Self-efficacy).

ABI is effective in reducing alcohol consumption among hazardous drinkers across a range of settings. In the United Kingdom facial injury disproportionately affects young men from deprived backgrounds and most injuries are sustained as a result of interpersonal violence while drinking. ABIs have been shown in several studies to help this cohort successfully reduce their alcohol intake; this effect is maintained at up to 1 year post intervention (Goodall et al. 2008; Smith et al. 2003).

ABIs are not particularly effective for those with alcohol dependence who require more intensive and individualized treatment programmes. However, they can be effective for those with high AUDIT scores whose pattern of alcohol consumption is intermittent heavy binge drinking and who do not display symptoms of dependence.

There is good evidence that BI following an injury will both decrease consumption and reduce the likelihood of a repeat injury (Gentilello et al. 1999). In the clinical setting alcohol screening and brief interventions are short, practical, and straightforward to deliver. With training, different members of the team (e.g. nursing staff) can provide these interventions very effectively.

Several authors have speculated that in some cases either the violent act, the injury, or the treatment required may make the individual more amenable to change (the Teachable Moment) or indeed may act as an intervention of sorts precipitating a change in behaviour. It has also been suggested that the screening process, during which patients may be asked detailed questions about their drinking, may also serve as an intervention by raising awareness (McCambridge and Day 2008).

While ABI seems to be effective in reducing drinking in the short-term, long-term effects of brief interventions are controversial. Some studies have shown little long-term benefit while others have shown a long lasting effect. In addition, little is known about the efficacy of such interventions in the criminal justice setting, although there is a body of evidence that confirms the need for alcohol interventions for offending populations and evidence is starting to emerge on their potential usefulness (Newbury-Birch et al. 2009).

Interventions that Address both Alcohol and Violence

There are few programmes that attempt to address both alcohol misuse and violence. One such programme is COVAID (Control of Violence for Angry Impulsive Drinkers). COVAID is a ten-session programme based on a cognitive behavioural model that aims to reduce the likelihood of alcohol related aggression and violence. It addresses both the emotions and behaviour associated with aggression and violence and some of the contextual factors such as the drinking environment and problem solving in the face of challenge. A recent randomized controlled trial of COVAID versus treatment as usual in a prison population showed a significant reduction in alcohol-related aggression scores in the COVAID group (Bowes et al. 2012). However, the trial was small and the potential of the intervention to actually affect alcohol related violence in the community is unclear. A single session version of

COVAID was developed for use in health settings and was very effective in helping patients to reduce their drinking but had no effect on alcohol-related aggression scores (Goodall et al. 2012).

Individual Level Interventions for Illicit Substance Abuse

The ASSIST (Alcohol, Smoking, Substance Involvement Screening Test) was developed by the WHO for use with a linked brief intervention strategy (Humeniuk et al. 2010). It was developed primarily to help those with substance abuse issues but recognizes that these do not always occur in isolation. The ASSIST screening and brief intervention identifies and concentrates on the primary substance of abuse and is most suitable for individuals who are not dependent on that substance. Like ABI the ASSIST BI is based on the FRAMES approach. A recent randomized controlled trial using the ASSIST BI for a variety of different substances showed a significant reduction in ASSIST scores at 3 months post intervention compared with controls (Humeniuk et al. 2012). The ASSIST BI can also be used with individuals who fall into the 'high-risk' category, for example those regularly injecting drugs, but as a means of encouraging them to seek further help rather than as a primary intervention. As with ABI there is little evidence of the efficacy of programmes such as the ASSIST BI in criminal justice settings or with offending populations, and their effect on actual levels of violence remains to be investigated.

Some longer programmes for substance abuse have been studied in criminal justice settings. The prison-based therapeutic community programme for female offenders in the United States (Sacks et al. 2012) showed significant reductions in substance abuse, exposure to trauma, and criminal activity in the year after release. This very intensive programme brought women with substance abuse issues together for several hours over five days of the week in a therapeutic community.

Alcohol Monitoring and its Potential Impact on Violence

Alcohol monitoring using transdermal technology is attracting considerable attention in the United Kingdom as a potential means to reduce violence through helping offenders to desist from drinking (Neville et al. 2013; Shaw et al. 2012). It has been widely used in the United States with individuals convicted of driving under the influence of alcohol. There is emerging evidence that supporting individuals to abstain from drinking may also reduce violence, specifically intimate partner violence (Kilmer et al. 2013).

Transportability of Programmes Nationally and Internationally

Policy level interventions for substance abuse have the potential to be implemented across high-, middle-, and low-income countries. There is evidence from a range of settings that they would impact positively on violence. However, they require a determined and coordinated approach and policy makers need to be willing to put the health and safety of the population above political and commercial concerns, as many of these measures are not popular with either the public or the alcohol industry.

Brief interventions for both alcohol and other substances were adopted by the WHO as an effective harm reduction strategy and have been widely used in many different settings and cultures worldwide. The ASSIST, for example, was trialled in Australia, Brazil, India, and the United States and found to be effective in all but the United States (WHO 2008). ABI was robustly trialled in Australia, Kenya, Mexico, Norway, United Kingdom, Russia, United States, and Zimbabwe and was effective across all these settings (WHO Brief Intervention Study Group 2006). Generally BIs are both effective and cost effective, they can be provided by a range of individuals (Oakey et al. 2008), and require only minimal training. Although they do not have a proven track record in reducing violence they do deal effectively with associated behaviours and in doing so may have some effect on the potential for injury.

Longer programmes such as COVAID and psychotherapy for alcohol and substance abuse are resource hungry, labour intensive, and need to be delivered by skilled personnel. This will inevitably limit their usefulness and scalability, particularly in low-income countries. Similarly, the use of transdermal alcohol monitoring to assist offenders and others in reducing their alcohol consumption is expensive in terms of the technology, personnel, and infrastructure required to provide 24/7 monitoring. It could be problematic to introduce such programmes in low-income countries where there may not be ready access to the Internet or mobile phone networks.

Finally, there may also be cultural issues around dealing with issues of substance abuse in certain countries, and policymakers and programme leaders would need to be sensitive to these.

Gaps in the Evidence

The efficacy of interventions for alcohol both at the policy and individual level is well researched and not in doubt. Similarly, several good and well-founded interventions address the abuse of other substances. The majority of individualized interventions for both alcohol and other substances of abuse have been tested in healthcare settings with very little evidence of efficacy in offending populations or in criminal justice settings. Although some studies in relation to alcohol are currently on-going in these settings in the United Kingdom, we cannot yet speculate as to the outcomes.

The majority of research on interventions for any substance of misuse focuses either on reduction in use of the substance or on a change in attitudes to violence or aggression as the primary outcome with very few showing a real reduction in levels of violence at either an individual or community level. While attributing a reduction in violence to any one factor is fraught with difficulty, in a well-designed and controlled study, using data from the criminal justice system would, in addition to the usual primary outcome measures, give those who seek to take interventions and scale them up some reassurance of a more rounded view of their efficacy.

Conclusions

Abuse of alcohol and other substances are behaviours which impact on both violence perpetration and victimization but the relationship between the substance misuse and violence is complex. This chapter has reviewed the evidence for interventions for both alcohol and other substances, and has found many well-researched interventions that are effective in reducing substance abusing behaviour. At the legislative level these interventions do seem to impact on levels of violence. What is less clear, however, is whether individual level interventions also have the potential to reduce or prevent violence. More work is needed, particularly in the criminal justice arena where successful interventions have the potential to reduce offending and recidivism and to impact significantly and in a positive way on society in general.

References

Anakwe, R. E., Aitken, S. A., Cowie, J. G., Middleton, S. D., and Court-Brown, C. M. (2011). The epidemiology of fractures of the hand and the influence of social deprivation. *Journal of Hand Surgery (European Volume)*, 36, 62–5.

Babor, T., and Higgins-Biddle, J. C. (2001). *Brief Interventions for Hazardous and Harmful Drinking. A Manual for Use in Primary Care.* Geneva: World Health Organization.

Bellis, M., and Hughes, K. (2011). Getting drunk safely? Night-life policy in the UK and its public health consequences. *Drug and Alcohol Review*, 30, 536–45.

Bien, T. H., Miller, W. R., and Tonigan, J. S. (1993). Brief interventions for alcohol problems: A review. *Addiction*, 88, 315–36.

Boden, J., Fergusson, D. M., and Horwood, L. J. (2012). Alcohol misuse and violence behavior: findings from a 30-year longitudinal study. *Drug and Alcohol Dependence*, 122, 135–41.

Bowes, N., McMurran, M., Williams, B., Siriol, D., and Zammit, I. (2012). Treating alcohol-related violence: intermediate outcomes in a feasibility study for a randomized controlled trial in prisons. *Criminal Justice and Behavior* 39, 333.

Chermack, S.T., and Blow, F. C. (2002). Violence among individuals in substance abuse treatment: the role of alcohol and cocaine consumption. *Drug and Alcohol Dependence*, 66, 29–37.

Conway, D. I., McMahon, A. D., and Graham, L. et al. (2010). The scar on the face of Scotland: deprivation and alcohol-related facial injuries in Scotland. *The Journal of Trauma, Injury Infection and Critical Care*, 68, 644–9.

Coulton, S., Newbury-Birch, D., and Cassidy, P. et al. (2012). Screening for alcohol use in criminal justice settings: an exploratory study. *Alcohol and Alcoholism*, 47, 423–7.

Degenhardt, L., and Hall, W. (2012). Extent of illicit drug use and dependence, and their contribution to the global burden of disease. *Lancet*, 379, 55–70.

Gentilello, L., Rivara, M., Donovan, F. P. et al. (1999). Alcohol interventions in a trauma center as a means of reducing the risk of injury recurrence. *Annals of Surgery* 230, 473–80.

Gmel, G., Bissery, A., and Gammeter, R. et al. (2006). Alcohol attributable injuries in admissions to a Swiss emergency room—an analysis of the link between volume of drinking, drinking patterns and pre attendance drinking. *Alcoholism, Clinical and Experimental Research*, 30, 501–9.

Goodall, C. A., Bowman, A., and Smith, I. et al. (2012). A randomized trial of brief intervention strategies in patients with alcohol-related facial trauma as a result of interpersonal violence. *Addiction Science and Clinical Practice*, 7, A66.

Goodall, C. A., Oakey, F., and Ayoub, A. F. et al. (2008). A prospective randomised controlled trial of nurse delivered brief interventions for alcohol misuse to hazardous drinkers with alcohol related facial trauma. *British Journal of Oral Maxillofacial Surgery*, 46, 96–101.

Hansel, B., Thomas, F., and Pannier, B. et al (2010). Relationship between alcohol intake, health and social status and cardiovascular risk factors in the Urban Paris-Ile-de-France cohort. Is the cardioprotective action of alcohol a myth? *European Journal of Clinical Nutrition*, 64, 561–8.

Houchin, R. (2005). *Social Exclusion and Imprisonment in Scotland. A Report.* Glasgow Caledonian University. Available at: http://www.scotpho.org.uk/downloads/SocialExclusionandImprisonmentinScotland.pdf [Accessed 1 August 2013].

Humeniuk, R. E., Babor, T., and Souza-Formigoni, M. L. et al. (2012). A randomized controlled trial of a brief intervention for illicit drugs linked to the Alcohol Smoking and substance Involvement Screening Test (ASSIST) in clients recruited from primary health-care settings in four countries. *Addiction*, 107, 957–66.

Humeniuk, R. E., Henry-Edwards, S., Ali R. L., Poznyak, V., and Monteiro M. (2010). *The ASSIST-linked Brief Intervention for Hazardous and Harmful Substance Use: Manual for Use in Primary Care.* Geneva: World Health Organization.

Ker, K., and Chinnock, P. (2008). Interventions in the alcohol server setting for preventing injuries. *Cochrane Database of Systematic Reviews*, Issue 3. Art. No.: CD005244.

Kilmer, B., Nicosia, N., Heaton, P., and Midgette, G. (2013). Efficacy of frequent monitoring with swift, certain, and modest sanctions for violations: insights from South Dakota's 24/7 Sobriety Project. *American Journal of Public Health*, 103, e37–43.

Leyland, A. H., and Dundas, R. (2010). The social patterning of deaths due to assault in Scotland, 1980-2005: population-based study. *Journal of Epidemiology and Community Health*, 64, 432–9.

MacAskill, S., Parkes, T., Brooks, O., Graham, L., McAuley, A., and Brown, A. (2011). Assessment of alcohol problems using AUDIT in a prison setting: More than an 'aye or no' question. *BMC Public Health*, 11, 865.

McCambridge, J., and Day, M. (2008). Randomized controlled trial of the effects of completing the Alcohol Use Disorders Identification Test questionnaire on self-reported hazardous drinking. *Addiction*. 103, 241–8.

McKinlay, W., Forsyth, A. J. M., and Khan, F. (2009). The McKinlay report: alcohol and violence among young male offenders in Scotland. *SPS Occasional Paper*, 1(9). Edinburgh: Scottish Prison Service.

Miller W. R., and Sanchez V. C. (1993). Motivating young adults for treatment and lifestyle change. In: G. Howard (ed.), *Issues in Alcohol Use and Misuse by Young Adults*. Notre Dame: University of Notre Dame Press, pp. 55–82.

Neville, F. G., Williams, D. J., Goodall, C. A., Murer, J., and Donnelly P. (2013). An experimental trial exploring the impact of continuous transdermal alcohol monitoring upon alcohol consumption in a cohort of male students. *PLoS ONE*, 8, e67386.

Newbury-Birch, D., Bland, M., and Cassidy, P. et al. (2009). Screening and brief interventions for hazardous and harmful alcohol use in probation services: a cluster randomised controlled trial protocol. *BMC Public Health*, 18, 418.

Scottish Emergency Department Alcohol Audit (SEDAA) Group. (2006). *Understanding Alcohol Misuse in Scotland: Harmful Drinking: One: The Size of the Problem.* Edinburgh: NHS Quality Improvement Scotland.

Oakey, F., Ayoub, A. F., and Goodall, C.A. et al (2008). Delivery of a brief motivational intervention to patients with alcohol-related facial injuries: role for a specialist nurse. *British Journal of Oral Maxillofacial Surgery*, 46, 102-6.

Pennings, E. J. M., Leccese, A. P., and Wolff, F. A. D. (2002). Effects of concurrent use of alcohol and cocaine. *Addiction*. 97, 773–83.

Prochaska, J. O., and DiClemente, C. C. (1998). Toward a comprehensive transtheoretical model of change. Stages of change and addictive behaviors. In: W. Miller and N. Heather (eds), *Treating Addictive Behaviors, 2nd edition*. New York: Plenum Press, pp. 3–25.

Sacks, J, Y, McKendrick, K., and Hamilton, Z. (2012). A randomized clinical trial of a therapeutic community treatment for female inmates: outcomes at 6 and 12 months after prison release. *Journal of Addictive Diseases* 31, 258–69.

Scottish Government (2011). *2010/11 Scottish Crime and Justice Survey: Main Findings*. Edinburgh: Scottish Government.

Shaw, D., McCluskey, K., Linden, W., and Goodall, C. A. (2012). Reducing the harmful effects of alcohol misuse: the ethics of sobriety testing in criminal justice. *Journal of Medical Ethics*, 38, 669–71.

Smith, A. J., Hodgson, R. J., Bridgeman, K., and Shepherd J. P. (2003). A randomized controlled trial of a brief intervention after alcohol-related facial injury. *Addiction*. 98, 43–52.

UNODC (2012). *World Drug Report*. New York: United Nations.

Warburton, A. L, and Shepherd, J. P. (2000). Effectiveness of toughened glassware in terms of reducing injury in bars: a randomised controlled trial. *Injury Prevention*, 6, 36–40.

Welte, J. W., and Wieczorek, W. F. (1998). Alcohol, intelligence and violent crime in young males. *Journal of Substance Abuse*, 10, 309–19.

WHO Brief Intervention Study Group (1996). A cross-national trial of brief interventions with heavy drinkers. *American Journal of Public Health*, 86, 948–55.

World Health Organization (2006). *WHO Facts on Alcohol and Violence. Youth Violence and Alcohol*. Geneva: World Health Organization.

World Health Organization (2008). *The Global Burden of Disease. 2004 Update*. Geneva: WHO.

World Health Organization (2008). The Effectiveness of a Brief Intervention for Illicit Drugs Linked to the Alcohol, Smoking and Substance Involvement Screening Test (ASSIST) in Primary Health Care Settings: A Technical Report of Phase III Findings of the WHO ASSIST Randomized Controlled Trial. Geneva: WHO.

World Health Organization (2010). *Global Strategy to Reduce the Harmful Use of Alcohol*. Geneva: WHO.

CHAPTER 32

Hospitals as a locus for violence intervention

Jonathan Purtle, Theodore J. Corbin,
Linda J. Rich, and John A. Rich

Introduction to Hospitals as a Locus for Violence Intervention

Non-sexual assault, hereafter referred to as 'violent injury', is a recurrent problem. It is estimated that up to 44 per cent of violently injured patients are violently reinjured within 5 years—20 per cent fatally (Goins et al. 1992; Kennedy et al. 1996; Morrissey and Byrd 1991; Reiner et al. 1990; Sims et al. 1989). Hospital-based violence intervention programmes (HVIPs) serve to interrupt cycles of violence.

We use 'HVIP' as an umbrella term to describe interventions which provide direct services to patients shortly after they have received hospital care for a violent injury. The primary aims of HVIPs are to prevent violent reinjury and retaliation. HVIPs vary in design, but typically involve a combination of brief intervention in the hospital, needs assessment, and intensive case management services. While not all HVIPs share a single theoretical framework or model of practice, they all operate from the assumption that violent injury is a chronic, recurrent problem and that hospitals are a promising locus for preventive intervention. Evidence of HVIP effectiveness is nascent, but methodologically rigorous evaluations have demonstrated their benefits across a range of outcomes that have translated into substantial cost savings for hospitals, healthcare systems, and society.

This chapter provides an overview of the HVIP model. The scope of the chapter is limited to HVIPs that provide direct services to victims of violence and does not include discussion about hospital-based programmes that do not provide direct services but work to prevent violence through information sharing with police—such as the Cardiff Model, which has demonstrated effectiveness (Alcohol Learning Center 2009).

Theoretical Overview

Violent Injury is a Recurrent Problem

Because most patients receive medical care for injuries only after an act of violence has occurred, hospitals may appear more appropriate settings for violence intervention than for violence prevention. The epidemiology of violence, however, indicates that violent injury is often not a one-time event. Many violently injured individuals are violently reinjured after they leave the hospital and some engage in retaliatory violence against those responsible for their injury (Kubrin and Weitzer 2003). HVIPs are grounded in the theory that violent injury is a recurrent problem and that reinjury and retaliation are preventable.

Estimates of violent reinjury vary dramatically, depending on study setting (e.g. urban or rural) and variation in study follow-up period, methods for assessing reinjury, and classifying what constitutes the initial injury. Despite these methodological issues, the extant research on hospital recidivism for violent injury allows some key findings to emerge. Rates of reinjury appear to be highest in urban areas. In U.S. cities, for example, studies suggest that the 5-year reinjury rate is between 33 per cent and 45 per cent (Goins et al. 1992; Kennedy et al. 1996; Morrissey and Byrd 1991). One study found the 5-year mortality rate to be 20 per cent (Sims et al. 1989). The risk of violent reinjury also appears to be highest when a patient first leaves the hospital and then attenuates over time. A study of violent injury among the entire New Zealand population found that 70 per cent of violent reinjuries that occurred within a year of the initial injury took place within 30 days of hospital discharge (Dowd et al. 1996).

By recognizing the recurrent nature of violent injury and risk of retaliatory violence, HVIPs can simultaneously span the domains of primary, secondary, and tertiary prevention. By helping secure follow-up medical care and mental health services, HVIPs are tertiary prevention for the physical and psychological sequelae of violent injury. Through the provision of needs assessments and intensive case management services which positively alter participants' risk profiles, HVIPs are secondary prevention for violent reinjury. By applying de-escalation and mediation techniques, HVIPs are primary prevention for retaliatory violence against individual(s) responsible for the initial injury.

Intervention at a Teachable Moment

'It [violent injury] was a wakeup call for me' (Liebschutz et al. 2010, p. 1376). This statement—provided by a young, violently injured man in a U.S. city—epitomizes the theory of the 'teachable moment' in HVIP practice. Teachable moments are instances when individuals are particularly responsive to behavioural change interventions (Cunningham et al. 2009). The effectiveness of interventions in healthcare settings (such as those aimed at reducing alcohol and tobacco use) provides empirical support for the teachable moment, and research suggests that it is applicable to violence prevention activities (Johnson et al. 2007). HVIPs apply the theory of the teachable moment to engage violently injured individuals in interventions to prevent reinjury and retaliation.

As the quotation from Liebschutz et al. illustrates, the experience of surviving a violent injury often causes one to evaluate the circumstances that led to one's injury. As the possible consequences of violence—such as disability and death—become more salient after violent injury, individuals may begin to think about what they can do to stay safe in the future. Such thoughts may include relocating to safer communities, ceasing involvement with antisocial peers or gangs, or where appropriate, moving away from involvement in the illicit economy. These changes, however, may be difficult to achieve in the absence of alternatives for social support and economic self-sufficiency. HVIPs supplement violently injured patients' desires to stay safe and alter their life course trajectory with concrete resources.

Intervention at a Reachable Moment

Unfortunately, the communities with the highest incidence of violent injury are often the most isolated from mainstream institutions of comprehensive healthcare, quality education, and sustainable employment. As a result, many of the systems and services capable of reducing risk for violent reinjury do not reach the communities that need them the most. Violent injury represents a 'reachable moment' when individuals from isolated, violent, communities are brought into contact with hospitals—institutions where a variety of resources are often concentrated (Holdsworth et al. 2012). HVIPs harness the power of the reachable moment by engaging patients from isolated communities and connecting them with systems and services, such as supportive housing, job training, and educational assistance, that help prevent reinjury by reducing risk factors and promoting protective factors.

Violent Injury is a Traumatic Experience

Many individuals experience psychological reactions from violent injury that persist long after they leave the hospital (Kilpatrick and Acierno 2003). Symptoms of posttraumatic stress, including nightmares, difficulties sleeping, and hypervigilance, may lead violently injured individuals to seek weapons or turn to using alcohol or illicit substances to restore feelings of safety. Paradoxically, these actions, which may seem logical to victims in the context of their neighbourhoods, may increase their risk for reinjury (Rich 2009; Rich and Grey 2005). Based on this understanding, many HVIPs actively address the mental health consequences of violent injury guided by the belief that behavioural health interventions are critical to preventing reinjury and retaliation.

Surveys in healthcare settings have demonstrated the traumatic effects of violent injury. A study of men hospitalized for violent injury found that 27 per cent had possible post-traumatic stress disorder (PTSD) at 3-month follow-up, and 18 per cent at 1-year follow-up (Jaycox et al. 2004). A study of adults seeking care for violent injury at a public, urban hospital found that 41 per cent met the criteria for acute stress disorder within 1 month of the injury (Greenspan and Kellermann 2002). A cross-sectional study of clients participating in a Philadelphia HVIP found that 75 per cent met the diagnostic criteria for PTSD 6 weeks after their injury (Corbin et al. 2013).

Despite the symptoms of posttraumatic stress that many patients experience after violent injury, the majority do not seek or obtain mental health services (Kilpatrick and Acierno 2003; New and Berliner 2000). The under-utilization of these services results from perceived stigma of mental illness, distrust of mental health professionals, and lack of knowledge about and logistical challenges to accessing care (Kelly et al. 2010; Liebschutz et al. 2010). Many HVIPs employ trauma-informed, culturally competent workers who break down these barriers. HVIPs provide patients with psychoeducation about the possible effects of traumatic stress, help them develop safe coping strategies, and connect them to mental health services.

Status of Evidence

HVIPs have demonstrated effectiveness across a range of outcomes in randomized controlled trials (Aboutanos et al. 2011; Cheng et al. 2008b; Cooper et al. 2006; Zun et al. 2006). The results from HVIPs conducting quasi-experimental evaluations, such as retrospective cohort designs and hospital chart reviews, also suggest that HVIPs prevent hospital recidivism for violent injury and produce positive outcomes (Becker et al. 2004; Gomez et al. 2012; Shibru et al. 2007; Smith et al. 2013b). Despite this body of research, a systematic review of HVIP outcome evaluations concluded that, while HVIPs represent a promising strategy for violence prevention, more randomized controlled trials were needed before they could be established as an 'evidence-based practice' (Snider and Lee 2009). The HVIP model has yet to reach the apex of the hierarchy of evidence in the health sciences, but questions regarding HVIP effectiveness must be considered within the context of *why* HVIPs have been implemented and *which* outcomes have been considered indicators of programme success.

Historically, HVIPs have not been implemented as research projects in the United States. Rather HVIPs have been implemented as service projects to address unmet, and urgent, community needs. As a result, outcomes research has been a secondary priority to that of providing direct services to victims of violence. The results of non-experimental evaluations and narrative accounts of programme success have been sufficient for many HVIPs to sustain funding and remain in operation. Only recently, however, have well-established HVIPs secured funding to conduct methodologically rigorous outcome evaluations. In Canada, conversely, HVIPs are being developed within a structured research paradigm, progressing sequentially through the phases of formative research and small-scale feasibility studies prior to full-scale HVIP implementation (Snider and Nathens 2012; Snider et al. 2010).

Unlike pharmaceutical treatments or medical procedures, for which target outcomes are clearly defined, there is substantial diversity in the types of outcomes which are considered indicators of HVIPs success. While preventing violent reinjury and retaliation are desired outcomes for all HVIPs, these programmes also produce other tangible benefits for clients, connecting them to housing, education, and legal services; providing psychoeducation, identifying mental health needs, and facilitating referrals to treatment; and offering social support during difficult transition periods. HVIP staff can provide empirical accounts of how these outcomes have saved the lives of HVIP clients and the lives of those against whom they would have otherwise retaliated. To date, however, few of these outcomes have been systematically captured in a way that allows for causal inference to be established. At present, the 'practice-based evidence' supporting the effectiveness of the HVIP model outweighs the research which supports it as an 'evidence-based practice'.

Intervention Procedures

HVIPs vary in the specifics of their design and scope, but typically include a combination of brief intervention soon after the injury occurs (often in the hospital), psychosocial needs assessment, and intensive community-based case management services. HVIPs work to identify and reduce risk factors, promote protective factors, and prevent violent reinjury, retaliation, and the mental health sequelae of violent injury. HVIPs are typically 'hospital-based' and operate out of emergency departments or trauma centres. They are sometimes also 'hospital-affiliated', operating in the community outside the organizational structure of the hospital and receiving referrals from departments that identify and refer patients.

HVIP services are provided by intervention specialists. Intervention specialists are highly trained professionals from the community who provide brief crisis intervention, linkages to community-based services, mentoring, home visits, follow-up assistance, and long-term case management. Some intervention specialists have been formally trained as social workers or community health workers, while others are paraprofessionals from the community. Intervention specialists are culturally competent; knowledgeable about the social norms and dynamics around violence in the communities where they work; have 'street credibility' and, often, shared knowledge of the norms of the urban environment with respect to violence (Anderson 2000). This skill set enables intervention specialists to establish rapport with and gain the trust of HVIP clients. Intervention specialists generally carry caseloads of 14–20 clients who receive services for an average of 6–12 months. Intervention specialists typically report to a supervisor with masters or doctoral level training in social work, clinical psychology/psychiatry, emergency medicine, or trauma surgery.

After enrolling the client in the programme, intervention specialists work with clients and their families to develop a discharge plan and to ensure that their immediate safety needs are met. Formal assessments are conducted to identify client needs, establish goals, and develop a service plan that is amended as the client progresses. Intensive case management is provided to connect clients with needed services. These services may include, but are not limited to, follow-up medical care, substance abuse treatment, mental health treatment for injury-related PTSD, academic support, job training, vocational programmes, and housing assistance. Intervention specialists also work with clients to identify their inherent skills, strengths, and interests and explore how these assets might best serve them in a career. Intervention specialists regularly conduct home visits and take clients to appointments.

As an example of HVIP intervention procedures, Figure 32.1 depicts the process and components of Healing Hurt People (HHP). HHP is an HVIP operating out of paediatric and adult hospitals in Philadelphia, Pennsylvania. After a patient is treated for violent injury and is medically cleared, hospital staff activates a referral to HHP. During his or her first interaction with the potential client, the intervention specialist introduces the programme, assesses the patient's immediate safety needs, and provides psychoeducation about the potential effects of traumatic stress (Corbin et al. 2011).

HHP comprises five major programmatic components, each of which is supported by evidence of effectiveness (Corbin et al. 2011). Assessment is first conducted to evaluate the client's short-term risks for reinjury and retaliation, history of traumatic experiences, and medical/psychosocial needs. Intensive case management and navigation services are then provided to ensure that the needs identified through assessment are met. Throughout this process, the intervention specialist serves as a mentor and helps the client develop effective coping strategies, engage in safe behaviours, and resist community pressure to retaliate. HHP clients also participate in trauma-informed psychoeducation groups. The groups provide clients with a safe environment, cognitive framework, and common vocabulary that promotes healing, growth, and change. At the paediatric hospital, youth with symptoms of PTSD are offered the Child and Family Traumatic Stress Intervention (CFTSI). CFTSI is an evidence-based, trauma-specific, caregiver–child psychotherapy intervention that can prevent development of chronic PTSD if provided within 30 days of the traumatic event (e.g. violent injury; Berkowitz et al. 2011). While not a direct service to clients, case review is held on a weekly basis. During case review, a multidisciplinary group meets to discuss challenges that clients and intervention specialists are facing, formulate solutions, and identify policy-level barriers to effectively serving victims of violence.

Research Outcomes

HVIPs have demonstrated promising results in methodologically rigorous evaluations across the domains of preventing violent reinjury and involvement with the criminal justice system, reducing risk factors, and cultivating protective factors. In a randomized controlled study, an HVIP serving violently injured youth aged 10–15 years in Baltimore, Maryland, was found to significantly reduce misdemeanour offending behaviour, decrease feelings of aggression, and improve self-efficacy at 6-month follow-up (Cheng et al. 2008a). A randomized evaluation found that youth and young adults participating in a Chicago, Illinois, HVIP were significantly less likely to be violently reinjured as measured by self-report (Zun et al. 2006). A randomized evaluation of an HVIP in Richmond, Virginia, found that those in the intervention group had better rates of hospital and community service utilization and lower rates of drug and alcohol use compared to those in the control group at 6-week and 6-month follow-up (Aboutanos et al. 2011). Differences in rates of reinjury were not observed. Caught in the Crossfire, an HVIP in Oakland, California, employed a retrospective cohort design and observed significant reductions in involvement with the criminal justice system (Shibru et al. 2007). These findings were consistent with an earlier evaluation of the HVIP (Becker et al. 2004). Neither evaluation, however, demonstrated significant reductions in reinjury. One randomized evaluation of an HVIP serving youth aged 12–17 years found that the programme had no statistically significant effects on reinjury rates (Cheng et al. 2008b).

A randomized evaluation of the Violence Intervention Program, an HVIP serving adult victims of violence in Baltimore,

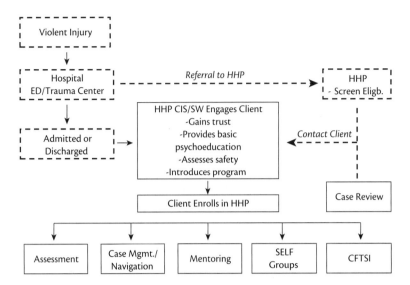

Fig. 32.1 The 'Healing Hurt People' HVIP model in Philadelphia, PA.

Maryland, demonstrated promising results which translated into substantial cost savings (Cooper et al. 2006). While differences in the number of arrests were not observed between the control and intervention groups, subjects in the intervention group were half as likely to be convicted of any crime and four times less likely to be convicted of a violent crime—differences that translated into approximately US$1.25 million in savings from prevented incarceration costs. The same evaluation found that the intervention group had a lower hospital recidivism rate (5 per cent vs. 26 per cent), saving an estimated US$598,000 in healthcare costs, and a higher employment rate (85 per cent vs. 20 per cent) than the control group.

Retrospective hospital chart reviews also provide evidence of positive HVIP outcomes. The Wraparound Project, an HVIP in San Francisco, California, found that the 6-year violent reinjury rate among HVIP clients was 4.5 per cent, compared to 16 per cent for a historical control group of violently injured patients who were treated at the same hospital (Smith et al. 2013b). Prescription for Hope, an HVIP in Indianapolis, Indiana, found that the 1-year reinjury rate for HVIP clients was 0 per cent compared to 8.7 per cent for a control group of violently injured patients (Gomez et al. 2012).

Transportability of Programmes

The HVIP model took root in the United States and has only recently been adopted internationally. Nationally, HVIPs have demonstrated transportability between regions of the United States with different sociodemographic profiles, norms, and dynamics around violence (e.g. presence vs. absence of gang culture) (Smith et al. 2013a). More than 20 HVIPs currently operate in the United States (National Network of Hospital-based Violence Intervention Programs 2013). The widespread implementation of HVIPs has highlighted features which are essential for successful transportability.

Violent injury is a potentially traumatic experience regardless of the country or region where it occurs. HVIP staff should be familiar with symptoms of posttraumatic stress and how these symptoms might influence clients' needs and affect behaviour. It is also imperative that HVIP staff be culturally competent. Violent injury often disproportionately affects men and boys, racial and ethnic minorities, and individuals with lower socioeconomic status. HVIP staff should have an understanding of how issues of gender, race, ethnicity, and class intersect to shape clients' perceptions of intervention and trajectories of recovery. HVIP staff should also be knowledgeable about the norms and dynamics of violence in the communities they serve. Some HVIPs exclusively hire members of the local community to serve as intervention specialists. Many violently injured individuals have extreme distrust in the mainstream institutions which have failed them, including healthcare, and may be resistant to intervention (Schwartz et al. 2010). HVIP staff must be aware of this possibility and approach clients in a sensitive manner.

It is also essential that HVIPs obtain 'buy-in' from the hospitals with which they are affiliated. Physicians, nurses, and other hospital staff not directly involved with the HVIP are critical to identifying victims of violence, providing referrals, and successfully implementing the programme. Buy-in from hospital administrators is aided by the fact that HVIPs are often implemented by paraprofessionals from the community and are thus a relatively low cost intervention. Using local paraprofessionals, and not relying on high cost and highly trained professionals, also supports programme transportability to setting where resources are limited.

Gaps in Evidence

Gaps in knowledge include if, when, how, and for whom HVIPs work. Some of these knowledge gaps are tied to methodological issues that are being addressed. One issue stems from the fact that HVIPs differ in their design and implementation procedures. With support from the United States Department of Justice, the National Network of HVIP (NNHVIP) has developed materials to standardize HVIP practice, such as a manual describing how to establish a programme (Karraker et al. 2011). Fidelity measures and adherence scales, however, are only now being developed (Smith et al. 2013a). Such instruments are important to building the HVIP evidence base because they will help ensure that HVIPs are implemented consistently and because they will promote internal validity in multisite evaluations.

Evaluations of HVIPs have also not been conducted uniformly. There is substantial variability in the outcomes assessed, assessment instruments used, data collection procedures employed, follow-up periods over which outcomes are observed, and population characteristics between studies. In the United States, NNHVIP is currently working to collect uniform data from different HVIPs and to prospectively track outcomes. More consistent data collection and evaluation design will also eventually permit a meta-analysis that would allow the HVIP model to advance on the hierarchy of evidence.

Given the sample sizes of HVIP evaluations most have not had the statistical power needed to detect all outcomes of interest or to identify variables which mediate and moderate programme outcomes. The individual-level characteristics which predict programme outcomes remain elusive. As the demand for HVIP services often exceeds programme capacity, such information would be valuable in providing an empirical basis for establishing HVIP eligibility criteria based on a risk profile. Lastly, the long-term benefits of HVIPs are unknown. HVIPs are designed to reach victims of violence at a critical point in their lives and provide them with social, emotional, and material resources that are capable of altering their life course trajectories. Controlled evaluations of HVIPs have not had follow-up periods exceeding 18 months.

Conclusions

Medical care provided in trauma centres and emergency departments has become effective in addressing the physical consequences of violent injury. Mortality has been reduced through the translation of biomedical research into practice and policies which codify evidence-based practices as standards of medical care. Similarly to the way that biomedical research has informed standards of medical care to treat the physical consequences of violent injury, public health research on violence can be integrated into the continuum of care for the violently injured patient to prevent violence and promote psychological recovery. HVIPs serve to meet this need.

References

Aboutanos, M. B., Jordan, A., and Cohen, R., et al. (2011). Brief interventions with community case management services are effective for high-risk trauma patients. *Journal of Trauma*, 71, 228–37.

Alcohol Learning Center (Public Health England). (2009). *The Cardiff Model—Effective NHS Contributions to Violence Prevention*. United Kingdom: Cardiff University.

Anderson, E. (2000). *Code of the Street: Decency, Violence, and the Moral Life of the Inner City*. New York: WW Norton.

Becker, M. G., Hall, J. S., Ursic, C. M., Jain, S., and Calhoun, D. (2004). Caught in the crossfire: the effects of a peer-based intervention program for violently injured youth. *Journal of Adolescent Health*, 34, 177–83.

Berkowitz, S. J., Stover, C. S., and Marans, S. R. (2011). The Child and Family Traumatic Stress Intervention: secondary prevention for youth at risk of developing PTSD. *Journal of Child Psychology and Psychiatry*, 52, 676–85.

Cheng, T. L., Haynie, D., Brenner, R., Wright, J. L., Chung, S. E., and Simons-Morton, B. (2008a). Effectiveness of a mentor-implemented, violence prevention intervention for assault-injured youths presenting to the emergency department: results of a randomized trial. *Pediatrics*, 122, 938–46.

Cheng, T. L., Wright, J. L., Markakis, D., Copeland-Linder, N., and Menvielle, E. (2008b). Randomized trial of a case management program for assault-injured youth: impact on service utilization and risk for reinjury. *Pediatric Emergency Care*, 24, 130–6.

Cooper, C., Eslinger, D. M., and Stolley, P. D. (2006). Hospital-based violence intervention programs work. *Journal of Trauma*, 61, 534–40.

Corbin, T. J., Purtle, J., and Rich, L., et al. (2013). The prevalence of trauma and childhood adversity in an urban, hospital-based violence intervention program. *Journal of Health Care for the Poor and Underserved*, 24, 1021–30.

Corbin, T. J., Rich, J. A., Bloom, S. L., Delgado, D., Rich, L. J., and Wilson, A. S. (2011). Developing a trauma-informed, emergency department-based intervention for victims of urban violence. *Journal of Trauma & Dissociation*, 12, 510–25.

Cunningham, R., Knox, L., and Fein, J., et al. (2009). Before and after the trauma bay: the prevention of violent injury among youth. *Annals of Emergency Medicine*, 53, 490–500.

Dowd, M. D., Langley, J., Koepsell, T., Soderberg, R., and Rivara, F. P. (1996). Hospitalizations for injury in New Zealand: prior injury as a risk factor for assaultive injury. *American Journal of Public Health*, 86, 929–34.

Goins, W. A., Thompson, J., and Simpkins, C. (1992). Recurrent intentional injury. *Journal of the National Medical Association*, 84, 431–5.

Gomez, G., Simons, C., and St. John, W., et al. (2012). Project Prescription for Hope (RxH): trauma surgeons and community aligned to reduce injury recidivism caused by violence. *American Surgeon*, 78, 1000–4.

Greenspan, A. I., and Kellermann, A. L. (2002). Physical and psychological outcomes 8 months after serious gunshot injury. *Journal of Trauma*, 53, 709–16.

Holdsworth, G., Criddle, J., Mohiddin, A., Polling, K., and Strelitz, J. (2012). Maximizing the role of emergency departments in the prevention of violence: developing an approach in South London. *Public Health*, 126, 394–6.

Jaycox, L. H., Marshall, G. N., and Schell, T. (2004). Use of mental health services by men injured through community violence. *Psychiatric Services (Washington, D.C.)*, 55, 415–20.

Johnson, S. B., Bradshaw, C. P., Wright, J. L., Haynie, D. L., Simons-Morton, B. G., and Cheng, T. L. (2007). Characterizing the teachable moment: is an emergency department visit a teachable moment for intervention among assault-injured youth and their parents? *Pediatric Emergency Care*, 23, 553–9.

Karraker, N., Cunningham, R., Becker, M., Fein, J., and Knox, L. (2011). *Violence is Preventable: A Best Practices Guide for Launching & Sustaining a Hospital-based Program to Break the Cycle of Violence*. Washington, D.C.: Office for Victims of Crime, U.S. Department of Justice, Office of Justice Programs.

Kelly, V. G., Merrill, G. S., Shumway, M., Alvidrez, J., and Boccellari, A. (2010). Outreach, engagement, and practical assistance: essential aspects of PTSD care for urban victims of violent crime. *Trauma, Violence & Abuse*, 11, 144–56.

Kennedy, F., Brown, J. R., Brown, K. A., and Fleming, A. W. (1996). Geographic and temporal patterns of recurrent intentional injury in south-central Los Angeles. *Journal of the National Medical Association*, 88, 570–2.

Kilpatrick, D. G., and Acierno, R. (2003). Mental health needs of crime victims: epidemiology and outcomes. *Journal of Traumatic Stress*, 16, 119–32.

Kubrin, C. E., and Weitzer, R. (2003). Retaliatory homicide: concentrated disadvantage and neighborhood culture. *Social Problems*, 50, 157–80.

Liebschutz, J., Schwartz, S., and Hoyte, J., et al. (2010). A chasm between injury and care: experiences of black male victims of violence. *Journal of Trauma*, 69, 1372–8.

Morrissey, T. B., and Byrd, C. R. (1991). The incidence of recurrent penetrating trauma in an urban trauma center. *Journal of Trauma*, 31, 1536–8.

National Network of Hospital-based Violence Intervention Programs. (2013). Available at: http://nnhvip.org/. [Accessed 18 November 2013].

New, M., and Berliner, L. (2000). Mental health service utilization by victims of crime. *Journal of Traumatic Stress*, 13, 693–707.

Reiner, D. S., Pastena, J. A., Swan, K. G., Lindenthal, J. J., and Tischler, C. D. (1990). Trauma recidivism. *American Surgeon*, 56, 556–60.

Rich, J. A. (2009). *Wrong Place, Wrong Time*. Baltimore: Johns Hopkins University Press.

Rich, J. A., and Grey, C. M. (2005). Pathways to recurrent trauma among young Black men: traumatic stress, substance use, and the 'code of the street'. *American Journal of Public Health*, 95, 816–24.

Schwartz, S., Hoyte, J., James, T., Conoscenti, L., Johnson, R. M., and Liebschutz, J. (2010). Challenges to engaging black male victims of community violence in healthcare research: lessons learned from two studies. *Psychological Trauma: Theory, Research, Practice and Policy*, 2, 54–62.

Shibru, D., Zahnd, E., Becker, M., Bekaert, N., Calhoun, D., and Victorino, G. P. (2007). Benefits of a hospital-based peer intervention program for violently injured youth. *Journal of the American College of Surgeons*, 205, 684–9.

Sims, D. W., Bivins, B. A., Obeid, F. N., Horst, H. M., Sorensen, V. J., and Fath, J. J. (1989). Urban trauma: a chronic recurrent disease. *Journal of Trauma*, 29, 940–7.

Smith, R., Dobbins, S., Evans, A., Balhorta, K., and Dicker, R. A. (2013b). Hospital-based violence intervention: risk reduction resources that are essential for success. *Journal of Trauma and Acute Care Surgery*, 74, 976–82.

Smith, R., Evans, A., Adams, C., Cocanour, C., and Dicker, R. (2013a). Passing the torch: evaluating exportability of a violence intervention program. *American Journal of Surgery*, 206, 223–8.

Snider, C. E., Kirst, M., Abubakar, S., Ahmad, F., and Nathens, A. B. (2010). Community-based participatory research: development of an emergency department-based youth violence intervention using concept mapping. *Academic Emergency Medicine* ,17, 877–85.

Snider, C., and Lee, J. (2009). Youth violence secondary prevention initiatives in emergency departments: a systematic review. *Canadian Journal of Emergency Medical Care*, 11, 161–8.

Snider, C., and Nathens, A. (2012). Hospital referral to a community programme for youth injured by violence: a feasibility study. *Injury Prevention*, 18, A63.

Zun, L. S., Downey, L., and Rosen, J. (2006). The effectiveness of an ED-based violence prevention program. *American Journal of Emergency Medicine*, 24, 8–13.

CHAPTER 33

Preventing violence through changing social norms

Fergus G. Neville

Theoretical Overview of Preventing Violence through Changing Social Norms

Whilst some attempts to tackle violence at an individual level have been effective (e.g. anger management, partner communication, and parenting skills), they do not address the broader social context in which violence is rooted and perpetuated (Berkowitz 2004). Social norms interventions represent a strategy for violence prevention at a social level. Interventions at the psychological level of groups are appropriate in several ways. For instance, 'interpersonal' violence perpetration and victimization are often framed by collective identities, even if an altercation only physically involves two people. Social norms are central to the way in which these collective memberships shape behaviour, and thus represent a potential opportunity for violence prevention. This chapter will not attempt to catalogue all violence prevention programmes which make use of social norms. Rather, the purpose will be to discuss initiatives which draw out key themes from which we can infer best practice. Before coming to these examples, it is necessary to first outline what social norms actually are, and why they are relevant to behaviour change, particularly with regards to violence prevention.

What are Social Norms?

Social influence research shows that people's behaviour is not determined simply by what they think, but by what they think other people like them think. In more technical terms, behaviour can be driven by the perceived social norms of fellow group members (Elcheroth et al. 2011; Smith and Louis 2009; Turner 1991). Although various definitions of social norms exist within the academic literature, there is general agreement that they refer to shared beliefs within a social unit about the appropriate ways to think, feel, and behave in a given context (Chekroun 2008; Turner 1991).

Injunctive and Descriptive Norms

Cialdini and colleagues (1990) further argue that there are two types of norms: injunctive norms refer to what members of a social unit ought (and ought not) to do, whilst descriptive norms refer to how most of them actually behave. Injunctive and descriptive norms can differ from one another. For example, whilst donating blood is generally seen as something one ought to do (an injunctive norm), regrettably few people actually do it (a descriptive norm). The distinction between these is of relevance to the design of social norm interventions. If a violence intervention only presents a group's descriptive norms (e.g. sexual assault statistics) then this may unintentionally increase the prevalence of the negative behaviour. This is because group members who did not originally act this way may begin to do so in an attempt to bring their own behaviour into line with the descriptive norm (Paul and Gray 2011). Misalignment of descriptive and injunctive norms may therefore explain the mixed efficacy of social norm campaigns.

Interventions that neglect social norms are also problematic. For example, Australian researchers demonstrated that a university 'sun-smart' drive could actually decrease sunscreen use if it failed to provide information regarding normative student behaviour (Smith and Louis 2009). This was because without normative information, students inferred from the need for a campaign that other students did not engage in, or approve of, sun protection—and they therefore used sun screen less, in order to fit in with their perceptions of the social norm. When participants were instead informed that the majority of students approved of sun protection behaviour, there was an increase in intended sunscreen use. The fact that the identity of the referent group in the second experimental condition was 'ingroup'—fellow students—is critical.

Social Norms and Social Identities

Social norms are important, because they are the means by which social categories can influence their members' behaviour (Cialdini et al. 1990). Social identity research has shown that people are in possession of multiple identities—at both personal and group levels of self—which become salient in different social contexts (Reicher et al. 2010). People inside one's social group become ingroup members, and those outside become outgroup. As one defines or 'self-categorizes' oneself in terms of different identities, one self-stereotypes and adopts the norms and behaviours associated with that relevant identity. For instance, in different situations I might think of myself as an academic, a father, or a football supporter. As each identity becomes more salient to me in different social contexts, my behaviour will be shaped by the social norms congruent with the relevant identity.

This body of work has contributed to social norm research by signifying that what is influential is not what just anybody thinks, but what others within one's salient social category thinks. This is because the normative position of fellow group members is recognized as subjectively valid (Duck et al. 1999; Turner 1991). This has particular practical relevance, because normative messages in public health interventions are typically from the perspective of outgroups (e.g. adults or health professionals), and not from salient and meaningful referent ingroups (Smith and Louis 2009; World Health Organization (WHO) 2009).

The recognition that groups have the ability to positively influence their members is a significant departure from classic group psychology, which viewed groups as inherently deleterious (e.g. Zimbardo 1969). Instead of being regarded as a threat, social group membership should instead be seen as an opportunity for positive social influence through social norms. This works both ways of course: social norms can drive negative behaviours as well as positive ones. Social groups should therefore be seen as neither intrinsically positive nor negative. The point is to be aware of the powerful role that social norms play in shaping behaviour, and to design violence prevention initiatives that can harness this power.

Norm Enforcement

Social groups are able to influence behaviour because there is pressure to conform to a social norm which is a criterion of group membership. Individuals can be included or excluded from a social category based upon the fit of their behaviour relative to the norms of the group (Turner et al. 1987). Social pressure to conform may also be exerted through ingroup members communicating their disapproval of counter-normative actions, and via a fear of disapproval (and desire for approval) by ingroup members (Chekroun 2008). Moreover, because social norms operate as a function of internalized social identities, group members' behaviour can continue to be shaped by group norms when they are alone and not under observation (Hogg and Vaughan 2008).

In practical terms, this suggests a key and efficacious role for ingroup members in 'self-policing' the behaviour of fellow category members. This prospect is exemplified by an anecdote from an ethnographic study of football supporters (Stott et al. 2001). When Scotland fans—who pride themselves upon being non-violent and convivial—witnessed one of their own assault a Tunisian supporter during the 1998 World Cup in France, they violently attacked the Scottish perpetrator and shunned him for the remainder of the tournament. Not only did this action prevent an escalation of intergroup violence, it reinforced the norm amongst Scottish fans that violence against supporters of other teams was socially unacceptable. Whilst violent intervention is hardly an ideal model of violence prevention, the example does illustrate the significant role that ingroup members play in regulating one another's behaviour.

The Status of the Evidence

There is a growing body of evidence which demonstrates that carefully designed social norm interventions can successfully reduce problematic social behaviours, and encourage desirable ones. However, at present social norm interventions with a view to violence prevention remain relatively under-evaluated. What little work has been done has generally focused upon gender violence interventions in universities. This is in large part due to ease of access to participants, particularly when the interventions have been designed by academics. These interventions can function as a useful starting point in the development of a roadmap for constructing thoroughly-evaluated social norms interventions into a variety of forms of violence.

Brief Description of Intervention Procedures

Gender and Sexual Violence

Gender and sexual violence social norm interventions are typically premised upon the influence of (mis)perception of peer attitudes and behaviours. Although the majority of men may disapprove of violence against women, this view is often not expressed if men do not gauge their peers as sharing this view (Fabiano et al. 2003). This can create a cognitive error such that lack of expressed peer disapproval is taken by perpetrators as tacit approval of their behaviour—by fellow ingroup members no less—thereby perpetuating future abuse (Baer et al. 1991). Indeed, in community samples of American men, perpetrators of gender violence typically overestimate both peers' support for forced sex (Abbey et al. 2007) and the prevalence of gender violence amongst other males (Neighbors et al. 2010), and individuals who perceive their peers to find sexual aggression acceptable also score highly on measures of sexual aggression (Loh et al. 2005). As Tharp and colleagues (2013) note, peer groups which contain at least one member who engages in sexual violence but is not challenged can lead to a group norm which supports and normalizes violent sexual behaviour.

Bohner and colleagues (2006) used an experimental paradigm to provide further evidence of the importance of perceived social norms in this context. Male university students were presented with false feedback indicating that their male peers had either very high or low rape myth acceptance. Participants in the first condition subsequently reported a significantly greater willingness to rape than participants in the second. This simple study illustrates the critical role that men who object to gender violence have to play in its prevention, through expression of their collective opposition and assertion that the behaviour is counter-normative.

This is because, whilst a perceived group norm supportive of gender violence can inhibit intervention, a belief that fellow group members share one's willingness to intervene can facilitate perpetrator confrontation (Brown and Messman-Moore 2009). For example, male undergraduates' self-reported willingness to intervene in sexual violence is significantly predicted by their perception of how likely other males (but not females, i.e. only a meaningful referent ingroup) are to intervene (Fabiano et al. 2003). The correction of misperceived ingroup norms concerning gender violence therefore presents an opportunity to design social norm violence prevention interventions. Moreover, this work points to the importance of designing interventions aimed at entire cohesive social groups, and not just known perpetrators (Gidycz et al. 2011).

An example of a successful social norms programme based upon this approach is described by Gidycz et al. (2011), who worked with male undergraduate students. In addition to strategies designed to increase empathy with females and promote understanding of consent, the programme presented normative feedback on campus-wide male discomfort with sexual assault and aggression, and encouraged male participants to express their own opposition to gender violence. This functioned to undermine mistaken perceptions of comfort with sexual assault, and validate a positive majority norm of intervention into the behaviour of a minority. Evaluation of the initiative concluded that relative to a control group, programme participants self-reported less sexual aggression at a 4-month follow-up, and a greater expectation that peers would intervene in incidents of gender violence.

Another illustrative example of a promising social norms programme is the Mentors in Violence Prevention initiative (MVP; Katz 1995). This was designed specifically to provide bystanders—who are often seen as peripheral to interpersonal violence—with the tools to intervene through discouragement, prevention, and interruption. To date MVP has been widely implemented in the United States with professional sports teams, the military, and high schools students, and is currently being piloted with young people in Scotland and Sweden. MVP is a form of peer-led learning such that ingroup members (e.g. players in one's sports team or students in one's class) are trained to deliver sessions to their peers. The sessions involve discussion of a variety of gender violence scenarios, and of options in how best to respond to them. Doing nothing is never seen as an acceptable strategy. Peer-group audiences are single-gender in order to facilitate an honest discussion of experiences and views without embarrassment.

The role of social norms is critical to MVP in at least three ways. First, participants are encouraged to discuss issues of gender violence with other ingroup members, and to reach a consensus position in opposition to it. Second, the programme aims to shift social norms to facilitate empowerment and intervention. Third, interventions should then reinforce and validate the social norm that gender violence is unacceptable, and that intervention is normative. MVP is also designed to deliver practical intervention strategies, and is thus congruent with Berkowitz's (2004) assertion that men are more receptive to positive practical messages rather than negative approaches which focus on blame. Evaluations to date suggest that MVP participants are more likely to intervene in situations of gender violence than non-participants (e.g. Katz et al. 2011).

One of the reasons why MVP appears to be successful is because the normative influence comes from ingroup peers and not outsiders. This notion is also central to the CeaseFire programme (alternatively named Cure Violence), a U.S.-based initiative designed to mediate street conflicts before they lead to serious violence (Whitehill et al. 2013). Outreach workers ('violence interrupters') are employed from the communities in which they work, and often have a personal history of gang involvement and incarceration. These individuals are seen as 'credible messengers', and have the contacts and skills to encourage protagonists' peers to assert influence to avoid violent outcomes. The prevention of one violent incident may then avert future retaliatory attacks, and also demonstrate that conflicts may be resolved without the use of force. Furthermore, CeaseFire encourages community events (marches, vigils, etc.) against violence, thereby explicitly communicating a collective desire for peace, and not tacit approval for street violence which may result from community silence. Initial evaluations of the approach indicate a promising decrease in gun crime and homicides (e.g. Webster et al. 2013), although it is difficult to isolate the specific role of social norms from the programme's various conflict mediation strategies.

Edutainment

Educational entertainment ('edutainment') campaigns have attempted to shift social norms and attitudes to violence through the media. For example, a radio soap opera in post-war Rwanda explored issues of tribalism, retaliation, and cooperation. Paluck (2009) demonstrated that over the course of a year listeners' personal attitudes towards these issues remained stable, but that they experienced positive change in their perceptions of ingroup norms. Participants listened to and discussed the shows in groups of peers, and it was this communication of other's normative positions which Paluck argued was crucial to the normative change.

Alcohol and Violence

Whilst excessive alcohol intoxication (and other forms of substance misuse) does not inevitably lead to violent behaviour, it is a risk factor for violence. Given this relationship, social norm interventions designed to attenuate alcohol intake may act as indirect violence interventions (WHO 2009). There are several ways in which social norms are relevant to alcohol and violence. For example, cultures which tolerate greater levels of alcohol abuse display a stronger link between violent behaviour and alcohol consumption, and a social belief that alcohol provides courage may lead to alcohol consumption before the perpetration of violence (WHO 2009). Interventions which correct mistaken perceptions of peer norms regarding excessive alcohol consumption (so called 'pluralistic ignorance' (Prentice and Miller 1993) can successfully reduce alcohol consumption, and therefore address a key risk factor in violence perpetration and victimhood (Moreira et al. 2009).

Community Social Norm Change: A Case Study

Deep-rooted cultural practices and beliefs can provide a potential challenge to a social norms approach to violence prevention. Interventions implemented by outsiders are often ineffective at changing behaviours which are seen as integral to a group's social identity. Female genital mutilation (FGM)—described as 'de facto violent' by United Nations Children's Fund (UNICEF) (2013)—in rural Senegal was regarded as one of these issues. Attempts to stop FGM as a cultural practice by non-community members failed, and an official law passed against the practice had little impact. Non-conformation with the circumcision norm could lead to exile from the social group, in part due to a cultural belief that not undergoing the operation could spiritually endanger both the individual and the community. Norm enforcement was therefore viewed as a form of individual and collective protection.

However, since 1998 a collective movement led by villagers at a community level has substantially reduced the practice using a social norms approach (Melching 2012). First, villagers came to a consensus around their community goals which included well-being and health. A sustained period of community discussion and reflection then concluded that FGM was incongruent with these goals. Crucially, a new norm of not circumcising was framed not as an attack upon tradition, but rather as a means of enacting long-standing community norms of health. Next, community members publically denounced FGM, and expressed commitment to the sanctioning of individuals who violated the new norm. It was this shift in social norms with community led sanctions that led to behaviour change. Despite FGM being outlawed in Senegal, it was only the change in 'community law' which allowed families to disregard the traditional practice without fear of community repercussion (Melching 2012).

This case study is a useful way of summarizing many of the key points outlined in this chapter. The first is that the social identity of the target population is crucial in a number of ways. A cohesive social group is necessary for intragroup social influence through public support for social norms of non-violence, and community-led 'self-policing' or sanctions for group members who act in defiance of collective norms. Second, the adoption of non-violent social norms must be congruent with a group's self-identity. Finally, the intervention only worked when it was owned by ingroup members and not outsiders. Whilst there can be a role for external organizations in implementing non-violence interventions, the very nature of social influence determines that social norm change must be driven by prototypical ingroup members.

Transportability of Programmes Nationally and Internationally

Common Process, Bespoke Content

In order for a social norms approach to be effective, it must articulate with the target group's social identity. Since a group's norms are embedded in social context, any initiative will need to account for this context. This means that although the processes of norm and behaviour change will remain constant between programmes, the content of the details will necessarily vary in order to be culturally relevant. Social norm interventions are therefore transportable nationally and internationally, so long as they are contextually sensitive. For instance, group-specific statistics are more powerful than general figures, and interventions must consider the culture and goals of the group.

The importance of designing bespoke norm interventions for different social groups was demonstrated in the evaluation of a social norms campaign regarding sexual consent for deaf and hard-of-hearing students (White et al. 2003). The implementation of a campus-wide initiative was initially unsuccessful for this sub-group. The programme was then redesigned to be specifically relevant for this population, including a consideration of their communication style and culture. There was a subsequent decrease in sexual assaults in this group only after the bespoke intervention was implemented.

Gaps in the Evidence

Whilst existing research offers preliminary hope for the utility of social norms interventions in violence prevention, there remains a need for high-quality evaluations of theoretically based programmes. At present, many interventions are not underpinned by theory (Paul and Gray 2011), and do not undergo rigorous evaluation. The evaluations that are conducted generally only employ self-report attitudinal measures which may not correspond to behaviour change outcomes around violence perpetration or bystander intervention (Paul and Gray 2011). This is partly because of demand characteristics around topics such as sexual assault (i.e. participants are unlikely to reveal support for sexual assault if they expect this response to be negatively evaluated by the researcher; Breitenbecher 2000), and also due to the relatively low perpetration rates in researchers' favourite population of choice—university undergraduates. Although this is a useful

group with which to pilot interventions (particularly around sexual assault and alcohol), the field should progress to populations at greater risk of violence perpetration, and also consider the addition of behavioural measures and routinely collected criminal justice data.

An improvement in evaluation design would also allow conclusions to be drawn with greater certainty about the efficacy of interventions. For example, at present many evaluations do not include suitable comparison groups. Evaluating attitude or behaviour change at a 1-year follow-up requires a non-intervention comparison group to determine whether any post-intervention differences are due to the programme, or other factors such as maturation effects (particularly likely with student populations) (Paul and Gray 2011). It is particularly important for future evaluations to measure what participants think their peers believe, in addition to their personal opinions. As this chapter has argued, change in the epistemic relationships between group members at a meta-representational level is central to normative and behavioural change, but is seldom measured.

Random assignment into research conditions would also improve the quality of evaluation. This is often practically challenging because violence prevention strategies are typically designed to target specific problematic groups. Although randomization at an individual level may be unrealistic, random allocation at the level of the group (e.g. school, neighbourhood, etc.) might be achievable (Paul and Gray 2011). Furthermore, a movement toward mixed-methods evaluations would also allow researchers to capture the qualitative richness that is inherent in social norms interventions, in addition to survey and routinely collected quantitative data.

A more thorough description of research methods and intervention implementation would also improve the evidence base. At present these sections of evaluations are often sparse, creating ambiguity about which elements of an intervention worked and why (Paul and Gray 2011). More precise description of intervention implementation and an effort to specifically evaluate all elements of this in a macro fashion will result in a clearer picture of the effectiveness of the social norms component (see Chapter 17 of this volume). Finally, many evaluations fail to include a long-term follow-up of intervention. This is in part a consequence of the ephemeral nature of research funding. Nonetheless, an effort to explore how social norms violence interventions affect attitudes, norms, and behaviours in the long-term is essential for the design of future programmes including their projected cost-effectiveness.

Conclusions

A social norms approach to violence prevention has gained traction is recent years, and incipient evaluations have yielded promising results. This chapter has reviewed the theory underpinning a social norms approach to violence prevention, and has discussed a variety of interventions in order to draw out key themes. The first point to note is that norms are the mechanism by which social categories influence their members. Psychological groups should therefore be reconceptualized as a resource—and not a threat—in violence prevention. Behaviour is also commonly driven at a meta-representational level by the perceived norms of ingroup members, and thus ingroup peers have a key role to play in preventing violence. The perceptive element of this is a fertile area for social norms interventions, through correction of misperceptions about others' attitudes and behaviours. This is good news for practitioners, because altering the epistemic relationships between group members is a substantially easier task than trying to simultaneously change everyone's personal attitudes. In practical terms, social norms violence interventions will work best when designed to target cohesive groups in order to encourage peer influence and 'self-policing'. Bespoke programmes should be designed for specific social units in order to be culturally relevant and efficacious, and both descriptive and injunctive norms should be utilized to prevent counterproductive effects. Interventions should also be delivered from the perspective of ingroup members, and behaviour change should be consonant with defining tenets of the target group's identity.

Acknowledgements

The author wishes to thank the editors and multiple colleagues for constructive comments on earlier drafts of this manuscript.

References

Abbey, A., Parkhill, M., Clinton-Sherrod, A., and Zawacki, T. (2007). A comparison of men who committed different types of sexual assault in a community sample. *Journal of Interpersonal Violence*, 22, 1567–80.

Baer, J. S., Stacy, A., and Larimer, M. (1991). Biases in the perception of drinking norms among college students. *Journal of Studies on Alcohol*, 52, 580–6.

Berkowitz, A. D. (2004). Working with men to prevent violence against women: program modalities and formats (part two). *Violence against Women Resource Network*. Available at www.vawnet.org. [Accessed 02 February 2013].

Bohner, G., Siebler, F., and Schmelcher, J. (2006). Social norms and the likelihood of raping: perceived rape myth acceptance of others affects men's rape proclivity. *Personality and Social Psychology Bulletin*, 32, 286–97.

Breitenbecher, K. H. (2000). Sexual assault on college campuses: is an ounce of prevention enough? *Applied and Preventive Psychology: Current Scientific Perspectives*, 9, 23–52.

Brown, A. L., and Messman-Moore, T. L. (2009). Personal and perceived peer attitudes supporting sexual aggression as predictors of male college students' willingness to intervene against sexual aggression. *Journal of Interpersonal Violence*, 25, 503–17.

Chekroun, P. (2008). Social control behavior: the effects of social situations and personal implication on informal social sanctions. *Social and Personality Psychology Compass*, 2, 2141–58.

Cialdini, R. B., Reno, R. R., and Kallgren, C. A. (1990). A focus theory of normative conduct: recycling the concept of norms to reduce littering in public places. *Journal of Personality and Social Psychology*, 6, 1015–26.

Duck, J. M., Hogg, M. A., and Terry, D. J. (1999). Social identity and perceptions of media persuasion: are we always less influenced than others? *Journal of Applied Social Psychology*, 29, 1879–99.

Elcheroth, G., Doise, W., and Reicher, S. D. (2011). On the knowledge of politics and the politics of knowledge: how a social representations approach helps us rethink the subject of political psychology. *Political Psychology*, 32, 729–58.

Fabiano, P. M., Perkins, H. W., Berkowitz, A., Linkenbach, J., and Stark, C. (2003). Engaging men as social justice allies in ending violence against women: evidence for a social norms approach. *Journal of American College Health*, 52, 105–12.

Gidycz, C. A., Orchowski, L. M., and Berkowitz, A. D. (2011). Preventing sexual aggression among college men: an evaluation of a social norms and bystander intervention program. *Violence Against Women*, 17, 720–42.

Hogg, M. A and Vaughan, G. M. (2008). *Social Psychology. 5th Ed.* Harlow: Pearson.

Katz, J. (1995). Reconstructing masculinity in the locker room: the Mentors in Violence Prevention Project. *Harvard Educational Review*, 65, 163–75.

Katz, J., Heisterkamp, H. A., and Fleming, W. M. (2011). The social justice roots of the mentors in violence prevention model and its application in a high school setting. *Violence against Women*, 17, 684–702

Loh, C., Gidycz, C. A., Lobo, T. R., and Luthra, R. (2005). A prospective analysis of sexual assault perpetration: risk factors related to perpetrator characteristics. *Journal of Interpersonal Violence*, 20, 1325–48.

Melching, M. (2012). *Creating Social Norms to Prevent Violence against Girls and Women*. UN Women Expert Group Meeting, Bangkok.

Moreira, M. T., Smith, L. A., and Foxcroft, D. (2009). Social norms interventions to reduce alcohol misuse in university or college students. The *Cochrane Database of Systematic Reviews*, 8, CD006748.

Neighbors, C., Walker, D. D., and Mbilinyi, L. F. et al. (2010). Normative misperceptions of abuse among perpetrators of intimate partner violence. *Violence Against Women*, 16, 370–86.

Paluck, E. L. (2009). Reducing intergroup prejudice and conflict using the media: a field experiment in Rwanda. *Journal of Personality and Social Psychology*, 96, 574–87.

Paul, L. A., and Gray, M. J. (2011). Sexual assault programming on college campuses: using social psychological belief and behavior change principles to improve outcomes. *Trauma, Violence, & Abuse*, 12, 99–109.

Prentice, D. A., and Miller, D. T. (1993). Pluralistic ignorance and alcohol use on campus: some consequences of misperceiving the social norm. *Journal of Personality and Social Psychology*, 64, 243–56.

Reicher, S. D., Spears, R., and Haslam, S. A. (2010). The social identity approach in social psychology. In: M. S. Wetherell, and C. T. Mohanty (eds), *Sage Handbook of Identities*. London: Sage, pp. 45–62.

Smith, J. R., and Louis, W. R. (2009). Group norms and the attitude–behaviour relationship. *Social and Personality Psychology Compass*, 3, 19–35

Stott, C., Hutchison, P., and Drury, J. (2001). Hooligans' abroad? Inter-group dynamics, social identity and participation in collective 'disorder' at the 1998 World Cup Finals. *British Journal of Social Psychology*, 40, 359–84.

Tharp, A. T., DeGue, S., Valle, L. A., Brookmeyer, K. A., Massetti, G. M., and Matjasko, J. L. (2013). A systematic qualitative review of risk and protective factors for sexual violence perpetration. *Trauma, Violence, & Abuse*, 14, 133–67.

Turner, J. C. (1991). *Social Influence*. Milton Keynes: Open University Press.

Turner, J. C., Hogg, M. A., Oakes, P. J. Reicher, S. D., and Wetherell, M. S. (1987). *Rediscovering the Social Group: A Self-Categorization Theory*. Oxford: Blackwell.

UNICEF (2013) *Child Protection from Violence, Exploitation and Abuse*. Available at: http://www.unicef.org/protection/57929_58002.html [Accessed 17 January 2013].

Webster, D. W., Whitehill, J. M., Vernick, J. S., and Curriero, F. C. (2013). Effects of Baltimore's Safe Streets program on gun violence: a replication of Chicago's CeaseFire program. *Journal of Urban Health*, 90, 1–14.

White, J. A., Williams, L. M., and Cho, D. (2003). A social norms intervention to reduce coercive sexual behaviors among deaf and hard-of-hearing college students. *The Report on Social Norms*, 2, 1–8.

Whitehill, J. M., Webster, D. W., Frattaroli, S., and Parker, E. M. (2013). Interrupting violence: how the CeaseFire program prevents imminent gun violence through conflict mediation. *Journal of Urban Health*, 90, 84–95.

World Health Organization. (2009). *Violence Prevention: The Evidence. Changing Cultural and Social Norms that Support Violence*. Available at: http://www.who.int/violence_injury_prevention/violence/4th_milestones_meeting/publications/en/ [Accessed 17 January 2013].

Zimbardo, P. G. (1969). The human choice: individuation, reason, and order versus deindividuation, impulse and chaos. *Nebraska Symposium on Motivation*, 17, 237–307.

CHAPTER 34

Community-engaged violence prevention: approaches and principles

Mohamed Seedat, Shahnaaz Suffla,
and Catherine L. Ward

Introduction to Community-Engaged Violence Prevention

Violence results from a complex interplay of individual and systemic risk factors, in which community-level risk plays an important part. Communities are contexts within which individuals, families, institutions, and interpersonal relationships are nested, and thus community-strengthening approaches to violence prevention promote specific community characteristics as mediators of violence prevention, with a view to enhancing community cohesion, connectedness, social capital, and organization (West et al. 2006). Community-level interventions may of course include behavioural or setting-level interventions as well as those at the community level, but are predicated on the mobilization of target populations and community groupings to lead on priority community issues.

There are many chapters in this volume that describe the logic, implementation, and assessment of specific behavioural, setting, and community strengthening approaches. In this chapter, we focus on the modes and mechanisms of engagement inherent to community-level violence prevention measures. We review select engagement approaches, provide illustrative examples, and evaluate the exemplars offered to draw out the critical elements of a framework for engagement. The engagement orientation to community strengthening assumes that communities are critical stakeholders for fortifying prevention efforts, and that tested and effective interventions will be better received, adopted, and sustained through initiatives that actively encourage community mobilization (Backer and Guerra 2011).

Engagement: Modes, Approaches and Principles

Three modes of engagement have been identified: *transactional*, *transitional*, and *transformational*, each of which results in different levels of interactions within communities (Bowen et al. 2010; see Table 34.1):

- *Transactional* engagement, characterized by uni-directional messaging, involves the transfer of financial donations, skills, technical expertise, and services from intervention agencies to communities. Engagement is occasional and may include the agency sharing information with the community, consent from the community for the intervention, consultation (limited to obtaining feedback, and so not involving community representatives in the development, implementation, or evaluation of the intervention), and involvement (at most, training community members to deliver the intervention); the agency maintains full influence over the engagement process even though communities earn benefits through the skills and resource transfers.

- *Transitional* engagements, framed by the notion of bilateral communication, encompass consent, consultations, and involvement, but preclude co-responsibility for resources or any form of joint meaning-making; while resources may be shared with community groups, they are controlled solely by the agency.

- *Transformational* engagement embraces participation through shared leadership and responsibility for learning, projects, and decision-making. Connections and trust are forged through personal relationships and shared understandings and organizational language that is thought to arise from dynamic dialogue, active listening, and critical reflectivity (Balmer et al. 2007).

Clearly, transformational engagement approaches encourage great breadth and depth of community mobilization.

Table 34.1 shows how these different modes are driven by different models or philosophies of community engagement, and use different methods. Recent South African work (Eksteen et al. 2012; Lazarus et al. 2012; Seedat 2012; Suffla et al. 2012) suggests that community engagement is a complex interactive process that is influenced by contextual specificities and that undergoes shifts over time. In one moment the community engagement may embrace actions to obtain community consent, consultation, and involvement for the initiation and development of interventions; in another moment community engagement may involve contestation, conflict, and resistance arising from differences related to institutional location, identity, and subject positions.

True transformational engagement advocates for meaningful participation. However, there is a danger that simply paying

Table 34.1 Categorization of engagement

Model/s	Degree of engagement	Mode and function	Methods
• Centralized	Low	• Transactional or transitional • *Information-sharing*: people are informed about decisions taken • Community has no influence over decision-making process	• Media releases • Fact/information sheets • Notification letters Newsletters • Websites
• Centralized	Low–Medium	• Transactional or transitional • *Consent*: aimed at securing community approval and endorsements	• Questionnaires • Surveys • Focus group discussions • Meetings
• Consultation/public participation	Medium	• Transactional or transitional • *Consultation*: invites input from community members on a proposal • No community participation in actual decision-making process	• Questionnaires • Surveys • Focus group discussions/community conversations • Meetings • Workshops
• Asset-based/social economy • Learning-led • Service development	Medium-High	• Transactional or transitional • *Involvement*: includes community in planning and decision-making processes • Community members are involved as volunteers or service users	• Advisory committees • Community workshops • Training and capacity building activities • Site meetings • Site visits • Volunteers/service users
• Community democracy • Community organizing • Local and national networks	High	• Transformational • *Participation*: invites active engagement from community members • Exchange of information • Integration of local knowledge • Coalition-building • Community influences decisions	• Community reference groups • Community design teams • Community forums • Community panels
• Critical	High	• Transformational • *Empowering*: addresses power differentials through opportunities for dialogue and agency • Engagement in collection action for change and justice • Politicization and co-creation of knowledge • Enhances critical consciousness • Encourages participatory governance	• Emancipatory action research • Participatory evaluation teams • Advocacy groups • Campaigns to influence policy

Source: data from Bowen, F., et al., When suits meet roots: the antecedents and consequences of community engagement strategy, *Journal of Business Ethics*, Volume 95, Issue 2, pp. 297–318, Copyright © 2010; Hashagen, S.,*Models of Community Engagement*. Scottish Community Development Centre, Scottish Community Development Centre, Copyright © 2002, available from http://www.dundeecity.gov.uk/dundeecity/uploaded_publications/publication_283.pdf; and Seedat, M., Community engagement as liberal performance, as critical intellectualism and as praxis, *Journal of Psychology in Africa*, Volume 22, Issue 4, pp. 489–500, Copyright © 2012

lip-service to the notion of participation can perpetuate the unfair and disingenuous exercise of power in engagement initiatives (Leal 2007). For violence prevention, then, true community participation aims to include marginal voices and knowledge, assure contextual congruence, and promote a shared ownership of the problem of violence and its solutions, among diverse community interest groups and professionals (Spinks et al. 2004).

Illustrative Engagement Approaches

In this section, we describe and examine two community engagement-based approaches to violence prevention that reflect an amalgam of the different strands represented in Table 34.1, and which support the implementation of evidence-based practices in violence prevention.

The Ukuphepha Engagement Approach

The Ukuphepha Engagement Approach has been used in five South African low-income communities, and aims to mobilize community action through defined community engagement pathways directed at supporting violence prevention and reduction, and safety, peace, and health promotion in high-risk settings (Eksteen et al. 2012; 'ukuphepha' means *to be safe* in isiZulu, one of South Africa's 11 official languages). Specifically, it underpins the delivery of a suite of interventions to family and extended social and living systems through community-wide interventions and home visitation. The former include education and sensitization, psycho-educational activities at early childhood development centres, outreach to play parks, and advocacy and emergency services offered by resource persons. Home visitation offers a health and safety curriculum delivered to primary caregivers that integrates child health, family functioning, and child abuse prevention components (Seedat et al. 2012). The Ukuphepha Engagement Approach delineates six interconnected community engagement pathways (see Figure 34.1). Each of these pathways is linked to specific activities which the approach views as cornerstones for mobilizing community action and co-ownership over community-based prevention and promotive initiatives.

i. *Relationship building*: The Ukuphepha Engagement Approach, informed by the principles of diversity and interactive processes (see Hashagen 2002), is predicated on building relationships with a wide range of organizational and individual stakeholders who are concerned with development and prevention issues. Connections with both individuals and organized structures are built through regular conversations and consultations, which are opportunities to raise awareness about intended projects, discuss challenges, priorities, and prevention approaches, and obtain consent and support for interventions.

ii. *Community-centred learning:* Inspired by Paulo Freire's (1970) emancipatory methods, the Ukuphepha Engagement Approach considers learning as a dialogue marked by reflection, recognition of personal experiences, meaning-making, questioning, and the participation of all stakeholders in the development of relevant and beneficial training programmes (Phiri et al. 2012). Community-centred learning is boosted through the recruitment and training of community members in aspects of the prevention sciences that contribute to both self-development and broader community safety.

iii. *Social justice and contextual congruence:* The Ukuphepha Engagement Approach maintains that assessment measures

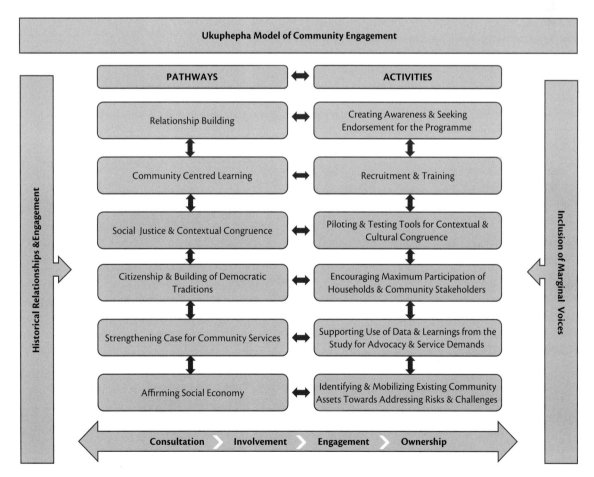

Fig. 34.1 The Ukuphepha engagement approach.

and interventions that are culturally embedded help assure social justice, programmatic efficacy, and social relevance. These are obtained by incorporating community voices and cultural expressions into the development and adoption of research questions, data collection processes, context sensitive assessment tools, risk prioritization, and selection and development or adaptation of the interventions.

iv. *Citizenship and democratic traditions*: These are built through the use of open discussion forums, acceptance of dissenting voices, and consensus-driven decision-making mechanisms and inclusivity (Viswanathan et al. 2004). The Ukuphepha Engagement Approach utilizes a variety methods (such as focus groups and community conversations), to engage community stakeholders as decision-makers in the formulation of intervention objectives, intervention selection, implementation, and evaluation.

v. *Strengthening cases for community services*: The Ukuphepha Engagement Approach places a special accent on community advocacy to pressure local authorities (see Viswanathan et al. 2004) to deliver municipal and recreational services such as refuse removal and street lighting. The approach identifies capacity-building exercises and the stimulating of critical consciousness as key to strengthening the community's advocacy efforts, and contributing to its ability to influence policy-makers.

vi. *Affirming social economy:* The community's social economy is affirmed by identifying and mapping community assets, which may be both tangible (e.g. educational and faith-based institutions,), and intangible (e.g. community resiliency). The mapping process identifies communities' enduring traditions and networks that support social solidarity, a culture of accountability, social exchange, and community connectedness. As a process-level intervention, community asset mapping may encourage engagement, agency, ownership, and inclusivity. Asset-mapping is not to be read as a dichotomization of 'needs' and 'assets'; rather, it offers generative methods to identifying and mobilising community resources to deal with priority issues, and corrosive discourses and practices (Fraser 1989).

The Ukuphepha Engagement Approach thus represents a multi-faceted engagement platform for the conceptualization and delivery of community-level interventions, and is grounded in a contextual interpretation of the fundamental principles of community engagement principles, which lends strongly to its value and utility. However, in its attunement to a very particular socio-historical milieu, the Ukuphepha Engagement Approach's applicability across contexts is yet to be established (Eksteen et al. 2012).

The Communities that Care Approach

Communities That Care (CTC) is a community engagement approach that has been extensively used in the United States, and adapted for use in the United Kingdom, the Netherlands, and Australia, to enable communities to identify and implement effective, ecologically valid preventive interventions, focused on youth social problems such as substance abuse, violence, and delinquency, and which may also be applied to various community injury and violence priorities (Fagan et al. 2008; Feinberg et al. 2004). It is based on a five-phase process (Gomez et al. 2005; Hawkins et al. 2002).

i. *Community readiness:* The focus is on assessing community readiness to utilize the CTC approach. Where the focus is on youth development, readiness is indicated when key community stakeholders prioritize youth development and the prevention of risky youth behaviours, and demonstrate commitment to working collaboratively towards consensually developed objectives.

ii. *Community mobilization*: The engagement process involves the facilitation and establishment of a coalition, and includes grassroots community members dealing with youth development and risky behaviours, as well as leaders who shape public opinion. Community stakeholders are supported to forge a futuristic vision for their community's youth and establish a community board that includes representatives of diverse sectors working in youth development and safety promotion. The board exercises oversight over the planning, implementation, and monitoring of prevention activities and mobilizes resources for the community's prevention vision and plans. This engagement promotes community ownership and direction over resource mobilization, and prevention planning and implementation. However, it is unclear how key stakeholders and grassroots actors are identified and enlisted to participate in the CTC approach and if any attempts are made to engage unorganized and marginal constituencies in the community.

iii. *Mapping community strengths*: Once formed, the board maps community strengths and challenges, using relevant data and survey instruments to delineate risk and protective factor profiles and problematic youth behaviours. The data-led profiling process helps to build consensus around priorities, focuses actions, and informs resource allocations.

iv. *Logical approach:* The board is encouraged to assume a logical approach to developing strategic plans that: address risk factors, capitalize on community strengths and protective aspects, curtail duplication in services, attend to identified gaps in community responses to youth development and safety promotion, and specify risk reduction and protective factor outcomes to be accomplished within an indicated time-frame. The CTC approach specifically engages the board to: review and select empirically tested approaches for strengthening youth development, reduce prioritized risks and enhance existing protective behaviours, and develop a monitoring and evaluation plan for assessing changes in risk and protection profiles.

v. *Implementation and evaluation:* The board is engaged to mobilize the requisite resources for the implementation of the plan; the implementation process is supported by information systems that facilitate regular inter-agency communications and regular monitoring of progress towards outcomes (Hawkins 1999).

Outcomes and process-based evaluations have indicated various benefits arising from the adoption and application of the CTC system. Twelve intervention communities in the United States were able to enact the CTC approach with high rates of implementation fidelity (Fagan et al. 2009; Hawkins et al. 2008). All the intervention communities successfully established coalitions, implemented prevention programmes, and sustained prevention service quality over the 5 years of the study (Brown et al. 2007). Other community-randomized trials revealed promising results with respect to reduction of risky youth behaviours, but longitudinal follow-up studies are required to establish whether CTC has significant enduring influences on violent, delinquent, and drug use behaviours (Brown et al. 2007; Quinby et al. 2008). Yet other studies have demonstrated that training in the CTC system helps community coalitions to use empirical approaches to prevention planning, and map their community's risks and protection profiles (e.g. Hawkins 1999).

Critical Assumptions

In this section we examine fundamental concepts that frame the logic of change and application of the two approaches reviewed: community and coalitions.

Notions of Community and Change

The Ukuphepha Engagement Approach constructs communities as vibrant entities with inherent capacities to identify and marshal resources towards containing risks and determinants of violence. Accordingly, for the Ukuphepha Engagement Approach, community is both geographical place and assets (Kramer et al. 2011). While the CTC approach has been applied in distinct geographical zones, it tends to place the emphasis on members of priority populations that share a particular experience, with specific attention to risk factors that predict violence and protective factors that buffer against risk. Communities are therefore viewed from both a threat and an assets perspective, and as possessing the potential to navigate from risk and threat to becoming healthy, productive, and contributing entities.

Thus, both approaches define communities as being inherently resourceful, solution-driven, and generative; geographical entities become communities when those who reside therein share norms, values, and aspirations; communities are underpinned by consensus, shared values, and visions and a sense of connectivity; and it is assumed that communities' social capital, sense of connectivity, and social cohesion imbue them with capacities for violence prevention and safety promotion. Cooperative and consensus-making capacities move groups of people towards commonalities and connections, myriads of networks and social exchanges, as well as generative interpersonal relationships. This notion of community emphasizes social capital and social cohesion as the elements that 'make' a community.

Despite its intention not to mask 'risks', 'needs', and 'challenges', the Ukuphepha Engagement Approach tends, in its emphasis on assets, to understate that communities are also characterized by hostilities, competition for scarce resources, conflict, and fierce struggles for identity and representation. The CTC approach also does not explicitly speak to the influences of contest and conflict in building coalitions and leadership competencies. It is critical to recognize that communities are not released of aggressive, overly competitive, and conflictual influences and impulses simply through a focus on assets (Homan 2004, Kramer et al. 2012).

Violence prevention programmes must therefore consider the influences of generative and conflict-driven forces in communities.

Coalitions: Enactments of Engagement

The CTC's conception of coalitions as mechanisms of change warrants an examination of the logic and nature of coalitions, which have increasingly come to be recognized as the coordinating structures driving community-centred prevention in many regions of the world (Wolff 2001). A coalition may be defined as:

> an organization of diverse interest groups that combine their human and material resources to effect a specific change that members are unable to bring about independently. (Brown 1984, p. 4)

Coalitions are quite distinct from networks and alliances. Networks tend to be loose, flexible arrangements that bring people or organizations together for purposes of sharing ideas and information. Alliances bring together associations and/or individuals who are centred on specific objectives for a short term. Coalitions are fixed on specific objectives, and involve long-term commitments and formalized structures (Brown 1984).

Coalitions themselves are not prevention strategies; instead, they represent a particular way of organizing, planning, and delivering multi-system and multi-dimensional prevention programmes, policies, and practices. In the case of violence and other health and social issues, coalitions may be regarded as vehicles for establishing structures and systems for engaging communities to determine, lead, and manage activities towards controlling and preventing violence; they can reduce inter-agency competitiveness, promote collaboration among different groups, and enhance the credibility and influences of their defined activities (Davis et al. 2006). Coalitions represent a collective enactment of power to pressure an external group and achieve agreed on objectives. As such, while coalitions are to be accountable to their constituent membership, they also require the autonomy to make independent decisions. Coalitions derive their collective power from the authority delegated to them by their constituent organizations.

Several factors lead to successful coalition-building and sustainability (Mizrahi and Rosenthal 2001). These include: optimal political and economic conditions, an accent on social change, availability of appropriate economic resources, history of affirming experiences with coalitions, and membership commitment, contributions, and competence. Coalitions require tangible resources such as money and staffing, as well as intangibles like specialized expertise, information, and access to contact lists. Further, an ideological purpose and social change focus offer coalitions the larger anchoring framework for formulating and following objectives, and defining interactional and decision-making processes (Mizrahi and Rosenthal 2001). Commitment is shaped by a range of motivational factors, including the search for resources and public influence on the one hand, and values related to the notions of public good or community interests on the other. Coalitions therefore need to understand and address motivations related to both self interest and public good. Finally, empirical work involving 41 social change coalitions in metropolitan New York and New Jersey in the United States indicate that leadership competency, 'the analytical and interactional skills needed to make a coalition work' (Mizrahi and Rosenthal 2001, p. 66), is the most critical factor in coalition-building and success.

CTC-related evaluation studies that have examined predictors of prevention-coalition success and sustainability have highlighted the importance of community readiness. Community readiness in the CTC system is indicated by the presence of democratic-minded community leadership that facilitates grassroots participation and leadership capacities to manage conflict as well as residents' sense of connection to the community. Readiness is often evident in the coalition's internal functioning (Feinberg et al. 2004), which is also strongly related to coalition sustainability. In addition to coalition internal functioning, sustainability of the CTC-aligned coalitions is contingent on coalition members' knowledge of prevention theory and practices, and implementation fidelity (Gomez et al. 2005). Thus, actual planning for sustainability is a notable influence on long-term coalition sustainability (Feinberg et al. 2008).

The preceding discussion suggests that it is important to invest early in technical assistance and regular training of key leaders in coalition functioning, development, and sustainability.

Conclusion

Community engagement may be marked by cooperation, contest, and struggle for resources and representation, and is thus a dynamic process that may be enacted through various approaches. Each of the approaches produces different kinds of engagement. For instance, consultation approaches aim to obtain community feedback and opinions without full participation in decision-making, and asset-based approaches emphasize both tangible and intangible community resources and promote community participation in the identification, implementation, and evaluation of prevention prescriptions. Participatory-oriented engagement, including asset-based approaches, help situate empirically tested violence prevention interventions within collaborative arrangements that mobilize communities to become involved and/or take ownership and control of the violence prevention agenda and associated initiatives. Meaningful and increased levels of participation serve to enhance prevention programme adoption and success.

Several systematic reviews (Chalk 2000; Guterman 2004; Sethi et al. 2006) help delineate the factors that enable community engaged prevention. The successful adoption and implementation of evidence-based prevention interventions is contingent on community readiness, which refers to preparedness to implement an intervention; cultivating community coalitions; relevance of intervention to the community's violence priorities and profile; implementation fidelity and availability of requisite resources; technical assistance; and regular training and on-going monitoring and evaluation (Sethi et al. 2006). In turn, coalition success is dependent on internal coalition functioning, leadership, and planning for sustainability (Fagan et al. 2009; Hawkins et al. 2008).

We draw on our descriptions to propose that community engagement is an eight-stage process that privileges the following considerations:

i. Comprehending community readiness and context

A facilitating environment is essential for communities to be engaged and effective in their support of evidence-based practices. Understanding the community's readiness to undertake collaborative violence prevention efforts therefore involves an assessment of community conditions, actors, and activities that may affect readiness.

ii. Building relationships

Building and sustaining collaborative relationships with community actors and other stakeholder groups that support the implementation of violence prevention interventions is a key priority for mobilizing communities towards the effective implementation of activities, advocacy, maximizing of resources and impacts, and fostering of coordinated networks, linkages, and partnerships. The relation-building process highlights that the development of trust is one of the central goals and benefits of engagement processes.

iii. Supporting and growing democratic leadership, structures, and practices

Representative governance and arrangements are a key strategic issue for community-level prevention initiatives. This process attaches significant value to the principles of participation, inclusiveness, interdependence, and collective choices and actions in violence prevention, while recognizing the diversity that exists among stakeholder groups and their respective agendas and resources.

iv. Participatory prioritization, planning, implementation, and evaluation:

Participatory community enquiry, prioritizing of interventions based on community needs, and planning, implementation, and assessment of subsequent actions are critical in influencing the ownership, credibility, and sustainability of interventions. Participatory processes that engage local voices, insights, and expertise represent a decentralized and partnership approach that embodies the ideals of collaboration, inclusiveness, and empowerment, and provide an opportunity for the disenfranchised particularly to be involved.

v. Community-centred capacitation and learning

Understanding that communities are frequently excluded from violence prevention efforts, capacity-building activities and support seek to strengthen the skills and competencies of communities to assume leading roles and effective action in promoting safety in their communities. The development of skills and access to knowledge resources is facilitated by dialogue between partners, provision of learning and training opportunities, and sharing through networks and mutual support.

vi. Resource mobilization and asset mapping

As an alternative to the traditional deficits-based approach, the identification of assets highlights communities' agenda-building and problem-solving capacities, and foster local knowledge, innovation, and control. The mobilization of community resources accords priority to maximizing the use of a community's resource base to promote safety, and to engaging people as citizens rather than merely recipients of interventions.

vii. Testing for cultural congruence

Prevention science that is grounded in a culturally and contextually relevant frame of reference enhances the effectiveness potential of violence prevention interventions, as well as signifies observance of the principle of social justice in research. Testing initiatives for their contextual and cultural fit and appropriateness subscribes to the view that communities have unique worldviews, social conditions, and discourses that warrant acknowledgement and integration into practices that involve them.

viii. Sustainability and advocating for routine services

The sustainability of violence prevention interventions in community settings is centrally connected to evidence-based practice, community mobilization, the enlistment of community assets, the strengthening of resources and capacities, and the on-going need for programme resources.

Since violence prevention interventions will be better received, adopted, and sustained through community participation (Backer and Guerra 2011), community mobilization initiatives should play an important part in violence prevention. Community mobilization needs to be carried out carefully and thoughtfully, with particular attention to community readiness; relationships within the community, and between the community and those leading the initiative; and the development and support of capacities and structures that can sustain the intervention into the future.

Acknowledgements

Work on this chapter has been supported in part by a grant from the University of Cape Town's Research Committee (URC) to the third author. The authors would also like to thank Najuwa Arendse for the support provided.

References

Backer, T. E., and Guerra, N. G. (2011). Mobilising communities to implement evidence-based practices in youth violence prevention: the state of the art. *American Journal of Community Psychology*, 48, 31–42.

Balmer, J. M. T., Fukukawa, K., and Gray, E. R. (2007). The nature and management of ethical corporate identity: a commentary on corporate identity, corporate social responsibility and ethics. *Journal of Business Ethics*, 76, 7–15.

Bowen, F., Newenham-Kahindi, A., and Herremans, I. (2010). When suits meet roots: the antecedents and consequences of community engagement strategy. *Journal of Business Ethics*, 95, 297–318.

Brown, C. (1984). *The Art of Coalition Building: A Guide for Community Leaders*. New York: The American Jewish Committee.

Brown, E. C., Hawkins, J. D., Arthur, M. W., Briney, J. S., and Abbott, R. D. (2007). Effects of Communities That Care on prevention services systems: findings from the community youth development study at 1.5 years. *Prevention Science*, 8, 180–91.

Chalk, R. (2000). Assessing family violence interventions: linking programs to research- based strategies. *Journal of Aggression, Maltreatment & Trauma*, 4, 29–53.

Davis, R., Parks, L., and Cohen, L. (2006). *Sexual Violence and the Spectrum of Prevention: Towards a Community Solution*. Enola, PA: National Sexual Violence Resource Centre.

Eksteen, R., Bulbulia, A., Van Niekerk, A., Ismail, G., and Lekoba, R. (2012). Ukuphepha: a multi-level community engagement model for the promotion of safety, peace and health. *Journal of Psychology in Africa*, 22, 501–510.

Fagan, A. A., Hanson, K., Hawkins, J. D., and Arthur, M. W. (2008). Bridging science to practice: achieving prevention program implementation fidelity in the community youth development study. *American Journal of Community Psychology*, 41, 235–49.

Feinberg, M. E., Bontempo, D. E., and Greenberg, M. T. (2008). Predictors and level of sustainability of community prevention coalitions. *American Journal of Preventive Medicine*, 34, 495–501.

Feinberg, M. E., Greenberg, M. T., and Osgood, D. W. (2004). Readiness, functioning, and perceived effectiveness in community prevention coalitions: a study of Communities That Care. *American Journal of Community Psychology*, 33, 163–76.

Fraser, N. (1989). *Unruly Practices: Power, Discourse, and Gender in Contemporary Social Theory*. Minneapolis: University of Minnesota.

Freire, P. (1970). *Pedagogy of the Oppressed*. New York: Herder and Herder.

Gomez, B. J., Greenberg, M. T., and Feinberg, M. E. (2005). Sustainability of community coalitions: an evaluation of Communities That Care. *Prevention Science*, 6, 199–202.

Guterman, N. B. (2004). Advancing prevention research on child abuse, youth violence and domestic violence: emerging strategies and issues. *Journal of Interpersonal Violence*, 19, 299–321.

Hashagen, S. (2002). *Models of Community Engagement*. Scottish Community Development Centre. Available at: http://www.dundeecity.gov.uk/dundeecity/uploaded_publications/publication_283.pdf [Accessed 28 February 2012].

Hawkins, J. D. (1999). Preventing crime and violence through Communities That Care. *European Journal of Criminal Policy and Research*, 7, 443–58.

Hawkins, J. D., Catalano, R. F., and Arthur, M. W. (2002). Promoting science-based prevention in communities. *Addictive Behaviors*, 27, 951–76.

Hawkins, J. D., Catalano, R. F. and Arthur, M. W. et al. (2008). Testing Communities That Care: the rationale, design and the behavioural baseline equivalence of the community youth development study. *Prevention Science*, 9, 178–90.

Homan, M. S. (2004). *Promoting Community Change: Making it Happen in the Real World*. 3rd ed. Belmont, CA: Brooks/Cole.

Kramer, S., Amos, T., Lazarus, S., and Seedat, M. (2012). The philosophical assumptions, utility and challenges of asset mapping approaches to community engagement. *Journal of Psychology in Africa*, 22, 537–46.

Kramer, S., Seedat, M., Lazarus, S., and Suffla, S. (2011). A critical review of instruments assessing characteristics of community. *South African Journal of Psychology*, 41, 503–16.

Lazarus, S., Taliep, N., Bulbulia, A., Phillips, S., and Seedat, M. (2012). Community-based participatory research: an illustrative case study of community engagement in one low-income community in the Western Cape. *Journal of Psychology in Africa*, 22, 511–8.

Leal, P.A. (2007). Participation: the ascendancy of a buzzword in the neo-liberal era. *Development in Practice*, 17, 539–48.

Mizrahi, T., and Rosenthal, B. (2001). Complexities of coalition building: leaders' successes, strategies, struggles and solutions. *Social Work*, 46, 63–78.

Phiri, L. L., Hendricks, N., and Seedat, M. (2012). Community-centred capacity development: a vehicle for engagement. *Journal of Psychology in Africa*, 22, 581–6.

Quinby, R. K., Hanson, K., Brooke-Weiss, B., Arthur, M. W., Hawkins, J. D., and Fagan, A. A. (2008). Installing the Communities That Care system: Implementation progress and fidelity in a randomised control trial. *Journal of Community Psychology*, 36, 313–32.

Seedat, M. (2012). Community engagement as liberal performance, as critical intellectualism and as praxis. *Journal of Psychology in Africa*, 22, 489–500.

Seedat, M., McClure, R., Suffla, S., and Van Niekerk, A. (2012). Developing the evidence-base for safe communities: a multi-level, partly randomised, controlled trial. *International Journal of Injury Control and Safety Promotion*, 19, 231–41.

Sethi, D., Racioppi, F., Baumgarten, I., and Bertolini R. (2006). Reducing inequalities from injuries in Europe. *Lancet*, 368, 2243–50.

Spinks, A., Turner, C., McClure, R., and Nixon, J. (2004). Community based prevention programs targeting all injuries for children. *Injury Prevention*, 10, 180–5.

Suffla, S., Kaminer, D., and Bawa, U. (2012). Photovoice as community engaged research: the interplay between knowledge creation and agency in a South African study on safety promotion. *Journal of Psychology in Africa*, 22, 519–28.

Viswanathan, M., Ammerman, A., and Eng, E. et al. (2004). *Community-based Participatory Research: Assessing the Evidence*. Evidence Report/Technology Assessment (2004) No. 99 (Prepared by RTI–University of North Carolina Evidence-based Practice Center under Contract No. 290-02-0016). AHRQ Publication 04-E022-2. Rockville, MD: Agency for Healthcare Research and Quality.

West, S., Wiseman, J., and Bertone, S. (2006). Mainstreaming change: learning from community strengthening in Victoria. *Just Policy: A Journal of Australian Social Policy*, 41, 34–40.

Wolff, T. (2001). Community coalition building—contemporary practice and research: Introduction. *American Journal of Community Psychology*, 29, 165–72.

SECTION 5

National and international policies to reduce violence

CHAPTER 35

Child protection policy

Robin J. Kimbrough-Melton and Gary B. Melton

Overview of Child Protection Policy

Societal efforts to protect children have existed in some form for centuries. During most of the nineteenth century, orphanages, sponsored by private, charitable organizations, cared for abandoned children (e.g. the Innocenti Centre in Italy). By the late 1800s, private organizations such as the New York Society for the Prevention of Cruelty to Children (NYSPCC) emerged to 'save' abused children (Schene 1998). As the first child protection agency in the world, the NYSPCC received and investigated complaints of child abuse and advocated for new laws to protect children. The NYSPCC also inspired analogous efforts in Great Britain in the late 1800s.

With origins in the United States, the formal child protection system that exists today in most of the developed democracies, and that is being emulated in the emerging democracies, is a relatively recent invention (dating from the early 1960s). In most countries, the system is organized around governmental intervention in families in response to allegations of child maltreatment. With some exceptions (e.g. Belgium, Russia, Switzerland), the central feature of the formal child protection system globally is mandated reporting of child abuse and neglect (Dubowitz 2012).

Mandated reporting emerged in the United States in the early 1960s after Denver paediatrician Henry Kempe and his colleagues 'discovered' the *battered child syndrome* (Kempe et al. 1962). Driven by a desire to prevent recurrence, Kempe and colleagues (1962) used the media to raise awareness of the problem while simultaneously advocating a mandated reporting policy to require health professionals to report suspected maltreatment to child protection authorities, who in turn would be responsible for investigating the allegations.

As intended, Kempe et al.'s (1962) advocacy generated unprecedented attention. In 1962, the U.S. Congress passed amendments to the Social Security Act that 'for the first time, identified Child Protective Services as part of all *public* child welfare' (De Francis 1967, p. 4). By 1967, every American state had adopted laws requiring professionals working with children, such as doctors and teachers, to report suspected child maltreatment. The shift of responsibility for child protection from the private sector to governmental agencies was solidified by 1974 when Congress passed the Child Abuse Prevention and Treatment Act.

Over the next 30 years, the evolution of child protection policy in the United States and globally was driven by the discovery of new problems (e.g. sexual abuse, psychological maltreatment), expansion of the definition of child abuse and neglect to encompass political realities and needs (e.g. Baby Doe regulations defining the withholding of 'medically indicated' treatment as child maltreatment) (Korbin 1994), and media attention to the most horrific failures of the system (Nelson 1986). High profile cases (e.g. Mary Ellen Wilson in New York; Maria Colwell in Great Britain) globally became the catalyst for increased state intervention to protect children from 'bad' parents.

Today the system that has evolved to protect children globally is widely, if not universally (see Drake and Pandey 1996; Mathews and Bross 2008), recognized as disastrous (Lonne et al. 2009; Melton 2005; Worley and Melton 2012). In that context, this chapter examines the evolution of child protection policy globally, the difficulties in implementing effective child protection systems, and possible directions for more humane and effective child protection systems designed to comport with international human rights law.

State of the Field

A System in Crisis

In 1990, after a generation of experience with the modern child protection system, the U.S. Advisory Board on Child Abuse and Neglect (U.S. ABCAN 1990) declared that child protection in the United States was in a state of emergency. The Board's declaration was based on astronomical growth in the number of child maltreatment reports, the growing complexity of family problems in the formal child protection system, and the misdirection of billions of dollars each year in a failing system. According to the Board, the most serious shortcoming of the child protection system was its reliance on a reporting and response process that is punitive in nature and that requires massive resources dedicated to the investigation of allegations of child maltreatment.

Analogous problems have been documented in other countries with systems oriented towards investigation (Lonne et al. 2009). However, as Lonne and colleagues have noted, the problems with child protection cannot be solved solely by getting rid of mandated reporting. The central problem in investigatory systems is the focus of the system on determining *what happened*, not *what can be done to help*.

What went Wrong?

The ineffectiveness of the child protection system can be tied to the initial assumptions underlying child protection policy, an overreliance on investigation, expansion of the scope of cases that come into the system, and significant social changes affecting children and families (Lonne et al. 2009; Melton 2005). Melton (2005, p. 10) has argued that the 'most fundamental mistake that the designers of modern child protection systems made was grossly to underestimate the scope of the problem of child abuse and neglect'. In contrast to the few hundred reports annually that Kempe et al. (1962) projected, each year millions (e.g. 3.4 million in 2011) of reports are made in the United States alone (U.S. Department of Health and Human Services 2012); a fact that has significant consequences for the effectiveness and the sustainability of the system and for the families who become involved with it.

Gradual expansion of the scope of cases to include issues of neglect related to such factors as poverty, intimate partner violence, poor parenting skills, and parental depression, has increased the numbers so significantly that it has become virtually impossible to help families with serious issues of maltreatment. The majority of the families involved in child protective services receive nothing other than an investigation (Lonne et al. 2009; Melton 2005). In the United States, approximately one-third of referrals to child protective services are 'screened out' as inappropriate for further action (Berrick 2011). Of the remaining two-thirds, only about one-quarter are 'substantiated' as likely that child maltreatment has occurred (Berrick 2011), and only about 40 per cent of these receive services. Similarly, in Australia, concern has been raised recently that only 30 per cent of the most serious child abuse cases in New South Wales are fully investigated (Power 2013). Thus, a common concern is that

> investigation occurs for its own sake, without any realistic hope of meaningful treatment to prevent the recurrence of maltreatment or to ameliorate its effects, even if the report of suspected maltreatment is validated. (U.S. ABCAN 1993, pp. 9–10)

Moreover, the over-inclusion of families for problems such as neglect has disproportionately affected children from minority groups often who live in low-income families. In the United States, children born to lower-income families have a referral rate that is more than 2.5 times higher than other children (Institute of Medicine 2012). As many as 35-40 per cent of children (White and African-American) living in low-income families may be reported to child protective services at some point (Wald 2014). However, African-American children are more likely than white children to be persistently poor (Wald 2014), and thus are more likely to be involved with the system. They are also disproportionately subjected to unsubstantiated re-reports of abuse or neglect (Worley and Melton 2012). The disproportionate impact of the child protection system on children from minority populations has been documented in other countries as well (Lonne et al. 2009).

The child protection system also is not well-equipped to help families who are referred for neglect because of 'inadequate parenting' that may negatively affect the child's development, but not safety (Wald 2014). Although evidence indicates that earlier intervention to help families produces better results, the allocation of resources primarily to investigation limits the capacity to provide services to most families. Moreover, the intrusiveness of the system and the stigma associated with referral to child protective services makes it less likely that families will engage in services provided by the state, even if services are voluntary.

International Policies

Because children are still developing, they have long been the recipients of special protection in international law. As early as 1924, the Geneva Declaration of the Rights of the Child recognized that states parties are obligated to ensure that children are 'protected against every form of exploitation' (Paragraph 4). In 1948, the Universal Declaration of Human Rights singled out children as being entitled to 'special care and assistance' (Article 25), a phrase that was later defined in the International Covenant of Economic, Social and Cultural Rights (1976) as meaning 'protection from economic and social exploitation' (Article 10, §3). Finally, in 1959, the Universal Declaration of the Rights of the Child further explicated the rights and needs of children, including the right to be protected from 'all forms of neglect, cruelty and exploitation' (Article 9). As precursors to the Convention on the Rights of the Child (CRC 1989), these documents were important for establishing a moral commitment to children. However, in contrast to the CRC, they are not legally binding in international law.

The CRC is a remarkably coherent and comprehensive statement of the basic rights that all children should enjoy and that governments should respect. Unanimously adopted by the United Nations General Assembly and quickly ratified by all but three governments (United States, Somalia, South Sudan), it has spawned a panoply of other documents. These include regional documents (e.g. African Charter on the Rights and Welfare of the Child, 1990; European Convention on the Exercise of Children's Rights, 1996), implementation strategies (e.g. Commission of the European Communities, 2006; South Asia Initiative to End Violence Against Children 2013), and General Comments from the Committee on the Rights of the Child (hereafter 'Committee').

Protecting Children Under the CRC

Article 19 of the CRC specifies the minimum obligations of states parties for the protection of children against *all forms of violence* while in the care of their parents or others. Articles 32, 33, and 34 expand on the protections of Article 19 by emphasizing the right to be protected from economic exploitation, illicit drugs, and sexual exploitation and sexual abuse, and Article 37 protects children from torture and cruel, inhuman, or degrading treatment or punishment. Finally two Optional Protocols on the involvement of children in armed conflict and on the sale of children, child prostitution, and child pornography address some of the worst forms of violence against children worldwide.

By requiring governments to take 'all appropriate legislative, administrative, social and educational measures' to protect the child, Article 19 places a high priority on child protection. Protective measures include prevention, but it is not enough that governments prevent child maltreatment. They must also provide support to the child and the child's caregivers to enable children to develop physically, mentally, morally, spiritually, and socially (Article 27) (Kimbrough-Melton 2014).

Article 19 focuses on the creation of a comprehensive child protection system including procedures for the 'identification, reporting, referral, investigation, treatment and follow-up of child maltreatment…and, as appropriate, for judicial involvement' (Article 19, §2). The inclusion of mandated reporting in the CRC is predictable since it was the principal component of child protection systems when the CRC was drafted. In monitoring reports, the Committee emphasizes the importance of a response system when egregious instances of child maltreatment occur (Hodgkin and Newell 2007). The Committee also has suggested that reporting mechanisms can be useful in raising awareness of abuse and neglect, especially in societies where strong social and cultural taboos prevent disclosure of abuse so that children who have been abused or neglected receive the help they need (Hodgkin and Newell 2007).

General Comment 13

Recognizing the inadequacy of governmental efforts in developing effective child protection systems, the Committee drafted General Comment 13 (Committee on the Rights of the Child 2011) to refocus implementation of Article 19 to align better with the original intent of the CRC. In addition to defining prohibited cultural and traditional practices, GC13 reminds governments of the obligation to implement preventive measures aimed at changing attitudes that perpetuate violence and targeting the root causes of violence (Paragraph 46).

National Policies

As a framework, the broad and constitutional nature of the language of the CRC, GC13, and related documents establishes norms and standards that can be useful in facilitating the development of more humane policies and practices at the national level. However, as noted by the Committee in GC13, the potential of the CRC in improving child protection policies at the national level has not been realized. Child protection systems and policies and the experience of governments in protecting children still vary widely across regions.

Gilbert (1997) compared child protection policies and practices in nine countries from North America and Western Europe. In the mid-1990s, countries could be classified based on the orientation of their child protection system. Regardless of whether they had voluntary or mandatory reporting, systems that were focused on investigating allegations of maltreatment had a child protection orientation (e.g. Canada, England, and the United States) while systems focused on providing services to maltreating families had a family service orientation (e.g. Nordic countries, Belgium, and Germany).

By the late 1990s, the policy context in these countries had changed. Media attention to high-profile failures, over-representation of minorities in child protective services, concern about the outcomes of children in out-of-home placement, the lack of services for families, and the unsustainable costs of operating child protective service systems, contributed to an environment focused on reform. Gradually, governments with a child protection orientation began to move towards a service orientation and those with a largely service orientation adopted more investigatory processes. For example, in the context of combatting social exclusion, England adopted an ambitious effort to 'modernize and broaden the role of children's services' (Parton and Berridge 2011, p. 63) that included child protection as an element. The terms 'protection' and 'abuse' were dropped from official documents and replaced by a duty 'to safeguard and promote the welfare of children…in need' (Parton and Berridge 2011, p. 63).

On the other hand, Belgium, which had a mostly family service orientation in the early 1990s, began to incorporate features of the child protection orientation. Historically, Belgium had had a public–private system where Confidential Centres handled reported cases of child maltreatment and private services, funded with public money, helped families in need. After the high-profile Dutroux case in 1996 involving extra-familial sexual abuse of six young girls, a series of reform proposals strengthened

legal protections for minors and allowed physicians to bypass the Confidential Centres and report suspected abuse directly to the authorities. Public opinion also changed in favour of detecting child abuse (Desair and Adriaenssens 2011). Despite these shifts in orientation, reforms have largely failed to produce significant improvements in the protection of children.

Child protection has not progressed any more rapidly in the developing world. Between 2007 and 2009, researchers surveyed 42 countries from Africa, the Americas, Asia, Europe, and the Middle East/North Africa to assess whether governments had incorporated Article 19 into their domestic law (Svevo-Cianci et al. 2010). Only 14 (33 per cent) of the 42 had established at least a basic child protection system, defined as having measures in each of the three primary areas (e.g. laws and policies; education, training, services and data management; monitoring and evaluation of progress related to the child's well-being) (Svevo-Cianci et al. 2010).

In the developing countries, legal systems, especially in formerly colonized countries that inherited a variety of legal traditions, have been a substantial barrier to incorporation of Article 19 into existing legislation (Goonesekere 2007). Many of the national plans of action adopted by some governments to implement the rights of the child include 'measures to prohibit, prevent and eliminate all forms of violence against children' (GC13, Paragraph 68). However, legal reform in the absence of social and economic reform is insufficient. Many of these efforts have been insufficiently connected to overall development policy, programmes, budget, and coordinating mechanisms to be very effective in protecting children (GC13 2013, Paragraph 68).

To promote the development of systems across government ministries and civil society, United Nations Children's Fund (UNICEF) and non-governmental organizations (NGOs) like Save the Children and World Vision have been working with countries in southeast Europe, Africa, Asia, and the Middle East to describe and analyse their existing child protection systems, including identifying strengths and best practices, and weaknesses and gaps, describing the policy context and reviewing the legal framework, and assessing services, staffing, and other resources that are required to serve children comprehensively (Wulczyn et al. 2010). The goal is to create a common understanding of existing structures, build public consensus, strengthen coordination among sectors (e.g. social protection, education, health) and between community networks and formal systems, and guide national decision-making.

Finally, regional human rights instruments and standards (e.g. the African Charter on the Rights and Welfare of the Child) have been used to facilitate integration of Article 19 into domestic law and advance child protection. Because the CRC has been viewed as too 'Western' in some regions, it was thought that regional instruments could contextualize the provisions of the CRC and address some of the practical problems in incorporating the rights into different legal traditions. However, the use of regional instruments to strengthen child protection generally has not led to significant law reform (Goonesekere 2007). In Eastern and Southern Africa, for example, nearly all of the countries have ratified the CRC and the African Charter. Regardless, only seven of the 21 countries have enacted a comprehensive Children's Act to bring their national child protection legislative framework into line with the CRC.

A Public Health Approach to Child Maltreatment

To address the deficiencies of current child protection schemes, national and sub-national governments and NGOs are gradually adopting a public health approach to child maltreatment. For example, the Centres for Disease Control and Prevention (http://www.cdc.gov/violenceprevention/overview/strategicdirec tions.html) in the United States has adopted a new strategy for child maltreatment prevention that emphasizes the promotion of safe, stable, and nurturing relationships between children and caregivers.

The attractiveness of the public health approach to child maltreatment prevention lies in its potential for focusing on prevention and health promotion not only at the individual and family levels but also at the community level. It acknowledges growing evidence of the importance of neighbourhoods to child safety and the desirability of intervening as early as possible to ensure that children reach their full potential. Moreover, because public health strategies address the underlying determinants of health (e.g. housing, income), which have been shown to be related to child abuse and neglect, a public health approach has the potential to engage a broader array of stakeholders (e.g. educators, law enforcement, business and religious leaders, civic organizations, local government) and professionals (e.g. paediatricians) in partnership with community members to provide advocacy and support to parents early to prevent child maltreatment.

Local Policies

The interest in public health strategies at the national and sub-national level is leading to experimentation with new strategies at the local level. In general, two types of reform efforts have emerged: (i) those stimulated by governmental agencies to improve outcomes for families who are already involved in the system, and (ii) those stimulated by NGOs and foundations to prevent child abuse and neglect.

Systems Changes

For the most part, efforts by child welfare agencies to engage community partners (e.g. faith communities, business sector, schools) generally have been focused on increasing the availability of services usually through community partnerships to families already involved with child protection and enhancing the likelihood that families will participate in services. Differential Response (also referred to as dual-track, multiple-track, and alternative response systems) and Family Group Conferencing are two such strategies. Other strategies have included collaboration between agencies, co-locating child welfare workers with health professionals, and better training of caseworkers.

Community Approaches

Research documenting the significance of community context and neighbourhood resources in child well-being led the U.S. ABCAN (1993) to call for a coordinated, comprehensive, community-based approach to child protection with a focus on supporting children in their environment—in the family, at school, in the neighbourhood and community. The U.S. ABCAN's approach was reinforced by GC13's emphasis on prevention and implementation of child protection strategies at the local level.

The few community-based approaches to protect children have varied widely in their goals, core components, comprehensiveness, and fundamental beliefs about how to enhance safety for children. Like Differential Response, most have sought to strengthen partnerships between child welfare agencies and local community agencies to enhance the availability of services for families. However, unlike Differential Response, they tend to be more preventative in reaching families before problems become serious.

Still another approach is represented by Strong Communities for Children (Melton 2014), which was implemented by the authors in selected counties of South Carolina. Based on the vision outlined by the U.S. ABCAN (1993), Strong Communities uses a principle-driven approach to community mobilization. The engagement of community residents in child protection is designed to lead to normative change and to foster an increased sense of community responsibility for 'keeping kids safe'. Grounded in a public health approach, Strong Communities emphasizes universal support to families combined with targeted support to higher need families. With more than 5,000 volunteers, Strong Communities demonstrated that ordinary citizens place a high priority on child protection and when engaged, will participate in ensuring that all families are part of the community. Substantiated cases of maltreatment for children aged 4 and under decreased by 41 per cent in the service area but increased by 49 per cent in the comparison area. Emergency room visits and inpatient stays attributable to neglect declined by 68 per cent for children of all ages in the service area but by only 19 per cent in the comparison area.

Conclusion

After more than 50 years of experience with the modern child protection system and abundant evidence that the system is overburdened, costly, and ineffective in achieving its intended outcomes, remarkably little has changed in the functioning of the system. Indeed, developing democracies are following the lead of the United States, the United Kingdom, Australia, and others in adopting child protection policies that have uniformly been shown to be ineffective.

Historically, child protection policy has been driven by horrific cases of child deaths, sexual exploitation, and other forms of abuse. Because serious child abuse is horrific, media attention often evokes an emotional response and desire for change. However, perhaps because the portrayal of child maltreatment is so lopsided, policy never really gets developed in the way it should. Rather, the most likely response after a bad case is tinkering with the investigative system (e.g. expanding the list of mandated reporters).

Nelson (1986) suggested that the lack of serious reform may result from the fact that child abuse is a valence issue—an issue that engenders a uniform visceral response among the public but often no consensus about how best to address the problem. In these instances, responses often tend to focus on strategies that are ultimately symbolic and likely to be acceptable to the public (e.g. strengthening mandated reporting laws after a scandal, or implementing better training of caseworkers after a child death) but that do little to remodel a system that is broken.

Although there is a consensus that significant reform is necessary, there is no agreement on the nature of the reform. Wald (2012) has called for a re-evaluation of the desired outcomes for children that are important to society. He argues that:

> framing the issue as maltreatment focuses on the wrong outcome; we should seek positive development, not just the absence of harm. (p. 184)

Others, like the authors, have argued for engaging the broader community in assuming responsibility for child safety and in generating new norms of support for families. The most likely scenario is a combination of both strategies—that is, reframing the problem to focus on developing a child's strengths and engaging communities to enhance the likelihood that families are supported in their day-to-day life. Although this approach is consistent with principles of international human rights law of treating people with dignity and respect, it is likely to require persistence and political will of the sort demonstrated by Kempe et al. (1962) 50 years ago.

References

African Charter on the Rights and Welfare of the Child, OAU Doc. CAB/LEG/24.9/49 (1990), *entered into force* 29 November 1999.

Berrick, J. D. (2011). Trends and issues in the U. S. Child Welfare system. In: N. Gilbert, N. Parton, and M. Skivenes (eds), *Child Protection Systems. International Trends and Orientations.* New York: Oxford University Press, pp. 17–35.

Centres for Disease Control and Prevention. Available at: http://www.cdc.gov/violenceprevention/overview/strategicdirections.html [Accessed 05 December 2013].

Commission of the European Communities. *Towards an EU Strategy on the Rights of the Child.* Brussels, 4 July 2006.

Committee on the Rights of the Child (2011). *General Comment No. 13: The Right of the Child to Freedom from all Forms of Violence.* 18 April 2011, CRC/C/GC/13. Available at http://www.refworld.org/docid/4e6da4922.html [Accessed 18 November 2013].

Convention on the Rights of the Child, G.A. res. 44/25, annex, 44 U.N. GAOR Supp. (No. 49) at 167, U.N. Doc. A/44/49 (1989), *entered into force* 02 Sept. 1990.

De Francis, V. (1967). *Child Protective Services: A National Survey.* Denver: American Humane Association.

Desair, K., and Adriaenssens, P. (2011). Policy toward child abuse and neglect in Belgium: shared responsibility, differentiated response. In: N. Gilbert, N. Parton, and M. Skivenes (eds), *Child Protection Systems. International Trends and Orientations.* New York: Oxford University Press, pp. 204–22.

Drake, B., and Pandey, S. (1996). Understanding the relationship between neighborhood poverty and specific types of child maltreatment. *Child Abuse & Neglect,* 20, 1003–18.

Dubowitz, H. (2012). *World Perspectives on Child Abuse.* 10th ed. Aurora: International Society for Prevention of Child Abuse and Neglect.

European Convention on the Exercise of Children's Rights, (Strasbourg, 25 January 1996; entered into force 1 July 2000).

Geneva Declaration of the Rights of the Child, adopted 26 September 1924, League of Nations, O.J. Spec. Supp. 21, at 43 (1924).

Gilbert, N. (1997). *Combatting Child Abuse: International Perspectives and Trends.* New York: Oxford University Press.

Goonesekere, S. (2007). Introduction and overview. In: UNICEF (ed.), *Protecting the World's Children. Impact of the Convention on the Rights of the Child in Diverse Legal Systems.* New York: Cambridge University Press, pp. 1–34.

Hodgkin, R., and Newell, P. (2007). *Implementation Handbook for the Convention on the Rights of the Child.* Geneva: UNICEF.

Institute of Medicine (IOM) and National Research Council (NRC). (2012). *Child Maltreatment Research, Policy and Practice for the Next Decade.* Washington, D.C.: National Academies Press.

International Covenant on Economic, Social and Cultural Rights, G.A. res. 2200A (XXI), 21 U.N. GAOR Supp. (No. 16) at 49, U.N. Doc. A/6316 (1966). 993 U.N.T.S. 3, entered into force 3 Jan. 1976.

Kempe, C. H., Silverman, F. N., and Steele, B. F. et al. (1962). The battered child syndrome.*Journal of the American Medical Association,* 181, 17–24.

Kimbrough-Melton, R. J. (2014). Child maltreatment as a problem in international law. In: J. E. Korbin, and R. D. Krugman (eds), *Handbook of Child Maltreatment.* Vol. 2. Dordrecht: Springer, pp. 541–51.

Korbin, J. E. (1994). Sociocultural factors in child maltreatment. In: G. B. Melton, and F. D. Barry (eds.). *Protecting Children from Abuse and Neglect. Foundations for a New National Strategy.* New York: Guilford, pp. 183–223.

Lonne, B., Parton, N., and Thomson, J., et al. (2009). *Reforming Child Protection.* Oxford: Routledge.

Mathews, B. P., and Bross, D. C. (2008). Mandated reporting is still a policy with reason: empirical evidence and philosophical grounds. *Child Abuse and Neglect,* 32, 511–6.

Melton, G. B. (2005). Mandated reporting: a policy without reason. *Child Abuse & Neglect,* 25, 9–18.

Melton, G. B. (2014). Strong Communities for Children: a community-wide approach to prevention of child maltreatment. In: J. E. Korbin, and R. D. Krugman (eds), *Handbook of Child Maltreatment.* Dordrecht: Springer.

Nelson, B. J. (1986). *Making an Issue of Child Abuse: Political Agenda Setting for Social Problems.* Chicago: University of Chicago Press.

Parton, N., and Berridge, D. (2011). Child protection in England. In: N. Gilbert, N. Parton., and M. Skivenes. (eds.). *Child Protection Systems. International Trends and Orientations.* New York: Oxford University Press, pp. 60–85.

Power, J. (2013). 'The system is failing the children of this state': most child abuse cases closed early, says PSA. *Sydney Morning Herald,* 26 June 2013. Available at: http://www.smh.com.au/nsw/the-system-is-failing-the-children-of-this-state-most-child-abuse-cases-closed-early-says-psa-20130625-2ovc3.html. [Accessed 28 June 2013].

Schene, P. A. (1998). Past, present, and future roles of child protective services. *The Future of Children,* 8, 23–38.

South Asia Initiative to End Violence against Children. Available at: http://www.saievac.org/. [Accessed 18 December 2013].

Svevo-Cianci, K. A., Hart, S. N., and Rubinson, C. (2010). Protecting children from violence and maltreatment: a qualitative comparative analysis assessing the implementation of U.N. CRC Article 19. *Child Abuse & Neglect,* 34, 45–56.

U.S. Advisory Board on Child Abuse and Neglect. (1990). *Child Abuse and Neglect: Critical First Steps in Response to a National Emergency.* Washington, D.C.: U.S. Government Printing Office.

U.S. Advisory Board on Child Abuse and Neglect. (1993). *Neighbors Helping Neighbors: A New National Strategy for the Protection of Children.* Washington, D.C.: U.S. Government Printing Office.

U.S. Department of Health and Human Services. (2012). *Child Maltreatment 2011.* Available at: http://www.acf.hhs.gov/programs/cb/research-data-technology/statistics-research/child-maltreatment. [Accessed 20 May 2013].

Universal Declaration of Human Rights, G.A. res. 217A (III), U.N. Doc. A/810 at 71 (1948).

Universal Declaration of the Rights of the Child, G.A. res. 1386 (XIV), 14 U.N. GAOR Supp. (No. 16) at 19, U.N. Doc. A/4354 (1959).

Wald, M. S. (2012). Preventing maltreatment or promoting positive development—where should a community focus its resources? A policy perspective. In: R. D. Krugman, and J. E. Korbin (eds.). *C. Henry Kempe: A 50 Year Legacy to the Field of Child Abuse and Neglect.* Dordrecht: Springer, pp. 182–95.

Wald, M.S. (2014). Beyond maltreatment: developing support for children in multiproblem families. In: J. E. Korbin, and R. D. Krugman (eds), *Handbook of Child Maltreatment.* Vol. 2, Dordrecht: Springer, pp. 251–80.

Worley, N., and Melton, G. B. (2012). Mandated reporting laws and child maltreatment: the evolution of a flawed policy response. In: R. D. Krugman, and J. E. Korbin (eds.). *C. Henry Kempe: A 50 Year Legacy to the Field of Child Abuse and Neglect.* Dordrecht: Springer, pp. 103–18.

Wulczyn, F., Daro, D., and Fluke, J. et al. (2010). *Adapting a Systems Approach to Child Protection: Key Concepts and Considerations.* New York: UNICEF.

CHAPTER 36

International, national, and local government policies to reduce youth violence

Margaret Shaw

Introduction to International, National, and Local Government Policies to Reduce Youth Violence

Policies on youth violence are often developed in the wake of a series of violent events, or in response to public concern about increasing violence involving young people. In that sense they are developed *after* problems have become evident. Governments and policymakers are placed in the difficult position of having to respond both to violent events themselves, and to public pressure to take strong and decisive action. This can often lead to the introduction of tough measures which satisfy public demands, and create an aura of control and stability. Yet youth violence, as is clear from other chapters in this book, has its roots in a complex series of causal factors which range from individual and family attributes, to social and economic conditions in local communities, and broader societal influences. Just being repressive can exacerbate the problems.

Toughening legislation and sentencing options for youth violence may have some immediate deterrent impacts, but can also be very counter-productive. They can reinforce criminal and violent lifestyles, and make it difficult for young people to be reintegrated back into their communities (Jutersonke et al. 2009; Ukeje and Iwilade 2012). They are costly—youth custody facilities, for example, require considerable funding and resources compared with alternative options. More importantly, toughening criminal justice options does not deal with the root causes of youth violence. It does not respond to the problems which led to the violent events, to the development of violent lifestyles, nor does it strengthen the protective factors which can help future young people find alternative ways of life. They may also violate young people's human rights.

Based on our accumulating knowledge of effective and evidence-based practice, we know that there are some very effective and cost beneficial programmes which have diverted young people from violence, or enabled them to exit violent lifestyles (Kennedy 2007; Organization for Economic Cooperation and Development (OECD) 2011; Savignac and Leonard 2011; Willman and Makisaka 2010; World Health Organization (WHO) 2010). They have helped reduce the influence of factors which facilitate violence, such as involvement in substance abuse and the presence of drugs and guns. Yet an effective programme in itself is only *one* response—an overall policy is needed—whether at the national, regional, or local level—and it is likely to be most effective if it is a policy which respects the rights of children and young people, and internationally agreed values about the treatment of young people and the reduction of youth crime. A coherent and comprehensive policy—based on careful analysis of the issues and their causal factors, and including a range of interventions responding to the specific needs identified—is more likely to bring about sustainable reductions in youth violence in the medium and long-term. This chapter reviews the emergence of youth violence prevention policies internationally, grounded in effective practice.

Policy Intervention and Evidence: A Problem of Youth or a Problem for Youth

In August 2011, the killing of a young black man by police in London, sparked an intense wave of rioting, looting, and destruction over 4 days, which subsequently spread to other parts of London and at least five major cities in the country. The immediate reaction from politicians was to blame 'the criminal classes', and gangs in particular, for coordinating the riots. The Minister of Justice Kenneth Clarke even referred to the rioters as coming from the 'feral underclass' (Newburn 2011). However, an in-depth study of the events, based on detailed interviews with rioters, victims, police, and lawyers, suggests that in fact there was very marginal gang involvement (*Guardian* and LSE 2011). It also showed that the rioters were overwhelmingly male (79 per cent) and young, two-thirds of them less than 21 years of age. They were primarily from poor and disadvantaged communities, often unemployed or on welfare supports, and almost half of them were students. The rioters felt a general sense of injustice and lack of opportunities and jobs, but the driving force appeared to be widespread anger and frustration at the police and their interactions with their communities, especially the use of aggressive stop and search policies targeting young (black) men. Subsequent government announcements promised there would be radical changes which would focus the penal system more concertedly on strong punishment to reduce offending. The United Kingdom government has, however, acknowledged that 'entrenched educational and social failures' (United Kingdom Government 2011 p. 7) underlay the violence, although they still identify gangs as a major concern.

The events and reactions in England could be applied to many other cities and countries, from the United States or El Salvador to South Africa. Young men—rather than young women—are primarily the instigators and victims of urban violence and homicide (United Nations Office on Drugs and Crime (UNODC) 2011). Urban youth violence is often concentrated in the poorest areas in cities, whether slums, public housing estates, decaying urban centres, or poorly served suburbs. In low- and middle-income countries the rapid growth of cities exacerbates the growth of slums and informal settlements with very poor living conditions, lack of facilities, transport, health, education or employment, and very little connection to the benefits of urban life. Gated communities and the expansion of private security in many countries reinforce the exclusion of those populations. The majority of the world's population now lives in cities, and the trend continues. Further, the majority of the expanding urban population are children and young people and it has been estimated that 60 per cent of urban populations will be under the age of 18 by 2030 (UN HABITAT 2010a). As with areas where armed youth violence is endemic, such as in Central America and the Caribbean, it is the persistent poverty, inequality, and social exclusion coupled with the presence of facilitators such as organized crime and trafficking in drugs and guns, which characterize many of the communities where youth violence occurs (Jutersonke et al. 2009).

The absence of meaningful employment is also a very common concern. A World Bank report concludes 'there is a strong perception in all of the communities studied that unemployment, especially of youth, is driving violence' (World Bank 2011 p. xv). Conversely UN HABITAT sees education as a driver for opportunity equality (UN HABITAT 2010a).

Finally, poor relations between the police and communities are characteristic of urban and youth violence. In spite of huge regional differences in political, cultural, social, and economic contexts, perceptions and trust in the police, and community strengths are almost universal concerns (Ward et al. 2012; World Bank 2011). Community perceptions are crucial in developing policies to respond to violence, in particular rebuilding trust between communities and the police, and building social capital.

Evolution in Policy Responses: Redirecting the Focus to the *Conditions* which Facilitate Youth Violence

Over the past 20 years the recognition that the root causes of youth violence must be tackled, and that youth and their communities are less the problem than part of the solution, has increased attention to prevention. This has led to significant changes in the kinds of policies being implemented. Whether they have emerged through a public health, a crime prevention and citizen security, a development, or an urban regeneration perspective, they have very similar characteristics and compatibility with the WHO ecological model (Shaw 2009, 2012). There has been a convergence of opinion on the importance of preventing violence using strategic planned interventions in cities and neighbourhoods. Such policies take account of the specific contexts in which violence emerges, undertake careful assessment of causal factors and needs, and utilize a multi-sector and multi-partnership approach, with close collaboration between institutions, communities, civil society, and young people themselves.

This evolution in policy has been coupled with changes in the delivery of international aid to low and middle income countries to increase effectiveness and sustainability. The 2005 *Paris Declaration on Aid Effectiveness* recognized the importance of country ownership in policy and programme development, and taking account of their own analysis of needs and timetables, rather than those of donor agencies (OECD 2005).

International Policies Guiding Youth Violence Policy: A Universal Consensus

A number of international norms and standards now guide national policy development on children and youth. They include the 1989 UN Convention on the Rights of the Child; the 1990 UN Guidelines for the Prevention of Juvenile Delinquency; and the 1997 UN Guidelines for action on children in the criminal justice system. These guidelines set out the principles on which relevant policies should be based, whether to prevent entry into the justice system, or on how the justice system should treat young people.

Further, the *prevention* rather than repression of youth violence is supported by the UN's 1995 Guidelines for Cooperation and Technical Assistance in the Field of Urban Crime Prevention, and the 2002 UN Guidelines for the Prevention of Crime. Both focus on the development of strategic plans at national, and at local government level where crime has its biggest impact. The basic principles for developing prevention policies in the 2002 UN Guidelines include:

◆ government leadership

◆ socioeconomic development and inclusion

◆ cooperation and partnerships

◆ sustainability and accountability

◆ use of a knowledge base

◆ Human rights and a culture of lawfulness

◆ interdependency

◆ differentiation.

The Guidelines identify a range of types of prevention approaches, from crime prevention through social development including early intervention, family and school programmes, community-based programmes, situational prevention, and rehabilitation (Box 36.1).

The principles underlying all of these international guidelines stress the importance of developing comprehensive approaches grounded in systematic analysis, working at different levels (with families, individuals, communities, and educational, health, social, and justice services) providing opportunities and engaging the active participation of children, young people, and their communities in the development of interventions. They are concerned not only with the *types* of programmes which can be used as part of a policy (what works), but with the ways in which they

Box 36.1 Characteristics of Effective Programmes to Prevent Armed Violence in Urban Areas

- Be rooted in the context in which they will be implemented
- Logically link problems to perceived drivers and to measurable outcomes
- Draw on the evidence base
- Address more than one risk factor
- Engage multiple sectors
- Intervene at multiple levels (OECD 2011, pp. 17–8).

Source: data from Organization for Economic Co-operation and Development (OECD), *Preventing and reducing armed violence in urban areas: programming note,* Conflict and Fragility, OECD Publishing, Paris, France, Copyright © 2011, http://dx.doi.org/10.1787/9789264107199-en

are *implemented* to ensure their effectiveness (how they work). They encourage collaborative partnerships between institutional services, local communities, and stakeholders which will help to sustain policies and programmes over time, and ensure accountability in terms of responsibilities and use of resources. They emphasize upholding the human rights of young people, non-discrimination, and the importance of tailoring policies to take account of gender, cultural, and ethnic differences and needs. For example, while boys are the main victims and perpetrators of violence, developing programmes for girls too recognizes that they may also lack alternative lifestyles, may condone or become involved in violence, be sexually abused, or become teenage mothers. In addition, the crime prevention guidelines emphasize the importance of government leadership at national and local levels, and of developing social and economic strategies which include, rather than exclude, individuals and groups in the community.

This consensus on the components for developing effective prevention is shared by many international agencies including UN HABITAT, UNODC, WHO, the World Bank, the Inter-American Development Bank (IDB), and the OECD. It has been the basis for UN HABITAT's Safer Cities Programme established in 1996, for the Inter-American Development Bank's Citizen Security Programme, and United Nations Development Programme's (UNDP) citizen security focus among others (UNDP 2012). A number of tools now exist to assist countries in developing policies which comply with these international norms (e.g. UNODC and UN HABITAT 2009; UNODC 2010).

National and State Policies

Many European countries and others including Brazil, Colombia, El Salvador, Mexico, South Africa, and Trinidad and Tobago, have adopted national or regional policies to reduce youth violence and promote healthy lifestyles based on these principles (Burton 2012; Jutersonke et al. 2009; Shaw and Carli 2011). They may be stand-alone youth policies, or form part of broader safety and security policy, but they all accept the central responsibility of the national government to support and facilitate action at the local level and base policy development on sound evidence. In Central

America, for example, there has been a shift in recent years from the repressive *mano dura* (hard hand) approach established in El Salvador in 2003 to respond to youth gangs and violence, to what is termed a *mano amiga* or *extendida* (friendly or extended hand) policy. In Honduras there has been a similar shift from the *cero toleranza* (zero tolerance) policy adopted in 2003 (Jutersonke et al. 2009).

Brazil has adopted policies to respond to endemic youth violence. Youth homicides in that country illustrate all the elements of the age, race, geography, and gender of urban youth violence. The homicide rate for those aged 0–18 years rose by 346 per cent from 1980 to 2010 (from a rate of 3.1 per 100,000 children and youth to 13.8 by 2010), to overtake all other causes of death for this age group (Waiselfisz 2012). Ninety per cent of homicide victims are male and the majority between the ages of 15 and 18. There are also very marked regional variations reflecting social and economic patterns across Brazil: from a rate of 5.3 per 100,000 children and adolescents in the city of Sao Paulo, to 79.8 per 100,000 in Maceio (Box 36.2).

While federal youth-directed policies existed previously, under the leadership of President Lula in 2007 the government launched a major national policy to respond to levels of violence, including youth violence. The *Programa Nacional de Seguridad Pública con Ciudadania* or PRONASCI—included structural interventions to improve the justice system and capacity of the police and other professionals, and funding to support states and municipalities in developing locally based interventions in high-risk areas (UNODC 2011). A significant funding requirement is that municipalities must create an integrated management department to be responsible for coordinating their projects. PRONASCI was partly modelled on the successful experience of the city of Diadema discussed under 'Local government policies'.

For the youth population, PRONASCI focuses on the social and economic exclusion of the most vulnerable youth. It encourages social and educational programmes which target root causes of violence, and recognizes the need for basic government services and good infrastructure in poor neighbourhoods (Perez 2009).

Trinidad and Tobago has also experienced very high rates of homicide resulting from changes in drug trafficking routes in the region. Its *Citizen Security Programme* under the Ministry of National Security was initiated in 2008 with the Inter-American Development Bank (IDB) as part of their broader Citizen Security initiative (Alvarado and Abizanda 2010; http://csp.gov.tt/). The

Box 36.2 The Open Schools Programme in Brazil

The Open Schools programme (Abrindo Espacos) initiated by UNESCO and adopted by the Brazil Ministry of Education in 2004, offered education, culture, sports, and work training to local youth at weekends. Evaluation of the programme in some 5,306 schools in Sao Paulo showed that between 2003 and 2006, crime in the surrounding areas of the schools involved was reduced by 45.5 per cent (Willman and Makisaka 2010, p. 37).

Source: data from Willman, A., and Makisaka, M., *Interpersonal violence prevention. A review of the evidence and emerging lessons,* World Development Report 2011 Background Paper, World Bank, Washington, DC, USA, Copyright © 2010 programme aims to reduce crime and violence by addressing key risk factors, and is focused on 22 high-need communities across the two islands, using a range of community-based prevention strategies. These include rapid impact projects which provide 'quick wins' enabling local communities and institutions to see results, grants to community organizations for micro projects, event sponsorship, community-based social interventions, public education, school-based violence reduction, training for community-based committees and organizations, and the creation of youth-friendly spaces. The programme also includes institutional strengthening of the Ministry of National Security and the Trinidad and Tobago Police Service. The overall programme and individual projects are being systematically monitored and evaluated.

In Europe, the Violence Reduction Unit, created in 2005, was established to focus on violent crime by youth, particularly knife crime and weapon carrying in Glasgow. Its core belief, adopting the WHO approach, is that violence is not a primarily a justice issue, but a public health one, which requires collaborative and long-term work among a wide range of institutions and communities to change social conditions and attitudes. The Glasgow *Community Initiative to Reduce Violence* combines targeted intervention and dissuasion for the most criminally engaged youth, with more general prevention programmes. The running of the project was handed over to the Strathclyde Police Force and it has achieved significant reductions in violent offending and weapon carrying. In 2006, the government of Scotland adopted the approach of the Violence Reduction Unit and extended its remit across the whole country (see United Kingdom Government 2011 and www.actiononviolence.com/CIRV).

In the United Kingdom since the late 1990s a number of prevention policies to support early childhood, family, and youth have been initiated on the premise that risk factors can be reduced, and policies require cross-government 'joined-up' collaboration (in particular the initiatives developed under the government of Tony Blair). Following the 2011 riots, a cross-government report on their plan of action proposes multi-agency and community partnerships in four areas: providing support to local authorities to tackle youth violence and gang problems; preventing young people from becoming involved in violence through early intervention; providing 'pathways out' of violent lifestyles especially through employment, skills, and education; and using extended judicial powers to suppress violence and gangs. The report acknowledges the problem of entrenched social and educational failure. New legislation will give local authorities greater autonomy to plan action and pool resources through 'Community Budgets' (United Kingdom Government 2011).

Local Government Policies

While national or state governments have a major leadership role, youth violence occurs at the local level and its root causes are primarily local. Many national and state policies focus on supporting local level policies and programmes. Regardless of the quality of a country's youth justice system, overall economic and social policies or endorsement of international standards, what happens at the local level is key. Municipal governments can make a very significant difference in the prevention of youth violence and this section provides some examples of effective interventions.

Such policies often combine a range of targeted social, educational, and health interventions, school-based curriculum programmes, sports, cultural, and recreation programmes, urban upgrading and situational crime prevention, with problem-oriented community policing and 'social urbanism' approaches (Shaw and Carli 2011; UNODC 2010). They work with local 'at risk' youth, both girls and boys, in participatory ways, and with neighbourhoods and civil society (including NGOs and the private sector) (Shaw, 2012; UN HABITAT 2010b). In most cases they are supported by higher levels of government, as in the case of Brazil's PRONASCI programme. This may include overall policy guidance, funding, and other support. Examples of city strategies with strong youth violence prevention components include the Boston Gun Project which has inspired many United States and other cities to apply similar approaches (Kennedy 2007); and a range of cities in Canada which have received funding from the federal government to implement 'model' youth violence and gang prevention programmes as part of broader youth strategies. They include the Abbotsford Youth Crime Prevention Project, and the Montreal *Programme de Suivi Intensif—Gangs de Rue*. Modelled on successful programmes developed elsewhere, they target specific high risk groups, working at the neighbourhood level, combining police, education, social, youth and environment services, and local community groups (Canada 2013).

The City of Diadema, Brazil developed an effective comprehensive policy to reduce the high level of homicides and prevent the involvement of young people in violence. Under the strong leadership of the mayor, the ten-point security plan integrated police operations and created neighbourhood policing; instituted geo-coding to map daily criminal activity; improved supports to schools; developed youth apprenticeship schemes for young people from the poorest favelas; supported environmental upgrading in the favelas, and public education on disarmament (Shaw and Travers, 2007; World Bank 2011). A municipal regulation, systematically enforced, closed all bars and restaurants between 11.00 pm and 6.00 am. Following the implementation of the plan in 2000, by 2004 there was an 80 per cent drop in homicides and other crimes. The process was participatory and inclusive, with regular consultations between city officials and citizens in each ward, and a participatory budgeting system enabling local citizens to allocate a percentage of municipal funds for area projects.

The *Fica Vivo* (Stay Alive) programme in Belo Horizonte, Brazil is a cost-effective state-municipal partnership which has achieved up to 47 per cent reductions in homicides in the areas where it has been implemented. Initially modelled on the Boston Gun Project but adapted to the Brazilian context, it involves partnerships between community police and municipal and state social programmes working together in the target sites and building the capacity of local residents and youth (World Bank 2011).

Evaluating and Building the Evidence Base: Current Weaknesses

What evidence is there of the impact of multi-sector partnership approaches? There is considerable evidence of the effectiveness of individual programmes, and some evidence of effective comprehensive strategies (Muggah 2012; World Bank 2011). However, evaluating youth violence prevention policies which use a range of interventions and multi-layered approaches is a complex process not amenable to randomized controlled trials. In addition, as Jutersonke et al. (2009) have stressed, crime and violence are highly heterogeneous within regions, and differences between countries in local conditions, socio-economic, political, and historical characteristics means that uniform impact cannot be expected. A further problem is the failure of many projects to invest in evaluation. In relation to Central America, for example, it is suggested that national governments are good at implementing and 'talking up' multi-sector prevention policies to attract international donor funding and aid, but little systematic evaluation is undertaken (Jutersonke et al. 2009). A review of community-policing in Latin America similarly reports a variable range of results, and identifies two crucial components for effectiveness: *support* for community policing by key actors from the national government (including presidents) to neighbourhood residents, and *continuity* in that support (Ungar and Arias 2012). Changes in government personnel, in governments, corruption, and insufficient resources can all threaten policy continuity in countries and cities, and longer-term outcomes.

A number of flexible approaches to evaluating complex community policy and programmes have emerged in recent years. They include mixed methods and 'RealWorld' approaches, 'theory of change', and performance management (Bamberger et al. 2006; Patton 2011). These approaches accept that policy must be adapted to context; that rapid results are not easily achieved and short-term interventions cannot be expected to produce long-term change; that problems are to be expected and solutions anticipated; and that investment in good data collection and monitoring is essential. They use mixed methods approaches to 'triangulate' data, collecting both qualitative and quantitative information on subject and comparison groups from a variety of sources, such as victimization, community satisfaction and internet surveys, case studies, observation, and data from a range of sources including police, justice, environmental, educational, and health systems. Some of the measures developed may be participatory in that they are developed by the subjects themselves.

Evaluation will usually be grounded in a logical framework such as a 'theory of change' approach matching inputs to expected outcomes in the given context. These will be measured by a set of agreed upon indicators, and assess not only whether a programme has been implemented as planned (process), but also its short-, medium-, and longer-term outcomes. These may include not only changes in levels of violence or gang membership, for example, but also changes in education and skills levels, social functioning, or attitudes among the youth involved, and community and police assessments of changes in local conditions.

Given that the evaluation of programmes requires considerable skills and resources, and the scaling up of projects is often unsuccessful, the use of performance management has also been suggested. This provides careful guidance on evaluating the overall effectiveness of a complex intervention programme, but allows for more rigorous evaluation of a specific group of programmes using, for example, quasi-experimental designs (Morgan and Homel 2013).

Conclusions

While it is not always easy to show precise links between youth violence policies and changes in levels of violence, there has been very wide application of comprehensive youth policies under good leadership in many countries, with a strong focus on tailoring them to the specific needs of communities and at-risk populations and areas. This includes early intervention, school-based programmes, and programmes promoting youth development through arts, media, sports, recreation, education, and skills training. For the most vulnerable young people—those in care, homeless, already exposed or involved in gang cultures and violence, or in the criminal justice system—targeted programmes to strengthen their capacities and provide them with alternative life skills are essential components, especially with the participation of young people themselves (UN HABITAT 2010b). At the national and city levels policies addressing employment opportunities and viable livelihoods; rebuilding community trust and relations between the state (especially the police) and the communities they serve; and investing in urban upgrading and the environment are equally important components.

All such policies help strengthen and protect young people and their families growing up. A strong component is the overarching support and responsibility shared by national and local governments, with adequate funding and resources over an extended period of time to build capacity and promote sustainability, and in particular to entrench robust evaluation approaches capable of measuring complex interventions.

References

Alvarado, N., and Abizanda, B. (2010). *Some Lessons Learned in Citizen Security by the IADB. Background Note for the World Bank's 2011 World Development Report*. Washington, D.C.: IDB.

Bamberger, M., Rugh, J., and Mabry, L. (2006). *RealWorld Evaluation: Working Under Budget, Time, Data, and Political Constraints.* Thousand Oaks: Sage Publications Inc.

Burton, P. (2012). *Country Assessment on Youth Violence, Policy and Programmes in South Africa.* Report no. 70733. Washington, D.C.: World Bank.

Canada (2013). *Youth Gang Prevention Fund Projects. Research Report: 2007-2012.* Ottawa: National Crime Prevention Centre, Public Safety.

Guardian and LSE. (2011). *Reading the Riots. Investigating England's summer of disorder.* London: *Guardian* and London School of Economics.

Jutersonke, O., Muggah, R., and Rodgers, D. (2009). Gangs and violence reduction in Central America. *Security Dialogue*, 40, 373–97.

Kennedy, D. M. (2007). *Making Communities Safer: Youth Violence and Gang Interventions that Work.* Prepared Testimony before the House Judiciary Subcommittee on Crime, Terrorism, and Homeland Security, 15 February 2007. Director, Center for Crime Prevention and Control, John Jay College of Criminal Justice New York.

Morgan, A, and Homel, P. (2013). Evaluating crime prevention: Lessons from large-scale community crime prevention programmes.*Trends and Issues No. 458.* Canberra: Australian Institute of Criminology.

Muggah, R. (2012). *Researching the Urban Dilemma. Urbanization, Poverty and Violence.* Ottawa: International Development Research Centre.

Newburn, T. (2011). Reading the Riots. *British Journal of Criminology Newsletter, No. 69, Winter 2011.* britsoccrim.org/new/newdocs/bscn-69-2011-TimNewburn.pdf

OECD. (2005). *Paris Declaration on Aid Effectiveness.* Paris: OECD Publishing.

OECD. (2011). Preventing and reducing armed violence in urban areas. Programming note. *Conflict and Fragility.* Paris: OECD Publishing.

Patton, M. Q. (2011). *Developmental Evaluation: Applying Complexity Contexts to Enhance Effectiveness and Use.* New York: The Guilford Press.

Perez, R. (2009). *Prevencion de la violencia armada juvenil. El cao do Brasil.* Presentation on the Prevention of Youth Violence in Latin America. Woodrow Wilson Centre, Washington, 27 October 2009.

Savignac, J., and Leonard, L. (2011). *Promising and Model Crime Prevention Programs Volume II.* Ottawa: Public Safety Canada.

Shaw, M. (2009). International models of crime prevention. In: A. Crawford (ed.), *Crime Prevention Policies in Comparative Perspective.* Cullompton, Devon: Willan Publishing, pp. 234–54.

Shaw, M. (2012). Addressing youth violence in cities and neighbourhoods. In C. Ward, A. van der Merwe, and A. Dawes (eds), *Youth Violence. Sources and Solutions in South Africa.* Cape Town: University of Cape Town Press, pp. 372–99.

Shaw, M., and Carli, V. (2011). *Practical Approaches to Urban Crime Prevention.* Proceedings of workshop 12th UN Congress on Crime Prevention and Criminal Justice, Salvador, Brazil, 12–19 April 2010. Montreal and Vienna: ICPC and UNODC.

Shaw, M. and Travers, K. (2007). *Strategies and Best Practices in Crime Prevention in Particular in Relation to Urban Areas and Youth at Risk.* Proceedings of the workshop held at the 11th UN Congress on Crime Prevention and Criminal Justice, Bangkok, Thailand, 18–25 April 2005. Montreal: ICPC.

United Kingdom Government (2011) *Ending Gangs and Youth Violence. A Cross-Government Report Including Further Evidence and Good Practice Case Studies.* London: Home Office.

Ukeje, C. U., and Iwilade, A. (2012). A farewell to innocence? African youth and violence in the twenty-first century. *International Journal of Conflict and Violence*, 6, 339–51.

UN Convention on the Rights of the Child 1989, UN Treaty Series Vol. 1577 No. 27531.

UN Guidelines for the Prevention of Juvenile Delinquency 1990, (Riyadh Guidelines) GA resolution 45/112, annex.

UN Guidelines for action on children in the criminal justice system 1997, (Vienna Guidelines) GA resolution 48/104.

UN Guidelines for Cooperation and Technical Assistance in the Field of Urban Crime Prevention 1995, ECOSOC resolution 1995/9 annex.

UN Guidelines for the Prevention of Crime 2002, ECOSOC resolution 2002/13 annex.

UNDP. (2012). *Caribbean Human Development Report 2012. Human Development and the Shift to Better Security.* New York: UNDP.

Ungar, M., and Arias, E. D. (2012). Reassessing community-oriented policing in Latin America. *Policing and Society*, 22, 1–13.

UN HABITAT. (2010a). *State of the Urban Youth 2010-2011. Leveling the Playing Field: Inequality of Youth Opportunity.* Nairobi: UN HABITAT.

UN HABITAT. (2010b). *Youth Resource Guide. Participate in Safer Cities!* Nairobi and Montreal: UN HABITAT and ICPC.

UNODC. (2011). *Global Study on Homicide 2011.* Vienna: UNODC.

UNODC. (2010). *Handbook on the Crime Prevention Guidelines: Making them Work.* New York: United Nations.

UNODC and UN HABITAT. (2009). Crime prevention assessment tool. *Criminal Justice Assessment Tool Kit.* New York: United Nations.

Ward, C, van de Merwe, A., and Dawes, A. (2012). *Youth Violence. Sources and Solutions in South Africa.* Cape Town: University of Cape Town Press.

Waiselfisz, J. J. (2012). *Mapa da Violencia 2012. Criancas e Adolescentes do Brasil.* Rio de Janeiro: FLACSO Brasil.

World Health Organization (2010). *Violence Prevention: The Evidence.* Geneva: WHO.

Willman, A., and Makisaka, M. (2010). Interpersonal violence prevention. A review of the evidence and emerging lessons.*World Development Report 2011 Background Paper.* Washington D.C.: World Bank.

World Bank (2011). *Violence in the City. Understanding and Supporting Community Responses to Urban Violence.* Washington, D.C.: World Bank, Social Development Department.

CHAPTER 37

International policies to reduce and prevent gender-based violence

Heléne Combrinck

Introduction

This chapter provides an overview of the development of gender-based violence as an international policy concern. International human rights law provides the normative framework for understanding gender-based violence and also imposes obligations on governments to address these violations at national level. International human rights law further sets up mechanisms such as regional human rights courts and treaty monitoring bodies to interpret and enforce this normative framework.

The chapter adopts a broadly historic approach rather than distinguishing between different aspects of gender-based violence such as sexual assault and intimate partner violence. This is necessitated because especially the earlier documents cover gender-based violence in a holistic manner; specialized instruments focusing on particular aspects have begun to emerge only relatively recently. Where possible, the chapter does however make reference to aspects of *sexual violence* and should be read to complement Chapter 38 (this volume) on policies to reduce intimate partner violence.

Emergence of Gender-Based Violence as an International Policy Concern

The early period of development of the international human rights system, from 1945 onwards, saw slow progress in the formal recognition of women's rights. Women's concerns gained prominence on the international agenda during the 1970s due to, amongst other factors, the declaration of the 'United Nations Decade for Women' from 1975 to 1985 (Fitzpatrick 1994; Wright 1993).

The major international human rights treaty on women's equality, the Convention on the Elimination of All Forms of Discrimination against Women, was adopted in 1979. Since this document does not make explicit reference to gender-based violence in the text itself, the body monitoring the implementation of the Convention, the Committee on the Elimination of Discrimination against Women (CEDAW), issued an interpretive comment in 1992 to address this shortcoming.

This comment (General Recommendation No. 19) explains that the general prohibition of gender discrimination in the Convention includes 'gender-based violence—that is, violence that is directed at a woman because she is a woman or that affects women disproportionately' (CEDAW 1992, para. 1). Gender-based violence is linked to each applicable Article of the Convention (for example, under 'employment', General Recommendation No. 19 addresses sexual harassment). A number of specific recommendations for governments to address such violence are listed (CEDAW 1992, paras 24(a)–(t)), which comprise 'all legal and other measures that are necessary to provide effective protection of women against gender-based violence' (para. 24(t)). These include preventive measures (such as public information programmes to change attitudes concerning the roles and status of men and women); and protective measures, for example, refuges and support services for women who are victims or at risk of violence.

General Recommendation No 19 clearly points out the connections between gender-based violence and women's health. It notes, in respect of Article 12 of the Convention, that violence against women puts their health and lives at risk and that states are required by this article to ensure equal access to healthcare (CEDAW 1992, para. 19). It further notes that specific instances of gender-based violence, such as family violence (para. 23), sexual harassment (para. 18), and compulsory sterilization or abortion (para. 22), hold particularly adverse health consequences for women.

In this interpretive comment, the CEDAW therefore lays down a strong foundation for understanding that the Convention imposes a duty on states to address gender-based violence as a health concern (in addition to a criminal justice or law enforcement priority).

The Recommendation further emphasizes that states may be responsible for acts of gender-based violence committed by private actors if they fail to act with due diligence to prevent violations of rights or to investigate and punish acts of violence, and to provide compensation (CEDAW 1992, para. 10). This entails that an illegal act which violates human rights and which is initially not directly imputable to a state (for example, because it is the act of a private person) can lead to the state's being held liable under international law. This is not because of the act itself, but because of the lack of due diligence on the part of the state to prevent the violation or to appropriately respond to it (for example, by investigating and punishing the perpetrator). This rule, initially formulated to cover individual instances where a government had failed to protect rights, has subsequently been expanded to impose much broader 'systemic' duties, as will be explained.

The CEDAW subsequently also adopted a General Recommendation on women's health to elaborate on Article 12 of the Convention. General Recommendation No. 24 confirms that the obligation to *protect rights* relating to women's health requires governments to take action to prevent and impose sanctions for violations of rights by private persons (CEDAW 1999, para. 15). Since gender-based violence is a critical health issue for women, governments should, amongst other measures, enact and enforce laws and formulate policies, including healthcare protocols and hospital procedures to address violence against women and abuse of girl children, and should provide appropriate health services.

Development of International Norms and Standards Relating to Violence against Women

The Declaration on the Elimination of Violence against Women

At the third World Conference on Human Rights, in 1993, women's rights advocates succeeded in placing women's rights, and particularly violence against women, firmly on the 'mainstream' human rights agenda (Mertus and Goldberg 1994). This was reflected in the outcome document of the conference, which proposed the introduction of a general declaration on the elimination of violence against women (Vienna Declaration 1993). The UN General Assembly accordingly adopted the Declaration on the Elimination of Violence against Women ('the Violence Declaration') in December 1993.

The Declaration defines the term 'violence against women' as any act of gender-based violence that results in, or is likely to result in, physical, sexual, or psychological harm or suffering to women, including threats of such acts, coercion, or arbitrary deprivation of liberty, whether occurring in public or in private life (Article 1).

Article 2 expands on this definition by setting out a non-exhaustive list of acts of violence against women occurring at three levels: in the family, in the community, and the state. In terms of the Declaration, governments are expected to condemn violence against women and to pursue by 'all appropriate means and without delay' a policy of eliminating violence against women (Article 4).

International Conference on Population and Development

The Programme of Action, which was the outcome of the International Conference on Population and Development held in 1994, confirmed the normative connection between gender-based violence, equality, and the right to health. Importantly, the Programme of Action notes that advancing gender equality, the empowerment of women, and the elimination of all kinds of violence against women, are cornerstones of population and development-related programmes (Principle 4).

The Programme of Action further states that everyone has the right to enjoyment of the highest attainable standards of physical and mental health, and requires states to take all appropriate measures to ensure, on a basis of equality of men and women, universal access to healthcare services (Principle 8). Violence against women, including intimate partner violence and rape, is specifically recognized as one cause of the rising number of women sustaining HIV and other sexually transmitted infections (para. 7.35).

The Beijing Declaration and Platform for Action

The UN Fourth World Women's Conference was held in Beijing in 1995. The Beijing Declaration and Platform for Action, adopted subsequent to the Conference, identifies twelve 'critical areas of concern' with concrete actions to be taken by various actors.

Section D of the Beijing Platform, which deals with violence against women, notably elaborates on the Violence Declaration, but also introduces a number of new themes. For example, it lists the violation of the human rights of women in situations of armed conflict as a further instance of violence against women (para. 114) and expands the groups of women who are particularly vulnerable to violence as recognized in the Violence Declaration to include (amongst others) women migrant workers and women living in poverty (para. 116).

The Beijing Platform identifies three strategic objectives in respect of violence against women, including taking integrated measures to prevent and eliminate such violence and studying its causes, consequences, and the effectiveness of preventive measures. A list of 'actions to be taken' is set out under each of these objectives (Strategic Objectives D1, D2, and D3). The actors include the UN, governments, trade unions, non-governmental organizations (NGOs), and international organizations.

Governments are expected to take measures with an emphasis on prosecution of offenders and ensuring access to justice for victims of violence (para. 124(d)). They are also required to formulate and implement 'plans of action to eliminate violence against women' (para. 124(j)). These include the duty to recognize and support the fundamental role of intermediate institutions, such as primary-healthcare centres and family-planning centres in the field of information and education related to abuse (para 125(f)); and to develop counselling, healing, and support programmes for girls and women who have been or are involved in abusive relationships, particularly those who live in homes or institutions where abuse occurs (para. 126(c)).

The area of inequalities in access to healthcare and related services is also delineated in the Beijing Platform as a critical concern. It is emphasized that gender-based violence places women at high risk of physical and mental trauma, disease, and unwanted pregnancy (para. 99). These situations often deter women from using health and other services. Actions to be taken (by a range of actors) include the training of primary health workers to recognize and care for girls and women who have experienced domestic violence or sexual abuse (para. 106(q)).

From Standard-Setting to Accountability

With the adoption of the Beijing Platform of Action in 1995, the development of international standards relating to violence against women reached a first phase of completion (Combrinck 2010). The next phase consisted of the further refinement of these principles through the adoption of regional instruments and the interpretation by treaty-monitoring bodies (notably, the Committee on the Elimination of Discrimination against Women) and the regional human rights courts such as the European Court of Human Rights and the Inter-American Court of Human Rights.

Interpretation by Treaty-Monitoring Bodies

The interpretation of international human rights instruments by the bodies monitoring these treaties is important to achieve clarity. This interpretation typically happens through complaints brought against states for violation of rights in terms of the complaints mechanism forming part of the instrument; in the case of the Women's Convention, this mechanism is the Optional Protocol (where states have ratified the Optional Protocol).

In this section, we will briefly examine the interpretation of the Women's Convention by the Committee on the Elimination of Discrimination against Women. Two instances are of specific importance, i.e., the Committee's inquiry into the murdered women of Ciudad Juarez (2005) and its views in the communication brought in *S.V.P. v. Bulgaria*.

From 1993 onwards, approximately 400 young women were brutally murdered in Ciudad Juárez, Mexico, a town in the state of Chihuahua on the border with the United States. About a quarter of the discovered bodies showed signs of serial sexual torture prior to death. Many more women had disappeared and remained missing. For a period of about 10 years (1993–2003), the Mexican authorities did little to investigate or bring an end to the murders. In 2002, two NGOs requested the CEDAW to conduct an inquiry under Article 8 of the Optional Protocol into the abduction, rape, and murder of the women in and around Ciudad Juárez. This inquiry started in July 2003.

The CEDAW found that that there had been serious shortcomings in the response of the Mexican state. In addition to the failure to properly investigate the disappearance and murder of the women in Ciudad Juárez, the policies adopted and the measures taken since 1993 to prevent, investigate, and punish crimes of violence against women had been ineffective and had fostered a climate of impunity and lack of confidence in the justice system. The Committee concluded that Mexico's actions constituted 'grave and systematic violations' of the provisions of the Women's Convention, as well as of General Recommendation No. 19, and expressed its concern that these violations had continued for more than 10 years (CEDAW 2005, paras 259–60).

Further clarity on the Committee's interpretation of state obligations can be found in *S.V.P. v. Bulgaria* (CEDAW 2012). The facts, briefly, were that the complainant's young daughter (then 7 years old) had been the victim of an act of sexual assault in 2004. Charges against the perpetrator were not brought until 17 April 2006, almost 2 years later. The case was closed in June 2006, following the approval by the court of a plea-bargaining agreement between the prosecutor and the accused, which provided for a suspended sentence and did not compensate the victim for her pain and suffering. As a result of the trauma she experienced due to the severe sexual assault, the victim was diagnosed with a psychiatric disorder and was, at the time of the complaint, attending a school for children with special needs.

The complainant submitted that the Bulgarian government did not act with due diligence for the effective protection of her daughter against the sexual violence suffered and its consequences. Her submission was based on the Bulgarian state's failures in respect of ensuring her daughter's right to effective compensation; ensuring her daughter's right to health; protecting the victim against the risk of further violence; and providing her daughter with proper rehabilitation services and counselling.

The Committee examined the Bulgarian Penal Code and noted shortcomings in the legislation, such as the fact that the punishment for sexual assault was still lower than the punishment for rape or attempted rape. The Committee also observed that the existing legislation did not appear to contain any mechanisms (such as protection orders) for protecting victims of sexual violence from re-victimization, since after the end of the criminal proceedings the perpetrators are released back into society (CEDAW 2012, para. 9.7). In this instance, the perpetrator was still living in the vicinity of the victim's home.

With regard to the complainant's claim that her daughter's health rights had been violated, the Committee concluded that Bulgaria had failed to in its obligation under Article 12 (read with General Recommendation No. 24) to enact and apply policies, including healthcare protocols and hospital procedures, to address the sexual violence experienced by the victim; and that it did not provide appropriate health services in her case.

Development of Regional Instruments

The Inter-American Human Rights System

In 1994, members of the Organization of American States adopted the Inter-American Convention on the Prevention, Punishment, and Eradication of Violence against Women (1994), also known as the 'Convention of Belém do Pará'. This Convention was the first document on violence against women with potentially legally binding effect (albeit only binding on states in the inter-American region). Similar to the international instruments already mentioned, it imposes duties on ratifying states to take a number of measures to address violence against women, including the provision of appropriate specialized services for women who have been subjected to violence (Convention of Belém do Pará 1994, Article 8(d)).

The Convention of Belém do Pará has been interpreted by the Inter-American Court for Human Rights (IACrtHR) in a number of key judgments, including the case of *González et al ('Cotton Field') v. Mexico*. In this matter, which follows on the inquiry into the Mexican government actions by the CEDAW (discussed earlier), the state was held liable for its failure to respond appropriately when three young women disappeared from the town of Ciudad Juarez. Their bodies were subsequently found in a cotton field outside the town.

The Court firstly revisited the general principles relating to due 'diligence' as these had developed in international law with reference to violence against women (IACrtHR 2009, paras 253–7). In particular, states parties should have an appropriate legal framework for protection that is enforced effectively, and prevention policies and practices that allow effective measures to be taken in response to complaints. The court remarked:

The prevention strategy should also be comprehensive; in other words, it should prevent the risk factors and, at the same time, strengthen the institutions that can provide an effective response in cases of violence against women. (IACrtHR 2009, para. 258)

The court accordingly found that the Mexican government had violated several rights set out in the American Convention on Human Rights and the Convention of Belém do Pará and had failed to comply with its obligations under these instruments. The Court's reparation order included the payment of damages to the victims' families; the completion of the investigation of the murders by specially trained investigators; the reform of criminal justice procedures; and the introduction of education and awareness campaigns.

The European Human Rights System

The European Court of Human Rights (ECHR) has developed a strong set of principles on the duties of states to respond to gender-based violence. Although the European Convention for the Protection on Human Rights and Freedoms does not have explicit provisions on gender-based violence as such, the Court has found these state obligations in Article 3 of the Convention (which provides protection against torture and inhuman or degrading treatment) and Article 8 (which guarantees the right to respect for private and family life).

Significantly, the Court has held governments responsible not only for the failure of state officials to appropriately intervene in individual cases of violence, but also for broader 'systemic' shortcomings in the legal system. While the majority of the cases before the Court have dealt with domestic violence, the case of *M.C. v. Bulgaria* is instructive in the context of sexual violence. The applicant had allegedly been raped by two male acquaintances and after a protracted investigation, the prosecution eventually declined to prosecute the two men based on the conclusion that there was insufficient evidence that the applicant had been forced to have sex.

The applicant alleged that the Bulgarian authorities had failed to provide her with effective legal protection against rape and sexual abuse, thus failing to comply with their duties under the European Convention. This claim was based firstly on the ineffective investigation of her rape case; the second ground included the claim that Bulgarian law and its application in rape cases contained an unduly strong expectation of active resistance on the part of the victim. The court found in the applicant's favour on both aspects, clearly demonstrating its willingness to measure systemic components (such as the substance of Bulgarian rape law) against the 'evolving convergence as to the standards to be achieved' by states (European Court of Human Rights 2003, para. 154).

An important recent development in the European context was the adoption in 2011 of the Convention on Preventing and Combating Violence against Women and Domestic Violence ('the Istanbul Convention'). This Convention draws on international developments over the past twenty years and is therefore in several ways a more 'advanced' instrument when compared to earlier documents such as the Violence Declaration. The Convention was adopted on 07 April 2011 and at the time of writing is not yet in operation.

The Convention calls for states to adopt and implement statewide, coordinated, and holistic policies to prevent and combat all forms of violence covered by the scope of this Convention (Article 7.1). Interestingly, the document notes that states are encouraged to apply the Convention 'to *all* victims of domestic violence' (Article 2.2; my emphasis); this would include male victims. At the same time, the Convention requires states to pay particular attention to women victims of gender-based violence in implementing its provisions (Article 2.2). This article reflects the growing international recognition accorded to men experiencing gender-based violence. At the same time, it takes a balanced approach by reminding states to pay particular attention to women victims of gender-based violence, given that women remain greatly over-represented in this group.

Governments are further required to ensure that victims have access to adequately resourced healthcare and social services; and that professionals are trained to assist victims (Article 20.2). Importantly, a separate article is devoted to support for victims of sexual violence: states must take the necessary measures to provide for the setting up of appropriate, easily accessible sexual violence referral centres for victims to provide for medical and forensic examination, trauma support, and counselling for victims (Article 25).

Given that the Convention is not yet in force, it is not possible to comment on its possible implementation; however, the document itself holds promise for expanding and clarifying the existing standards in the future.

The African Human Rights System

The Protocol to the African Charter on Human and Peoples' Rights on the Rights of Women in Africa ('the Maputo Protocol') was adopted in 2003 and came into operation in 2005.

The Protocol deals with violence against women mainly under two rights, that is the right to dignity (Article 3) and the rights to life, integrity, and security of the person (Article 4). State obligations to address violence against women are specifically addressed under the latter and include the duty to enact and enforce laws to prohibit all forms of violence against women including unwanted or forced sex (Article 4.2(a)). Importantly, the Protocol highlights the issue of sexual violence in respect of two groups of marginalized women, viz. elderly women and women with disabilities, and enjoins states to ensure the freedom from violence of each group of women (Articles 22(b) and 23(b)).

At a subregional level, mention may be made of the recently adopted Southern African Economic Development Community ('SADC') Protocol on Gender and Development. Although the Protocol contains detailed provisions on gender-based violence (Article 20), its delayed coming into force makes the achievement of the time-bound objectives highly unlikely. The target date for these objectives is 2015.

Finally, the Protocol on the Prevention and Suppression of Sexual Violence against Women and Children was agreed on by 11 countries in the Great Lakes region in 2006. This Protocol, which came into force in 2008, was developed in the specific context of sexual violence against women and children during and after the protracted armed conflict in this Central African region (Great Lakes Protocol 2008).

Ensuring Compliance

The brief overview summarizes how the main international and regional human rights documents conceptualize gender-based violence, and gives a 'snap-shot' of the legal and policy measures that governments subscribing to these treaties are required to adopt and implement. Valuable guidelines for this policy formulation are provided at the international level by bodies such as the World Health Organization (WHO). For example, the WHO Guidelines for Medico-Legal Care for Victims of Sexual Violence

(2003) establish treatment norms for the assessment and examination of adult victims of sexual violence, as well as special measures for the examination of child victims.

What are the consequences when states fail to comply with these international standards, despite being legally bound to do so? As noted, one option may be to bring a complaint to the relevant treaty monitoring body, as illustrated by the two examples of alleged violations brought before the CEDAW. However, in terms of the Optional Protocol to the Women's Convention, the CEDAW can only issue 'recommendations' to states to take remedial action. It is not a 'court of law' as such and its findings regarding complaints are referred to as 'views' rather than judgments (Steiner et al. 2007).

Compliance with these recommendations largely depends on the country's investment in being seen by the international community to be observing its international human rights obligations. For this reason, successful complaints before the CEDAW have in certain instances led to significant legal and policy reform at national level; in other instances, state action remains lacking. However, this is symptomatic of the UN treaty system generally, and is not specific to the Women's Convention.

Judgments from the regional human rights courts have more legal cogency and are regarded as binding on the state in question. Again, while implementation of a judgment against a government may prove problematic in the absence of domestic 'political will', advocates have successfully used favourable judgments by the regional courts as leverage to achieve law and policy reform (Roure 2009; Santos 2007).

Conclusion

The current position can therefore be summarized as follows: international and regional human rights law imposes obligations at international level that governments have to implement at national level. These duties include the enactment of laws, the formulation of policies and other measures to ensure that perpetrators of such violence are prosecuted and punished, and also the introduction of measures towards the *prevention* of gender-based violence.

Recent application of these international principles in specific instances of sexual violence has provided governments with more concrete guidance. For example, the case of *S.V.P* v. *Bulgaria* shows how policy measures to address sexual violence against women and girls should include healthcare protocols and hospital procedures.

It can therefore be said that the international framework is currently moving into a third phase of further clarification of the standard of 'due diligence' in state responses to gender-based violence. Additional sophistication is emerging around multiple and intersecting discrimination (for example, gender-based violence against women with disabilities), an understanding of men and boys as victims, and the importance of identifying good practices in comprehensive violence prevention strategies.

References

Beijing Declaration and Platform of Action A/Conf.177/20 and A/Conf.177/20/Add.1 (15 September 1995), endorsed by the UN General Assembly on 8 December 1995 (A/RES/50/42).

CEDAW. (1992). *General Recommendation No 19: Violence against Women.* UN Doc CEDAW/C/1992/L.1/Add.15 (1992).

CEDAW. (1999). *General Recommendation No 24: Women and Health.*

CEDAW. (2005). *Report on Mexico produced by the Committee on the Elimination of Discrimination against Women under Article 8 of the Optional Protocol to the Convention, and reply from the Government of Mexico.* UN Doc CEDAW/C/2005/OP.8/MEXICO (dated 27 January 2005).

CEDAW. (2012). *S.V.P. v Bulgaria. Communication No. 31/2011. Views adopted by the Committee at its fifty-third session, 1-19 October 2012.* UN Doc CEDAW/C/53D31/2011 (dated 24 November 2012).

Combrinck, H. (2010). *The Role of International Human Rights Law in Guiding the Interpretation of Women's Right to be Free from Violence under the South African Constitution.* LL D. South Africa: University of the Western Cape.

Convention on the Elimination of All Forms of Discrimination against Women. Adopted 18 Dec 1979, GA Res 34/180, UN GAOR, 34th Session, UN Doc A/34/46 (1980), entered into force 3 September 1981.

Convention on Preventing and Combating Violence against Women and Domestic Violence. 11.V.2011 (Adopted by the Council of Europe Committee of Ministers on 7 April 2011, Istanbul, Turkey).

Declaration on the Elimination of Violence against Women GA Res 48/104 UN Doc A/48/104 (adopted 20 December 1993).

European Court of Human Rights. 2003. *M.C. v Bulgaria Application no. 39272/98* (Judgment dated 4 December 2003); 40 EHRR 20.

Fitzpatrick, J. (1994). The use of international human rights norms to combat violence against women. In: R. J. Cook. (ed.), *Human Rights of Women: National and International Perspectives,* Philadelphia: University of Pennsylvania Press, pp. 532–71.

Great Lakes Protocol on the Prevention and Suppression of Sexual Violence against Women and Children (2008). Entered into force in June 2008.

IACrtHR. (2009). *González et al ('Cotton Field') v Mexico* (Unreported judgment dated 16 November 2009).

Inter-American Convention on the Prevention, Punishment and Eradication of Violence against Women ('Convention of Belém do Pará') OAS/Ser.L.V/II.92/doc31 rev.3 (1994) (signed on 9 June 1994, entered into force 3 March 1995).

Mertus, J., and Goldberg, P. (1994). A perspective on women and international human rights after the Vienna Declaration: the inside/ outside construct. *New York University Journal of International Law & Politics, 26,* 201–34.

Optional Protocol to the Convention on the Elimination of All Forms of Discrimination against Women GA Resolution A/RES/54/4 of 6 October 1999.

Programme of Action of the International Conference on Population and Development A/CONF.171/13 (dated 18 October 1994).

Protocol to the African Charter on Human and Peoples' Rights on the Rights of Women in Africa CAB/LEG/66 6/Rev 1 (2003), entered into force on 25 November 2005.

Roure, J. G. (2009). Domestic violence in Brazil: Examining obstacles and approaches to promote legislative reform. *Columbia Human Rights Law Review, 41,* 67–97.

SADC Protocol on Gender and Development, adopted 17 August 2008.

Santos, C. M. (2007). Transnational legal activism and the State: reflections on cases against Brazil in the Inter-American Commission on Human Rights. *SUR -International Journal on Human Rights, 7,* 29–59.

Steiner, H. J., Alston, P., and Goodman, R. (2007). *International Human Rights in Context: Law, Politics, Morals.* 3rd ed. Oxford: Oxford University Press.

Vienna Declaration (1993) Programme of Action Adopted by the World Conference on Human Rights on 25 June 1993 UN Doc A/Conf.157/23 (dated 12 July 1993).

World Health Organization (2003). *Guidelines for Medico-Legal Care for Victims of Sexual Violence.* Geneva: World Health Organization.

Wright, S. (1993). Human rights and women's rights: an analysis of the United Nations Convention on the Elimination of All Forms of Discrimination against Women. In: K. E. Mahoney, and P. Mahoney (eds), *Human Rights in the Twenty-first Century.* Dordrecht: Martinus Nijhoff Publishers, pp. 75–88.

CHAPTER 38

National and international policies to reduce domestic violence

Lillian Artz

Introduction to National and International Policies to Reduce Domestic Violence

Debates surrounding the development and application of international laws, norms, and policies pertaining to domestic violence have largely been dominated by Anglo-American and European literature. In order to bring a fresh angle to these policy discussions, as well as to highlight the perspectives of developing contexts, this chapter will reflect on developments from developing and transitional states, particularly South Africa, as a unique departure point for a discussion of international and domestic legal and policy-based measures aimed at addressing domestic violence.

A systematic examination of policies and laws aimed at addressing gender equality and acting against gender-based violence is beyond the scope of this chapter. A useful analysis of international human rights standards, the status of international treaties, and the application of international law on domestic law can be found in the work of Combrinck (Chapter 37, this volume). Here she describes the framework they provide for the development of progressive domestic legislation. These international policies will therefore not be revisited in detail.

The term 'domestic violence', as opposed to the more commonly used 'intimate partner violence', will be adopted here. Domestic violence not only captures the broader family contexts in which domestic violence occurs (including violence *against women* by other, non-intimate, members of the family), but it is also commonly used in international human rights instruments and country level legislation. It is a term that also recognizes the diverse range of cultural, institutional, civil, and other domestic arrangements within developing world contexts in which domestic violence may occur.

Advancing Rights: International Frameworks

Much of the foundational work of advancing the rights of persons subject to domestic violence has taken place through the establishment of international treaties and conventions which recognize domestic violence as a fundamental violation of human rights. Despite criticism for having little measurable impact on violence

prevention, international instruments provide frameworks from which to advocate for treatment policies, services, and resources. Simply put, once member states sign, ratify, or accede to international and regional human rights treaties, they commit to the development of national laws that instil important international norms and standards. Moreover, each international instrument has measures for state reporting to international bodies like the United Nations (U.N.), on the implementation of treaty obligations. Although not all of these instruments are binding, their contents 'have significant political value, in addition to some legal authority' and 'in many instances...have resulted in the initiation of important administrative and legislative measures aimed at protecting victims' rights and interests' (Artz and Smythe 2013, p. 271).

One of the first universal declarations that expressly recognized the rights of 'domestic' victims of crime was a U.N. General Assembly Resolution: Declaration of Basic Principles of Justice for Victims of Crime and Abuse of Power (1985). Previously, international instruments had largely focused on actions of 'states' rather than 'individuals'. This Declaration established important principles in relation to the treatment of individual victims of crime as well as individual perpetrators. This included access to justice and fair treatment, restitution, compensation, and victim assistance, as well as promoting domestic law to address abuses of power, and providing remedies to victims of such abuses. Also of significance was the definition of 'a victim':

> 'Victims' means persons who, individually or collectively, have suffered harm, including physical or mental injury, emotional suffering, economic loss or substantial impairment of their fundamental rights, through acts or omissions that are in violation of criminal laws operative within Member States, including those laws proscribing criminal abuse of power (s. 1).

The Declaration also promoted redress through judicial and administrative mechanisms, such as the adoption of domestic law (s. 5) and reinforced this through the promotion of information to victims (s. 6a), victim participation in judicial and administrative proceedings, where appropriate (s. 6b), victim support (s. 6c), victim protection of privacy or from intimidation or retaliation (s. 6d), expedient management and disposition of cases (s. 6 e).

Although early treaties only provided protection against domestic violence implicitly, the 1990s surfaced a series of conventions that gave more explicit attention to domestic violence (see Chapter 37, this volume):

◆ General Recommendation No. 19 by the Committee on the Elimination of Discrimination against Women (1992)

◆ Declaration of Elimination of Violence Against Women (1993)

◆ Vienna Declaration and Programme of Action adopted by the World Conference on Human Rights (A/CONF.157/24 (Part I), Chap. III)

◆ Beijing Declaration and Platform for Action adopted by the Fourth World Conference on Women (1995)

◆ Programme of Action of the International Conference on Population and Development (1994).

The past two decades have also seen numerous resolutions from the U.N. General Assembly on all aspects of violence against women and girls. One that is particularly noteworthy in relation to domestic violence is the General Assembly Resolution on the Elimination of Domestic Violence against Women (2003) which reasserts the U.N.'s commitment to establishing appropriate mechanisms to address domestic violence in criminal justice systems. Section 7 of this Resolution unambiguously calls upon states to:

◆ adopt, strengthen, and implement legislation that prohibits domestic violence (s. 7(a));

◆ make domestic violence a criminal offence and to ensure proper investigation and prosecution of perpetrators (s. 7(b));

◆ provide legal and social assistance to victims of domestic violence (s. 7(c));

◆ intensify measures aimed at preventing domestic violence against women (s. 7(d));

◆ provide or facilitate the provision of assistance to victims of domestic violence in lodging police reports and receiving treatment and support (s. 7(g))

More recently, in 2011, the Council of Europe adopted the Convention on Preventing and Combating Violence against Women and Domestic Violence ('the Istanbul Convention'). It specifically promotes the criminalization of domestic violence, which is viewed as a triumph of the Convention. To give effect to the Convention, state parties must introduce a number of offences where they currently do not exist in national legislation. Article 1 sets out the purpose of the Convention, which promotes (a) protection, prevention, and prosecution; (b) empowerment; (c) the design of a comprehensive framework, policies, and measures for the protection of victims; (d) the promotion of international cooperation; (e) providing support and assistance to organizations and law enforcement agencies to effectively cooperate in order to adopt an integrated approach to eliminating violence against women and domestic violence. Section 2 of this Article states that 'in order to ensure effective implementation of its provisions by the Parties, this Convention establishes a specific monitoring mechanism'. The convention also emphasizes international cooperation and requires state parties to 'take the necessary legislative and other measures to exercise due diligence to prevent, investigate,

punish and provide reparation for acts of violence covered by the scope of this Convention that are perpetrated by non-State actors' (Article 5). In addition to what are standard obligations on states who have adopted international treaties—changes to substantive and procedural laws, including the creation of a wide variety of civil protections and remedies—more novel provisions of the Convention include duties on state parties to:

◆ ensure that appropriate financial and human resources are allocated for the implementation of integrated policies (Article 8)

◆ support and cooperate with non-governmental organizations (Article 9)

◆ collect relevant statistical data at regular intervals on all forms of violence covered by the scope of the Convention; and to support research on the causes and effects, incidences, and conviction rates, and to ensure these are made publically available (Article 11)

◆ to prevent violence against women through awareness-raising (Article 13), education (Article 14), training of professionals (Article 15), preventative intervention and treatment programmes (Art 16.), and participation of the private sector and media

◆ protection and support through information (Article 19), general and specialist support services (Article 20 and 22), and the provision of shelters (Article 23)

There is a range of other major international human rights instruments that have bearing on domestic violence. Some of these have drawn less attention than others as frameworks for law and health policy reform, but include important principles and provisions for the prevention of domestic violence. In addition to the declarations and treaties that have been signalled as the cornerstones of legislative developments for domestic violence in every region of the world, conventions such as the Convention against Torture and Other Cruel, Inhuman or Degrading Treatment or Punishment ('CAT' 1984) have particular relevance. For instance, although it has been reasoned that one of the challenges of treating domestic violence as a human rights violation is that international human rights law does not apply to 'private' (non-state) forms of violence, Coomaraswamy explains that it could be argued that:

> Domestic violence involves the very four critical elements that constitute torture: (a) it causes severe physical and or mental pain, it is (b) intentionally inflicted, (c) for specified purposes, and (d) with some form of official involvement, whether active or passive. (2000, p. 10)

The [UN] Committee Against Torture further states that 'States parties' failure to prevent and protect victims from gender-based violence, such as rape, domestic violence, female genital mutilation, and trafficking' is a violation of CAT (General Comment No 2, 2007, paragraph 18). In reviewing country compliance with CAT, the Committee and the Special Rapporteur on Torture routinely request information on the prevalence of domestic violence in a country.

There are also several important regional instruments, such as the South African Development Community's (SADC's) Protocol on Gender and Development for the Prevention and Eradication of Violence against Women (1997) and the Protocol to the African Charter on Human and Peoples' Rights on the

Rights of Women in Africa (the 'African Women's Protocol' 2005) that have emerged as more contextually relevant instruments in the African context. The African Women's Protocol marked a milestone in the protection and promotion of women's rights in Africa by explicitly setting out the reproductive rights of women. The SADC's Protocol on Gender and Development (1997) however has been the most forthright in imposing duties on states to eradicate violence against women. These are contained within Article 20 of the protocol and include committing states to enacting and enforcing legislation that prohibits all forms of violence (s. 1(a)), and to ensuring that perpetrators of gender based violence are tried by a court of competent jurisdiction (s. 1(b)). It also commits states to reviewing and reforming criminal laws and procedures applicable to cases of gender-based violence (s. 3), as well as establishing special counselling services, and legal and police units to provide dedicated services to survivors of gender-based violence.

As international public health policies have largely taken a backseat to legal and jurisprudential developments, the SADC's Protocol on Gender and Development (1997) is progressive in its emphasis on healthcare responses to gender-based violence. Section 2 of the Protocol is unambiguous about state duties in this regard:

> 2. State Parties shall, by 2015, ensure that laws on gender based violence provide for the comprehensive testing, treatment and care of survivors of sexual offences, which shall include:

> (a) emergency contraception;

> (b) ready access to post exposure prophylaxis at all health facilities to reduce the risk of contracting HIV; and

> (c) preventing the onset of sexually transmitted infections.

In the Addendum to the 1997 Declaration on Gender and Development (1998), state parties are further obliged to undertake the following specifically in relation to domestic violence:

◆ enact laws such as sexual offences and domestic violence legislation, making various forms of violence against women clearly defined crimes, and taking appropriate measures to impose penalties and other enforcement mechanisms for the prevention and eradication of violence against women and children (s. 8);

◆ adopt legislative measures to ensure the protection and removal of all forms of discrimination against, and empowerment of, women with disabilities, the girl-child, the aged, women in armed conflict, and other women whose circumstances make them especially vulnerable to violence (s. 9);

◆ introduce, as a matter of priority, legal and administrative mechanisms for women and children subjected to violence, effective access to counselling, restitution, reparation, and other just forms of dispute resolution (s. 11); and

◆ adopt such other legislative and administrative measures as may be necessary to ensure the prevention and eradication of all forms of violence against women and children (s. 12).

Amongst other obligations, this addendum further provides for accessible information on services (s. 16), accessible, effective, and responsive police, prosecutorial, health, social welfare, and other services including establishing specialized units (s. 17) and specialized legal services (s 18). It also commits states to 'allocating the necessary resources to ensure the implementation and sustainability of the above programmes' (s. 24).

Country-specific health-driven protocols for the management of victims of domestic violence have struggled to gain traction within most major public health systems. Although domestic violence has been demonstrated to impact seriously on the general, reproductive, and mental health of victims of domestic violence, policy and treatment interventions have tended to focus narrowly on forensic medical examinations instead of preventative and comprehensive care protocols.

Domestic Violence Legislation: Global Trends, Local Views

Domestic law reform has been an integral part of international violence prevention projects to secure the protection of women and their families from domestic violence. Notwithstanding their limitations as measures for addressing domestic violence, the legal and criminal justice systems are powerful sites from which to challenge the social and legal understanding of women's experiences of domestic violence, and to ensure that these experiences are embodied within substantive law and criminal justice practice (Artz, 2008). In 2011, U.N. Women reported that 'as of April 2011, 191 countries have passed legislation on domestic violence, including almost all countries in Latin America and the Caribbean' but many of these still do not explicitly criminalize or prohibit rape within marriage (2011, p. 33).

Despite disparate legal systems and protective measures available in different jurisdictions, as countries around the world begin to adopt legislation to address domestic violence, they are inclined to opt for protection order-based responses to domestic violence. Protection orders—variously referred to as restraining orders, no contact orders, assistance orders, or interdicts—are generally court-issued orders that prevent *future* acts of domestic violence. There is significant variation in the contents and the application of protection order legislation across regions. For instance, there are considerable regional differences in relation to the criteria surrounding who qualifies for a protection order and under what conditions, the range of abuses that constitute domestic violence, the specific remedies available in relation to protection orders, the determination and consequences of violating orders, and the manner in which they are enforced. Legal differences also include varying definitions of domestic violence as well as of which relationships qualify for protection from domestic violence. The extent of protection provided by protection orders, including (for instance) provisions relating to the removal of weapons, prohibition of contact by abusers, alternative housing arrangements, and child support is also applied variously (Eigenberg et al. 2003; Finn 1989).

Most countries do not have a specific *criminal offence* in their criminal or penal codes which codify 'domestic violence', although either common law or these very codes do codify specific acts that may constitute domestic violence like assault, sexual assault, uttering threats, and criminal harassment (stalking). Separate civil statutes tend to complement these codes or common laws. While countries like India, New Zealand, Canada, and the United Kingdom have similar civil law approaches to domestic violence through the use of protection orders, other countries such as Brazil's Maria de Penha Law (Restrain Domestic and Family Violence against Women, No. 11.340, 2006) and South Africa's

Domestic Violence Act 116 of 1998, introduce additional protective measures such as the weapons removal, preventative arrest, interim custody arrangements, and emergency monetary relief. Tajikistan law specifically provides for free medical and legal assistance to victims of domestic violence (U.N.Women 2013). Nepal's Domestic Violence (Crime and Punishment) Control Act, 2066 (2009), Namibia's Combating of Domestic Violence Act, No. 4 of 2003 and Turkey's new Penal Code (2004; Law No. 6284) all include provisions criminalizing domestic violence. Turkey's domestic violence law also provides for services such as financial aid and psychological and legal services (Advocates for Human Rights 2011). In 2004, the United States introduced federal legislation on violence against women—the Violence Against Women Act (VAWA). Here, however, the legal system, which involves legislation and jurisdiction at the federal, state and even 'tribal' levels, the implementation of federal legislation with respect to domestic violence is to some extent dependent on whether individual states have a specific crime of domestic violence.

These Acts and penal code offences signal a distinct shift away from the traditional 'hands off' approaches taken in the past. In large part international legislation on domestic violence: (i) has created broad definitions of what constitutes domestic violence, to include physical, sexual, and psychological/emotional abuse, verbal abuse and threats as well as damage to property; (ii) includes some form of temporary removal of the accused or occupation of the residence by the victim; (iii) allows a third party to apply for a protection order on behalf of the victim, should she be incapacitated to do so; (iv) restricts access to victims and in some instances creates temporary custody arrangements for children; and (v) creates arrest policies for cases where protection orders are breached by those who these orders were issued against. Some jurisdictions, as outlined, have included additional dimensions to their domestic violence legislation and protection order remedies.

A Case in Point: South Africa's Domestic Violence Act

South Africa's Domestic Violence Act (DVA) was promulgated in 1998 with the aim of ensuring that 'victims of domestic violence received the maximum protection from domestic abuse that the law could provide' (Preamble of the DVA). As in many jurisdictions, the protection order granted in terms of the DVA is a civil order prohibiting an alleged abuser from committing certain acts of violence. However, it does not *criminalize* domestic violence per se. It only criminalizes the violation of the protection order. This legal remedy is meant to be preventative and involves a two-step process:

> The victim of domestic violence applies for an interim protection order (IPO) which is granted if the court is satisfied that there is *prima facie* evidence that the 'respondent' (the alleged abuser) has committed an act of domestic violence and that the applicant (the victim) would suffer undue hardship if a protection order was not issued immediately. Where urgency can be shown, an IPO is issued. The second part of the process involves finalizing the order. Once the IPO is served on the respondent, the applicant and the respondent are required to return to court on a certain date—referred to as the 'return date'—for a hearing during which the respondent is afforded the opportunity to present to the court reasons why the protection order should not be finalised. If the court is satisfied, on a balance of probabilities, that the respondent has committed or is committing an act of domestic violence, the protection order can be finalised (or varied in some way). (Artz 2011, p. 3)

In theory, the DVA provides a remedy that is specifically created for the applicant depending on his/her circumstances. When acts of domestic violence constitute recognized offences—such as common assault, rape, or malicious damage to property—criminal charges can be laid (in addition to the protection order). This binary system was established in South Africa to ensure that victims of domestic violence had recourse to the criminal system, the civil system, or the combination of both.

The South African Domestic Violence Act was also careful to define what constitutes a 'domestic relationship' and what amounts to 'domestic violence', both of which have been considered highly progressive in their ambit, even from an international perspective. In terms of section 1(viii) of the DVA, domestic violence means: physical abuse; sexual abuse; emotional, verbal and psychological abuse; economic abuse; intimidation; harassment; stalking; damage to property; entry into the complainant's residence without consent, where the parties do not share the same residence; or *any other controlling or abusive behaviour* towards a complainant, where such conduct harms, or may cause imminent harm to, the safety, health, or well-being of the complainant. Cognisant of the diverse civil, cultural, and 'by necessity' family arrangements in South Africa, it defines a domestic relationship as:

> a relationship between a complainant and a respondent in any of the following ways—they are or were married to each other, including marriage according to any law, custom or religion; they (whether they are of the same or of the opposite sex) live or lived together in a relationship in the nature of marriage, although they are not, or were not, married to each other, or are not able to be married to each other; they are the parents of a child or are persons who have or had parental responsibility for that child (whether or not at the same time); they are family members related by consanguinity, affinity or adoption; they are or were in an engagement, dating or customary relationship, including an actual or perceived romantic, intimate or sexual relationship of any duration; or they share or recently shared the same residence (s 1(vii)).

In another bold move, the South African Domestic Violence Act introduced provisions that placed positive legal duties on state role-players for implementing the Act. For instance, in an effort to redress the historical disinclination of the police to intervene in what they viewed as domestic private affairs (Artz 1999; Combrinck 1998; Combrinck and Artz 1999; Parenzee et al. 2001), Section 2 of the Act places a duty on the police to assist and inform complainants of their rights, including (i) assisting or making arrangements for the complainant to find a suitable shelter and to obtain medical treatment; (ii) handing a notice containing information to the complainant in the official language of the complainant's choice; and (iii) explaining to the complainant the content of such notice and the remedies at his or her disposal in terms of the Act and the right to lodge a criminal complaint (Artz 2003). Positive duties on the South African Police Service (SAPS) also include making an arrest without a warrant if the police reasonably suspect a person has committed domestic violence (s. 3) and arresting persons who have breached the conditions of a protection order (s. 8(b)). The Act also provides that the court may order the police to seize any arm or dangerous weapon in the possession of a person accused of domestic violence (s. 9) and to assist the complainant with arrangements regarding the collection of personal property (s. 7(2)(b)). Failure to comply with the duties set out in the Act constitutes misconduct, which must be reported to the Independents Complaints Directorate of the Police (s. 18(4)(a)).

Challenges to Domestic Violence Legislation: Implications for the Health Sector

There are universal implementation problems with domestic violence legislation. Research from around the world attests to the challenges enforcing protection orders, non-compliance of the law by state officials, the inconsistent application of the law across jurisdictions as well as the lack of laws that provide for support services that complement the legal process. This latter issue is of significance for health sector responses to domestic violence. Despite the progressive nature of international laws and policies relating to domestic violence, the absence of duties on the healthcare sector is not only a critical omission in relation to the potential provision of services that could be assured through substantive and procedural law and policies, but it also misses the opportunity to amplify the role of the health sector in violence prevention, through detection.

It is widely accepted that if victims of gender-based violence report to any formal state institution, it will be firstly to a health facility, and then to a criminal justice agency. Medical attention for domestic violence is more typically sought from, or identified in, emergency/trauma rooms, outpatient centres and general hospital admissions, primary healthcare settings, and other health facilities such as obstetrics and gynaecology units. Yet injuries and other consequences of domestic violence-related trauma and abuse (such as HIV transmission) are rarely documented and treated *as* domestic violence cases by attending healthcare practitioners. In health settings, women tend to report the *secondary effects* of domestic violence and rape (gynaecological issues, unresolved physical injuries, and acute or chronic symptoms such as abdominal pain, gastric complaints, headaches and fatigue, anxiety and depression, 'unexplained' injuries, and so on) which can signal health practitioners to the possibility of domestic violence.

Aschman et al. (2012) argue that while domestic violence has been established as an epidemic of global proportions—and international bodies such as the U.N., the World Health Organization, and the Federation for International Gynaecologists and Obstetricians have been highlighting the health implications of domestic violence (WHO 2013), the benefits of proactive health-centred approaches to domestic violence as well as the need for concentrated and systematic action in the health sector for over two decades—there is still resistance to standardized screening, examination, and treatment protocols for domestic violence in healthcare settings. There is no current (accessible) international policy framework for healthcare services for victims of domestic violence that sets treatment and care norms.

Domestic laws on domestic violence merely imply a role for healthcare workers through the provision of medico-legal services (Artz 2013). Duties on healthcare workers to detect and systematically treat victims of domestic violence are largely absent in both international and national domestic violence laws and policies. For instance, in South Africa's Domestic Violence Act, while the police are obliged to assist victims with seeking medical assistance, there is no legal duty on healthcare workers to provide any particular kind of assistance to victims. Healthcare workers are only implicated in the Act in that they are one of the list of professionals that can make an application for a protection order on behalf of a patient (s. 4(3)). Of course, as in most contexts, victims of domestic violence are entitled to medico-legal services just as any other victim of violence is entitled to these services. There are no duties on the health sector, however, 'to inquire about, screen for or holistically treat DV-related injuries and other health-related consequences of DV' (Aschman et al. 2012, p. 51).

Universally, the (legal) duties of health workers in domestic violence cases are mostly limited to the mandatory reporting of (child) sexual offences, abuse, and neglect. Comprehensive healthcare protocols, that promote basic standards for domestic violence cases, must be established and eventually feature—*as a human right*—in international instruments promoting the rights of victims of violent crime. For the moment, universal norms regarding the documentation, examination, treatment, and referral of domestic violence cases are far from being realized.

Acknowledgements

Text extracts from Artz, L., Fear or failure? Why victims of domestic violence retract from the criminal justice process, *South African Crime Quarterly*, Volume 37, pp. 3–10, Copyright © 2011, reproduced with permission from the publisher.

Text extracts from United Nations, *Declaration of Basic Principles of Justice for Victims of Crime and Abuse of Power* (1985 A/Res/40/34), reproduced with permission from the United Nations.

Text extracts from Department of Justice and Constitutional Development, Republic of South Africa, *Domestic Violence Act, 116 of 1998* (adopted 20th November 1998), reproduced under Government Printers Authorization No. 11680, dated 24 March 2014, available from http://www.justice.gov.za/legislation/acts/1998-116.pdf

Text extracts from Southern African Development Community's (SADC's) Protocol on Gender and Development for the Prevention and Eradication of Violence against Women (1997), reproduced under Government Printers Authorization No. 11680, dated 24 March 2014.

References

Advocates for Human Rights. (2011). *Stop Violence against Women: Turkey.* Available at: http://www.stopvaw.org/Turkey.html [Accessed 19 November 2013].

Artz, L. (2003). *Magistrates and the Domestic Violence Act: Issues of Interpretation.* South Africa: Institute of Criminology, Faculty of Law, University of Cape Town & the Open Society Foundation.

Artz, L., and Smythe, D. (2013). South African legislation supporting victim's rights. In: L. Davis and R. Snyman (eds), *South African Handbook of Victimology.* South Africa: Van Schaik Publishers, pp. 131–51.

Artz, L. (2008). *An Examination of the Attrition of Domestic Violence Cases in the Criminal Justice System on Post-Apartheid South Africa.* PhD Dissertation. Belfast: Queen's University.

Artz, L. (2011). Fear or failure? Why victims of domestic violence retract from the criminal justice process. *South African Crime Quarterly, 37,* 3–10.

Artz, L. (2013). *Medico-legal Centres: The Policing/Health Care Nexus.* Independent strategy paper written for the South Sudan Safety and Access to Justice Programme.

Aschman, G., Meer, T., and Artz, L. (2012). Behind the screens: domestic violence and health care practices. *Agenda, 26,* 51–64.

Beijing Declaration and Platform of Action A/Conf.177/20 and A/Conf.177/20/Add.1 (15 September 1995), endorsed by the UN General Assembly on 8 December 1995 (A/RES/50/42).

Coomaraswamy, R. (2000). Combating domestic violence: Obligations of the state. *Innocenti Digest,* 10–11.

Combating of Domestic Violence Act, No. 4. (Adopted by Namibian Parliament 24 June 2003). Available online at http://www1.chr.up.ac.za/undp/domestic/docs/legislation_16.pdf.

Committee Against Torture, General Comment 2, Implementation of article 2 by States Parties (2007). U.N. Doc. CAT/C/GC/2/CRP. 1/Rev.4 Para. 18.

Convention on Preventing and Combating Violence against Women and Domestic Violence. 11.V.2011 (Adopted by the Council of Europe Committee of Ministers on 7 April 2011, Istanbul, Turkey).

Declaration of Basic Principles of Justice for Victims of Crime and Abuse of Power (1985 A/Res/40/34).

Declaration on the Elimination of Violence against Women GA Res 48/104 UN Doc A/48/104 (adopted 20 December 1993).

Domestic Violence (Crime and Punishment) Act, 2066 (Adopted April 27 2009, Nepal). Available online at http://www.lawcommission.gov.np/en/documents/prevailing-laws/prevailing-acts/func-startdown/424/

Domestic Violence Act, 116 of 1998 (Adopted 20 November 1998). Available online at http://www.justice.gov.za/legislation/acts/1998-116.pdf

General Recommendation No. 19 by the Committee on the Elimination of Discrimination against Women. UN. (1992) Available online at http://www.un.org/womenwatch/daw/cedaw/recommendations/recomm.htm. [Accessed 9th December 2013]

Law to protect family and prevent violence against women, No. 6284 (Accepted on 8th March 2012). Available online at http://www.stopvaw.org/Turkey.html.

Maria da Penha Law, Retrains Domestic and Family Violence against Women, No. 11.340 (Adopted 7 August 2006).

Programme of Action of the International Conference on Population and Development, A/CONF.171/13 (18 October 1994).

,U.N. Convention Against Torture and other Cruel, Inhuman or Degrading Treatment or Punishment. General Comment No. 2 (2007): Implementation of article 2 by States parties, UN Doc. CAT/C/GC/2, para. 18.

U.N. Women (2013) *Tajikistan moves towards a law to prevent domestic violence.* Available online at http://www.unwomen.org/co/news/stories/2013/3/tajikistan-moves-towards-a-law-to-prevent-domestic-violence. [Accessed 9th December 2013]

U.N. Women (2011). *In pursuit of Justice: 2011/2012 Progress of the world's women.* UN Women.

Vienna Declaration and Programme of Action adopted by the World Conference on Human Rights (1993) OHCHR. Available online at http://www.ohchr.org/en/professionalinterest/pages/vienna.aspx/

VAWA Reauthorisation Act, HR 3402 / 109th Congress (2005). Adopted 30th June 2005. Available online at http://www.gpo.gov/fdsys/pkg/BILLS-109hr3402enr/pdf/BILLS-109hr3402enr.pdf.

WHO (2013) *Research: Addressing violence against women among women in antenatal care.* Available at: http://who.int/reproductive-health/topics/violence/prevention/en/index.html. [Accessed 9th December 2013].

CHAPTER 39

National and international policies to prevent elder abuse

Bridget Penhale

Issues in Responding to Mistreatment

Before considering the existence, or otherwise, of policies to prevent violence towards older people, it is necessary to briefly explore several relevant issues concerning the mistreatment (abuse and/or neglect) of older people. The first of these relates to the question of whether mistreatment occurs because it is an ageing issue. Put simply, do situations of elder abuse and neglect occur primarily or only as a consequence of the ageing process? From what is known, this appears unlikely. As an example, domestic violence in later life may be a continuation of long-standing patterns of behaviour (Brandl and Horan 2002; Fisher and Regan 2006), and which has existed throughout a relationship (Penhale and Goreham 2013), rather than something that only occurs due to ageing. However, it is apparent that there are several different forms of elder mistreatment and some of these types may be more related to the ageing process than others.

The second issue is a question about whether elder abuse happens as an outcome of the complexities of caregiving. Since it is known that situations of mistreatment do not just occur within a caregiving environment, this also does not appear to provide an answer, albeit that both abuse and neglect may result from failure(s) in caregiving. However, it does not appear that there is any direct causal link between caregiving and abuse or caregiving and neglect. If this were the case then pretty much all caregiving situations would be likely to be or to become abusive or neglectful. As work undertaken on the satisfactions of caregiving evidences (see, for example, Nolan 1997), this is clearly not the situation. Additionally, the available statistical evidence also does not correlate or substantiate this assumption, in that there are far more caregivers providing care to elderly people (usually relatives or partners) than situations of elder abuse or neglect that occur (those that are either reported or not).

Furthermore, if we employ a family violence perspective, which is relevant in this area (Lowenstein 2009), then our focus in terms of responding to such issues likely concentrates on the relevant systems of prevention, protection, and punishment. Yet even in this domain, there are apparent tensions, on the one hand between a service and welfare orientation, and on the other hand a justice and criminalization orientation. Overall, this means that the orientation taken towards prevention of mistreatment may be quite different, depending on which approach is taken, and whether the orientation is fundamentally based on either protection or punishment. Adoption of the latter orientation may well lead to an emphasis on criminal justice approaches rather than on welfare, care, and treatment. However, approaches that are premised on welfare and care are perhaps more likely in systems that are concerned with prevention (or at times also protection). In the development of responses to elder mistreatment, whether these are related to prevention, or to intervention, such aspects require additional attention and exploration.

Protection and Prevention

Prior to deliberating interventions and responses to elder abuse further, we must also consider the concept of protection. As a starting point, we must acknowledge that protection may be:

◆ preventive: to prevent something from occurring

◆ reactive: after an event has occurred but to prevent it from happening again (Browne and Herbert 1997).

There are several protective actions that might be taken concerning elder mistreatment. Such actions include rules, regulations and laws, policies, procedures, and guidance, which have developed in different countries over time as part of frameworks devised to protect older individuals who have experienced mistreatment or are at risk of it happening. Action taken to protect individuals generally includes some attention to systems of risk reduction. This requires accurate assessment and management of risk and these are usually continuing processes. As levels and even types of risk affecting individuals will likely change and alter over time, this means that the assessment process will also need to be dynamic and not seen as something that happens on one occasion. It also means that appropriate management of risk and risky situations needs to include such aspects as monitoring, review, and even regular reassessment of the situation in relation to affected individuals. In addition to assessment and management of risk, in a number of developed countries there is now consideration of risk enablement, through which individuals are supported to take risks in ways in which threats to their overall safety are minimized but that also acknowledges that individuals wish to take risks as part of their everyday lives.

Issues of vulnerability are also an important matter when considering protection; this may relate to vulnerability of the individual themselves due to their situations, or any vulnerability and potential risk of harm to others by an individual (Penhale and Parker 2008). In recent years in the United Kingdom there has been a change of emphasis in relation to vulnerability to recognize that an individual is not vulnerable because of any underlying condition or personal attributes, but that they may become vulnerable due to the situations or circumstances that they find themselves in; this is also known as 'situational vulnerability' (Penhale and Parker 2008).

In terms of levels of prevention, there are three distinct levels at which prevention may occur:

◆ action(s) at community-level that support individuals and prevent harm

◆ action(s) at the individual level to reduce risk of harm

◆ action(s) again at the individual level to prevent re-occurrence of event, once it has occurred (a more reactive approach, to prevent the situation happening again).

Principles of Assessment

Generally, at the level of the individual who is, or may be, affected by mistreatment, before any plan for future care, or full consideration of intervention is developed, the professional should undertake a comprehensive and full assessment of an individual's needs for those who are involved in the situation (perhaps particularly for the victim of the mistreatment). Whilst this assessment ought to be holistic and consider the whole person and their situation, it should also be abuse-focused (Bennett et al. 1997). There should be some initial determination about whether the situation merits an assessment or an investigation of the individual and their circumstances, as an investigation may be somewhat inquisitorial and adversarial in nature. In recent decades several brief tools to assist the assessment process have been developed (see, for example, Bomba 2006; Reis and Nahmiash 1995), and these should be seen as an addition to and part of the process of determining what has happened.

In any event, the care plan that is developed with the individuals concerned as a result of the assessment should include aspects relating to safety planning, and the needs of the individual for protection, in addition to other needs for support that the person may have (Manthorpe 1997). As well as an assessment of the apparent risks in the situation, or which might develop later, there needs to be consideration of how the risk(s) will be managed at that time or in future. The concept of 'protective responsibility' developed by social work academics Stevenson and Parsloe (1993) may also be relevant, as they proposed that professional practitioners should know about how to act responsibly concerning the service users they work with. This perspective recognizes that professionals may sometimes need to act to make sure that individuals have sufficient protection and are kept safe (Stevenson and Parsloe 1993). This might include actions taken to remove a person from a situation (where this is legally possible), but such action(s) would need to be achieved ethically. They must also be in accordance with the

responsibilities of the professional's organization, and their codes of professional conduct and practice as well as any relevant societal conventions that need to be observed.

Intervention Types

A number of different types of intervention exist that might be used in situations of elder mistreatment. These will likely differ from each other in terms of the approach taken and overall orientation. This will depend in part on whether mistreatment is considered to be predominantly a social, health, or criminal justice problem. Some potential types of intervention are:

◆ practical: for example, domiciliary support at home or to reduce apparent caregiver stress

◆ legal: for example, use of relevant legal systems, where these exist

◆ therapeutic: for instance, counselling and therapy to improve relationships

◆ focus on protection and safety: to keep the individual affected by mistreatment safe and to prevent further harm from occurring

◆ focus on autonomy and empowerment to enable the victim to survive and make necessary changes to their situation and lives (the nature of such changes to be determined by the individual)

◆ victim oriented approaches: techniques of intervention designed to assist the victim

◆ abuser oriented approaches: techniques of intervention to assist the abuser.

Decisions about appropriate interventions are based on the situation and type of mistreatment that has taken place. For instance, practical assistance in the home may support the individuals involved in situations where the abuse and/or neglect results from caregiver stress, but such help may not be suitable for financial abuse situations. At present, not enough is known about which intervention strategies work best in which types of situation in order to be able to state with certainty that a particular intervention is most suitable for a specific type of mistreatment. We need more work in future to clarify this issue.

Developing Frameworks for Protection

There has been long-standing discussion and debate in many countries about legislation in relation to adult abuse. The focal point of the debate has concerned whether there should be specific legislation relating to elder abuse or adult protection, which would be comparable to that which exists for children and young people (Penhale 1997). The alternative view is that there is sufficient protection within existing powers and statutes for all adults in many countries and that a separate law for vulnerable adults (which includes many older people) is therefore not necessary (Phillipson 1993). Furthermore, there is a view that were such legislation to develop this would be discriminatory towards vulnerable adults (Slater 1994), as they would not be accorded access to the range of laws normally afforded to all adults and this might be viewed as oppressive. The view is that such measures would create an 'othering' of this group, although they would have access to 'special legislation' designed specifically to protect them from abuse. From the United States have come suggestions that specific laws in relation to vulnerable adults may lead to infantilization and an over-simplistic linkage between protection of adults and the protection of children (Salend et al. 1984). In Canada, it seems that many people have taken a stance that laws intended for the general public are adequate for cases of abuse of older adults, that is family law and laws dealing with physical assault, financial abuse, neglect, mental cruelty, consumer protection, and housing can all be used to assist elders when necessary (Spencer 2006, personal communication).

The contrary view to the suggestions by Phillipson and Slater, outlined earlier, is that provision of specific laws relating to protection of adults at risk of abuse would serve individuals most in need more appropriately than the normal panoply of laws which may be difficult for disadvantaged and excluded individuals to access. Moreover Stevenson (1995) suggested, in connection with this debate in England and Wales, that there is an apparent lack of confidence by health and social care practitioners in the range of existing laws that might be used to assist in abusive or neglectful situations, which leads to views expressed by such professionals that it is not really possible to obtain legal solutions to situations of abuse of vulnerable adults. This could result in situations where existing provision may not even be considered by practitioners, due to this lack of confidence in the present system. Furthermore, there is a sense that practitioners may not provide information about legal provision to the individuals they work with, as they may not wish to raise expectations that a legal solution might be possible.

Legislation to Protect

Older people with impairments (physical and/or cognitive) may be situationally vulnerable and at risk of abuse from others. At times they may also put others at risk of harm by their actions. It is important to note that as in many, if not most countries, there is no single piece of legislation concerning protection of vulnerable adults (of any age) in England and Wales, although this may develop in future. Instead there are a number of different pieces of legislation, different elements (or specific 'sections') of which may be used by individuals who are in need of protection.

However, in Scotland there is specific legislation concerning adult protection, enacted in 2007. The Adult Support and Protection (Scotland) Act was implemented from autumn 2008. The development of legislation followed a period of consultation and a decision to introduce specific, unified legislation to protect adults at risk of harm (Scottish Office 1997). This law is based on a fundamental set of principles and aims to provide the means by which intervention can prevent harm from continuing, to develop stronger measures to protect individuals at risk of harm and to improve inter-agency co-operation and inter-disciplinary practice.

In general, international legislation to protect older people from the victimization of abuse is very scarce. Nevertheless, some countries have passed laws including provision to protect elders, such as Costa Rica, Ecuador, the United States, Finland, and Mexico (García 2010). Japan and South Africa also enacted specific legislation concerned with elder abuse in 2006. We shall specify a few of these.

In Costa Rica, the Law for the Elderly Adult Person was passed in 1999. This states that elders have the right to improve their quality of life through provision of legal and psychological protection in cases of physical, sexual, psychological, and property violence.

In Ecuador, the Elder Law of 1991 aims to guarantee an elder's right to live with dignity. Furthermore, Article 21 lists the administrative penalties in cases of abandonment, abuse, lack of attention in care homes, and psychological maltreatment.

In the United States the Older Americans Act passed in 1965, amended in 1992 and 2000, was created to ensure an older person's equal opportunities and to safeguard their rights. More recently the Elder Justice Act, which contains provisions relating to elder abuse has been enacted, although implementation is slower than hoped for.

In January 1999 the Finnish Act on Restraining Orders came into effect; this may be applied when an adult child extorts money from their elderly parent(s), so can be used in cases of financial abuse.

The 2002 Law for the Rights of Elderly Adults developed in Mexico is worth noting here. This aims to ensure the exercise of an older person's rights and Article 9 charges family members 'with preventing any family member from committing acts of discrimination, abuse, exploitation, isolation, violence or legal acts which endanger the elderly person, their property or their rights'. Article 50 of the Act further stipulates that anyone who knows of a case of abuse or maltreatment against an elderly person is legally obliged to inform the relevant authorities.

Spain does not have a specific crime against elders stipulated in law (although this exists for women and children). Instead elder abuse is covered in other Civil Penal Codes for the protection of this group. Furthermore, in cases of elder abuse advanced age is not considered an aggravating factor. The only explicit reference to older people appears in Organic Law 1/2004 on Integrated Protection Measures against Gender Violence, with Article 28 establishing:

> Women victims of gender-based violence will be considered a priority regarding access to protected housing and public residences for the elderly, under the terms of the applicable legislation.

Law 39/2006, for the Promotion of Personal Autonomy and Assistance to Persons in Situations of Dependence (Dependency Law), offers dependent people (elderly or others) the resources to address their situation. Although there is no explicit reference to abuse, such measures form part of primary and secondary prevention.

It is also important to recognize that in many countries there is no mandatory requirement to report (and act on) situations relating to abuse of either older people or adults who might be considered as vulnerable to mistreatment, although this does exist in a few countries such as Mexico, Israel, and the United States.

The Importance of Protection and Risk

The previous section relating to the use of legislation is a necessary consideration anywhere in the development of good management systems. This is perhaps especially relevant to protection, when it is fundamental to ensure as far as possible that individuals are not further disadvantaged or disempowered by the systems that should assist them. Organizations such as health and social care need to be concerned with more than just provision of direct care and support (including protection) to individuals. The delivery of such care needs to be based on clear policies, procedures, and guidance, which should be particularly developed to ensure that the care and support services provided are the most appropriate and resource-effective.

In order to be effective, perhaps particularly in the area of protection, health and care practitioners need to have a sound working knowledge of the policies and procedures of whichever agency they work for and relevant underpinning legislation. Any policy requires clear lines of responsibility and accountability, so that any decisions taken within that framework are authorized by those persons with necessary training and experience to make them. Social workers and others in the helping professions should begin to learn protective practice when they are undertaking qualifying training. Relevant training in the assessment and management of risk and risky situations, especially concerning violence and abuse should form part of this, as should education relating to the prevention of violence.

In the United Kingdom the general approach taken in this area appears to be based on the concept that provision of regulation and a clear regulatory framework will provide the necessary foundations from which professional practice can be developed, and, furthermore, that such provision will assist in providing protection to vulnerable individuals when required. Other countries may not necessarily have such a concerted approach to the development and establishment of regulation detailing professional practice, workforce issues, and relating to the provision of care and support to individuals.

National Guidance, Local Approaches

In general terms in many countries, guidance from governments in relation to elder abuse does not appear to have been a priority area of concern until relatively recently. Yet this is likely to be an important aspect of prevention of abuse and violence towards vulnerable individuals. The World Health Organization report on violence and health (WHO 2002) included some consideration of elder abuse, and the World Health Assembly held in Madrid in the same year (2002), from which the Madrid International Plan of Action on Ageing (MIPAA) was developed, also paid some attention to elder abuse, although few specific actions on mistreatment resulted at this time. More latterly, issues of safety and protection, indeed of elder abuse, have received rather more international attention in consideration of perspectives relating to the human rights of older people and work undertaken in this area concerning the question of whether there should be a convention on the human rights of older people, operational at United Nations level. In 2011, the UN also endorsed a UN International Day: World Elder Abuse Awareness Day, which is held annually on (or around) 15 June, which was initially introduced by the International Network for the Prevention of Elder Abuse (for further information, see http://www.inpea.net).

Generally, individual countries have been left to develop their own policies concerning the development of responses to elder abuse and this includes attention paid to issues relating to prevention. The provision of such policy guidance in these areas, albeit somewhat limited in many places, is, of course, both important and necessary. In particular, we need to be cognisant of the fact that health and care practitioners do not operate in a vacuum from the wider society in which they live and therefore need the direction of national government and relevant organizations, and where appropriate employing bodies in order to ensure that standards of practice are clearly set at appropriate levels. However, despite some national-led initiatives in relation to abuse, it may often be the case that more localized developments occur concerning this area, in regions or localities.

In a number of places, local organizations began work in the area of abuse and protection some time ago and did not wait for national initiatives to develop and improve practice in this area. In general it is now agreed that the frameworks developed should be inter-agency in approach (Pritchard 1999). Policies and procedures can be shared across agencies, or separate procedures developed by agencies, which then work to a shared, overarching policy, that is multi-agency in nature and scope. We must recognize that policies and procedures are important to inform practitioners of the actions that should be taken at particular points in the process of responding to a situation that is potentially related to abuse and/or neglect. However, policies and procedures on their own cannot ensure good practice and it is essential to explore how these are put into practice (Penhale 1993).

At local level most policies and procedural documents provide detail about what should happen from initial referral, or notification of alleged abuse and the successive stages of investigating, or assessing the circumstances and determining whether abuse has occurred or not. The subsequent stage consists of decisions to be taken about what actions may be necessary, and whether there is, or may be, a need for on-going work or monitoring and review of the situation. Within such procedural documents, specific strategies of intervention are not likely to appear, as this is left to professional decisions about individual situations. In the coming years, improving practice needs to move beyond the development of policies, regulation, and procedures that appear largely designed to guide practitioners through a sequence of processes.

Multidisciplinary Approaches to Protection

As in other areas of violence and abuse, the situations that result in elder abuse are often difficult, complex, and sensitive, and effective collaboration needs to take place between agencies across the range of different types of abuse that may occur. For such collaboration to be successful there needs to be effective multidisciplinary working; even within a relatively discreet area such as elder abuse it is unlikely that any one single profession or specialty would have sufficient expertise to deal with all potential situations. This requires participation and collaboration between different specialties on an inter-disciplinary basis, and is where a coordinated approach to protection, including a specific post of coordinator, can be of particular value. Since the implementation of policy guidance from 2001 in England and Wales (Department of Health 2000; Welsh Assembly Government 2000), an increasing number of local authorities have developed coordinator posts. It is not, however, at this stage a mandatory requirement. This is contrasted with the situation in the United States, where policies derived following implementation of the Older Americans Act,

1965, saw the development of Adult Protective Services teams consisting of specialist social workers with expertise in this area, whose remit includes coordination of responses at the local level. It is essential for such practitioners to have knowledge, understanding, and clear communication skills in dealing with professionals from across the range of professions.

Professionals working with older and vulnerable adults need to have a basic understanding of legal frameworks relating to protection. They also need ready access to expert assistance where necessary. Vulnerable individuals may require help to gain access to appropriate legal support, and increasingly, independent advocacy. This aspect can add unnecessary stress to an already difficult situation. Obtaining appropriate advice from professionals can help to alleviate situations for distressed individuals and may prevent future abuse occurring, at tertiary level.

Good Practice Matters

The development of appropriate responses to situations of elder abuse is at relatively early stages in many countries. In general, most work appears to be in relation to developing responses and procedural systems for professionals. This seems particularly apparent concerning identification and assessment of potentially abusive or neglectful situations, and awareness raising campaigns to assist recognition of mistreatment. Such campaigns may also have a preventative function, as well as sending a clear message of zero tolerance about abuse and violence wherever it occurs.

Institutional and service settings are key areas where attention is needed to afford vulnerable older service-users protection if necessary. However, there also needs to be emphasis on partnership and collaborative working to improve protection for individuals, as an essential prerequisite to development of effective policies and responses (Penhale et al. 2000). Effective inter-agency working is likely to be required within many situations; this may be supported through the development of well-defined inter-agency working arrangements and protocols.

Concluding Comments

At present, not enough is known about elder mistreatment irrespective of the setting in which it occurs. There needs to be better recognition of such situations and more understanding about potential causes. We need to know more about which approaches to prevention and intervention are most successful. For people dealing with situations, standards, both professional and to an extent personal, need to be identified, explored, and extended. Work needs to continue on establishing effective systems of public accountability nationally and internationally. This includes developing clear lines of support for individuals and well-defined expectations of what is required of professionals and para-professionals in such situations. Interventions need to be appropriate and sensitively tailored to meet the needs of the individuals involved. There is also a need to further develop the different levels at which prevention may be targeted in different national contexts.

Awareness and knowledge of the problem, including for the general public, needs to be increased worldwide. To achieve this, systems and approaches to education and training must develop further. This would serve as the framework from which appropriate and effective responses to prevention can then evolve. There is also a critical need for more research in this whole area to improve our knowledge and understanding of elder mistreatment and how to prevent it (Penhale 1999). Commitment and action by individuals and governments are both required in future to follow this agenda as far as necessary.

Acknowledgement

The author would like to acknowledge the assistance of colleague Dr Isabel Iborra for her contribution to the chapter.

References

Adult Support and Protection (Scotland) Act. (2007). TSO (The Stationery Office), London.

Bennett, G., Kingston, P., and Penhale, B. (1997) *The Dimensions of Elder Abuse: Perspectives for practitioners.* Basingstoke: Macmillan.

Bomba, P. (2006). Use of a single page elder abuse assessment and management tool: a practical clinicians approach to identifying elder mistreatment. *Journal of Gerontological Social Work, 46,* 103–22.

Brandl, B., and Horan, D. (2002). Domestic violence in later life: an overview for health providers. *Women & Health, 35,* 41–54.

Browne, K., and Herbert, M. (1997). *Preventing Family Violence.* Chichester: Wiley.

Department of Health (2000). *No Secrets: The Protection of Vulnerable Adults-Guidance on the Development and Implementation of Multi-Agency Policies and Procedures,* London: HMSO.

Fisher, B., and Regan, S. (2006). The extent and frequency of abuse in the lives of older women and their relationship with health outcomes, *The Gerontologist, 46,* 200–9.

García, Y. (2010). Normativa de protección de la violence sobre las personas mayores: derecho comparado. In: M. Javato, and M. de Hoyos (eds), *Violencia, Abuso y Maltrato de Personas Mayores. Perspectiva Jurídico Penal y Procesal,* Valencia: Tirant lo Blanch, pp. 239–50.

International Network for the Prevention of Elder Abuse (INPEA). (2013). Available at: www.inpea.net [Accessed 19 December 2013].

Lowenstein, A. (2009). Elder abuse and neglect –'old phenomenon': new directions for research, legislation, and service developments. *Journal of Elder Abuse & Neglect, 21,* 278–87.

Manthorpe, J. (1997). Developing social work practice in protection and assistance. In: P. Decalmer, and F. Glendenning (eds), *The mistreatment of elderly people.* 2nd ed. London: Sage, pp.163–74.

Nolan, M. (1997). Sustaining meaning: a key concept in understanding elder abuse. In: P. Decalmer, and F. Glendenning (eds), *The mistreatment of elderly people.* 2nd ed. London: Sage, pp.199–209.

Penhale, B. (1993). The abuse of elderly people: considerations for practice. *British Journal of Social Work, 23,* 95–112.

Penhale, B. (1997). Legal dimensions and issues In: G. Bennett, P. Kingston, and B. Penhale (eds), *The Dimensions of Elder Abuse: Perspectives for Practitioners,* Basingstoke: Macmillan, pp.116–52.

Penhale, B. (1999). Research on elder abuse: lessons for practice. In: M. Eastman, and P. Slater (eds), *Elder Abuse: Critical Issues in Policy and Practice,* London, Age Concern Books, pp. 1–23.

Penhale, B., and Goreham, W. (2013). *Mind the Gap: UK National Report,* Norwich: University of East Anglia

Penhale, B., and Parker, J. (2008) *Working with Vulnerable Adults.* London: Routledge.

Penhale, B., Parker, J., and Kingston, P. (2000) *Elder Abuse: Approaches to Working with Violence.* Birmingham: Venture Press.

Phillipson, C. (1993). Abuse of older people: sociological perspectives. In: P. Decalmer, and F. Glendenning (eds), *The Mistreatment of Elderly People.* London: Sage, pp. 102–15.

Pritchard, J. (1999). *Elder Abuse Work: Best practice in Britain and Canada,* London: Jessica Kingsley Publishers.

Reis, M., and Nahmiash, D. (1995). *When Seniors are Abused: A Guide to Intervention.* Quebec: Captus Press.

Salend, E., Kane, R., Satz, M., and Pynoos, J. (1984). Elder abuse reporting: limitations of current statutes, *Gerontologist, 24,* 61–9.

Scottish Office (1997) *Scottish Law Commission Report No 158. Report on Vulnerable Adults.* Blackwell: Edinburgh.

Slater, P. (1994). Social work and old age abuse: laying down the law. In M. Eastman (ed.). *Old Age Abuse: A New Perspective.* London: Chapman Hall, pp.179–98.

Stevenson, O. (1995). Abuse of older people: principles of intervention. In: Department Of Health/Social Services Inspectorate (eds), *Abuse of Older People in Domestic Settings: A report on two SSI seminars.* London: HMSO, pp.20–9

Stevenson, O., and Parsloe, P. (1993). *Community Care and Empowerment.* York: Joseph Rowntree Foundation.

Welsh Assembly Government (WAG) (2000). *In Safe Hands: Implementing Adult Protection Procedures in Wales.* Cardiff: Welsh Assembly Government.

World Health Organization (2002). *World Report on Violence and Health.* Geneva: WHO.

CHAPTER 40

National and international policies to prevent and reduce armed violence

Guy Lamb

Introduction to National and International Policies to Prevent and Reduce Armed Violence

The literature on armed violence prevention and reduction has briskly expanded in recent years, spurred on by various arms control diplomatic efforts and renewed interest in the topic by international organizations, such as the World Health Organization (WHO) and intergovernmental agencies like the United Nations Development Programme (UNDP) and the Organization for Economic Development and Cooperation (OEDC). Some civil society organizations have also refocused their work from arms control and disarmament to violence prevention and reduction and launched international campaigns in this area.

Many of the publications on the topic have sought to provide evidence-based recommendations of 'best practice' and 'what works'. However, as is readily acknowledged, the evidentiary foundation of armed violence prevention and reduction (AVPR) interventions is threadbare, with significant, in-depth, multi-country studies being a rarity. This is astounding as the United Nations Disarmament Research Institute (UNIDIR) calculated that the international donor community contributed close to US$900 million to small arms control interventions between 2001 and 2009 (Maze 2010), of which only an inconsequential amount was earmarked for research.

This chapter seeks to make a modest contribution to the AVPR literature by providing a synopsis of the noteworthy international and national armed violence prevention and reduction processes and initiatives. In addition, it critically reflects on the prevailing manner in which armed violence and AVPR has been conceptualized.

Defining Armed Violence and Armed Violence Prevention: Probing for Precision

The 'armed violence' community of researchers and policy recommenders is relatively small and is mainly associated with think tanks and United Nations (UN) agencies that operate out of Geneva, Switzerland. The Geneva Declaration on Armed Violence and Development (2006), a document devised by diplomatic consultations, chiefly informs this scholarship and publications. This Declaration, which has been signed by over 100 states, asserts that armed violence weakens development and results in insecurity.

Currently there is no consensus on the definition of 'armed violence'. The first report on the *Global Burden of Armed Violence* defined the term as:

> the intentional use of illegitimate force (actual or threatened) with arms or explosives, against a person, group, community, or state, that undermines people-centred security and/or sustainable development. (Krause et al. 2008, p. 2)

A year later a paper by the OECD on armed violence reduction, which was penned by some of the same authors that compiled the *Global Burden of Armed Violence*, defined the term as 'the use or threatened use of weapons to inflict injury, death or psychological harm, which undermines development' (2009, p. 21).

Also in 2009, the UN's Armed Violence Prevention Programme adopted a more nuanced definition of armed violence as:

> the intentional use of physical force, threatened or actual, with arms, against oneself, another person, group, community or State that results in loss, injury, death and/or psychosocial harm to an individual or individuals and that can undermine a community's, country's or region's security and development achievements and prospects. (p. 1)

The inclusion of the disclaimer of undermining development and people-centred security is conceptually problematic, as the connection between violence involving arms at all levels, particularly with respect to interpersonal violence in non-war contexts and high-income countries, and declining levels of development, is not supported by conclusive evidence. Of interest, the *World Development Report 2011*, which considered the nexus of conflict, security, and development in detail, only made a few passing references to 'armed violence' (World Bank 2011).

The term 'arm' is relatively broad, and can effectively include anything from craft firearms to weapons of mass destruction. Therefore, for the purposes of this chapter a more explicit interpretation of armed violence will be adopted, namely violence that involves the use of small arms (or firearms). The main motivation is that firearms are arguably the most prolific and lethal instruments used in incidents of armed violence.

The widely used definition of small arms is included in the *International Instrument to Enable States to Identify and Trace, in a Timely and Reliable Manner, Illicit Small Arms and Light Weapons* (UN 2005), which defines small arms as:

> any man-portable lethal weapon that expels or launches, is designed to expel or launch, or may be readily converted to expel or launch a shot, bullet or projectile by the action of an explosive. (p. 3)

More specifically, small arms are:

> weapons designed for individual use...[and] include, inter alia, revolvers and self-loading pistols, rifles and carbines, sub-machine guns, assault rifles and light machine guns. (p. 3)

Armed Violence Prevention and Reduction

As with the term armed violence, AVPR is of recent vintage. In the growing body of literature on this topic a combination of two approaches have been used to delineate the explicit methods of AVPR, namely: the restating of traditional techniques of small arms control (arms-specific), peace-building, and crime prevention; and the application of an armed violence 'lens' to the existing literature on more general violence reduction and prevention.

Consequently, most publications on AVPR have interpreted the concept to be highly inclusive, where many of the validated and established methods of more general violence prevention and reduction have been expeditiously redefined as armed violence prevention reduction techniques (Bellis et al 2010; Krause et al 2008; Krause et al 2011; OECD 2009; OECD 2011). For analytical purposes many publications make a distinction between 'direct' and 'indirect' AVPR approaches. Direct interventions focus on 'the instruments, actors and institutional environments' that enable armed violence, while indirect interventions focus on the 'proximate and structural risk factors' that result in armed violence (OECD 2011, p. 22).

Adopting an inclusive interpretation of AVPR may be intellectually beneficial as it reveals the inter-connectedness of the various forms of violence and violence prevention and reduction. However, such an approach dilutes the focus on the potential effectiveness of strategies that specifically relate to arms. Hence, for the purpose of this chapter, a less ambiguous approach to AVPR will be adopted, one that considers: measures that seek to control or limit access to small arms; and measures that directly target people in possession of small arms.

International and Intergovernmental Initiatives to Reduce Armed Violence

Multilateral Arms Embargoes

The chief international (UN) instrument to reduce and prevent further intensifications of armed violence is the UN Security Council (UNSC) arms embargoes. The UNSC often imposes mandatory arms embargoes against states or insurgent groups that are considered to pose a significant threat to international peace and security. Arms embargoes are based on the assumption that the transfer of arms and military material into the embargoed territories will contribute to an escalation of armed violence and instability (Lamb 2007). Some intergovernmental organizations have a mandate to impose arms embargoes in relation to its member states, such as the European Union.

The effectiveness of arms embargoes is a moot point, as such measures are entirely dependent on the extent to which states can put partisan interests aside and implement the embargo at the national level (Lamb 2007). A study by the Stockholm International Peace Research Institute suggests that embargo implementation increases where there is: the presence of a peace-keeping mission in the embargo area; and the full support for the embargo by the Permanent Five member of the UNSC and states that share borders with the embargoed area (Fruchart et al. 2007). To date there are no rigorous studies that have empirically linked the imposition of UNSC arms embargoes to reductions in armed violence, as arms embargoes are usually implemented in environments where conflicting parties are specifically looking to use violence as a means to achieve a particular set of objectives.

International Arms Control Instruments

Internationally, the reduction and prevention of violence perpetrated by small arms is pursued by means of two principal international agreements: UN Programme of Action to Prevent, Combat and Eradicate the Illicit Trade in Small Arms and Light Weapons in all its Aspects (2001); and the UN Protocol against the Illicit Manufacturing of and Trafficking in Firearms, their Parts and Components and Ammunition (2001).

The Programme of Action is a non-binding framework to guide states in combating small arms (and light weapons) proliferation. Through this initiative, states have committed themselves to a range of small arms and light weapons (SALW) control measures. Related to this, the UN has also developed International Small Arms Control Standards, which includes a module on AVPR. The legally binding UN Protocol asserts that the illicit manufacturing of and trafficking in firearms and ammunition has detrimental effects for security and well-being.

The UN General Assembly adopted the text of an Arms Trade Treaty (ATT) in April 2013. It seeks to establish standards for the conventional arms trade (which includes small arms) and will prohibit transfers of arms that will be used to perpetrate crimes against humanity, war crimes, genocide, attacks against civilians, and other grave breaches of the Geneva Conventions. The ATT, however, will only enter into force after 50 states have ratified it.

Regional Instruments and Agreements

There are a variety of regional declarations, plans of action, and instruments that relate to the control of SALW. These agreements have sought to, amongst other objectives: make the illicit production and possession of SALW a criminal offence; ensure/promote the destruction of stocks of surplus weapons; and introduce tighter control measures over weapon stockpiles and arms transfers. To assist in the implementation of these agreements, the relevant regional organizations have established a secretariat or implementation support unit. Detailed plans of action and various guidelines have also been devised to put into practice the provisions of the agreements.

Measures to Control or Limit Access to Arms

Various studies have suggested that there is a higher probability of armed violence, particularly firearm homicide, where there are elevated levels of firearm possession combined with risk factors for violence. Studies that have been conducted on arms control in Austria, Australia, Brazil, Colombia, El Salvador, and New Zealand indicate that the introduction of more stringent firearm controls can result in a reduction, or an accelerated reduction, in firearm injuries and homicides (WHO 2009). However, the body of evidence on the correlation between specific arms control mechanisms and AVPR is significantly limited. Consequently, the AVPR utility of most of these measures can only be partially determined, mainly in situations where such measures have been inadequately implemented or are completely absent.

Manufacturing and Dealer Controls

Governments typically use policy and legislation to control the types of arms and ammunition that are manufactured and traded. Manufacturers and dealers are usually required to: be licenced; maintain records of their stock; as well as implement safety and security measures in order to prevent loss and theft. Government authorities can promote and enforce compliance through regular inspections and pursuing criminal justice action when manufacturers and dealers do not adhere to legislative requirements. However, the effectiveness of such controls is largely dependent on the enforcement capacity of the authorities.

The United States is one of the few countries where there is publicly available case study data linking loss/theft of firearms from manufacturers and dealers to armed violence. For example, in 1999 an employee of an arms manufacturer, Kahr Arms (Worcester, MA), stole a handgun from his employer and used it to shoot two men, one fatally. Kahr Arms was charged with negligence due to inadequate security measures. In another case in 2002, John Allen Muhammad, also known as the 'Beltway sniper', and an accomplice shot ten people with an assault rifle that had either been misplaced by or stolen from the Bull's Eye Shooter Supply firearm dealership (Tacoma, Washington; Gerney and Parsons 2013).

Arms Transfers and Arms Brokering Controls

There is recognition by some arms exporting states that under certain circumstances, arms transfers have the potential to contribute to violence, as well as undermine international peace and security. Consequently, these arms exporting states have established arms export criteria with the objective of mitigating the possibility that their arms transfers may directly result in the occurrence or exacerbation of armed violence. The key aspects of such criteria commonly consider the human rights record, the state of internal stability of the recipient state, as well as the risk that the arms may be diverted to a conflict hotspot.

It appears that in many cases, governments that export arms without due consideration for the negative consequences of such transfers have contributed to armed violence (or an escalation thereof) in the recipient states. This has been the case in Darfur (an area subject to UNSC arms embargo), where Chinese and Russian arms were allegedly used by the Sudanese government to attack civilians, either directly through indiscriminate aerial bombardments, or by means of supplying arms to aggressive militia groups who in turn committed grave human rights abuses (Amnesty International 2007).

In relation to arms transfers, effective border control in transit states can significantly contribute to violence prevention in countries with a high risk of armed violence. There have been numerous cases where competent and alert border control and customs officials have seized illicit arms and ammunition shipments bound for conflict zones (Seniora and Poitevin 2010). However, where government border control is weak or absent, arms have flowed to repressive governments and violent insurgent groups, (Seniora and Poitevin 2010).

Effective control over arms brokers (who largely facilitate arms transfers) can only be achieved through establishing and implementing national legislation. However, only a few governments, such as the United States, South Africa and Member States of the European Union have instituted effective arms brokering regulations, which has meant the constraining and prosecution of arms brokers responsible for weapons smuggling has been a rarity, particularly as such individuals have been skilled in relocating their operations to circumvent new national control measures. The capture and prosecution of Viktor Bout, arguably one of the most notorious arms brokers, is an exceptional case, and required dynamic criminal justice cooperation between the authorities in the United States and Thailand (*The Economist* 2008).

Arms Stockpile Management

In the small arms literature it is a truism that where weapons stockpiles are securely maintained, well organized, and effectively managed, the risk is reduced that the arms and ammunition from such stockpiles will be lost or stolen. Recommended stockpile management techniques include: physical security, such as fencing, robust armouries with sturdy locks, access control, guarding, and patrolling; weapons registration systems, which can include the marking of the arms with unique codes and then recording detailed information about each firearm in a database, which can include the ballistic 'fingerprint' of the firearm; and weapon accountability systems. Regular audits and stocktaking are also recommended. In circumstances where arms are stolen or lost, information from the database can assist in determining where the weaknesses in the security and accountability measures exist.

Research undertaken by UN investigators into arms embargo violations reveals that insurgent groups have been able to source arms and ammunition from inadequately secured weapons stockpiles held by governments and peacekeepers in conflict hotspots (Lamb and Dye 2009a). This has reportedly been the case, for example, in the eastern Democratic Republic of Congo (DRC), Ivory Coast, Mali, and Sierra Leone. In all four countries, arms and ammunition for the insurgent groups were in short supply, and consequently the stolen and captured weapons from government or peacekeeping stocks arguably contributed to a perpetuation of armed violence in these contexts (Lamb and Dye 2009a).

Firearm Licensing

Firearm licensing typically entails background checks (of firearm licence applicants), waiting periods, minimum age stipulations, and limitations on the number and type of firearms and ammunition that an individual may possesses. In some countries, such as Australia, Mauritius, and South Africa, firearm competency testing (both knowledge of the law and practical proficiency regarding firearm handling and safety) exist as an additional licensing requirement. Some governments require licensed firearms to be marked, as well as undergo a ballistics test, with the marking and ballistic 'fingerprint' being recorded in a database. Such information is essential in police investigations and criminal justice action relating to firearm crime.

Evidence from public health research in the United States and Canada has indicated that background checks have the potential to reduce firearm homicides and injuries. It was found that U.S. states with less stringent background checks were significantly linked with relatively high levels of firearm homicides (Ruddell and Mays 2005). Another study suggested that the denial of legal firearms to persons with a prior felony conviction might lower their rate of subsequent criminal activity (Wright et al. 1999).

Minimum age licensing requirements (often between 18 and 21) for the possession of firearms have been introduced in a significant number of countries in an attempt to reduce the access of children and youth to firearms, and therefore diminish the possible occurrence of suicides, homicides, and unintentional shootings among children and youth (Sorenson and Berk 1999).

Measures that Directly Target People in Possession of Small Arms

Firearms have considerably greater lethality potential compared to sharp-force and blunt-force instruments, as a person with a firearm is able to injure or kill multiple individuals while maintaining a non-intimate distance with a minimal degree of effort. Unintentional fatal injuries from firearms also considerably surpass those that arise from other instruments. Consequently a series of measures have been devised to: regulate the manner in which legal firearms must be stored or secured, carried, used, and disposed of; and remove firearms from high risk and potentially violent individuals and groups, as well as criminals.

Disarmament and Weapons Collection

There are two general approaches to disarmament and weapons collection according to the UN's Integrated Disarmament, Demobilization and Reintegration Standards (IDDRS), namely: 'directed' and 'cooperative' disarmament (UN Inter-Agency Working Group on Disarmament, Demobilization and Reintegration 2006).

Directed programmes typically use legal or official instruments to compel those in possession of arms and ammunition to surrender them to the relevant authorities. They can be implemented by means of military and police operations, and/or through the creation of enforced weapons-free zones. The implementation of some directed programmes has been highly controversial, such as in Uganda and South Sudan where excessive lethal force was used, resulting in deaths and injuries (Lamb and Dye 2009b). Firearm amnesties are a less forceful means of directed disarmament, where immunity from prosecution is offered to those who surrender illegal firearms. In South Africa, for example, the police implemented an amnesty in 2005, which resulted in over 100,000 firearms being handed to the police (Kirsten 2007).

In Mozambique, a multi-year disarmament, arms collection, and destruction programme titled Operation Rachel was initiated in 1995 by the government in partnership with the South African police. A parallel civil society incentivized arms collection initiative was also established. These disarmament and arms collection processes resulted in the collection of more than 50,000 firearms and close to 10 millions rounds of ammunition. Studies of non-natural deaths in Maputo, the Mozambican capital, suggests that these disarmament and arms collections could possibly have contributed to the reduction in firearm-related deaths in Maputo (Francisco and Zacarias 2010; WHO and Small Arms Survey 2009).

Cooperative disarmament programmes entail the use of incentives to encourage voluntary disarmament, such as cash, food, goods, or development. Participation in cooperative disarmament processes is, however, largely influenced by perceptions of insecurity. If individuals feel unsafe, then it is unlikely that significant numbers of serviceable firearms and ammunition will be surrendered (Lamb and Dye 2009b).

Armed Government and Private Security Personnel

UN and non-governmental investigations of arms and ammunition supply and use in conflict zones reveals that armed government personnel are among the main sources of arms for rebel, militia, and high-risk groups. In many instances, soldiers voluntarily sell the arms and ammunition. Some country-specific examples include Albania, the eastern DRC, Libya, Sierra Leone, and Somalia.

Members of the security forces are often amongst the principal perpetrators of armed violence. Codes of conduct, standing orders, and human rights training can lessen the incidents of excessive use of lethal force. However, research has shown that such measures have the potential to prevent violence only in circumstances where armed government personnel are continually held to account for their actions and where disciplinary and criminal justice action is objectively pursued when transgressions occur (Lamb 2002).

Armed private security personnel have also been implicated in acts of violence in a variety of locations (including stable democracies), but particularly in war zones and volatile environments. The most infamous example has been the human rights abuses and extrajudicial killings committed by Blackwater employees in Iraq (Devereaux 2012). Regulations and codes of conduct for private security operators have been established in some contexts, but, as with armed government personnel, these systems will only be effective if properly and impartially enforced (Perrin 2006).

Legally Armed Civilians

Governments have imposed a range of controls on licensed civilian firearm owners. The nature and extent of these controls however varies between countries, and even within countries. There is case study evidence that suggests that some of these licencing requirements can contribute to AVPR.

In terms of safe storage, the WHO suggests that firearms in the home pose a risk for both intimate femicide and suicide (Krug et al. 2002). Evidence from public health research in the United States and Canada has indicated that safe storage of firearms in homes and businesses has the potential to reduce firearm homicides, suicides, and injuries. For example, a 2005 study of public health data from various states in the United States found that firearm prevalence and lax firearm storage practices, such as leaving firearms loaded and unlocked, were linked to firearm deaths in the home (Miller et al. 2005).

The WHO (2009) points to the violence reduction potential of targeted firearm carrying restrictions, and highlights initiatives in Colombia and El Salvador. In certain Colombian cities, firearm owners were prohibited from carrying firearms on high-risk days, such as weekends and public holidays. In El Salvador, firearms were banned from schools and a variety of public spaces in some municipalities. There is evidence to suggest that both initiatives contributed to the reduction in firearm homicides in the respective areas.

Specialized Criminal Justice and Policing Action

There is evidence that indicates that confiscating firearms from convicted perpetrators of violence can dramatically reduce homicides (and related perpetrator suicide). Bellis et al. (2010) points to potential benefits of specialized firearm courts (based on experiences in the United States and Jamaica), where firearm-related cases (particularly those committed by juveniles) are fast-tracked through the criminal justice system. In some instances, offenders of certain firearm crimes were placed in rehabilitation programmes, which contributed to reducing the rate of reoffending.

Policing action that specifically targets individuals and groups that possess illegal weapons have been pursued in many countries. These operations are typically intelligence-driven and involve the apprehension of illegal firearm owners, and the confiscation of the firearm. Such strategies have been linked to organized crime reduction strategies (particularly gangsterism), as well as community policing initiatives. Such policing operations can result in the reduction firearm violence in the short to medium term (Bellis et al. 2010).

Demobilization and Reintegration of Former Combatants

The demobilization and reintegration of individuals associated with military or armed formations into civilian society are widely viewed as an essential violence reduction measure in the aftermath of armed conflict. This is based on the basic assumption that the risk of post-war violence will be reduced if armed groups are disbanded, and those individuals that have been trained in the use of violence and/or possess firearms are able to pursue a civilian livelihood, and no longer have access to firearms in a post-war environment.

Those being demobilized are either disarmed prior to or during the demobilization process. In some countries, only individuals with firearms were permitted to participate in the demobilization process. However, logistical, infrastructural, and political dynamics may result in the implementation of sub-standard disarmament and demobilization procedures. There is case study evidence to suggest that such conditions may result in violence within the cantonment areas (such as in Zimbabwe in the early 1980s). In some cases ex-combatants absconded with their weapons and engaged in banditry activities (eastern DRC in the 2000s), or reignited armed conflict (Angola in the early 1990s; Lamb et al. 2012; Lamb 2013).

To date there are no reliable, multi-country studies that have considered the connection between reintegration processes and armed violence. However, relatively recent evidence from Mozambique and Zimbabwe indicate that party political expediency can contribute to the remobilization of reintegrated combatants, who then engage in violent acts (Lamb 2013).

Conclusion

Armed violence is likely to remain a priority concern for states, civil society, and international donors for the foreseeable future. Hence, there is an imperative for both a deeper and wider empirical base for AVPR programming and interventions, as in most cases existing research findings are not generalizable. This problem is compounded by the pursuit of all-encompassing definitions of AVPR. In order to make progress in understanding the strengths and weaknesses of AVPR there needs to be a more succinct focus on armed violence, and further rigorous qualitative and quantitative research should be undertaken (preferably comparable). In addition, donor governments and agencies should consider including research and in-depth evaluation as core components of their support for arms control and AVPR processes and activities.

References

Amnesty International and International Peace Information Service. (2007). *Sudan: Arms Continuing to Fuel Serious Human Rights Violations in Darfur*. London: Amnesty International.

Bellis, M. A., Jones, L., Hughs, K., and Hughs, S. (2010). *Preventing and Reducing Armed Violence: What Works?* New York and Oslo: United Nations Development Programme and Norwegian Ministry of Foreign Affairs.

Devereaux, R. (2012). Blackwater guards lose bid to appeal charges in Iraqi civilian shooting case. *The Guardian*, 5 June 2012. Available at: http://www.theguardian.com/world/2012/jun/05/blackwater-guards-lose-appeal-iraq-shooting [Accessed 17 December 2013].

Francisco, V. C., and Zacarias A. E. (2010). The burden of deaths caused by guns in Maputo City, Mozambique. *Injury Prevention, 16,* A167.

Fruchart, D., Holtom, P., Wezeman, S. T., Strandow, D., and Wallensteen, P. (2007). *United Nations Arms Embargoes. Their Impact on Arms Flows and Target Behaviour*. Solna: SIPRI.

Gerney, A., and Parsons, C. (2013). *Lost and Stolen Guns from Gun Dealers*. Center for American Progress 18 June. Available at: http://www.americanprogress.org/issues/guns-crime/report/2013/06/18/66693/lost-and-stolen-guns-from-gun-dealers/ [Accessed 20 November 2013].

Kirsten, A. (2007). *Simpler, Better, Faster Review of the 2005 Firearms Amnesty*. ISS Paper 134. Pretoria: Institute for Security Studies.

Krause, K., Muggah, R. and Gilgen, E. (2011). *Global Burden of Armed Violence*. Cambridge: Cambridge University Press.

Krause, K., Muggah, R., and Wenmann, A. (2008). *Global Burden of Armed Violence*. Geneva: Geneva Declaration Secretariat.

Krug, E. G. Dahlberg, L. L Mercy, J. A., Zwi, A. B., and Lozano, R. (2002). *World Report on Violence and Health*. Geneva: World Health Organization.

Lamb, G. (2002). Debasing democracy: security forces and human rights abuses in post-liberation Namibia and South Africa. In: Y. D. Davids, C. Keulder, G. Lamb, J. Pereira, and D. Spilker (eds), *Measuring Democracy and Human Rights in Southern Africa*. Discussion Paper 18. Uppsala: Nordic Africa Institute, pp. 30–49.

Lamb, G. (2007). Beyond 'shadow-boxing' and 'lip service'. The enforcement of arms embargoes in Africa. *ISS Paper 135*. Pretoria: Institute for Security Studies.

Lamb, G., and Dye, D. (2009a). Africa in the 21st Century: African solutions to an international problem: arms control and disarmament in Africa. *Journal of International Affairs, 62,* 69–83.

Lamb, G., and Dye, D. (2009b). *Security Promotion and DDR: Linkages between ISM, DDR, and SSR within a Broader Peacebuilding Framework*. First International Congress on Disarmament, Demobilization and Reintegration, Cartagena, 4–6 May 2009.

Lamb, G., Alusala, N., Mthembu-Salter, G., and Gasana, J-M. (2012). *Rumours of Peace, Whispers of War. Assessment of the Reintegration of Ex-Combatants into Civilian Life in North Kivu, South Kivu and Ituri, Democratic Republic of Congo*. Washington, D.C.: World Bank.

Lamb, G. (2013). *Historical Review of the Long-term Impact of Post-independence DDR in Southern Africa*. Washington, D.C.: World Bank.

Maze, K. (2010). *Searching for Aid Effectiveness in Small Arms Assistance*. Geneva and New York: UNIDIR.

Miller, M., Azrael, D., Hemenway, D., and Vriniotis, M. (2005). Firearm storage practices and rates of unintentional firearm deaths in the United States, *Accident Analysis and Prevention, 37,* 661–7.

OECD. (2009). *Armed Violence Reduction: Enabling Development*. Paris: OECD.

OECD. (2011). *Investing in Security: A Global Assessment of Armed Violence Reduction Initiatives, Conflict and Fragility*. Paris: OECD.

Perrin, B. (2006). Promoting compliance of private security and military companies with international humanitarian law, *International Review of the Red Cross, 88,* 613–36.

Ruddell, R., and Mays, G. L. (2004). Risky behaviour, juveniles, guns, and unintentional firearms fatalities, *Youth Violence and Juvenile Justice, 2,* 342–58.

Ruddell, R., and Mays, G. L. (2005). State background checks and firearms homicides. *Journal of Criminal Justice, 33,* 127–36.

Seniora J., and Cédric Poitevin, C. (2010). *Managing Land Borders and the Trafficking of Small Arms and Light Weapons*. Brussels: Groupe de recherche et d'information sur la paix et la sécurité.

Sorenson, S. B., and Berk, R. A. (1999). Young guns: an empirical study of persons who use a firearm in a suicide or a homicide. *Injury Prevention, 5,* 280–3.

The Economist. (2008). *International Man of Mystery. Flying Anything to Anybody*, 18 December 2008. Available at: http://www.economist.com/node/12795502 [Accessed 02 December 2013].

United Nations. (2001). *Programme of Action to Prevent, Combat and Eradicate the Illicit Trade in Small Arms and Light Weapons in All Its Aspects*. A/CONF.192/15. New York: UN.

United Nations. (2005). *International Instrument to Enable States to Identify and Trace, in a Timely and Reliable Manner, Illicit Small Arms and Light Weapons*. A/CONF.192/15. New York: UN.

United Nations. (2009). *Promoting Development through the Reduction and Prevention of Armed Violence*, A/64/228. New York: UN.

United Nations. (2013). *Arms Trade Treaty*. New York: UN.

UN Inter-Agency Working Group on Disarmament, Demobilization and Reintegration (UN IAWG–DDR). (2006). *Integrated Disarmament, Demobilization and Reintegration Standards*. New York: UN.

UN Security Council. (2013). *Final Report of the Panel of Experts established pursuant to Resolution 1973 (2011) concerning Libya*, S/2013/99. New York: UN.

Wright, M. A., Wintemute, G. J., and Rivara, F. P. (1999). Effectiveness of denial of handgun purchase to persons believed to be at high risk for firearm violence. *American Journal of Public Health, 89,* 88–90.

World Bank. (2011). *World Development Report. Conflict, Security and Development*. Washington, D.C.: World Bank.

World Health Organization. (2009). *Guns, Knives and Pesticides: Reducing Access to Lethal Means*. Geneva: WHO.

WHO and Small Arms Survey. (2009). *Firearm-related Violence in Mozambique*. Geneva: Small Arms Survey.

CHAPTER 41

Alcohol and violence

Peter Anderson

Introduction to Alcohol and Violence

Alcohol is an intoxicant drug that affects a wide range of structures and processes in the central nervous system which, interacting with personality characteristics, associated behaviour, and sociocultural expectations, is a causal factor for intentional and unintentional injuries and harm to people other than the drinker; including interpersonal violence, suicide, homicide, and crime (Anderson and Baumberg 2006; Anderson et al. 2009).

Essentially, the more alcohol is consumed, the more frequently it is consumed, and the more that is consumed on a drinking occasion, the greater the risk of injury and violence, with no level of consumption that is risk free (Shield et al. 2012). One-third of all the health harm from alcohol comes from injuries, and about one in five of all unintentional injuries and one in four of all intentional injuries are due to alcohol (Taylor et al. 2011). Some one-quarter of all crime, one-half of all violent crime, two-fifths of all sex offences, and two-fifths of all family violence are estimated to result from alcohol (Anderson and Baumberg 2006).

The most extensive study investigating the harm done by alcohol to people other than the drinker has been undertaken in Australia (Laslett et al. 2010). Seventy per cent of respondents had been affected by a stranger's drinking, experiencing nuisance, fear or abuse, two-fifths of respondents seriously so. Thirty per cent of respondents had been affected by the drinking of someone close to them, one in ten seriously so. The costs to society resulting from someone else's drinking were essentially as much as the costs attributable to individual drinkers alone.

All evidence-based alcohol policies that reduce the harm done by alcohol also reduce alcohol-related injuries and violence, although not all studies provide separated estimates of the impact on violence. These include environmental policies that increase the price of alcohol and reduce its availability and marketing, and policies that are implemented in the community, including those that affect the design of drinking establishments. All of these actions have immediate effect in reducing alcohol-related violence and injury.

The surprising thing is that, in general, the world has failed to take the harm done by alcohol seriously, including violence and injuries, which affect people other than the drinker, and to implement the action that is needed. An illustration of the failure is the fact that over the 20-year period from 1990 to 2010, ill-health and deaths from alcohol have increased by one-third (Lim et al. 2012). This situation is likely to get worse over the coming years, since, whilst only two-fifths of the world's adults are current drinkers, with economic development in Africa and Asia, more non-drinking people will start to drink alcohol (Shield et al. 2011).

This chapter describes alcohol's impact on injuries and violence. It then outlines those policies at the level of the government and the community that can be put in place to reduce alcohol-related injuries and violence. The chapter concludes with a call for an international binding agreement to manage alcohol, the only psychoactive drug not covered by such an agreement.

Alcohol and Personal Violence

Injuries

The risk of injury and violence is related to both the volume of alcohol consumed and the frequency of drinking. Risks increase non-linearly with increasing alcohol consumption, with no risk free level of consumption (Taylor et al. 2010). For non-motor vehicle injury, when considering the amount of alcohol consumed during a previous 3-hour period, the odds ratios (OR) for an injury compared with not drinking increase from 1.30 (95 per cent CI: 1.26–1.34) at 10g of alcohol (one standard drink) consumed during the previous three hours to an OR of 24.2 (95 per cent CI: 16.2–36.2) at 140g (14 standard drinks) consumed during the previous 3 hours.

Alcohol-attributable fractions for death by injury are estimated as 0.13 for death by falls, 0.20 for death by fires, 0.22 for death by drowning, 0.27 for self-inflicted injuries, and 0.28 for homicides (Taylor et al. 2011). The lifetime risk of death from an alcohol related injury increases with both the amount drunk per day and the frequency of drinking (National Health and Medical Research Council 2009). Perhaps surprisingly, at any given volume or frequency of consumption, the risks are greater for men than for women. A man who drinks more than 20g of alcohol five or more times a week has a more than 1 in 100 lifetime risk of dying from an alcohol-related injury.

Violence

A substantial proportion of incidents of aggression and violent crime involves one or more participants who have been drinking, with episodic heavy drinking, frequency of drinking, and drinking volume all independently associated with the risk of aggression (Anderson and Baumberg 2006). The relationship between alcohol consumption and the risk of involvement in violence, including homicide, is stronger for intoxication than for overall consumption. A large number of studies have demonstrated a significantly increased risk of involvement in violence among heavy drinkers, who are also more likely to be the recipients of violence.

There is an overall relationship between greater alcohol use and criminal and domestic violence, with particularly strong evidence from studies of domestic and sexual violence (Anderson and Baumberg 2006). The relationship is attenuated when other characteristics, such as culture, gender, age, social class, criminal status, childhood abuse, and use of other drugs in addition to alcohol, are taken into account. Generally the higher the level of alcohol consumption, the more serious is the violence. Alcohol-related sexual assaults by strangers seem to be more likely to occur the greater the alcohol consumption of the victim, whereas the risk of alcohol-related sexual assaults by partners or spouses seems to be independent of the alcohol consumption of the victim (Anderson and Baumberg 2006).

Aside from epidemiological and experimental research relating intoxication and violence, there is also research indicating specific biological mechanisms that link alcohol to aggressive behaviour (Alcohol and Baumberg 2006), which are moderated by situational and cultural factors. The pharmacological effects of alcohol include increased emotional lability, focus on the present, less self-awareness, decreased ability to consider consequences or reduced ability to solve problems, and impaired self-regulation. However, these biological pathways are mediated by people's expectations about how people act after drinking, including how acceptable it is to act drunkenly and how accepted certain behaviours are when drunk. Alcohol also appears to interact with personality characteristics and other factors related to a personal propensity for violence, such as impulsivity. In addition to alcohol consumption and drinking pattern, the social context of drinking is also important for alcohol-related aggression, especially for young people whose drinking behaviour is influenced strongly by peers.

Public drinking establishments are high-risk locations for alcohol-related aggression. However, drinking contexts by themselves do not explain the relationship between alcohol and aggression, since the impact of alcohol also acts independently of the context or setting in which drinking is taking place. The environment for alcohol-related aggression is also not independent of drinking. Although a few incidents that occur in bars involve interpersonal conflict between friends or couples that might have occurred in another setting, almost all incidents of aggression that occur in bars are unplanned, emerge from the social interaction in the bar, and often involve strangers. The Comparative Risk Assessment study of the World Health Organization (WHO) concluded that it seems reasonable to assume that almost all incidents of violence occurring in bars and other environments where drinking is the main activity should be considered attributable to alcohol, either directly through the pharmacological effects of alcohol or indirectly through the social norms related to drinking (Rehm et al. 2004).

In the European Union, it has been estimated that between 7 and 47 per cent of all crimes, between 24 and 86 per cent of all violent crimes, between 19 and 53 per cent of all robberies, and between 29 and 60 per cent of all sex offences are linked to alcohol (Anderson and Baumberg 2006). Links are found between alcohol and crime across the European Union, but the proportion of crimes that are alcohol related are higher in northern as opposed to southern European countries. Some four out of ten homicides and two out of ten suicides in the European Union are estimated to be due to alcohol. Alcohol is estimated to cost the European Union some €155 billion a year (Shield et al. 2012), of which over one-quarter is due to costs of crime, excluding traffic accident-related costs (Anderson and Baumberg 2006).

Family Harm and Violence

A large number of cross-sectional studies and a few longitudinal studies on alcohol consumption and marital aggression have shown that husbands' heavy drinking increases the risk of marital violence, in a dose-dependent manner (Anderson and Baumberg 2006). Parental drinking can affect the environment in which a child grows up through financial strain, poor parenting, marital conflicts, and negative role models. A large number of studies have reported a variety of childhood mental and behavioural disorders to be more prevalent among children of heavy drinkers than others, although many of these studies have been criticized for inadequate methodology (Anderson and Baumberg 2006). A few recent reports from well-designed studies have shown a higher risk of child abuse in families with heavy drinking parents. Systematic reviews have suggested that alcohol is a cause of child abuse in 16 per cent of cases (Ridolfo and Stevenson 2001).

Goals and Approaches to Reducing Alcohol-Related Violence

Given that alcohol-related violence results from each of drinking volume, frequency of drinking, and frequency and volume of episodic heavy drinking, any measures that reduce the amount of alcohol consumed on average and during a drinking occasion are likely to reduce alcohol-related violence, with immediate effect, that is no time lag. Relationships between changes in per capita alcohol consumption and changes in death rates for a range of injuries (and other diseases) have been studied throughout the world, but particularly in Europe, where a reduction of one litre of pure alcohol per capita per year in medium-consuming countries was associated with a 3 per cent reduction in deaths from accidents, a 1.5 per cent reduction in deaths from suicide, and a 7 per cent reduction in deaths from homicide (Norström et al. 2001).

Impact of Environmental Policies

Alcohol's global harm, including alcohol-related violence, is preventable. There is a very extensive evidence base to inform the implementation of effective alcohol policy that can reduce alcohol-related violence (Anderson et al. 2009; Babor et al. 2010). Not all alcohol policy measures and actions that have been evaluated have specifically portioned out separate impacts on violence.

Price Increases

According to WHO estimates, tax increases represent the most cost-effective response to reduce alcohol-related harm, including violence, in countries with a high prevalence of heavy drinking (Anderson et al. 2009). In lower-prevalence contexts, where alcohol use by women is relatively infrequent, population-level effects drop off and cost-effectiveness ratios rise accordingly. The effect of alcohol tax increases stands to be mitigated by illegal production, tax evasion, and illegal trading. Reducing this unrecorded consumption via concerted tax enforcement strategies by law enforcement and excise officers is estimated to cost more than a tax increase but produces similar levels of effect. In settings with higher levels of unrecorded production and consumption such as India, increasing the proportion of consumption that is taxed (and therefore more cost to the price-sensitive consumer) may represent a more effective pricing policy than a simple increase in excise tax (which may only encourage further illegal production, smuggling, and cross-border purchases).

Systematic reviews find that price increases reduce alcohol consumption across all beverage types and across all types of drinkers from light to heavy drinkers and across all jurisdictions (Österberg 2012a; Sornpaisarn et al. 2013). Price increases also reduce mortality rates, deaths form violence, crime, use of illegal drugs, and incidence of sexually transmitted diseases (Wagenaar et al. 2010), as well as rape, robberies, family violence, and homicide (Anderson and Baumberg 2006). A reduction in alcohol taxation in Finland in 2004 had substantial effects in increasing alcohol-related sudden deaths, overall alcohol-related mortality, and criminality and hospitalizations (Österberg 2012a). In Alaska, United States, excise duty increases in 1983 and 2002 were associated with substantial reductions in alcohol-related disease mortality (Wagenaar et al. 2009).

A specific pricing policy that targets particularly cheap alcohol is to set a minimum price per gram of alcohol sold. This option also has many other advantages, in that, even more than tax increases, which also do the same, introducing a minimum price per gram of alcohol sold targets heavy-drinking occasions and heavy drinkers, much more so than lighter drinkers, leading to reductions in unintentional and intentional injuries, including alcohol-related assaults (Purshouse et al. 2010). Minimum alcohol prices in British Columbia, Canada, have been adjusted intermittently over the years 1989–2010. Time series and longitudinal models of aggregate alcohol consumption with price and other economic data as independent variables found that a 10 per cent increase in the minimum price of an alcoholic beverage reduced its consumption relative to other beverages by 16 per cent, and acute alcohol attributable deaths, including intentional injuries and homicide (for which the specific impact was not portioned out) by 29 per cent (Zhao et al. 2013).

Limits on Availability

The WHO's estimates include reducing access to retail alcohol as a highly cost-effective policy option to reduce alcohol-related harm, including alcohol-related violence (Anderson et al. 2009). Increasing the availability of alcohol sales times by two or more hours increases alcohol-related harm (Hahn et al. 2010). With the international trend towards increased bar opening hours, few studies have examined the impacts of reduced alcohol service hours in bars. However, in Newcastle, Australia, pub closing times were restricted in 2008 following police and public complaints about violence, disorderly behaviour, and property damage related to intoxication. The restrictions led to a reduction in recorded assaults of 37 per cent (Kypri et al. 2010).

Greater alcohol outlet density is associated with increased alcohol consumption and harms, including injury, violence, crime, and medical harm (Bryden et al. 2012; Osterberg 2012b). One form of alcohol sales regulation used in many countries is for the government to monopolize ownership of one or more types of retail outlet. In addition to limiting outlet density and the hours and days of sale, such monopolies remove the private profit motive for increasing sales. There is substantial evidence that such monopolies reduce alcohol consumption and alcohol-related harm (Österberg 2012b).

Homicide is one of the leading causes of death in Brazil. Local policy measures were introduced in response to the city of Diadema having one of the highest murder rates. These included a new licensing law in 2002 prohibiting on-premise alcohol sales after 23.00 hours. Homicide and assault data from local police archives were analysed to evaluate the effect of restricting alcohol availability through limiting opening hours. Models were adjusted for contextual conditions, municipal efforts, and law enforcement interventions that took place before and after adoption of the closing-time law. Homicide rates in Diadema dropped by 44 per cent following the introduction of limited opening hours (Duailibi et al. 2007).

Bans on Advertising

The WHO's estimates include bans on alcohol advertising as a highly cost-effective policy option to reduce alcohol-related harm (Anderson et al. 2009). Studies on alcohol advertising have not normally reported a separate impact on alcohol-related violence. However, since advertising has been shown to increase risk of drunkenness, it is likely to impact alcohol-related violence (Swahn et al. 2011). A meta-analysis of 132 studies found a small but significant positive association between alcohol advertising and alcohol consumption, although only for spirits advertising (Gallet 2007). Looking at alcohol advertising expenditure data across the United States, Saffer and Dave (2006) found, when controlling for alcohol price, income, and a number of socio-demographic variables, that advertising expenditure had an independent yet modest effect on the monthly number of adolescents drinking and binge-drinking. It was estimated that a 28 per cent reduction in alcohol advertising would reduce the monthly share of adolescent drinkers from 25 per cent to between 24 and 21 per cent. For binge-drinking, the reduction would be from 12 per cent to between 11 and 8 per cent. In a more recent study, the effect of partial bans was reported not to have affected alcohol consumption in 17 countries over 26 years (Nelson 2010). There are methodological difficulties with these econometric studies, primarily due to alcohol advertising expenditure being used as approximate measures of the effectiveness of alcohol marketing.

In contrast, evidence from longitudinal observational studies shows that commercial communications, particularly through social media and electronic communication outlets, encourages non-drinkers to start drinking and existing drinkers to drink more and to drink more hazardously (de Bruijn 2012). Even simply watching a one hour movie with a greater number of drinking scenes, or viewing simple advertisements, can double the amount drunk over the hour's viewing period (Engels et al. 2009). In many jurisdictions, much store is put on self-regulation of commercial communications and withdrawal of communications that are found to breach self-regulatory codes. However, these approaches are irrelevant, since extensive evidence shows that withdrawn commercial communications simply live on, accessible to all, in social media, which are, in any case, heavily financed by global alcohol producers (de Bruijn 2012).

Community-Based Policies

Community-Based Programmes and Indigenous Communities

Community-based programmes include education and information campaigns, media advocacy, counter-advertising and health promotion, controls on selling and consumption venues, and other regulations reducing access to alcohol, enhanced law enforcement and surveillance, and community organization and coalition development (Anderson et al. 2009). Interventions that have controlled access, which have included the environmental contexts of selling and distribution and which have involved enforcement, are effective in reducing alcohol-related assault injuries.

Members of indigenous communities are more likely than members of the general community to be non-drinkers; however, those who do drink are more likely to drink at harmful levels (Brady 2000). Restricting alcohol supply appears to have been effective in reducing alcohol-related harms in such communities. A community intervention project in the Northern Territory in Australia aimed to reduce higher levels of alcohol-related harm to national levels by use of a range of strategies, including a levy on alcoholic beverages with more than 3 per cent alcohol to fund education for preventing alcohol-related harm, increased controls on alcohol availability, and expanded treatment and rehabilitation services. The intervention led to a significant preferential reduction in acute alcohol-related deaths from injuries (alcohol-related violence was not partitioned out) in the Northern Territory compared with the control areas, largely due to the tax levy (Chikritzhs et al. 2005).

Drinking Places

Drinking places are high risk locations for aggressive behaviour, with risks increasing with intoxication (Graham and Homel 2008). Preventing intoxication in drinking places through responsible alcohol service training and policies, and implementation of regulations to prohibit service to intoxicated persons, tend to be ineffective in reducing alcohol-related violence (Graham et al. 2014). However, strong research evidence links alcohol-associated harm in on-premise licensed venues to late night trading and to venue capacity (Hughes and Bellis 2012). In any crowded environment the probability of conflict and aggression between individuals is considerably increased. In general, the design of an alcohol sales place can make a considerable difference in the likelihood of trouble and problems (Seabury 2007). Features of an establishment's physical design have an impact on the risk of aggression and violence, though studies documenting this have been relatively few. One study found that the low-risk venues had fewer cross-flows of streams of customers caused by physical design than the high-risk venues, thereby providing reduced opportunities for patrons to intrude accidentally on one another's personal space and for violent incidents to ensue (Graham and Homel 2008).

Globally Binding Framework

Given the extent of alcohol's global harm, including violence, there have been many calls for an international convention on alcohol (Casswell 2012), the only major 'psychoactive drug of abuse' not covered by a legal binding agreement, similar to the Framework Convention on Tobacco Control, or even the United Nations Conventions on drugs. There are many reasons to justify alcohol's inclusion in a legally binding agreement (Room 2006): alcohol's global damage is extensive and substantial over most of the world (Lim et al. 2012); damage transcends national borders, alcohol being an important commodity in international

trade, with smuggling and informal cross border trade practised all across the world; alcohol-related harm is not something that can be managed by countries alone—this is not just a matter of illegal trade or communication by digital media, but also a principle of comity between nations, in which countries should honour and support existing evidence-based alcohol control policies of other countries, such as those that relate to price, advertising, and availability; and, alcohol is not yet covered by an international legal agreement.

As a psychotropic substance, alcohol could be scheduled under the 1971 drugs convention if a WHO Expert Committee finds that the substance has the capacity to produce a state of dependence *and* impairs central nervous system functioning, *or* produces similar abuse and ill effects as a substance already covered by the Convention, *and* that there is sufficient evidence that the substance is likely to be abused so as to constitute a public health and social problem warranting the placing of the substance under international control (Room 2006). By these criteria, it would be difficult for an expert committee not to recommend alcohol for scheduling under the convention.

Alcohol could also be the subject of a framework convention as is the case for tobacco. A legally binding convention could provide trade liberalization that is both sustainable in relation to alcohol and respectful of comity of nations. It would provide the needed global governance architecture, resources, and institutional policy support to further policy development at the country level, particularly in low and middle income counties, and be free from the actions of the vested interests of the alcohol industry (Casswell 2013). There are different roads to take with building such architecture. Instead of routing from convention to protocol, as has been done with tobacco, one could route protocol to convention and start with a protocol on commercial communications (Casswell 2012).

Conclusions

Alcohol causes harm to people other than the drinker, including physical, mental, sexual, and family violence, as well as violent crime and murder. Since the more alcohol is consumed, the more frequently it is consumed, and the more that is consumed on a drinking occasion, the greater the risk of injury and violence, with no level of consumption that is risk free, any policy or action that reduces the volume of alcohol consumed and the amount drunk on a drinking occasion will reduce alcohol-related violence, with no time lag. At a government level, nationally and locally, the most cost-effective policies to do this include price increases, restrictions on availability, and bans on advertising. Not all analyses measuring the impact of such policies have portioned out specific effects on violence and more general harm to people other than the drinker, and this is an area for more targeted reporting. Local policies can be supplemented with targeted action on drinking places, in particular their design. Alcohol related violence is set to increase as greater proportions of the world's population start to drink alcohol, subsequent to economic development, fuelled by the marketing strategies of the alcohol industry. To help mitigate these increases, there is an urgent need to put in place a global legally binding agreement, similar to the framework convention on tobacco control, to reduce the harm done by alcohol, including alcohol-related injury and violence.

References

Anderson, P., and Baumberg, B. (2006). *Alcohol in Europe: A Public Health Perspective. A Report for the European Commission*. London: Institute of Alcohol Studies.

Anderson, P., Chisholm, D., and Fuhr, D. C. (2009). Effectiveness and cost-effectiveness of policies and programmes to reduce the harm caused by alcohol. *Lancet*, 373, 2234–46.

Babor, T., Caetano, R., and Casswell, S. et al. (2010). *Alcohol: No Ordinary Commodity: Research and Public Policy*. 2nd ed. Oxford: Oxford University Press.

Brady, M., (2000). Alcohol policy issues for indigenous people in the United States, Canada, Australia and New Zealand. *Contemporary Drug Problems*, 27, 435.

Bryden, A., Roberts B., and McKee, M. et al. (2012). A systematic review of the influence on alcohol use of community level availability and marketing of alcohol. *Health and Place*, 18, 349–57.

Casswell, S. (2012). Current status of alcohol marketing policy—an urgent challenge for global governance. *Addiction*, 107, 478–85.

Casswell, S. (2013). Vested interests in addiction research and policy. Why do we not see the corporate interests of the alcohol industry as clearly as we see those of the tobacco industry? *Addiction*, 108, 660–85.

Chikritzhs T., Stockwell, T., and Pascal, R. (2005). The impact of the Northern Territory's Living with Alcohol program, 1992–2002: revisiting the evaluation. *Addiction*, 100, 1625–36.

De Bruijn, A. (2012). The impact of alcohol marketing. In: P. Anderson, L. Møller, and G. Galea (eds), *Alcohol in the European Union: Consumption, Harm and Policy Approaches*. Copenhagen: WHO Regional Office for Europe, pp. 89–95.

Duailibi, S., Ponicki, W., and Grube, J. et al. (2007). The effect of restricting opening hours on alcohol-related violence. *American Journal of Public Health*, 97, 2276–80.

Engels, R. C., Hermans, R., and van Baaren, R. B. et al. (2009). Alcohol portrayal on television affects actual drinking behaviour. *Alcohol and Alcoholism*, 44, 244–9.

Gallet, C. A. (2007). The demand for alcohol: a meta-analysis of elasticities. *Australian Journal of Agricultural and Resource Economics*, 51, 121–35.

Graham, K., and Homel, R. (2008). *Raising the Bar: Preventing Aggression in and around Bars, Pubs and Clubs*. Devon: Willan Publishing.

Graham, K., Miller, P., and Chikritzhs, T. et al. (2014). Reducing intoxication among bar patrons: some lessons from prevention of drinking and driving. *Addiction*, 109, 693–98.

Hahn, R. A., Kuzara, J. L., and Elder, R. et al. (2010). Effectiveness of policies restricting hours of alcohol sales in preventing excessive alcohol consumption and related harms. *American Journal of Preventive Medicine*, 39, 590–604.

Hughes, K., and Bellis, M. (2012). Drinking environments. In: P. Anderson, L. Møller, and G. Galea (eds), *Alcohol in the European Union: Consumption, Harm and Policy Approaches*. Copenhagen, WHO Regional Office for Europe, pp. 83–8.

Kypri, K., Jones, C., and McElduff, P. et al. (2010). Effects of restricting pub closing times on night-time assaults in an Australian city. *Addiction*, 106, 303–10.

Laslett, A-M., Catalano, P., and Chikritzhs, Y. et al. (2010). *The Range and Magnitude of Alcohol's Harm to Others*. Fitzroy, Victoria: AER Centre for Alcohol Policy Research, Turning Point Alcohol and Drug Centre, Eastern Health.

Lim, S. S., Vos, T., and Flaxman, A. D. et al. (2012). A comparative risk assessment of burden of disease and injury attributable to 67 risk factors and risk factor clusters in 21 regions, 1990–2010: a systematic analysis for the Global Burden of Disease Study 2010. *Lancet*, 380, 2224–60.

National Health and Medical Research Council (2009). *Australian Guidelines to Reduce Health Risks from Drinking Alcohol*. Canberra: NHMRC.

Nelson, J. P. (2010). Alcohol advertising bans, consumption, and control policies in seventeen OECD countries, 1975–2000. *Applied Economics*, 42, 803–23.

Norström, T. Ö. Hemström, M., and Ramstedt, I. et al. (2001). Mortality and population drinking. In: T. Norström (ed.), *Alcohol in Postwar Europe: Consumption, Drinking Patterns, Consequences and Policy Responses in 15 European Countries*. Stockholm: National Institute of Public Health, European Commission, pp. 157–76.

Österberg, E. (2012a). Pricing of alcohol. In: P. Anderson, L. Møller, and G. Galea (eds), *Alcohol in the European Union: Consumption, Harm and Policy Approaches*. Copenhagen: WHO Regional Office for Europe, pp. 96–102.

Österberg, E. (2012b). Availability of alcohol. In: P. Anderson, L. Møller, and G. Galea (eds), *Alcohol in the European Union: Consumption, Harm and Policy Approaches*. Copenhagen: WHO Regional Office for Europe, pp. 83–8.

Purshouse, R., Meier, P. S., and Brennan, A. et al. (2010). Estimated effect of alcohol pricing policies on health and economic outcomes in England: an epidemiological model. *Lancet*, 375, 1355–64.

Rehm, J., Room, R., and Monteiro, M. et al. (2004) Alcohol. In: WHO (ed.). *Comparative Quantification of Health Risks: Global and Regional Burden of Disease Due to Selected Major Risk Factors*. Geneva: WHO, pp. 959–1108.

Ridolfo, B., and Stevenson, C. (2001). *The Quantification of Drug-Caused Mortality and Morbidity in Australia, 1998*. Canberra: Australian Institute of Health and Welfare.

Room, R. (2006). International control of alcohol: alternative paths forward. *Drug Alcohol Rev*, 25, 581–95.

Saffer, H., and Dave, D. (2006). *Alcohol advertising and alcohol consumption by adolescents. Health Economics*, 15, 617–37.

Seabury, O. (2007). *The Carlisle State Management Scheme*. Carlisle: Bookcase.

Shield, K. D., Kehoe, T., and Gmel, G. J. et al. (2012). Societal burden of alcohol. In: P. Anderson, L. Møller, and G. Galea (eds), *Alcohol in the European Union: Consumption, Harm and Policy Approaches*. Copenhagen: WHO Regional Office for Europe, pp. 10–28.

Shield, K. D., Rehm, M., and Patra, J. et al. (2011). Global and country specific adult per capita consumption of alcohol, 2008. *Journal of Addiction Research and Practice*, 57, 99–117.

Sornpaisarn, B., Shield, K., and Cohen, J. et al. (2013). Elasticity of alcohol consumption, alcohol-related harms, and drinking initiation in low- and middle-income countries: a systematic review and meta-analysis. *International Journal of Alcohol and Drug Research*, 2, 45–58.

Swahn, M., Ali, B., and Palmier, J. B. et al. (2011). Alcohol marketing, drunkenness, and problem drinking among Zambian youth: findings from the 2004 Global School-Based Student Health Survey. *Journal of Environmental and Public Health*.

Taylor, B., Irving, H. M., and Kanteres, F. et al. (2010). The more you drink, the harder you fall: a systematic review and meta-analysis of how acute alcohol consumption and injury or collision risk increase together. *Drug and Alcohol Dependence*, 110, 108–16.

Taylor, B. J., Shield, K. D., and Rehm, J. (2011). Combining best evidence: a novel method to calculate the alcohol-attributable fraction and its variance for injury mortality. *BMC Public Health*, *11*, 265.

Wagenaar, A. C., Maldonado-Molina. M. M., and Wagenaar, B. H. (2009). Effects of alcohol tax increases on alcohol-related disease mortality in Alaska: time-series analyses from 1976 to 2004. *American Journal of Public Health*, *99*, 1464–70.

Wagenaar, A. C., Tobler, A. L., and Komro, K. A. (2010). Effects of alcohol tax and price policies on morbidity and mortality: a systematic review. *American Journal of Public Health,* 2270–8.

Zhao, J., Stockwell, T., and Martin, G., et al. (2013). The relationship between minimum alcohol prices, outlet densities and alcohol attributable deaths in British Columbia, 2002 to 2009. *Addiction*, *108* 1059–69.

CHAPTER 42

Violence and drug control policy

Mark A. R. Kleiman, Jonathan P. Caulkins,
Thomas Jacobson, and Brad Rowe

The Drugs–Violence Connection

Violence by and against drug dealers causes havoc, from the streets of United States cities to source and transit countries including Afghanistan, Mexico, Honduras, and Colombia. About two-thirds of those arrested for violent crimes in the United States test positive for illicit drugs or have a history of substance abuse or dependence (U.S. ONDCP ADAM II Annual Report 2012), and we have no reason to assume that the United States is an anomaly in this regard (Parry et al. 2004). Though the association between drug consumption and violent crime does not, by itself, demonstrate causality, the overlap is breath-taking.

Those facts point to drug policy as a potentially important element of a violence-control strategy. But the academic literature largely focuses on distilling the drugs–violence connection to the minimal quantity of violence that can safely be *directly* attributed to drugs. That leads to an understatement of the actual causal linkages, because it ignores many indirect or delayed pathways. Paul Goldstein's widely used tripartite framework (1985) for distinguishing between different types of drug violence illustrates alike the power and the limits of such partial analysis.

Goldstein's category of 'psychopharmacological violence' includes violence perpetrated by users due to intoxication or withdrawal. To this might be added the indirect consequences of changes in behaviour patterns and social connections resulting from substance abuse disorders. Intoxication of victims can be a factor in interpersonal violence, and intoxication is also involved in a large fraction of intentional self-injury.

'Economic-compulsive violence' traditionally includes robberies committed to pay for drug purchases; logically, the category should be extended to income-producing crimes committed to pay for other things, such as food and rent, by persons whose licit employment opportunities are diminished by habitual intoxication, a phenomenon that can arise with licit as well as illicit drugs.

'Systemic violence' arises from illicit drug markets. It includes crimes against dealers (e.g. robberies), crimes by dealers (against customers, employees, suppliers, competitors, law enforcement agents, or witnesses), and the lawful (or, sometimes, lawless) violence by law enforcement against participants in drug markets. Arrest and incarceration for drug law violations could be, though it generally is not treated as a form of systemic drug-related violence. The transactional nature of drug dealing forces drug enforcement to rely on unusually intrusive enforcement techniques including 'dynamic entry' raids on suspected dealers, with sometimes fatal results to innocent victims of police error (Balko 2006). The practice of enticing or coercing some drug-market participants to testify against others can also sow the seeds of violence.

The Goldstein taxonomy, while well-established, is less than comprehensive (Caulkins and Kleiman 2013; Office of National Drug Control Policy 2013). Focusing on contemporaneous effects, it omits important developmental, neighbourhood, and inter-generational phenomena: for example, violence committed as a result of foetal exposure to alcohol; violence committed later in life as result of childhood exposure (personal or vicarious) to drug-related crime, including domestic violence; violence by and against people made homeless by substance abuse, even if they are not current consumers; violence by and against people whose life-courses were influenced by their own incarceration or by the incarceration of a parent; and gun violence among those who are not dealers but who arm themselves in response to weapons possession among drug dealers in their neighbourhoods. Much of drug dealers' violence turns out, on close examination, to be more interpersonal than directly business related (Atkinson et al. 2009), excluding it from Goldstein's tripartite taxonomy; but when drug selling gives a dealer the money and incentive to acquire firearms and the motivation to cultivate a reputation for toughness, and that dealer then shoots someone in a dispute over an affront, that incident ought to be counted as drug-related violence.

How much Violence is Attributable to Drugs?

By analogy with the literature on disease causation, the 'attributable fraction' of drug-related violence could be defined as the incidence of violence perpetrated or suffered by the drug-involved subpopulations (users and dealers) minus the incidence of violence that would be perpetrated or suffered by the same subpopulation were drugs not a factor. That is, in a hypothetical world where drugs did not exist but all else were the same, how much less violence would there be? Unfortunately, existing methods are nowhere nearly sophisticated enough, nor existing data rich enough, to calculate such an attributable fraction (Caulkins and Kleiman 2013). Not all of the observed difference between drug-involved and non-drug-involved individuals can be attributed to drug-related activities as opposed to personal and social characteristics correlated with both drugs and violence, or causation running from violence to drug use rather than the other way around. Furthermore, even if the drug-attributable fraction were measurable, there is no reason to think that reducing drug activity by a given fraction would lead to a proportional reduction in drug-related violence (by contrast with, for instance, tobacco-related disease, where a 10 per cent reduction in pack-years ought to lead to roughly a 10 per cent reduction in attributable morbidity and mortality) (Caulkins 2013). In addition, drug-dealing might—for an individual or an organization—substitute for predatory acquisitive crimes such as theft, robbery, kidnapping, or extortion, or it might facilitate such crimes; the net effect might not be the same in the long run as it is contemporaneously. As a result, the fraction of violence attributable to drug dealing in historical terms might not be the same as the fraction by which violence could be reduced by eliminating drug dealing going forward (Kleiman et al. 2013). That suggests a focus on marginal rather than total or average quantities: How much less (or more) violence could we expect to see as the result of a given change in drug policy?

While much of the drugs violence discussion focuses on drug legalization, the details of both prohibitory and regulatory control regimes also matter. Prohibition regimes differ in enforcement practices, sentencing patterns, treatment policies, prevention and treatment efforts, and the management of drug-involved offenders. Likewise, the example of alcohol illustrates that the amount of drug-related violence can vary substantially among different regimes of legal availability (Cook 2007). Undue concentration on legal status can distract from opportunities for gain from less dramatic policy shifts.

Violence-Minimizing Enforcement Strategy

Prohibition tends to decrease consumption, thereby decreasing psychopharmacological violence from the prohibited drug. It also decreases all forms of violence generated indirectly by dependence: for example, subsequent violence by children abused by their intoxicated parents. Furthermore, inasmuch as poly-drug abuse is the norm, reduced dependence on the prohibited drug (e.g. cocaine) might indirectly lead to reduced abuse of other criminogenic drugs (e.g. alcohol). However, other effects might diminish or conceivably even reverse any such beneficial effect. For example, there may be substitution away from the prohibited drug and into other, more violence-inducing drugs; this may be a particular issue with marijuana prohibition. More generally, prohibition creates risky, high-price markets that foment economic-compulsive and systemic violence.

Enforcement involves its own set of policy choices. Prohibition by itself suppresses prevalence by making consumption risky and establishing abstinence as the implicit societal norm. But there is little evidence that further increases in the general intensity of enforcement have been very effective at raising prices (Caulkins 2000; Caulkins and Chandler 2005). Even if prices do increase, the effect on violence is ambiguous; psycho-pharmacological violence would be expected to decrease, but economic-compulsive violence might go up or down depending on how strongly consumers respond to price changes. If an increase in price produces

a more-than-proportional decrease in volume consumed (a situation economists call 'elastic demand') the result is a decrease in total expenditure and thus, presumably, users' need for crime-derived income. In that case, enforcement-driven drug price increases would be expected to reduce non-drug crime. But if demand is relatively 'inelastic,' so that a price increase creates a less-than-proportional decrease in quantity, the result will be an increase in total expenditure, with possibly perverse effects on acquisitive crime.

Imagine, for example, a drug whose consumption is financed entirely from criminal proceeds, and whose demand is relatively inelastic, so that a 20 per cent increase in price is associated with only a 10 per cent decrease in quantity purchased. Then the total expenditure after such a price increase will be 8 per cent greater $(1.2 \times 0.9 = 1.08)$ than it was before.

At first blush, the same analysis applies to systemic crime. However, even if that were true in the long run, in the short run any change may increase violence as individuals and organizations contest who will gain and who will lose from the new circumstances (Beittel 2012). The overall outcome may depend on the nature of that additional drug enforcement. Vigorous but unselective enforcement may exacerbate violence in drug markets by increasing the benefits accruing to those best able to wield it. Conversely, enforcement targeted at especially violence-prone dealers may reduce the amount of violence per kilogram or per million dollars of illicit revenue.

Whatever resources are devoted to drug law enforcement cannot be devoted to enforcement against predatory crime (though of course the population of dealers overlaps with the population of predatory criminals, so incarcerating drug dealers may incapacitate away some violent acts unrelated to their dealing). Thus increased violent crime might be among the opportunity costs of the drug enforcement effort.

Retail drug markets can be 'flagrant' or 'discreet'. An open-air market is flagrant; so is a market characterized by dedicated drug sales locations, such as 'smoke shops' or 'crack houses'. By contrast, both indoor selling in multi-purpose locations (e.g. bars) and sales mediated by cell phone or on-line order and consummated by delivery to the user's home can be nearly invisible to non-participants.

Flagrant markets create violence because both buyers and sellers offer attractive robbery targets (as they hold cash and valuable inventory and are reluctant to call the police) and because dealers therefore have a strong incentive to arm themselves. Flagrant drug dealing also tends to create local disorder. Which discourages licit commerce and thereby reduces licit economic opportunity

It follows that, if enforcement focused on unusually violent flagrant retail markets can force displacement into more dispersed and discreet retail patterns such as home delivery, the result can be to reduce violence, even without reducing the volume of sales (Caulkins 1992): that is, the 'drug market intervention' approach represented by the successful crackdown on the crack market in the West End of High Point, North Carolina and subsequently elsewhere (Kennedy 2011). An alternative approach to violence-minimized drug enforcement would concentrate on the most violent actors (individuals or organizations) while relaxing enforcement against less-violent dealers, thus both incapacitating the most violent and creating a disincentive for violence (Caulkins and Reuter 2009).

Heterogeneity Among Drugs

The extent to which reducing consumption reduces violence varies enormously from drug to drug. (Ironically, alcohol, which remains legal, is responsible for more violence than all the illegal drugs combined, although not necessarily the most per user.)

Psycho-pharmacologically, the central nervous system stimulants (cocaine and the amphetamines) seem to be at least as dangerous as alcohol on a dosage unit basis, albeit with a much smaller consumer base. The effects of alcohol and the stimulants are hard to disentangle in part because they are frequently used together; they appear to be consumption complements, and there are specific chemical mechanisms—such as the formation of coca-ethylene in the bloodstream of people who consume alcohol and cocaine together—that make combination use especially violence inducing (Pennings et al. 2002). Cocaine, unlike alcohol, is expensive enough for economic-compulsive violence to be a significant problem. Especially in the form of crack, cocaine—more, for example, than methamphetamine—tends to be a drug of frequent purchase, generating violence-prone patterns of illicit retail trade (Kleiman and Young 1995).

The sedative effect of the opiates, including heroin, may reduce psycho-pharmacological violence among those currently under their influence, but the strong drug seeking generated by withdrawal symptoms generates considerable income-producing crime (some of it violent). In the United States, heroin dealing, but not apparently dealing in diverted pharmaceutical opiates, is associated with retail-level violence, perhaps because of the flagrancy of open heroin dealing compared with discreet dealing in pills (SAMHSA 2007).

Cannabis, now probably the largest illicit drug market in the United States, does not seem to generate much violence by users or dealers; while a large share of U.S. arrestees test positive for recent cannabis use, that appears to reflect the demographics of its user population rather than any pharmacological effect. In part because it is relatively inexpensive, cannabis tends to be purchased in bulk, and thus usually does not support the sort of violence-prone open markets characteristic of crack or heroin.

With the exception of illicit drug production and trafficking in Mexico, the largest effects of cannabis on violence may be indirect, through its effects on the consumption of other drugs. The substitution of cannabis for alcohol or the stimulants would tend to decrease violence. However, there is no theoretical reason why cannabis should be a substitute for alcohol rather than a complement to it, and current empirical evidence is mixed and equivocal. If cannabis were to prove to be a complement, then increasing cannabis use might be violence increasing through its impact on drinking. The actual relationships might well vary over time and across populations, based on social as well as purely pharmacological factors. The question of 'cross-elasticity of demand' across drugs—broadly construed to include lagged, and not just contemporaneous, effects—deserves more research attention.

International Drug-Trafficking Violence

The most dramatic drug-related violence takes place in some low- and middle-income countries where illicit drugs are produced, processed, and exported as well as being consumed, and where the combination of large illicit economies and weak states can make drug trafficking a serious threat to public authority. That problem is an artefact of drug prohibition, and ill-designed drug enforcement can make it worse (Caulkins et al. 2010).

Mexico has drawn much attention in recent years for the ghastly violence perpetrated by its drug trafficking organizations. Some of those groups have been around for decades, at least since Mexico first began producing marijuana and heroin for U.S. consumption. But their dramatic rise in wealth and violence occurred after Mexico became the primary corridor for South American cocaine passing into the U.S. market, which in turn came after U.S. law enforcement succeeded in clamping down on the old Caribbean cocaine smuggling routes in the 1980s and early 1990s (Paul et al. 2011).

The current spike in drug violence in Mexico is at least partially correlated with the crackdown that began with former President Calderon sending federal troops into several Mexican states to suppress drug trafficking and violence in 2006. The period from 2006 to 2012 saw a massive increase in dealer-on-dealer, dealer-on-official, and dealer-on-citizen violence, leading to the creation of an estimated 1.6 million refugees from the bloodshed.

A harm reduction or realpolitik approach might consider the ways in which different enforcement tactics could shift trafficking routes to minimize violence. A policy that tacitly allowed the traffic to flow via sea routes and through smaller, less-populated countries might lead to less total violence, but there is obvious difficulty in writing off some smaller countries, even if in a cold-hearted calculus that might reduce the body count.

Even within a given country, drug-trafficking enterprises vary widely in their propensity for violence. Law enforcement can modulate its efforts with an eye toward eliminating the most violent actors, thus both creating disincentives for violence and exerting selective pressure to reduce, over time, the average violence propensity of surviving organizations and individuals. This would extend to the international arena the successful violence reduction strategies typified by the Boston Gun Project and the High Point intervention (Kennedy 2011).

One approach that has been speculated about, but not yet put into practice, would be to selectively focus enforcement on the distributors in consumer countries supplied by the most violent organizations in source and transit countries. For example, the United States might thus make a policy of attacking U.S. wholesale and retail dealers buying from the one or a few of the most violent organizations. By announcing such a strategy, it might be possible to induce a 'race to the bottom' in Mexican gangs' use of violence, with each seeking to appear less violent than its rivals (Kleiman 2011). Such an approach has great theoretical appeal but faces formidable operational obstacles (Chi et al. 2013).

Demand Reduction

As mentioned, suppressing the supply of violence-linked drugs has ambiguous effects on violence levels. By contrast, reducing demand is purely violence reducing: less intoxication, less money spent by users, and less money made by dealers means less violence, without much in the way of caveats or offsetting effects.

However, the validity of the oft-repeated claim that 'demand reduction' is generically superior to 'supply reduction' depends in part on the efficacy of demand-reduction measures. Success at preventing or delaying drug initiation—the usual measure of efficacy for prevention programmes—may or may not translate into genuine value in reducing drug abuse. Only a minority of those who use any drug become habitual or problematic users, and those few account for the vast bulk of drug consumption, revenues of the illicit-drug industries, and drug-related harm. Thus a prevention programme could dramatically reduce the prevalence of drug consumption without having great social benefit if it prevented use only by those who would not have used much anyhow. Alternatively, prevention may reduce consumption and violence by a greater proportion than it reduces prevalence if it reduces the conditional probability of progressing to abuse. Community-based prevention is an entirely distinct intervention, with far fewer high-quality evaluations; it may offer still-untapped opportunities to reduce demand, but the scale of those benefits is hard to estimate with any confidence.

A variety of drug treatment programmes have been shown to improve outcomes for participants who remain in them for a period of months. That is grounds for expanding treatment funding, but the effective demand for treatment—meaning the willingness of persons suffering from substance abuse disorder to enter treatment, remain in treatment, and adhere to therapeutic guidance—may pose a stronger constraint than the supply of paid treatment programmes. The federal Centre for Substance Abuse Treatment routinely reports that the 'need for' treatment greatly exceeds the supply, but the mere fact that someone is in clinical need of treatment does not necessarily mean he or she will seek treatment, or even accept it if offered. Indeed, some findings suggest that group self-help on the model of the Twelve-Step fellowships (Alcoholics Anonymous and groups based on similar principles) may be as beneficial to those who continue in them as are professional counselling and other interventions, but this is not generally taken to have solved the 'treatment gap' (Kaskutas 2009). This issue of insufficient demand despite widespread need may become more acute as recent policy changes (mental health parity legislation and the Affordable Care Act) make treatment more available.

With treatment, as with prevention, it is important to distinguish two questions: whether the programmes are beneficial, or even have benefits in excess of their costs, and whether they are highly effective in the sense of dramatically reducing drug use. Relapse is the norm, and the reduction in consumption achieved by making community-based treatment more readily available relative to a no-treatment baseline is not overwhelmingly large. (NIDA 1999; Ritchie et al. 2011). Both treatment and prevention tend to be cost-justified because the problems they ameliorate are so costly, rather than because they are highly effective.

Opiate substitution therapy seems to be an exception in three respects. First, the evidence concerning its effectiveness, including effectiveness at reducing crime and violence, is much stronger than for other forms of treatment. Second, opiate substitution treatment slots are in short supply. Third, it is only relevant for opiate dependence; there are no comparably effective pharmacotherapies for other drugs—and the vast bulk of illicit drug-related violence comes from stimulants, notably cocaine and methamphetamine.

One answer to the problem of inadequate treatment demand is to make treatment mandatory. The evidence suggests that, other things being equal, a spell of coerced treatment is as likely to prove beneficial as is a spell of voluntary treatment. And a large fraction of people with serious substance abuse problems comes into frequent contact with the criminal justice system, making criminal justice referral a potential means of getting treatment to those most in need, even when that need is not accompanied by desire.

But in addition to concerns about civil liberty and personal autonomy, actually coercing people into drug treatment turns out to be difficult. Even in semi-voluntary 'drug diversion' programmes, where offenders elect to undergo treatment in lieu of criminal punishment, actual attendance often falls far short of nominal requirements, with typical completion rates of 50 per cent or lower (Belenko 2001). In principle, those who fail to complete are subject to sanctions, including incarceration, but in practice overworked probation officers and judges tend to let violations slide, even when the treatment provider reports a subject's non-attendance. A programme can thus easily find itself in a 'death spiral', with high non-compliance rates swamping the capacity of the criminal justice system to enforce the mandate and low sanctions probabilities fostering high non-compliance rates (Kleiman 2009). Coerced treatment can also put a strain on treatment resources, leading to dilution of effort and loss of efficacy, and potentially demoralize treatment staff who confront unwilling, and even hostile, clients (Urada et al. 2008).

Mandated treatment is not the only option. The same authority that imposes a treatment mandate could also impose a mandate to desist from the use of drugs, without specifying treatment as a means to that end. If it were true that persons with substance abuse disorders act involuntarily—in the sense that their behaviour does not respond to contingencies—then such an approach would be bound to fail. However, the empirical evidence, both in experimental settings and in practical experience, shows otherwise. Seriously drug-involved criminal offenders dramatically reduce drug use, new arrests, and days behind bars if subjected to properly administered programmes of frequent random drug testing backed by swift, certain, and proportionate sanctions—typically, starting with a few days behind bars and escalating with repeated violations—even without a treatment mandate (Hawken et al. 2013). Sobriety 24/7, a programme pioneered in South Dakota for drunken drivers which requires two alcohol breath tests per day for a few months, with the threat that any non-zero result will lead to an immediate overnight jail stay, has been demonstrated to substantially reduce driving under the influence recidivism even after offenders are no longer subject to testing, and, as an unexpected side-benefit, to reduce domestic violence to an extent observable in county-wide crime data (Kilmer et al. 2012). It appears that—just as Caesare Beccaria claimed in the eighteenth century—swiftness and certainty make punishments effective even without severity (Beccaria 1764/1767), and that principle holds as much for drug-involved offenders as for others (Hawken et al. 2013).

Conclusion

Most of the money now spent on drug abuse control is devoted to constraining supply. Unfortunately, untargeted supply control often finds itself at cross-purposes with violence control. That has led to calls for shifting resources from supply to demand control programmes. That might represent an improvement for countries, such as the United States, that have pushed supply control efforts into the region of diminishing returns. But it is not a panacea. Even treatment on demand does not 'solve' the drug problem;

some European countries have been offering more or less unlimited access to treatment for decades. With the notable exception of opiate substitution therapies such as methadone, conventional treatment does more to reduce the misery of those treated than it does to reduce their drug consumption. Likewise, exposing young people to prevention messages does not protect them from drug use to anywhere near the degree that vaccination protects them from mumps or measles.

There are, however, more promising approaches. Enforcement could recognize and exploit the heterogeneity across individuals, markets, and dealing practices in tendency to produce violence. Drug dealers collectively commit horrific amounts of deadly violence, but when one remembers that well in excess of a million people participate in drug dealing in the United States each year, while drug-related homicides are in the thousands, it becomes clear that the majority of dealers do not. Focusing enforcement on the people, organizations, and market practices that are most violence-prone, putting them at a competitive disadvantage, might displace the market into less destructive forms.

Charging drug law enforcement with the manageable task of enhancing public safety by mitigating the collateral damage—and especially the violence—created by drug markets would make more sense than asking it to pursue the Quixotic goal of greatly reducing the use of drugs with well-established mass markets by making them more expensive or less available.

On the demand side, the most promising option seems to be coercive demand reduction among drug-using offenders. Drug testing, with swift and certain sanctions for detected drug use, can reduce consumption more dramatically than can any currently available drug-treatment regimen. If such programmes can be successfully operated at full scale, their use in consumer countries could put a significant dent in the demand for drugs which—unlike constraining supply in ways that drive up price—reduce all the varieties of drug-related violence, in consumer, transit, and source countries alike.

References

ADAM II (Arrestee Drug Abuse Monitoring Program) (2012). *Annual Report*. Washington, D.C.: United States Office of National Drug Control Policy.

Atkinson, A., Anderson, Z., Hughes, K., Bellis, M. A., Sumnall, H., and Syed, Q. (2009). *Interpersonal Violence and Illicit Drugs*. Liverpool: Centre for Public Health, Liverpool John Moores University, WHO Collaborating Centre for Violence Prevention.

Balko, R. (2006). *Overkill, The Rise of Paramilitary Police Raids in America*. Washington, D.C. The Cato Institute.

Belenko, S. (2001) *Research on Drug Courts: A Critical Review, 2001 Update*. Columbia: The National Center on Addiction and Substance Abuse (CASA), Colombia University.

Beccaria, C. (1764). *Dei Delitti e Delle Pene*. English trans. (1767): An_Essay_on_Crimes_and_Punishments. Available at: http://en.wikisource.org/wiki/An_Essay_on_Crimes_and_Punishments [Accessed 19 December 2013].

Beittel, J. S. (2012). *Mexico's Drug Trafficking Organizations: Source and Scope of the Rising Violence*. Washington, D.C.: Congressional Research Service.

Caulkins, J. (1992). Thinking about displacement in drug markets: why observing change of venue isn't enough. *Journal of Drug Issues, 22,* 17–30.

Caulkins, J. (2000). Do drug prohibition and enforcement work? *What Works? White Paper Series*. Arlington, VA: Lexington Institute.

Caulkins, J. (2013). *Drug Control and Reductions in Drug-attributable Crime*. Washington, D.C.: U.S. Department of Justice, National Institute of Justice.

Caulkins, J., and Kleiman, M. (2013). *How Much Crime is Drug-related? History, Limitations and Potential Improvements of Estimation Methods*. Washington, D.C.: U.S. Department of Justice, National Institute of Justice.

Caulkins, J., Kleiman, M., and Kulick, J. (2010). *Drug Production and Trafficking, Counterdrug Policies, and Security and Governance in Afghanistan*. New York: Center on International Cooperation, New York University.

Caulkins, J., and Chandler, S. (2005). Long-run trends in incarceration of drug offenders in the U.S. Pittsburgh, PA: Heinz College Research. Paper 21.

Caulkins, J., and Reuter, P. (2009). Towards a harm-reduction approach to enforcement. *Safer Communities, 8,* 9–23.

Chi, J., Hayatdavoudi, L., Kruszona, S., and Rowe, B. (2013). *Reducing Drug Violence in Mexico: Options for Implementing Targeted Enforcement*. Los Angeles: Luskin School of Public Affairs, University of California Los Angeles.

Cook, P. (2007). *Paying the Tab: The Costs and Benefits of Alcohol Control*. Princeton: Princeton University Press.

Goldstein, P. (1985). The drugs/violence nexus: a tripartite conceptual framework. *Journal of Drug Issues, 15,* 493–506.

Hawken, A., Davenport, S., and Kleiman, M. (2013). *Managing Drug-involved Offenders*. Washington, D.C.: U.S. Department of Justice, National Institute of Justice.

Kaskutas, L. A. (2009). *Alcoholics Anonymous Effectiveness: Faith Meets Science*. Washington, D.C.: NIH Public Access.

Kennedy, D. (2011). *Don't Shoot: One Man, a Street Fellowship, and the End of Violence in Inner-City America*. New York: Bloomsbury.

Kilmer, B., Nicosia, N., Heaton, P., and Midgette, G. (2012). Efficacy of frequent monitoring with swift, certain, and modest sanctions for violations: insights from South Dakota's 24/7 Sobriety project. *American Journal of Public Health, 103,* e37–e43.

Kleiman, M., and Young, Y. (1995). Factors of production in retail drug dealing. *Urban Affairs Review, 30,* 730–48.

Kleiman, M., Caulkins, J., and Gehred, P. (2013). *Measuring the Costs of Crime*. Washington, D.C.: U.S. Department of Justice, National Institute of Justice.

Kleiman, M. (2009). *When Brute Force Fails: How to Have Less Crime and Less Punishment*. Princeton: Princeton University Press.

Kleiman, M. (2011). Surgical strikes in the drug wars: smarter policies for both sides of the border. Foreign Affairs. Available at: http://www.foreignaffairs.com/articles/68131/mark-kleiman/surgical-strikes-in-the-drug-wars [Accessed 19 December 2013].

National Institute on Drug Abuse (1999),*Principles of Drug Addiction Treatment*. Washington, D.C.: National Institute on Drug Abuse.

Office of National Drug Control Policy (2013). *Improving the Measurement of Drug- Related Crime*. Washington, D.C.: Executive Office of the President.

Parry, C. D. H., Plüddemann, A., Louw, A., and Leggett, T. (2004). The 3-metros study of drugs and crime in South Africa: findings and policy implications. *The American Journal of Drug and Alcohol Abuse, 30,* 167–85.

Paul, C., Gereben Schaefer, A., and Clarke, C. (2011). *The Challenge of Violent Drug-Trafficking Organizations: An Assessment of Mexican Security Based on Existing RAND Research on Urban Unrest, Insurgency and Defense-Sector Reform*. Santa Monica: RAND Corporation.

Pennings, E. J. M., Leccese, A. P., and Wolff, F. A. D. (2002). Effects of concurrent use of alcohol and cocaine. *Addiction, 97.* 773–83.

Ritchie, L., Martin, S. S., Wexler, H. K., and Dillard, D. L. (2011). *Program Profile: Delaware KEY / Crest Substance Abuse Programs*. Washington, D.C.: National Institutes of Justice. Available at http://www.CrimeSolutions.gov.

Substance Abuse and Mental Health Services Administration (SAMHSA). (2007). *Results from the 2006 National Survey on Drug Use and Health: National Findings*. Washington, D.C.: Office of Applied Studies, NSDUH Series H-32, DHHS Publication No. SMA 07-4293. Rockville, MD.

Urada, D., Hawken, A., and Bradley, T. et al. (2008). *Evaluation of Proposition 36: The Substance Abuse and Crime Prevention Act of 2000*. Los Angeles: Department of Alcohol and Drug Programs, California Health and Human Services Agency. University of California Los Angeles. Integrated Substance Abuse Programs.

CHAPTER 43

How does policy transfer support the uptake of violence prevention policy?

Alison Morris-Gehring and Peter D. Donnelly

Introduction to Policy Transfer Support and the Uptake of Violence Prevention Policy

Policymakers are burdened with many issues, have limited resources, and conflicting political imperatives. Matters advancing improved public health compete for policy attention, resources, and priority. The political nature of the policy process renders the evidence base alone insufficient to give rise to the adoption of a preventative solution to the problem of interpersonal violence. The conditions influencing the formulation of policy determine the mobilization of political priority and resources for violence prevention.

As presented in this book, there is an accumulation of evidence on the causes and manifestations of violence and how these can be reduced. However, in comparison relatively little is known about how political priority is generated for violence prevention in terms of the policy agenda. The advancement of a public health-based preventative approach towards violence is framed in the processes shaping the development and implementation of policy. An understanding of the policy environment therefore informs action to increase the uptake of violence prevention policy.

Public policy processes are complex, involving innumerable individual and organizational actors, conflicting ideas, values, and beliefs about how to define problems and what to do about them. An analytical approach grounded in political science has been widely applied across disciplines within the social sciences including health policy and systems research (Gilson and Raphaely 2008; Shiffman 2007; Tantivess and Walt 2008). Health policy analysis takes a multidisciplinary approach to explain the interaction between institutions, interests, and ideas in the development of health policy. However, examples of its application to the issue of interpersonal violence remain scarce. The process of putting the issue of violence on the agenda and formulating the solution of prevention at a country level has largely gone without investigation.

The influence of experiences from other contexts on the development of policy is a component of the policy process (Dolowitz and Marsh 2000). The subject of this chapter is the transfer across domains of knowledge and ideas drawn from the experience of developing violence prevention policy and how this supports the uptake of a strategy of prevention in different countries. This chapter aims to (i) outline the concept of policy transfer; (ii) understand how knowledge of violence prevention policy drawn from one context shapes the development of violence prevention policy in another context, and (iii) describe the mechanisms that facilitate the transfer of violence prevention policy.

A growing awareness of the scale and consequences of violence has seen an increase in the number of countries that recognize the importance of prevention. However, until recently there have been few countries where this is reflected through policy. Thus the attention of this chapter is how drawing lessons from several countries has helped spread the conceptualization of interpersonal violence as a global health problem and how this sharing of knowledge and ideas could be further strengthened to promote the adoption of a preventative approach.

What is Policy Transfer?

Policy transfer is not a simple copy-and-paste exercise to move a policy from one context to another. Rather, it encapsulates the influence of policy experience in other countries on developing policy. A standard definition of policy transfer is the transfer of insight and information produced within one context to a policy area located elsewhere in space or time (Rose 1991). Policymakers draw lessons from the policies, institutions, and ideologies of their counterparts, both within and across countries, and across time, to guide the development of policy solutions to the problems in their own domain. For example, in the late 1990s there was a proliferation of policy transfer activity between Britain and the United States. Under the Blair and Clinton administrations these common policy initiatives included reduction of school class sizes; crime zero-tolerance and anti-truancy drives; welfare-to-work approaches to limiting welfare, and the creation of work incentives (Evans 2009). An understanding of both the occurrence of policy transfer and the processes involved in transferring policy is important for a number of reasons (Stone 1999). In the case of interpersonal violence examination of how violence prevention policy experience is shared between countries sheds light on how the issue of violence and a strategy of prevention might be prioritized on the policy agenda.

There has been a considerable growth in interest in policy transfer. The field of social policy presents a number of approaches to studying the processes involved in the transfer of policy and practice between countries (Grin and Loeber 2007). Within the literature, policy transfer sits alongside lesson-drawing, policy diffusion, and exporting ideas; however, although there is considerable overlap, these concepts are not interchangeable. Policy transfer is a mechanism of influence where policy experience in one context shapes the development of policy in another context. The experience of developing and implementing violence prevention policy therefore generates knowledge and ideas that can support the mobilization of interest and resources for violence prevention in other countries.

As part of the wider policy process, the transfer procedures involve the selection of policy ideas, interpretation of the environment, and adoption of the policy. There are different degrees of transfer ranging from the copying or synthesis of policy, legislation or practice, to simply inspiring solutions (Dolowitz and Marsh 1996). The voluntary transfer of insight and information from experiences elsewhere can facilitate the identification of proven effective policy solutions as well as legitimizing decisions. One example is the influence on the introduction of smoking in public places restrictions in Scotland and England in 2006 and 2007 of similar policies adopted in other English-speaking jurisdictions, particularly the Republic of Ireland (Asare and Studlar 2009). However, policies can also be imposed on policymakers (Bennett 1991). This coercive transfer is typified by tying financial loans to policy conditions. For example, the implementation of Structural Adjustment Programmes (SAPs) in return for investment from the International Monetary Fund or the World Bank that characterized the political economy of developing countries throughout the 1980s and 1990s.

The supply of proven effective policy solutions is not a sufficient condition to produce policy transfer (Rose 1991). Political desirability and demand for a solution to a policy problem are necessary for there to be a sharing of insight and information from another context. The transfer of a technically proficient solution does not inevitably result in successful policy outcomes. Policy compatibility, implementation feasibility, and cultural acceptability principally determine the effectiveness of the transfer process (Evans and Davies 1999).

Policy transfer primarily involves the state and international organizations, with key actors being bureaucrats and politicians. However, non-state entities, in particular think tanks, foundations, and the university sector, can also be agents of transfer. These organizations then fulfil the role of importer, exporter, and facilitator of best practice and a common perspective. The external leverage of international institutions in particular can facilitate policy dialogue and the spread of ideas. A transnational policy community of state agencies, international organizations, and non-state entities forms around a common issue. Experts, professionals, policymakers, and advocates coalesce to collectively present conceptual notions and empirical findings. The network of concerned organizations facilitates the transfer of policy ideas as it takes forward a shared consensus (Stone 2000). These networks of transfer regularly interact through conferences, working groups, and newsletters and enable the exchange of expertise and experience—for example, the 'Roll Back Malaria Initiative' that involves the World Health Organization (WHO), the World Bank, the United Nations Children's Fund (UNICEF), the United Nations Development Programme, bilateral development agencies, businesses, NGOs, and the media with the shared aim to reduce mortality due to malaria by 75 per cent by 2015 (Reinicke and Deng 2000).

There is an increasing understanding of the processes involved in transferring policies and practices from exporter to importer and how agents of policy transfer facilitate this process. However, this chapter first turns to the occurrence of policy transfer and the bank of violence prevention policy experience.

The Transfer of Violence Prevention Policy Experience

Awareness and acceptance of a public health approach to interpersonal violence is fairly widespread. However, conflicting perceptions of violence prevention challenge a preventative solution's gaining traction on the policy agenda. Lessons drawn from the formulation and delivery of violence prevention policy elsewhere can address these challenges. Violence prevention policy experience provides information about the effectiveness of violence prevention policy as well as insight into cultivating political desirability and cultural acceptability for a strategy of prevention.

As more governments around the world come to recognize that injuries and violence can and must be prevented, many are attempting to ascertain an understanding of the problem in their countries as a basis for designing, implementing, and monitoring effective prevention strategies. Nationally there are indicators to suggest violence prevention has emerged as a priority in some states; there are over 100 officially appointed Health Ministry focal persons for the prevention of violence; over 50 countries have had national launches of the *World Report on Violence and Health*; and over 25 countries have developed reports and/or action plans on violence and health (WHO 2007), such as the Integrated Provincial Violence Prevention Policy Framework adopted in the Western Cape Province of South Africa (Box 43.1). In the WHO European Region, 23 per cent of countries reported to have a holistic national violence prevention policy (WHO Regional Office for Europe 2008). As violence prevention rises up the policy agenda this mobilizes resource allocation for violence prevention programmes and research.

Escalating country activity and strengthening scholarship presents an expanding pool of knowledge of what violence prevention policy is and how it can be implemented. This bank of violence prevention policy experience provides insight and information on the factors that help to drive the issue of violence prevention up the political agenda as well as those determinants that constrain the formulation of violence prevention policy. It informs both an understanding of how a preventative solution is adopted as well as instructing action to galvanize reform of violence prevention policy in other countries.

A core presumption of public health is the strong influence of objective reality on public health outcomes. The evidence-based public health approach to interpersonal violence attributes principal weight to the measurement and severity of the problem and the availability of effective interventions (WHO 2002). The bank of violence prevention programme evidence is predominant over the bank of violence prevention policy experience. The emergence of violence prevention databases providing access to scientific studies measuring the impact of interventions demonstrates

Box 43.1 Western Cape Province of South Africa violence prevention policy

In the Western Cape Province of South Africa a preventative strategy to reducing violence has been adopted by the Western Cape Government. The Integrated Provincial Violence Prevention Policy Framework institutionalizes an intersectoral framework that supports and sustains multi-dimensional prevention strategies. It adopts a comprehensive intersectoral approach that balances short-term evidence-based interventions, with longer-term interventions to holistically address the complex social norms that support violence. The framework establishes a long-term policy commitment to violence prevention.

One of the main objectives of the policy framework is to enhance collaboration between health, criminal justice, and educational and social development sectors to prevent violence through the adoption of shared strategies. Government departments coordinate activity to adopt policies designed to address upstream dimensions of violence, such as income inequality and early childhood development, as well as investing in immediate interventions focused on reducing the availability and harmful use of alcohol (such as the Western Cape Liquor Act of 2009 that regulates liquor outlets).

The Integrated Provincial Violence Prevention Policy Framework is in response to the large-scale problem of interpersonal violence experienced in the province. In the Western Cape Province of South Africa the levels of violent behaviour is significantly higher than the national average and is a major cause of mortality and physical injury in the province (South African Police Service 2011). Research institutions within the Western Cape Province, such as the four universities and two science councils as well as independent research institutes, generate data and research on the scale and nature of the problem of violence in the province. There is an extensive spectrum of government and non-government agencies involved in responding to the problem of interpersonal violence. An active violence prevention policy community, advanced through the Violence and Injury Prevention Cross-Ministry Working Group, has taken forward this preventative public health approach.

Source: data from Alison Morris Gehring, *International studies in violence prevention: A policy analysis* (PhD), University of St Andrews, School of Medicine, UK, Copyright © 2013.

the significance of the evidence base for violence prevention. Examples of initiatives to promote the evidence base include Violence Prevention the Evidence Base and Resources, hosted by the Centre for Public Health at Liverpool John Moores University and found at http://www.preventviolence.info/, and the Blueprints for Healthy Youth Development, launched by the Centre for the Study and Prevention of Violence at the University of Colorado Boulder http://www.blueprintsprograms.com/. A data-led understanding of the problem of violence and the availability of effective interventions is valuable in conceptualizing the problem of violence and designing policy solutions. However, the receptiveness of decision-makers to the data varies. Thus additional communication strategies complimenting the evidence-base are required

to gain political traction for violence prevention on the policy agenda (Shiffman 2009).

The political nature of developing violence prevention policy requires greater consideration of other factors such as the power of networks, ideas, and opportunities in attaining public health outcomes (Shiffman and Stone 2007). The lessons drawn from the development of violence prevention policy in one context can guide the achievement of political desirability and cultural acceptability for violence prevention in another context, as well as ensuring technical feasibility. The sharing of violence prevention policy experience thus provides insight into the political processes of violence prevention policy that are not widely addressed by the current evidence base.

As outlined in other chapters, a public health-based strategy of preventing violence has been advocated over the last 30 years as an alternative, or at least complementary, approach to interpersonal violence. The mounting global movement for violence prevention supports a growing conceptualization of prevention as an effective solution to the global health problem of violence. The emergence of violence prevention on national policy agendas and expanding volume of research presents a wealth of knowledge and ideas. Lessons drawn from this widening bank of violence prevention policy experience influence the development of violence prevention policy in other contexts—for example, the utilization of policy experience in other countries to inform the development of violence prevention policies and programmes in Lithuania (Box 43.2).

The transfer of information and insight shared through violence prevention policy experience provides guidance on how to promote the uptake of violence prevention policy in countries where the issue is struggling to progress. There are examples of states and international institutions acting as agents of policy transfer to facilitate the creation of consensual knowledge and conceptual notions drawn from violence prevention policy experience in other countries. This chapter now considers the mechanisms that support the sharing of best practice and spreading of ideas.

The Processes of Transferring Violence Prevention Policy Experience

Along with the bank of violence prevention evidence and experience, the global violence prevention field contains agencies and structures that facilitate the sharing of this knowledge across countries. Comprising states, international institutions, and non-state entities, these agents of policy transfer facilitate policy dialogue and encourage the exchange of ideas. The following section outlines principal examples of these agencies and structure, and considers how this activity progresses the uptake of violence prevention policy.

International institutions play a significant role as policy transfer agents. Over recent decades an increasing number of international agencies have acknowledged the momentous problem violence poses to global health. This growing concern is reflected through the body of work undertaken to document the scale of the problem and the intersection of violence with other major global issues. This includes reports such as the United Nations Office of Drugs and Crime (UNODC) 2011 *Global Study on Homicide*, the World Bank Report on *Violence in the City* 2010, the UN-HABITAT/WHO *Hidden Cities Report* 2010, and the

---

Box 43.2 Lithuania violence prevention policy and programme development

In Lithuania government and non-government agencies have adopted widely accredited interventions to reduce the levels of violence-related injury. For example, the Action Plan for the Prevention of School Violence (2007), led by the Ministry of Education, rolled out programmes that had been implemented and evaluated in other countries such as the violence reduction programme, Zippy's Friends for pre-school children, the Second Step Programme for primary school children, and the Olweus Bullying Prevention Programme for secondary school students.

State agency participation in cross-country collaborative projects further supports the sharing of best practice in Lithuania. An example is the Child and Adolescent Mental Health in Enlarged EU (CAMHEE) project, launched in January 2007. In Lithuania the child and adolescent mental health indicators, including the prevalence of suicides, bullying, and number of children living in state institutions, are among some of the highest in Europe. Cross-country collaboration facilitated an exchange of experiences and knowledge between Lithuania and the other partner countries. This project presented the opportunity to raise public awareness of interpersonal violence issues and generate political support for relevant national policies and programmes (Puras 2009).

International institutions and global governance exercise external leverage in Lithuania in shaping the conceptualization of the problem of violence and the policy solutions adopted. In Lithuania support for violence prevention policies and programmes is framed by the human rights and equal opportunities agenda. The issue of human rights was advanced as a component of Lithuania's accession into the European Union and increasing international role. Under the National Human Rights Action Plan for Lithuania, the United Nations Development Programme (UNDP) worked with the relevant government ministries to support the development and implementation of measures necessary for Lithuania to meet its international human rights obligations (UNDP 2005). Foreign embassies are also engaged in this area and facilitate policy dialogue across ministries and sectors to help build political desirability and demand for violence prevention.

Source: data from Alison Morris Gehring, *International studies in violence prevention: A policy analysis* (PhD), University of St Andrews, School of Medicine, UK, Copyright © 2013.

United Nations Secretary-General's *World Report on Violence against Children*, 2006. This proliferation of documentation and awareness-raising by international institutions follows on from the WHO's original *World Report on Violence and Health* (2002).

International institutions provide access to best practice, technical assistance, and the opportunity to engage in collaborative projects. Agencies such as WHO, UNDP, and the World Bank collect empirical findings to establish global best practice and build conceptual notions. International institutions utilize a global pool of experts and advocates to transmit knowledge and information about violence prevention policy and practice from one context to another.

Technical assistance projects illustrate vertical policy transfer between international institutions and states. This involves the tailoring of best practice to the context while maintaining programme fidelity. International agencies also facilitate collaborative projects that allow countries to work together to directly share experience and enhance violence prevention initiatives. Through advocacy, information dissemination, and supporting implementation these institutions facilitate the spread of innovative violence prevention policies.

Violence prevention has also benefited from the horizontal transfer of policies, institutions, and ideas between countries. Cross-country collaborative projects have shared knowledge and experience that has shaped violence prevention policy development. Such projects can help to recast violence as a preventable public health problem and change expectations as to what is possible. One example of this is the Violence Prevention Policy Development Collaboration between the University of St Andrews, Scottish Government, and WHO (Box 43.3).

Cross-country collaborative projects enable both the exchange of expertise and experience of a public health approach to violence as well as acting as a catalyst for further advancing violence prevention policy. Shared learning is also supported through international networks. Several international alliances now exist on interpersonal violence, including the WHO Violence Prevention Alliance and the Geneva Declaration on Armed Violence Reduction.

The Violence Prevention Alliance is a global network of experts and professionals, sharing expertise and information and forming common patterns of understanding regarding violence prevention policy. Members are coalesced around a shared consensus to strengthen support for data-driven violence prevention programmes based on the public health approach. This mechanism supports policy transfer by providing a bank of information, advocating policy solutions, spreading ideas and information, and synthesizing credible research (Violence Prevention Alliance 2012).

Agents of transfer within the network work both collectively at the global level, and, as individuals, locally, to proactively promote the idea of violence prevention and the use of evidence-based practice. This enables state and non-state entities to advance the ideas of violence prevention beyond the domestic context and

---

Box 43.3 Violence Prevention Policy Development Collaboration

This project aimed to build a holistic policy response to interpersonal violence through shared learning, technical assistance, and capacity development. Through country visits and on-going communications this sought to raise the political priority of violence. Working with three countries that struggle with very high levels of violence and have the political will to change that situation, a collaborative initiative was established to support the development and implementation of violence prevention policies. This produced important new insights into what helps and hinders the development of violence reduction policy.

Source: data from Alison Morris Gehring, *International Studies in Violence Prevention: A Policy Analysis* (PhD), University of St Andrews, School of Medicine, UK, Copyright © 2013.

into the global arena, thus presenting a means for the international diffusion and dissemination of the idea of violence prevention and the policy alternatives. Moreover a global network of experts provides intellectual authority to reinforce and legitimate the conceptualization of interpersonal violence as a public health problem and the presentation of prevention as best practice.

Transnational policy communities facilitate the stimulation, collection, and spread of knowledge and ideas between contexts that supports the advancement of a preventative approach towards violence. This global network provides the platform and structural framework for sharing knowledge and best practice, building consensus, and spreading ideas. Along with states and international institutions as agents of policy transfer, the transnational policy community enables the sharing of experience in other countries to ultimately spread the uptake of violence prevention policy.

Conclusion

Policy transfer is a mechanism of influence where policy experience in one context shapes the development of policy in another context. Lessons drawn from the formulation and delivery of violence prevention policy guide the achievement of political desirability and cultural acceptability; and the uptake of proven effective policy solutions in another country. The emergence of violence prevention on national policy agendas and expanding volume of research presents a bank of knowledge of what violence prevention policy is and how it can be implemented.

The comprehensive evidence base for violence prevention is an established tool in articulating the problem of violence and designing policy solutions. However, the political nature of the policy process renders the evidence base alone insufficient to gain political traction for violence prevention on the policy agenda. Insight and information provided by the experience of developing violence prevention policy informs an understanding of how the issue of violence and a strategy of prevention are prioritized on the policy agenda. Therefore both evidence and experience have a role to play in spreading awareness and acceptance of interpersonal violence as a global health problem.

The violence prevention community is integral in facilitating the collection and exchange of violence prevention expertise and experience. Transnational policy networks in particular support the transferring of violence prevention policy by sharing best practice and spreading a common perspective. This role could be further strengthened by the coalescing and informed engagement of the violence prevention policy community in the web of institutions, interests, and ideas that underpin the public health policy process.

Health policy development is a process that interweaves research and politics. As with any other health issue, the processes that determine the adoption of violence prevention policy are inherently political. The experience of developing and implementing violence prevention policy provides insight into the conditions that determine the mobilization of political priority and resources for violence prevention. Policy transfer thus instructs action to promote the uptake of violence prevention policy in countries where the issue is struggling to progress.

References

Asare, B., and Studlar, D. (2009). Lesson-drawing and public policy: secondhand smoking restrictions in Scotland and England. *Policy Studies*, 30, 365–82.

Bennett, C. (1991). Review article: what is policy convergence and what causes it? *British Journal of Political Science*, 21, 215–33.

Dolowitz, D., and Marsh, D. (1996). Who learns from whom: a review of the policy transfer literature. *Political Studies*, 44, 343–57.

Dolowitz, D., and Marsh, D. (2000). Learning from abroad: the role of policy transfer in contemporary policy making. *Governance*, 13, 5–24.

Evans, M. (2009). Policy transfer in critical perspective. *Policy Studies*, 30, 243–68.

Evans, M., and Davies, J. (1999). Understanding policy transfer: a multi-level, multi-disciplinary perspective. *Public Administration*, 77, 361–85.

Gilson, L., and Raphaely, N. (2008). The terrain of health policy analysis in low-and middle-income countries: a review of published literature 1994-2007. *Health Policy and Planning*, 23, 294–307.

Grin, J., and Loeber, A. (2007). Theories of policy learning: agency, structure and change. In: F. Fischer, G. Miller, and M. Sidney (eds), *Handbook of Public Policy Analysis: Theory, Politics and Methods*. New York: Taylor and Francis Group, pp.201–23.

Puras, D. (2009). *CAMHEE Project: The General Overview of Preliminary Conclusions and Recommendations*. Vilnius: State Mental Health Centre.

Reinicke, W., and Deng, F. (2000). *Critical Choices: The United Nations, Networks and the Future of Global Governance*. Ottawa: International Development Research Centre.

Rose, R. (1991). What is lesson-drawing? *Journal of Public Policy*, 11, 3–30.

Shiffman, J. (2007). Generating political priority for maternal mortality reduction in five developing countries. *American Journal of Public Health*, 97, 796–803.

Shiffman, J. (2009). A social explanation for the rise and fall of global health issues. *Bulletin World Health Organization*, 87, 608–13.

Shiffman, J., and Stone, S. (2007). Generation of political priority for global health initiatives: a framework and case study of maternal mortality. *Lancet*, 370, 1370–9.

South African Police Service. (2011). *Crime Report 2010/2011*. Pretoria: South African Police Service.

Stone, D. (1999). Learning lessons and transferring policy across time, space and disciplines. *Politics*, 19, 51–9.

Stone, D. (2000). Non-governmental policy transfer: the strategies of independent policy institutes. *Governance*, 13, 45–70.

Tantivess, S., and Walt, G. (2008). The role of state and non-state actors in the policy process: the contribution of policy networks to the scale up of antiretroviral therapy in Thailand. *Health Policy and Planning*, 23, 328–38.

The World Bank. (2010). *Violence in the City: Understanding and Supporting Community Responses to Urban Violence*. Washington D.C.: The World Bank.

United Nations Development Programme. (2005). *Human Rights in Lithuania*. Vilnius: UNDP.

United Nations Office on Drugs and Crime. (2011). *Global Study on Homicide 2011*. Vienna: UNODC.

United Nations Secretary-General's Study on Violence against Children. (2006). *World Report on Violence against Children*. Geneva: United Nations Secretary-General's Study on Violence against Children.

Violence Prevention Alliance. (2012). *Plan of Action for 2012-2020*. Available at: http://www.who.int/violence_injury_prevention/violence/global_campaign/gcvp_plan_of_action.pdf [Accessed 22 November 2013].

World Health Organization/United Nations Human Settlement Programme. (2010). *Hidden Cities: Unmasking and Uncovering Health Inequities in Urban Settings*. Geneva: WHO/UN-HABITAT.

World Health Organization. (2007). *Third Milestones of a Global Campaign for Violence Prevention Report 2007*. Geneva: WHO.

World Health Organization. (2002). *World Report on Violence and Health*. Geneva: WHO.

World Health Organization Regional Office for Europe. (2008). *Progress in Preventing Injuries in the WHO European Region*. Copenhagen: WHO Regional Office for Europe.

CHAPTER 44

The history and role of international agencies in violence prevention

Alexander Butchart and Christopher Mikton

Introduction to the History and Role of International Agencies in Violence Prevention

According to the World Health Organization's (WHO) Global Burden of Disease estimates for 2011, over half of all global deaths caused by violence were due to suicide (797,823), over a third due to homicide (486,493), and under a tenth (86,307) due to war and other forms of collective violence (WHO 2013). International organizations have traditionally played a major role in the prevention of collective violence (Krug et al. 2002). For instance, the United Nations (UN) Charter (United Nation 1945), the UN peacekeeping activities, and the 1949 Geneva Conventions and their Additional Protocols (International Committee of the Red Cross 1949), all aim to prevent collective violence and promote international peace. By contrast, the role of international organizations in preventing interpersonal and self-directed violence (which account for the overwhelming majority of deaths due to violence) has been much less prominent. This, however, is changing with the emergence in the last 30 years of the global interpersonal violence prevention field, to which several international organizations have been making important contributions.

Ultimately, violence is prevented by taking concrete measures on the ground. These may include implementing programmes to prevent violence and developing services for victims; formulating and implementing violence prevention policies; enacting and enforcing laws; and developing human and institutional capacity. It is primarily at national and sub-national—including municipal level—that such measures are taken. However, international organizations can contribute to violence prevention directly by providing funding, policy advice, or operational assistance to countries and, indirectly, by contributing to the global violence prevention field and the global public knowledge it produces, which can then be applied by national and sub-national actors.

This chapter aims to sketch the history of international organizations' involvement in violence prevention and, in the process, point out the main roles, characteristics, and approaches adopted by some of the most influential international organizations in violence prevention. Throughout, the chapter focuses on interpersonal violence—one of the two forms of violence (along with self-directed violence) in relation to which the role of international organizations has rarely been examined.

Defining International Organizations, their Roles, and the Global Violence Prevention Field

Archer (2001) defined international organization as:

> a formal, continuous structure established by agreement between members (governmental and/or nongovernmental) from two or more sovereign states with the aim of pursuing the common interest of the membership. (p. 33)

Archer (2001) further emphasizes three features of this definition: membership—it must draw its membership from two or more sovereign states; aim—it must pursue a common interest and not just the interests of a single member; and structure—it should have its own formal structure of a continuous nature established by an agreement. Two broad types of international organizations can be distinguished: those whose members are governments and states (international governmental organizations or IGOs), and those whose members are non-governmental (international non-governmental organizations or INGOs).

Many different concepts have been used to understand the roles and functions of international organizations within the international system. For instance, Archer (2001) describes international organizations as *instruments* inasmuch as they are used by members to pursue their own particular ends; *arenas* in that they 'provide meeting places for members to come together to discuss, argue, co-operate, and disagree' (p. 73); and *actors* when they act within the international system with varying degrees of autonomy from their constituent members. Archer (2001) identifies the following key functions of international organizations: interest articulation and aggregation; establishing and changing norms; socialization by seeking to affect peoples' systems of belief and patterns of behaviour; generating information, in the form, for instance, of statistical data on health and populations; and, finally, operational activities such as providing aid.

A prominent role of international organizations is rule making through the formulation and adoption of resolutions and conventions on behalf of member states. Rule application and adjudication is less prominent a role as this is largely left to sovereign states in the absence of a central world authority with the power of enforcement. IGOs role as autonomous actors depends largely on the resolutions and recommendations they produce. Although these are rarely legally binding on member states and generally not supported by enforcement mechanisms, they can nonetheless influence governments to act differently (Archer 2001). Examples relevant to violence prevention include: the Convention on the Rights of the Child (General Assembly of the United Nations 1989); the Convention on the Elimination of All Forms of Discrimination Against Women (United Nations 1979); UN General Assembly Resolution 62/141 establishing the mandate of the Special Representative of the Secretary General on Violence against Children (United Nations General Assembly 2008a); and resolution 63/23 entitled Promoting Development through the Reduction and Prevention of Armed Violence (United Nations General Assembly 2008b).

Following Morris et al. (2008), we define the global violence prevention field as consisting of international actors which are financially, intellectually, institutionally, and personally interlinked to varying degrees and share a common focus on preventing interpersonal and self-directed violence. These include IGOs and INGOs, international development banks, regional cooperation organizations, bilateral aid agencies, charitable foundations, universities, and research institutions with an international reach. The global violence prevention field can be viewed as having several purposes: supporting national actors in countries with high burdens of violence and which lack the resources to address it; producing global public knowledge such as standards, regulations, and the identification of priorities; mobilizing, pooling, and distributing financial resources; providing technical assistance when required; and strengthening human and institutional resources.

History, Roles, and Approaches of International Organizations in Violence Prevention

The history of international organizations' involvement in violence prevention can be divided into three broad phases. From around the mid-1970s until the late 1990s was the 'formative' phase, when organizations declared their interest in addressing the problem, and the main sectoral divisions within the global violence prevention field were staked out. The late-1990s until around 2010 was the 'normative' phase dominated by efforts to build global consensus on the definition and scope of the global violence prevention field and approaches to preventing violence. From 2011 to date there are signs that the field is entering an 'operational' phase where the emphasis is less on developing norms about how to prevent violence and more on implementing what is known.

The Formative Phase: 1970–1999

In this period, international organizations started to register their interest in addressing the challenges of preventing interpersonal

violence. Perhaps the first to do so was the International Society for the Prevention of Child Abuse and Neglect formed in 1976 (Box 44.1). In the early 1980s, the UN Educational, Scientific, and Cultural Organization adopted the 'Seville statement on violence' (1986) asserting that violent behaviour is not genetically programmed into human nature and therefore that it is preventable. In 1989 the General Assembly of the UN adopted the Convention on the Rights of the Child (UNCRC), which obliges governments 'to protect the child from all forms of physical or mental violence, injury or abuse, neglect or negligent treatment, maltreatment or exploitation' (General Assembly of the United Nations 1989, Article 19, paragraph 1), followed in 1990 by publication of the United Nations Guidelines for the prevention of Juvenile Delinquency which stated that 'the prevention of juvenile delinquency is an essential part of crime prevention in society' (General Assembly of the United Nations 1990, Article 1, paragraph 1).

In 1993, the UN General Assembly adopted the Declaration on the Elimination of Violence against Women (United Nations General Assembly 1994), and WHO devoted World Health Day 1993 to preventing violence and injuries with the slogan 'Handle life with care: prevent violence and negligence' (World Health Forum 1993). In 1994 the United Nations Development Programme's (UNDP) Human Development Report introduced the 'new concept of human security', including 'personal security' (United Nations Development Programme 1994, pp. 30–1), and the WHO Regional Office for the Americas convened the Inter-American Conference on Society, Violence and Health (World Health Organization, n.d.). The International Centre for the Prevention of Crime (Box 44.2) was also established in 1994, in part to provide support for local policies to deal with urban violence and insecurity. In 1996 and 1997, the World Health Assembly (WHA) adopted resolutions calling on WHO to support a science-based public health approach to violence prevention (World Health Assembly 1996, 1997). In 1996, United Nations Development for Women established its Trust Fund to Eliminate

Box 44.1 The International Society for the Prevention of Child Abuse and Neglect (ISPCAN)

ISPCAN is a non-profit membership INGO whose mission is to support individuals and organizations working towards the prevention and treatment of child abuse, neglect, and exploitation worldwide. Its main objectives are to increase awareness of the extent, the causes, and possible solutions for all forms of child abuse; disseminate academic and clinical research to those in positions to enhance practice and improve policy; support international efforts to promote and protect the Convention on the Rights of the Child; improve the quality of current efforts to detect, treat, and prevent child abuse; facilitate the exchange of best practice standards being developed by ISPCAN members throughout the world; and design and deliver comprehensive training programmes to professionals and concerned volunteers engaged in efforts to treat and prevent child abuse.

Source: data from *International Society for the Prevention of Child Abuse and Neglect* (ISPCAN) *website*, Copyright © 2014, available from http://www.ispcan.org/.

Box 44.2 International Centre for the Prevention of Crime (ICPC)

ICPC is an INGO that acts as an international forum for national governments, local authorities, public agencies, specialized institutions, and non-government organizations to exchange experience, emerging knowledge, and policies and programmes in crime prevention and community safety.

ICPC's mission is to promote safer and healthier societies and communities through the application of strategic and evidence-led programmes and initiatives which aim to reduce and prevent offending and victimization and to support international norms and standards.

Source: data from *International Center for the Prevention of Crime (ICPC) website*, Copyright © ICPC-CIPC 2014, available from http://www.crime-prevention-intl.org/

Violence against Women (which has now been taken over by UNWomen—Box 44.3), and UN Habitat launched the first 'Safer Cities' programme.

In declaring their interest in violence prevention, these initial commitments by international organizations also specified how they understood and portrayed the problem of violence and its prevention. For the UN General Assembly, both in respect of violence against children and violence against women, acts of violence were framed as human rights violations, and violence prevention as a challenge for criminal justice and legal systems, best addressed by translating international human rights instruments (e.g. the Convention to Eliminate all Forms of Discrimination Against Women, and the UNCRC) into national law and ensuring its enforcement. By contrast, the 1996 and 1997 WHA resolutions prioritized a scientific approach to

Box 44.3 UN Women

Established in 2010, UN Women is a UN programme dedicated to gender equality and the empowerment of women. It merges four previously distinct parts of the UN system, which focused exclusively on gender equality and women's empowerment. Ending violence against women by addressing gender inequality is one of UN Women's priority areas. In this area it focuses on programme and technical assistance, policy and normative support, and managing the UN Trust Fund to End Violence against Women. As part of programme and technical assistance, for instance, UN Women's Global Programme on Safe Cities Free of Violence against Women focuses on reducing sexual harassment and violence in urban public spaces, through community empowerment and partnerships with local authorities. To bring about normative change, UN Women coordinates the UN Secretary-General's UNiTE to End Violence against Women campaign and supports widespread social mobilization through its Say NO—UNiTE to End Violence against Women platform.

Source: *United Nations Entity for Gender Equality and the Empowerment of Women (UNWomen) website*, Copyright © 2011–2014 UN Women, available from http://www.unwomen.org/.

understanding and preventing violence, in which acts of violence were seen as an outcome of the interaction between individual (including biological), close relationship, community, and societal factors, and violence prevention as a multi-sectoral challenge requiring policies and programmes that could address underlying causes and risk factors.

The formative phase thus set in place the two dominant frames of reference (human rights and public health) that continue to inform the international violence prevention field, and, which, during the normative phase, became more sharply delineated.

The Normative Phase: 2000–2010

With some exceptions, the work of international organizations during the formative phase was directed towards advocating for increased attention to the problem of violence, and there were few efforts to produce normative and technical guidance documents for stakeholders at national and local levels. By contrast, the normative phase from around 2000–2010 was characterized by intensive efforts to provide such guidance, as international organizations began establishing dedicated programmes to address interpersonal violence.

In 2002 WHO (Box 44.4), with technical support from the United States Centers for Disease Control and Prevention (CDC), published the *World Report on Violence and Health* (Krug et al. 2002). This established the role of public health, alongside other sectors, in understanding and preventing violence, and in 2003 was the subject of a WHA Resolution on implementing its recommendations (World Health Assembly 2003). Since then WHO has

Box 44.4 World Health Organization (WHO) and the Violence Prevention Alliance (VPA)

The WHO is a specialized agency of the UN (which has a 194 Member States), and which acts as the directing and coordinating authority for health within the United Nations system. The WHO Prevention of Violence Unit's aim is to spearhead global action to address violence as a major threat to public health using advocacy, data collection, trend monitoring, evaluation, dissemination of evidence-based practices in prevention, and to support countries to define, measure, describe, and monitor violence as a public health problem, and to develop science-based approaches to violence prevention and services for victims and perpetrators. In addition, the Unit launched the Global Campaign for Violence Prevention and the Violence Prevention Alliance (VPA) in 2004 and has been leading these since then. The VPA is a network of international, governmental and non-governmental organizations, private foundations, research institutions, and universities committed to preventing interpersonal violence using an evidence-based public health approach (Violence Prevention Alliance 2012).

Source: data from World Health Organization (WHO) website, Copyright © WHO 2014, available from http://www.who.int/en/ and Violence Prevention Alliance, Violence Prevention Alliance/Global *Campaign for Violence Prevention: Plan of action for 2012-2020*, Copyright © WHO 2012, *available from* http://www.who.int/violence_injury_prevention/violence/global_campaign/actionplan/en/index.html regularly published policy and technical guidelines, and training materials, covering the prevention of several types of interpersonal violence. WHO guidance materials and policy documents assert that all violence prevention activities, from policy formation, through prevention programming, to the provision of services for victims and perpetrators, should be science based.

Other science-based public health initiatives established during this normative phase included the Sexual Violence Research Initiative (SVRI). Launched in 2003 by the Global Forum for Health Research, the SVRI was initially hosted by the WHO before moving to the Medical Research Council, South Africa in 2006. The CDC's Division for Violence Prevention, which pioneered the public health approach to violence prevention within the United States (Rosenberg and Fenley 1991), has since the late 1990s played a pivotal role in many of the normative developments described. For example, CDC experts helped draft the WHA resolutions on violence prevention, and were among the editors of the *World Report on Violence and Health*. CDC provides on-going technical support to countries for the development of science-based violence prevention policy, surveillance systems, and programmes, including, for instance, supporting Brazil and South Africa in the development of national injury surveillance systems, and working with United Kingdom scientists to evaluate the City of Cardiff's approach to violence prevention (Florence et al. 2011). CDC also made substantial contributions to the *World Report on Violence against Children*, and was one of the founding partners of Together for Girls (see section 'The operational phase').

In 2006, drawing on technical input from the Office of the High Commissioner for Human Rights, the United Nations Children's Fund (UNICEF), WHO, and others, the *World Report on Violence against Children* was published (Pinheiro 2006; United Nations 2006a), and informed the UN Secretary General's Report on Violence against Children in the same year. At the same time, the UN *Secretary General's In-depth Study on all Forms of Violence against Women* (United Nations 2006b) was published. Both reports prioritized a human rights approach. In 2009, the *UN Secretary General's Report on Violence against Children* was followed up by a *Lancet* article setting out the tenets of a rights-based approach to prevention (Reading et al. 2009). This noted that:

> the definition of child maltreatment as a violation of rights implies that the responsibility and accountability of policy makers to intervene is an international legal obligation based on standards upheld universally, and that nearly every government in the world has ratified. (p. 337)

It also noted that in making the child an individual with rights, the UNCRC makes:

> the state directly responsible to the child to promote his or her rights. The child has the right to make a direct call on the state and to be heard in the development of legislation and policy, besides receiving protection. (p. 335)

Accordingly, normative guidance based on the UNCRC consists of a series of 'general comments' that detail UNCRC articles relevant to violence against children and then explain what governments are obliged to do in order to operationalize these articles (United Nations Committee on the Rights of the Child 2011, 2013).

The *World Report on Violence against Children* led in 2009 to appointment of the Secretary General's Special Rapporteur on

Violence against Children, and led UNICEF to re-evaluate its child protection activities, and scale up its participation in international efforts to support the prevention of violence against children in non-conflict settings, and in relation to violence that occurs within the family (Box 44.5).

These public health-, human rights-, and child protection-oriented activities were complemented by several more eclectic international programmes that draw upon scientific, human rights, and political analyses. For example, in 2006, the Geneva Declaration on Armed Violence and Development was launched, followed in 2008 by a UN General Assembly Resolution on 'Promoting development through the reduction and prevention of armed violence' (United Nations General Assembly 2008b), and in 2009 by establishment of the Armed Violence Prevention Programme, an effort by six UN agencies to provide joint violence prevention programming in countries directly affected by armed violence. In 2007, the World Bank established its Social Cohesion and Violence Prevention Team.

The Operational Phase: 2011 to Date

Movement into the operational phase began with observations in 2009 and 2010 by several international organizations that, based upon scientific findings from high-income countries (HIC), sufficient knowledge about how to prevent violence now existed. This message was reinforced by a number of international foundations that, through their experience in funding governments and NGOs, recognized a major gap between the poor technical knowledge and capacity of the partners they were funding, and the by now well-developed stock of global public knowledge, such as the evidence base for violence prevention, guidance documents, and training materials. This led to priorities for the international violence prevention field being re-defined as ensuring that national and local partners in low- and middle-income countries (LMIC) be better supported to act on the evidence for prevention, and that large-scale, high-quality outcome

---

Box 44.5 United Nations Children's Fund (UNICEF)

UNICEF aims to provide humanitarian, health, and development assistance to children and mothers in low- and middle-income countries. It is mandated by the UN General Assembly to advocate for the protection of children's rights, to help meet their basic needs, and to expand their opportunities to reach their full potential, and is guided in its activities by the Convention on the Rights of the Child (General Assembly of the United Nations 1989). Within UNICEF's five focus areas, violence prevention comes mainly under 'child protection'. UNICEF's Child Protection Strategy (2008) contains two main pillars: (i) strengthening child protection systems—including laws, policies, regulations, and services across all social sectors, especially social welfare, education, health, security, and justice; and (ii) supporting the social changes that strengthen the protection of children from violence, exploitation, and abuse. Its approach is explicitly human rights-based, and emphasizes that successful child protection begins with prevention.

Source: data from *United Nations Children's Fund (UNICEF) website*, Copyright © UNICEF 2014, available from http://www.unicef.org/

evaluation trials in of a small set of particularly promising violence prevention strategies be strongly encouraged in LMIC.

Three major initiatives typify the role of international organizations in the operational phase. First, Together for Girls (TfG) is a global public–private partnership dedicated to eliminating violence against children, with a focus on sexual violence against girls. It includes UN agencies (including UNAIDS, UNICEF, UN Women, and WHO), the private sector, the United States Department of State, and the CDC. TfG country projects mainly involve the conduct of nationally representative epidemiological surveys of violence against children as a basis for subsequent policy and programme development, and have been completed or are underway in Botswana, Kenya, Malawi, Nigeria, Rwanda, Swaziland, Tanzania, Zambia, Zimbabwe, Haiti, and several countries in East Asia and the Pacific. Second, the Children and Violence Evaluation Challenge Fund, established in 2010, aims at reducing the prevalence of violence against children by funding high-quality evaluations of violence prevention and child protection interventions in LMIC. These evaluations are expected to help generate a solid evidence base that will be used to strengthen programmes and policies for preventing violence against children.

Box 44.6 United National Office on Drugs and Crime (UNODC)

The UNODC is an IGO that is a UN programme, rather than specialized agency, and as an integral part of the UN can claim universal membership. It is mandated to assist Member States address the interrelated issues of drug control, crime prevention, and international terrorism in the context of sustainable development and human security. Most of the issues that UNODC addresses overlap with violence prevention. For instance, UNODC's work to establish legal and institutional frameworks for drug control through effective implementation of international drug control conventions has an important bearing on violence prevention. The global homicide statistics it produces and the Global Study on Homicide (2011) are important tools for monitoring of homicide trends and formulating violence prevention policies. UNODC's crime prevention and criminal justice reform work is also highly relevant to violence prevention at the national level.

Source: data from *United Nations Office on Drugs and Crime (UNODC) website,* Copyright © UNODC 2014, available from https://www.unodc.org/.

Third, the WHO, with UNODC (Box 44.6) and UNDP, initiated in 2011 a global survey of national efforts to prevent violence that is documenting the existence and extent of policies, programmes, and laws addressing all forms of interpersonal violence. Known as the *Global Status Report on Violence Prevention,* it is anticipated that the survey will provide baseline data on country-level violence prevention progress which can then be used to set national violence prevention priorities and monitor subsequent national, regional, and global progress in violence prevention.

Conclusion

Over the last 20 years, the global field of violence prevention has become better established, evolving—with international organizations playing a central role—through a formative, a normative, and, more recently, an operational phase. It has begun to successfully produce global rules and knowledge for violence prevention, embodied in various conventions, resolutions, global reports, international guidelines, and compilations of evidence of what works. Disparate international actors have started to coalesce into networks and to harmonize their approaches to violence prevention. Priorities for the field have begun to be identified at both international and national levels, and concerted efforts are being made to generate high-quality data about the scale and the severity of the problem, particularly in LMIC.

However, despite these substantial strides, the global violence prevention field has yet to attract political and financial support commensurate with the scale and severity of the problem. For instance, whereas other new areas of global public health concern, such as tobacco control and road traffic injury prevention, each receive hundreds of millions of dollars in funding each year, the total value of funds available for interpersonal violence prevention probably amount to just tens of millions of dollars. To gain insight into why interpersonal violence prevention is struggling to 'take off', one of the concluding chapters to this volume (Chapter 45) identifies several policy and practice issues, which, if successfully addressed, could help the field to achieve greater global prominence and stronger local impact.

Acknowledgement

Text extracts from *The Lancet,* Volume 373, Issue 9660, Reading, R. et al., Promotion of children's rights and prevention of child maltreatment, pp. 332–43, Copyright © 2009, reproduced with permission from Elsevier, http://www.sciencedirect.com/science/journal/01406736

References

Archer, C. (2001). *International Organizations*. 3rd ed. New York: Routledge.

Florence, C., Shepherd, J., Brennan, I., and Simon, T. (2011). Effectiveness of anonymised information sharing and use in health service, police, and local government partnership for preventing violence related injury: experimental study and time series analysis. *British Medical Journal*, 342.

General Assembly of the United Nations. (1989). *Convention on the Rights of the Child*. General Assembly Resolution 44/25 of 20 November 1989. Geneva: Office of the High Commissioner for Human Rights.

General Assembly of the United Nations. (1990). *United Nations Guidelines for the Prevention of Juvenile Delinquency (The Riyadh Guidelines)*. A/RES45/112. New York: General Assembly of the United Nations. Available at: http://www.un.org/documents/ga/res/45/a45r112.htm [Accessed 03 June 2006].

ICPC (2013) International Center for the Prevention of Crime. Available at: http://www.crime-prevention-intl.org/ [Accessed on 03 June 2013]

International Committee of the Red Cross (ICRC) (1949) *Geneva Conventions of 1949 and their Additional Protocols*. Geneva: ICRC. Available at: http://www.icrc.org/eng/war-and-law/treaties-customary-law/geneva-conventions/ [Accessed 19 December 2013].

ISPCAN (2013) International Society for the Prevention of Child Abuse and Neglect. Available at: http://www.ispcan.org/ [Accessed on 03 June 2013]

Krug, E., Dahlberg, L., Mercy, J., Zwi, A., and Lozano, R. (2002). *World Report on Violence and Health*. Geneva: World Health Organization.

Morris, S. S., Cogill, B., and Uauy, R. (2008). Effective international action against undernutrition: why has it proven so difficult and what can be done to accelerate progress? *Lancet*, 371, 608–21.

Pinheiro, P. S. (2006). *World Report on Violence against Children*. Geneva: United Nations.

Reading, R., Bissell, S., and Goldhagen, J. et al. (2009). Promotion of children's rights and prevention of child maltreatment. *Lancet*, 373, 332–43.

Rosenberg, M. L., and Fenley, M. A. (1991). *Violence in America: A Public Health Approach*. New York: Oxford University Press.

UNICEF (2013) United Nations Children's Fund. Available at: http://www.unicef.org/ [Accessed 03 June 2013]

United Nations (1945) *Charter of the United Nations and Statute of the International Court of Justice*. San Francisco: United Nations.

United Nations. (1979). *Convention on the Elimination of All Forms of Discrimination against Women*. New York: United Nations. Available at http://treaties.un.org/Pages/ViewDetails.aspx?src=TREATY&mtdsg_no=IV-8&chapter=4&lang=en [Accessed 16 December 2013]

United Nations. (2006a). *Report of the Independent Expert for the United Nations Study on Violence against Children* (A/61/299). New York: United Nations. Available at: http://srsg.violenceagainstchildren.org/un_study [Accessed 03 June 2013].

United Nations. (2006b). *In-depth Study on all Forms of Violence against Women: Report of the Secretary-General*. New York: United Nations.

United Nations Committee on the Rights of the Child. (2011). *General Comment Number 13. The Right of the Child to Freedom from all Forms of Violence*. Geneva: Office of the High Commissioner for Human Rights. Available at: http://www2.ohchr.org/english/bodies/crc/comments.htm [Accessed 03 June 2011].

United Nations Educational, Scientific and Cultural Organization. (1986). *Seville Statement on Violence, Spain* (subsequently adopted by UNESCO at the twenty-fifth session of the General Conference on 16 November 1989). Rome: United Nations Educational, Scientific and Cultural Organization. Available at: http://portal.unesco.org/education/en/ev.php-URL_ID=3247&URL_DO=DO_TOPIC&URL_SECTION=201.html [Accessed 03 June 2013].

United Nations General Assembly. (1994). *Declaration on the Elimination of Violence against Women*. A/RES/48/104. New York: United Nations. Available at: http://daccess-dds-ny.un.org/doc/UNDOC/GEN/N94/095/05/PDF/N9409505.pdf?OpenElement [Accessed 16 December 2013].

United Nations General Assembly. (2008a). *Rights of the child*. A/RES/62/141. New York: United Nations. Available at: http://srsg.violenceagainstchildren.org/document/a-res-62-141_133 [Accessed 16 December 2013].

United Nations General Assembly. (2008b). *Promoting development through the reduction of armed violence*. A/RES/63/23. New York: United Nations. Available at: http://www.violenceanddevelopment.org/docs/unga_resolution_avd_2008_final_english.pdf [Accessed 16 December 2013].

United Nations Development Programme. (1994). *Human Development Report 1994: New Dimensions of Human Security*. New York, Oxford University Press. Available at: http://hdr.undp.org/en/reports/global/hdr1994/chapters/ [Accessed 03 June 2013].

United Nations Office on Drugs and Crime (2011) *Global Study on Homicide*. Vienna: United Nations Office on Drugs and Crime.

Violence Prevention Alliance. (2012). *Violence Prevention Alliance/Global Campaign for Violence Prevention: Plan of action for 2012-2020*. Available at: http://www.who.int/violence_injury_prevention/violence/global_campaign/actionplan/en/index.html [Accessed 07 June 2013].

World Health Assembly. (1996). *Prevention of Violence: A Public Health Priority*. (Forty-ninth World Health Assembly, Resolution WHA49.25). Geneva: WHO.

World Health Assembly. (1997). *Prevention of Violence*. (Fiftieth World Health Assembly, Resolution WHA50.19). Geneva: WHO.

World Health Assembly. (2003). *Implementing the Recommendations of the 'World Report on Violence and Health'* (Fifty-Sixth World Health Assembly, Resolution WHA56.24). Geneva: WHO.

World Health Forum (1993). World Health Day 1993. *World Health Forum*, 14, 331–2.

World Health Organization. (2013). *Global Health Estimates Summary Tables: Deaths by Cause, Age and Sex, by WHO Region*. Geneva: WHO. Available at: http://www.who.int/healthinfo/global_burden_disease/en/ [Accessed 27 August 2013].

World Health Organization. (n.d.) *Report of the WHO global consultation on violence and health*, Geneva, 2–3 December 1996. Unpublished report.

Challenges and priorities for researchers, practitioners, and policymakers

CHAPTER 45

Challenges and priorities for practitioners and policymakers

Alexander Butchart, Christopher Mikton, Catherine L. Ward, and Peter D. Donnelly

Introduction to Challenges and Priorities for Practitioners and Policymakers

The very existence of this book, and the volume of content within it, demonstrates that a great deal of scientific effort has been devoted to understanding and preventing interpersonal violence. There *is* evidence that interpersonal violence can be prevented. Despite this growing evidence base, violence continues at very high rates, and clearly much remains to be done in terms of putting this evidence base into practice.

The volume contains much to which those who commission, design, and implement programmes should attend. Many authors (see Chapters 18–34) echo similar themes: the need for programmes that decrease risk factors and increase protective factors that have been identified as salient in a particular context; the need for programmes to have a clearly conceptualized theory of change that is grounded in the evidence; allowing programme participants plenty of opportunity to practise new skills; providing participants sufficient 'dose' of the programme to achieve behaviour change; and ensuring that programmes are evaluated, particularly if they are being implemented in new contexts. That violence prevention initiatives are often weak in these areas is not unique in the broad arena of prevention science; but all prevention programmes are more likely to be successful if they attend to these elements (Nation et al. 2003).

It is clear, however, that there are programmes that are effective in preventing violence. But the context in which programmes must operate is also key, and this lies more within the realm of government and policy interventions than at the level of programmes. For instance, Mitis and Sethi (Chapter 8), and Gebo and colleagues (Chapter 29) argue that structural risk factors such as socioeconomic deprivation and concentrated urban poverty are strongly associated with male violence and with the existence of gangs, and that while individuals in those contexts may desist from violence through careful programming, violence and gangs will continue as long as those contexts continue to exist.

At the policy level, violence prevention has yet to become central to either the international agenda or, in many cases, those of states, which is a critical problem—rates of violence will not reduce without significant resources and attention being paid to violence, its associated risk and protective factors, and making the necessary changes. This includes attending to the issue at a number of levels: establishing and maintaining systems for the routine collection of data, such as national systems capable of accurate counts of homicides (see Chapter 2, this volume); implementing prevention programmes nationally (or, at least, in high-risk areas; see Chapters 18–34, this volume); and changing policies to create the kind of environment that will enable prevention and intervention programmes to achieve success (see Chapters 35–42, this volume). The scale of the resources required to carry out this agenda, and particularly the need for policy changes, puts government firmly in the position of necessarily being the chief actor (Coie et al. 1993). Further, successful prevention frequently needs inter-sectoral implementation (Coie et al. 1993)—for instance, ensuring that policies across health, education, and social services are coherent with each other, or that the governance structures for multi-sectoral programmes link, for instance, health and policing (see Chapter 23, this volume)—and that can only be achieved through strong leadership within government that actively works to overcome the silos within which government departments tend to work.

Globally the field of violence prevention has struggled to achieve the unification and success of other prevention fields, such as tobacco control and the reduction of road traffic injuries (see Chapter 44). The remainder of this chapter addresses the challenges faced by violence prevention as a broad field, and suggests a way forward.

Why Global Violence Prevention has Struggled to Take Off

Shiffman and Smith's (2007) framework is helpful for understanding why the field of global violence prevention has so far struggled to develop the necessary political will and financial strength. As shown in Table 45.1, this framework for examining efforts to

Table 45.1 The four categories for the framework on determinants of political priority for global initiatives

	Description	Factors shaping political priority
Actor power	The strength of the individuals and organizations concerned with the issue	1. Policy community cohesion: the degree of coalescence among the network of individuals and organizations that are centrally involved with the issue at the global level 2. Leadership: the presence of individuals capable of uniting the policy community and acknowledged as particularly strong champions for the cause 3. Guiding institutions: the effectiveness of organizations or coordinating mechanisms with a mandate to lead the initiative 4. Civil society mobilization: the extent to which grassroots organizations have mobilized to press international and national political authorities to address the issue at the global level
Ideas	The ways in which those involved with the issue understand and portray it	5. Internal frame: the degree to which the policy community agrees on the definition of, causes of, and solutions to the problem 6. External frame: public portrayals of the issue in ways that resonate with external audiences, especially the political leaders who control resources
Political contexts	The environments in which actors operate	7. Policy windows: political moments when global conditions align favourably for an issue, presenting opportunities for advocates to influence decision makers 8. Global governance structure: the degree to which norms and institutions operating in a sector provide a platform for effective collective action
Issue characteristics	Features of the problem	9. Credible indicators: clear measures that show the severity of the problem and that can be used to monitor progress 10. Severity: the size of the burden relative to other problems, as indicated by objective measures such as mortality levels 11. Effective interventions: the extent to which proposed means of addressing the problem are clearly explained, cost effective, backed by scientific evidence, simple to implement, and inexpensive

generate political priority for global initiatives identifies 11 factors, grouped into four categories, that determine the political priority accorded global initiatives—'actor power', 'ideas', 'political contexts', and 'issue characteristics'.

Actor Power

Actor power in relation to interpersonal violence is reduced by inadequate policy cohesion and leadership among international organizations, the lack of guiding institutions, and weak civil society mobilization in some areas of global violence prevention. International organizations and networks that address violence prevention have struggled to coalesce around a shared agenda, in part because of the different approaches they adopt to violence prevention. These approaches can—somewhat crudely—be characterized as the evidence-based, the human rights, and the criminal justice approaches. Each has to some degree its own universe of experts, lead organizations, and networks, and derives its violence prevention ideas from its own frame of reference.

Most prominent among those adopting an evidence-based approach are criminological and public health organizations such as the World Health Organization (WHO), United Nations Office on Drugs and Crime (UNODC), and the American and British Criminological Societies, which give priority to evidence-based and scientific approaches to understanding and preventing violence. Organizations giving priority to a human rights approach in their activities draw on human rights treaties, conventions, and other official documents developed by the Office of the High Commissioner for Human Rights (OHCHR), and include OHCHR

itself, the United Nations Children's Fund (UNICEF), and the United Nations Entity for Gender Equality and the Empowerment of Women (UNWomen). The criminal justice approach includes associations of police officers and justice officials whose main task is to 'do justice' (i.e. ensure that offenders are properly identified, that the degree of their guilt is as accurately ascertained as possible, and that they are punished appropriately), although increasingly criminal justice and law enforcement sectors in high-income countries are involved in evidence-based violence prevention efforts. None of these three groups, and no organizations within them, has a strong mandate to lead on the prevention of violence (i.e. a UN General Assembly resolution explicitly allocating leadership across different agencies to a single one), and there is considerable competition both between and within them for financial resources and political backing.

Civil society mobilization with the aim of pressurizing national authorities and international agencies to do more to address interpersonal violence is limited. Among such efforts is the White Ribbon Campaign to stimulate opposition to violence against women. As of late 2013, efforts by campaigns such as these had not mobilized substantive and sustained upward pressure on governments and international agencies to do more by way of violence prevention.

What is clearly needed, therefore, on the dimension of 'actor power', is a coordinating body strong enough to increase cohesion within the policy community to the point where all stakeholders are aiming to achieve a shared set of prevention goals and supporting a uniform set of evidence-informed policies and programmes to reach those goals. Strength could be increased from within the UN system, through a UN General Assembly Resolution that mandates a single agency to lead, and/or from without the UN system, by having a donor provide substantial funding to an appropriate agency to take charge. In the meantime there are efforts on several fronts (e.g. by WHO's Violence Prevention Alliance and the Geneva Declaration) to unify the violence prevention field but these have so far lacked the traction required.

Ideas

Prior to the 2002 publication by WHO of the *World report on violence and health* (Krug et al. 2002) it is difficult to gauge the degree of agreement between agencies centrally involved in the problem on the definition of, causes of, and solutions to interpersonal violence. By contrast, since 2002 there has been widespread uptake of WHO's conceptual and operational definitions of violence, and of the *Report's* ecological model for understanding the risk and protective factors for, and underlying causes of, violence and organizing prevention strategies. Consequently, there is now substantially greater agreement across agencies, at least on the definitions and risk factors for interpersonal violence, and increasingly so in respect of solutions.

The role of WHO in helping to build stronger agreement on these ideas about violence was spelt out in a 1996 World Health Assembly Resolution which requested the Organization to 'characterize different types of violence, define their magnitude and assess the causes and the public health consequences of violence' (WHA49.25, 1996). Building on definitions of violence formulated in the mid-1980s by the CDC, the 2002 *World Report on Violence and Health* defined violence as 'the intentional use of physical force or power, threatened or actual, against oneself, another person, or against a group or community, that either results in or has a high likelihood of resulting in injury, death, psychological harm, maldevelopment or deprivation' (Krug et al. 2002). It provided a typology of violence which distinguished between three high-level types of violence—self-directed, interpersonal, and collective—each of which was in turn divided into sub-types, and an ecological model that located the risk factors for violence within a nested model made up of the levels of the individual, relationships, the community, and wider society (Krug et al. 2002). Ensuring that WHO definitions remained close to the definitions developed by the US Centers for Disease Control (United States Centers for Disease Control and Prevention, 2013a; Rosenberg and Fenley 1991) helped multiply the number of violence prevention stakeholders exposed to these ideas, and accelerated agreement across agencies. This was further reinforced by the 2006 *World Report on Violence against Children* (Pinheiro 2006), which adopted the WHO definitions and typology of violence, and its ecological model.

The biggest challenge in relation to the dimension of 'ideas' is better reconciliation of the essentially individualizing, ethical, and legalistic approach of criminal justice and human rights with the population-based, scientific, and multi-level approach adopted by criminology and public health. In theory, these different approaches should complement each other—the criminal justice and human rights approaches providing the moral framework and goals towards which a more value-free scientific approach could help to work towards. However, in practice these two approaches seem too often to work at cross-purposes

Political Contexts

Policy Windows

The post-2015 development agenda, which will replace the Millennium Development Goals (MDGs), constitutes the most significant policy window in respect of efforts to increase the political priority of global initiatives. Freedom from interpersonal violence was not among the original MDGs, and interpersonal violence does not receive significant attention as an impediment to achieving the goals, despite the negative impact of violence on achieving the MDGs (Bowman et al. 2008). There is reason to believe, however, based on a recent report by the high-level panel of eminent persons on the post-2015 development agenda that violence prevention will figure more prominently in the global development goals currently being formulated (see United Nations, 2013).

The 2012 scandal surrounding child sexual abuse by the deceased U.K. media celebrity Jimmy Savile; the December 2012 school shooting in Newton, United States, and the rape and murder in Delhi of a young woman traveling on a bus in India, are good examples of events that, owing to extensive global media coverage, present opportunities for violence prevention advocates to influence decision-makers. More than the events themselves, it is media coverage of the responses to the events by heads of state and other high-level decision-makers when they promise to reform laws and institute prevention measures that constitute windows of opportunity for international organizations to advocate for increased violence prevention efforts.

The capacity of international organizations to utilize these policy windows is varied. On the one hand, some international NGOs are quick to publish opinion pieces in newspapers and on high-profile blogs, appealing to readers to seize the opportunity for advancing violence prevention created by these events. On the other hand, strong advocacy statements from UN agencies in major newspapers and journals are largely absent. For example, while both the UNICEF and WHO corporate websites and Facebook pages carried items that referred to the U.S. shootings and the rape in India, no Director-level statements on these topics were reported in the media. If a coordinating body for policy were to be established, then it should include personnel dedicated to communication efforts, both to take advantage of communications 'windows' when they open, and to sustain and coordinate communications around violence prevention so that the issue is constantly on the global agenda.

In relation to the dimension of 'political contexts' it is therefore hard to imagine that a moment will arise 'when global conditions align favourably' (Shiffman and Smith 2007, p. 1371) for violence prevention policy, owing to the great variance in the frequency and consequences of violence within and between countries. The circumscribed effects of interpersonal violence compound this, as it is generally concentrated within specific communities.

Global Governance Structure

An important consequence of the different approaches adopted by organizations involved in violence prevention is that they inhibit the development of coherent global governance structure that can serve as a platform for collective action, since each group takes its mandate from different and at times contradictory normative documents and governing body directives. To date, the most concerted effort to establish such a structure is the VPA (the Violence Prevention Alliance led by WHO—see Chapter 44, this volume, for more details). However, while the VPA has succeeded in having participants using all three approaches agree on a global plan of action (Violence Prevention Alliance 2012), the VPA's informal status as a voluntary network of organizations means that it lacks the formal authority necessary to bring other UN agencies fully on board.

Issue Characteristics

International agencies adopting an evidence-based approach, most notably WHO, the Institute of Health Metrics and Evaluation (IHME), and the CDC, play a dominant role in establishing the severity of interpersonal violence relative to other problems.

Deaths due to Violence

Inclusion of the categories 'violence' (which refers to interpersonal violence), war, and self-inflicted injuries in the first *Global Burden of Disease Study* (GBD; Murray and Lopez, 1996) allowed deaths due to interpersonal violence to be compared to these other types of violence and other leading causes of death (e.g. tuberculosis, heart disease, cancers). This report estimated that for the year 1990, violence was the sixteenth leading cause of death (just below stomach cancers and diabetes mellitus) and that by the year 2020 it would rise to the fourteenth leading cause of death (just below liver cancer and above war). Given that the GBD study examined a total of 109 major diseases and injuries, these rankings propelled violence close to the centre of the global public health stage, where it has remained since, appearing as the twentieth leading cause of years of life lost in the IHME's 2012 GBD revision (Lozano et al. 2012). These estimates are disaggregated by geographical region, sex and age, and provide the only global and regional source of information about the size the violence problem relative to other conditions.

Non-fatal Violence

In the last 15 years or so an increasing number of high-quality population-based surveys and meta-analyses synthesizing their results have become available, often conducted by international organizations. These include, for instance, such multi-country surveys as the Demographic and Health Surveys carried out by MEASURE DHS; national baseline surveys on violence against children conducted by CDC and UNICEF, and others funded by the UBS Optimus Foundation; and the Global School-based Student Health Survey carried out by WHO. Their findings have clearly established that the prevalence of non-fatal violence—such as child maltreatment, youth violence, intimate partner and sexual violence, and elder maltreatment—is high, and often higher in low- and middle-income countries than in high-income countries. WHO has recently published the first global systematic review of scientific data on the prevalence of two forms of violence against women and found that globally one in three women has been a victim of intimate partner and/or sexual violence (WHO, 2013). Furthermore, CDC and UNICEF surveys on violence against children in Southern and Eastern Africa have, for instance, found prevalence rates of child sexual abuse in girls of 27.9 per cent in Tanzania and 33.3 per cent in Swaziland, and of child physical abuse in boys of 71.7 per cent in Tanzania (Reza et al. 2009; UNICEF et al. 2011).

Violence as a Risk Factor for other Conditions

While individual studies dating back to the 1970s have measured the effects of violence on non-injury physical and mental health outcomes and high-risk behaviours, it was only in the mid-1990s that the CDC's studies on Adverse Childhood Experiences (United States Centers for Disease Control and Prevention 2013b), and the WHO's World Mental Health Survey (WMHS, 2013) and others began promoting international efforts to assess the effects of violent victimization on short and long-term health and behavioural outcomes. In so doing, they added a new dimension to the characteristics of violence, which now came to be understood as both a problem in itself, and a risk factor for some of the leading contributors to the global burden of disease, such as cancer, cardiovascular disease, diabetes and HIV/AIDS.

Evidence for Effective Interventions

There is good evidence about the extensive toll that violence takes in low- and middle-income countries. There is also good evidence showing that interventions to prevent most forms of interpersonal violence are effective in high-income countries. Despite this, the resources to develop the capacity for implementing and evaluating these interventions in low- and middle-income countries remain insufficient. However, the evidence base for violence prevention is growing rapidly, and, the Latin American and sub-Saharan Africa regions are especially prominent sources of new outcome evaluation studies demonstrating the preventability of violence in low- and middle-income countries (see WHO and Liverpool John Moores University, http://www.preventviolence.info/evidence_base.aspx).

In relation to the dimension of issue characteristics, the current success by international agencies in demonstrating the size and consequences of the violence problem relative to other problems has yet to be matched by equivalent success in showing what works to prevent violence in low- and middle-income countries. This has resulted in a David and Goliath situation where proposed solutions seem trivial in the face of a towering problem.

And yet as Alison Morris-Gehring (Chapter 43) has shown, progress in assisting administrations in adopting violence reduction strategies is possible. In part this involves informed facilitation as well as a willingness to work within their particular historical context. Mostly however it involves overcoming what she describes as 'compartmentalised conceptualisation': in other words, bringing all of the main actors and agencies to share a common enough view of the problem that action becomes possible.

Conclusion: The Way Forward

This chapter suggests that four main areas where the global violence prevention field needs strengthening are (i) the development of a coordinating body; (ii) reconciling different normative approaches; (iii) shifting interpersonal violence from being viewed as a local problem with few international effects, to a view of it as a global problem; (iv) and the perceived weakness of the evidence base relative to the magnitude and consequences of the problem. Strengthening the global violence prevention field and successfully achieving widespread reductions in violence thus demands the intensification of efforts to address these weaknesses.

The inadequacy of current efforts to coordinate global violence prevention activities could be resolved through following the example of road traffic injury prevention, which in 2004 was the subject of a UN General Assembly Resolution that mandated a single UN agency (WHO) to take the lead in coordinating a UN-wide response to the problem. Prior to this, responsibility for road traffic injury prevention was dispersed between several different agencies and the issue attracted little high-level policy attention. Subsequently, because leadership was now consolidated within a single agency that had already demonstrated a clear will to address the problem, high-level advocacy became more focused and compelling, technical guidance on how to prevent road traffic injuries more consistent across different agencies, and political and financial support for the field grew substantially. However, the extent to which violence prevention would be similarly boosted by consolidating leadership within a single UN agency is dependent on different agencies agreeing to work from a common normative framework. Failing this, strengthening the role of the VPA, for instance by having national governments clearly endorse its status as the global violence prevention coordinating body, may be the next best alternative.

The need to reconcile human rights and public health as the dominant normative approaches to violence prevention is probably best met by continuing to highlight their complementarity, while emphasizing how rights-based aspirations to a life free from violence can only ultimately be realized through implementation on the ground of evidence-based approaches. To paraphrase comments made in a similar debate around HIV/AIDS (De Cock et al. 2002), the portrayal of violence against a background of either human rights, poverty, gender, or public health elicits different responses, but the measure of each response must be its ability to curtail violence, and at what social cost. Philosophical and technical approaches to violence prevention must interrupt the underlying causes and risk factors, mitigate the acute and long terms effects on individuals and populations, reduce stigma and vulnerability, and promote the rights and welfare of all children and adults. Success in doing so requires thinking in terms of both prevention and mitigation and demands attention to rights, justice and evidence.

The geographically circumscribed nature and consequences of violence means the largest windows of opportunity to develop policies for addressing it are likely to be at the local level. Rather than viewing this as a barrier, global violence prevention efforts should thus highlight the extreme variability in violence rates between places as evidence for its preventability. For example, Lozano et al. (2012, p. 2124) note that

> violence as a cause of death is one of the most heterogeneous across different regions…The huge variation…raises important questions about the origins and socio-political context of violence, the drivers of change in violence-related mortality, and the effectiveness of public health strategies in reducing deaths from violence.

From this perspective, the more the world's violence hotspots become geographically concentrated, the more compelling are arguments for its prevention. Of course, efforts to establish global windows of opportunity for violence prevention should not be neglected, and it is notable that a report by the high-level panel of eminent persons on the post-2015 development agenda (United Nations, 2013) included as proposed goals 'to prevent and

eliminate all forms of violence against girls and women' (United Nations, 2013, p. 30), and 'to reduce violent deaths per 100,000 by x and eliminate all forms of violence against children' (United Nations, 2013, p. 31). Stakeholders within the global violence prevention field thus stand much to gain by ensuring that these suggested goals are ultimately included when in the final set of post-2015 development are adopted by the UN General Assembly.

A remaining challenge in the global violence prevention field is the perception that it is held back because the evidence base for preventing violence is underdeveloped in comparison to the evidence underlying efforts to address other social and health problems where investments in prevention are many times greater. This should be addressed by coordinated efforts on the part of violence prevention experts to make two key observations. First, that the evidence base is in all likelihood not the most important factor in determining whether an issue becomes a global policy priority. Rather, as Shiffman (2009) notes, the rise and persistence of global issues may best be explained by how the policy community comes to understand and portray them and establish institutions that can sustain this portrayal.

> This explanation emphasizes the power of ideas, and challenges interpretations of issue ascendance and decline that place primary weight on material, objective factors such as mortality and morbidity levels and the existence of cost-effective interventions. (Shiffman 2009, p. 608)

The second key observation concerns the violence prevention evidence base, which although it may not be the primary determinant of how far violence prevention ascends the global priority ladder, remains an important factor. Accordingly, it is instructive to note that not only is the existing evidence base for violence prevention just as strong as the evidence base underlying many other public health and social issues which do enjoy greater political priority (alleviating poverty, reducing health inequalities or promoting primary healthcare), but that the violence prevention evidence base is also one of the fastest growing.

Attending to these four areas must be a matter of priority for the international scientific, advocacy and policymaker communities, if any real reductions in interpersonal violence are to be achieved. At the global level, the first two of these—the development of a coordinating body for violence prevention and the need to reconcile different normative approaches—should be priorities. The first depends on key international actors—the main international organizations and their member states, large international NGOs, and the main donors in the field—working together in a concerted fashion to establish such a coordinating body, and as importantly, providing it with sufficient resources and a strong enough mandate to fulfil its role. The second requires all actors in the field to recognize that a scientific, evidence-based approach has a major contribution to make towards the realization of the human right to live life free of violence.

Acknowledgements

Writing this chapter was supported in part by a grant from the University of Cape Town's Research Committee (URC) to the third author.

References

Bowman, B., Matzopoulos, R., Butchart, A., and Mercy, J. A. (2008). The impact of violence on development in low- to middle-income countries. *International Journal of Injury Control and Safety Promotion*, 15(4), 209–19.

Coie, J. D., Watt, N. F., West, S. G., Hawkins, J. D., Asarnow, J. R., Markman, H. J., Ramey, S. L., Shure, M. B., and Long, B. (1993). The science of prevention: A conceptual framework and some directions for a national research programme. *American Psychologist*, 48(10), 1013–1022.

De Cock, K. M., Mbori-Ngacha, D., and Marum, E. (2002). Shadow on the continent: public health and HIV/AIDS in Africa in the 21st century. *Lancet*, 360(9326), 67–72.

Krug, E., Dahlberg, L., Mercy, J., Zwi, A., and Lozano, R. (2002). *World Report on Violence and Health* Geneva: World Health Organization.

Lozano, R., Naghavi, M., Foreman, K., Lim, S., Shibuya, K., Aboyans, V., et al. (2012). Global and regional mortality from 235 causes of death for 20 age groups in 1990 and 2010: a systematic analysis for the Global Burden of Disease Study 2010. *Lancet*, 380(9859), 2095–128.

Murray, C., and Lopez, A. (eds) (1996). *Global Burden of Disease: A comprehensive assessment of mortality and disability from diseases, injuries, and risk factors in 1990 and projected to 2020.* Cambridge, MA: Harvard University Press.

Nation, M., Crusto, C., Wandersman, A., Kumpfer, K. L., Seybolt, D., Morrissey-Kane, E., and Davino, K. (2003). What works in prevention: Principles of effective prevention programs. *American Psychologist*, 58(6/7), 449–56.

Pinheiro, P. S. (2006). *World report on violence against children.* Geneva: United Nations Secretary-General's Study on Violence Against Children.

Reza, A., Breiding, M. J., Gulaid, J., Mercy, J. A., Blanton, C., Mthethwa, Z., et al. (2009). Sexual violence and its health consequences for female children in Swaziland: a cluster survey study. *Lancet*, 373(9679), 1966–72.

Rosenberg, M. L., Fenley, M. A. (1991). *Violence in America: A Public Health Approach.* New York: Oxford University Press

Shiffman, J. (2009). A social explanation for the rise and fall of global health issues. *Bulletin of the World Health Organization*, 87, 608–13.

Shiffman, J., and Smith, S. (2007). Generation of political priority for global health initiatives: a framework and case study of maternal mortality. *Lancet*, 370(9595):1370–79.

United Nations Children's Fund, U.S. Centers for Disease Control and Prevention, and Muhimbili University of Health and Allied Sciences (2011). Violence against children in Tanzania: Findings from a National Survey 2009. Dar es Salaam, Tanzania: United Republic of Tanzania.

United Nations. (2013). A new global partnership: eradicate poverty and transform economies through sustainable development. New York: United Nations Publications. http://www.un.org/sg/man agement/pdf/HLP_P2015_Report.pdf (accessed 6 January 2014).

United States Centers for Disease Control and Prevention. (2013a). Violence Prevention —from http://www.cdc.gov/violenceprevention/

United States Centers for Disease Control and Prevention. (2013b). Adverse Childhood Experiences Study. Centers for Disease Control and Prevention—from http://www.cdc.gov/ace/

Violence Prevention Alliance (2012). Violence Prevention Alliance Global Campaign for Violence Prevention: Plan of Action for 2012-2020. Geneva, Switzerland: Violence Prevention Alliance.

WMHS. (2013). World Mental Health Survey, Harvard University—from http://www.hcp.med.harvard.edu/wmh/

World Health Assembly. Prevention of violence: a public health priority. (Forty-ninth World Health Assembly, Resolution WHA49.25). Geneva, World Health Organization, 1996.

WHO. Global and regional estimates of violence against women: Prevalence and health effects of intimate partner violence and nonpartner sexual violence. Geneva: Switzerland, 2013.

CHAPTER 46

Violence prevention: challenges and priorities for researchers

Catherine L. Ward and Peter D. Donnelly

Introduction to Challenges and Priorities for Violence Prevention Researchers

This volume serves as a compendium of the current state of the science of violence prevention, and therefore also provides an opportunity to reflect on the state of that science. This chapter attempts that reflection: on the data we have, the methods we use, what we know and do not know about what works to prevent violence, and concludes with ideas about how scientists can contribute to knowledge translation for better implementation of what does work.

The traditional cycle of prevention science is a five-step one (Mrazek and Haggerty 1994):

i. First, information on incidence and prevalence of the particular type of violence must be collected, collated and analysed in order to identify the extent of the problem.

ii. Second, risk and protective factors that affect incidence and prevalence must be identified, as effective prevention programmes will need to target these.

iii. Then programmes must be designed, based on a clear theory of change that suggests how the programme actions will target the risk and protective factors and achieve the outcomes. These programmes must then be piloted, and, if the pilot test is successful, then tested using the most rigorous methods possible.

iv. Once efficacy has been established (i.e. it has been demonstrated that the programme works under ideal conditions), effectiveness trials must be run to determine whether the programme still achieves effects under real-world conditions.

v. Finally, if effective, the programme should be taken to scale.

The many chapters in this book make it clear that there is a great deal that the field has achieved. We have, for instance, a fair amount of prevalence data on homicide (see Chapter 2, this volume) and increasingly on child maltreatment and intimate partner violence (see Chapters 3 and 6). There is enough evidence of programme effect that several bodies now exist to rank prevention programmes according to their demonstrated efficacy and effectiveness for examples, (see Table 46.1).

These bodies help identify effective programmes, many of which programmes are reviewed in Section 4 of this book. Several of these programmes have even been taken to scale, in the sense that they have been rolled out widely. For instance, the Incredible Years parent training programme (see Barlow, Chapter 18, this volume) has been made widely available through Sure Start services in Wales (Hutchings and Bywater 2010).

But gaps remain—in data, in theory, in programme development, in programme evaluation, and in taking programmes to scale. And although there are gaps throughout these areas of violence prevention in every context, the chapters in this volume make it very clear that those gaps are overwhelmingly located in low- and middle-income countries (LMIC).

What Data are Still Needed?

A consistent theme throughout the epidemiology chapters (Chapters 2–11) is the need for both more data and better quality data. Even with homicide data, probably the most easily accessible of all violence-related data, there are gaps—particularly in low- and middle income countries (LMIC); as Matzopoulos and colleagues (Chapter 2, this volume) point out, the least data, and the least reliable data, comes from areas where the problem is probably most prevalent. Data on non-fatal violence from administrative sources (such as police and hospital data) are also scarce, but would be relatively easy to collect if appropriate data collection systems were put in place (Mitis and Sethi, Chapter 8, this volume). In some areas such as elder maltreatment, there is very little data at all (Penhale and Iborra, Chapter 9, this volume).

Where there are gaps in the data, some of the problems can be addressed simply by further studies, but attention also needs to be paid to how the phenomenon is measured. Merrick and colleagues (Chapter 3, this volume), and Penhale and Iborra (Chapter 9), both call for better measurement tools to identify child and elder maltreatment, respectively, as well as for standardization of measures so that results can more easily be compared across studies (another gap common to all forms of violence addressed in this volume). In some areas (such as youth violence) measurement could be improved by ensuring that violent behaviour is reported separately from other more general data (such as delinquency; Ward, Chapter 4, this volume). Variations in the way violence

Table 46.1 Bodies reviewing and ranking prevention programmes

Country	Name	Website
USA	Blueprints for Healthy Youth Development	http://www.blueprintsprograms.com/
	National Registry of Evidence-Based Programs and Practices (maintained by the U.S. Substance Abuse and Mental Health Services Administration)	http://nrepp.samhsa.gov/
	Model Programs Guide of the Office of Juvenile Justice and Delinquency Prevention	http://www.ojjdp.gov/mpg/
U.K.	National Institute for Health and Clinical Excellence	http://www.nice.org.uk/

is defined and measured also seriously undermine the ability to determine costs of violence (Corso and Taylor, Chapter 15); which is an essential part of building an argument for policymakers to invest in prevention initiatives.

Attention to methods for collecting prevalence data is also required. Careful, thorough, population-based studies are necessary; but as Merrick and colleagues (Chapter 3) point out with regard to child maltreatment, these have pitfalls: official sources tend to under-report the problem, and problems with self-report surveys range from selecting a biased sample (for instance, school-based surveys will exclude all those not in school) to the fact that respondents' memories for events may not be accurate. Similar problems pertain to other forms of violence, for instance, elder maltreatment (Penhale and Iborra, Chapter 9, this volume).

Where are the Gaps in Understanding Risk and Protective Factors for Violence?

Gaps in our understanding of risk and protective factors and how they influence violent behaviour echo gaps in the prevalence data. In elder abuse, for instance, very little is known about risk and protective factors at all (Penhale and Iborra, Chapter 9, this volume). Where we do know a great deal, it is usually about risk factors (for instance, for youth violence—Ward, Chapter 4, and Tremblay, Chapter 5) rather than protective factors, which are woefully under-researched. In addition, most of what we know about risk and protective factors is at the individual rather than the community and societal levels—and it is clear, from the evidence that we do have, that there are structural drivers of violence such as long-term deprivation (Ceccato, Chapter 11, this volume; Gebo et al., Chapter 29; Hagedorn, Chapter 30). Nor do we understand how these structural drivers influence risk and protection at the individual level. And at a very fundamental level, given that the same risk and protective factors seem to influence male and female aggression, it is a glaring gap in the evidence base that we still do not fully understand why men and boys are so much more

likely to be physically aggressive than women and girls (Ward, Chapter 4; Mitis and Sethi, Chapter 8; this volume).

The lack of data on risk and protective factors (particularly from LMIC) has a number of consequences for theory-building. For instance, different risk and protective factors may be more influential in different contexts (Matzopoulos et al., Chapter 2, this volume), and this should play a significant role in what preventive interventions are implemented. Second, more nuanced, detailed understandings of pathways to violence would be possible with more cross-cultural research—for instance, developmental pathways to aggression may differ across different cultural contexts where norms (such as women's and men's social roles) may differ from Western contexts where the most research has taken place (Stöckl et al. Chapter 6, this volume). This kind of theory development requires more longitudinal studies, particularly in LMIC. And thirdly, there are standard criminological theories, such as social disorganization theory (Shaw and McKay 1942), which may or may not apply in high-violence contexts where organized crime plays a significant role (Ceccato, Chapter 11, this volume)—but until we have a better understanding of risk and protective factors that are influential in those contexts, we cannot build better theory.

All of these data deficits make understanding the consequences of violence, and hence the associated costs, very difficult indeed (Corso and Taylor, Chapter 15, this volume). Both of these are crucial for any advocacy agenda—for convincing policymakers that prevention does pay (Aos et al. 2011)—again underlining the importance of getting the epidemiological work done, and done well.

Where are the Gaps in Interventions?

When it comes to interventions, as with prevalence data, we need more evidence, and better quality evidence. The first need is, quite simply, for more randomized controlled trials (RCTs) of the very many different intervention programmes reviewed in Chapters 18–34. In addition, all evaluation studies should have long-term follow-ups, as it is sustainable change that is needed and should be assessed (Barlow, Chapter 18, this volume); in fact, the Blueprints for Healthy Youth Development group now require a one-year follow-up as a basic standard of quality evidence (http://www.blueprintsprograms.com/resources/Blueprints_Checklist.pdf). In many areas, there are not enough high-quality evaluations that meet criteria for inclusion in systematic reviews and meta-analyses, and until we have this quantity of evidence, the evidence base will remain limited.

It is not only quantity that is needed, but the authors in this volume also consistently call for better quality trials, and deeper analysis of the data generated by trials. Within RCTs, we need great complexity of analysis. For instance, RCTs should attempt a sufficiently large sample size so that they are adequately powered to test effects on sub-groups, to assess whether the programme is equally effective for all groups, or perhaps has iatrogenic effects for some (Fagan and Catalano, Chapter 20, this volume; Haegerich and Massetti 2012). Large sample sizes will also allow for the testing of mediating variables, which will allow tests of programme theory—to ask the question whether reductions in violent outcomes are really achieved via the new skills that the programme seeks to develop in participants (Fagan and Catalano, Chapter 20; Rothman, 2012); for instance, in a parent training programme, are reductions in child maltreatment achieved via improved positive parenting and reduced use of harsh punishment, or is there some other mechanism at play? Many authors mentioned the lack of good programme theory as a weakness in violence prevention interventions—for instance, Feder and Sardinha (Chapter 26), Flood (Chapter 27), and Neville (Chapter 33). A focus on assessing programme theory as well as outcomes during evaluations can help both to develop an understanding of theories of change across programmes, thus boosting the field as a whole; and help programme staff to understand and improve their programme from the basis of a strong theory of change (Birckmayer and Weiss 2000).

Another necessary element of quality in evaluation studies is to ensure that the outcomes measured are the actual outcomes desired, rather than proxies or mediating variables. This is a particular problem, for instance, in norms interventions, where attitudes rather than behaviour are more likely to be assessed (Neville, Chapter 33). Every effort should of course be made to measure the actual desired outcome, but it must also be recognized that many of the outcomes that interventions aim to prevent (such as child maltreatment) may have a low base rate in the population, which makes demonstrating a reduction very complex. Further, measuring these mediators is typically far easier and therefore cheaper to assess, which is likely to make such assessments more affordable in LMIC, where we lack evidence for almost any prevention programme. Nonetheless, where possible, actual outcomes should be measured.

Many interventions that appear to make common sense (De Donder, Chapter 28), such as public information and awareness-raising campaigns, and helplines (common interventions not only in elder abuse but also in intimate partner violence and child maltreatment) are not amenable to RCTs. However, thoughtful, rigorous evaluations are much needed. Currently most of these initiatives go completely unevaluated, and there is thus no evidence of whether they achieve their goals or not. Similarly, another glaring gap is the development and testing of interventions to shift norms. Norms of violence and of masculinity have been implicated as fundamental in many forms of violence (Flood, Chapter 27, this volume), but few interventions in this area have been thoughtfully developed or evaluated (Flood, Chapter 27; Neville, Chapter 33).

Other Areas Needing Investigation

There are two other areas that urgently need the attention of scientists: the need to measure the impact of structural changes or differences in structure across contexts, and the evaluation of complex initiatives.

Both Gebo and colleagues (Chapter 29) and Hagedorn (Chapter 30) point out that gang violence and violence carried out by young marginalized men will persist unless fundamental structural changes are made—such as reductions in racism, inequality and social marginalization. There is mounting evidence, although again from high-income countries, that violence is related to inequality in society (Wilkinson and Pickett 2009). Intuitively that seems likely to hold true in LMIC, but that needs more thorough investigation—and where it does hold true, appropriate interventions need to be identified. The approaches reported by Shaw (Chapter 36), which include attention to education and employment opportunities, provide some sense that these changes can be

made, and can successfully be evaluated. But more interventions and quality evaluations are necessary in this critical area.

Many violence prevention interventions, including structural interventions, are complex, and necessarily so—see, for instance, the multi-level programmes reviewed by Fagan and Catalano (Chapter 20), and the community interventions described by Seedat and colleagues (Chapter 34). Evaluation of complex initiatives is itself complicated, and this is a developing area of evaluation science (Williams et al., Chapter 17). More attention to methods for effective evaluation of such initiatives is urgently required.

Of course, increasing the number of RCTs (and the sample size and quality of RCTs), or any other kind of evaluation, will take funds. Here the donor community has a role to play in prioritizing the funding of evaluation alongside the funding of interventions. Without this, good science cannot go forward.

It is not only the lack of evaluations that is problematic in the field, but also that many interventions are implemented without being based in good programme theory. Programmes are unlikely to achieve an effect without a sound theory of change that is informed by the evidence—and may even do harm, as witness the now infamous 'Scared Straight' programmes which actually increased rather than decreased delinquency (Petrosino et al. 2003). Often, of course, interventions are not implemented as research projects, but rather in response to need—and the chapters dealing with epidemiology in Section 2 of this volume clearly demonstrate that there is a need, and that it is substantial. One intriguing approach to developing programme theory after the fact is described by Purtle and colleagues (Chapter 32, this volume), who describe how hospital-based intervention programmes in the United States have come together to form a national network, which is beginning to develop a common standardized manual, fidelity measures, and the like. This initiative will assist in surfacing programme theory and so aiding both effective implementation and evaluation of such programmes across sites. It provides an interesting model for strengthening the field that might well be emulated by other groups of interventions.

It is perfectly understandable that interventions develop in advance of evidence: developing an intervention and garnering sufficient evidence for it to be considered a model programme can take 20 years; and even where there are model, effective, evidence-based programmes, none has achieved population coverage (Rotheram-Borus et al. 2012). In the face of huge need, service providers are likely to move to meet that need even if evidence is lacking. Yet rolling out untested interventions is not the answer: it is not only that programmes might do harm, but that inadequate evaluations might over- or underestimate effect, and the limited resources available in any community for violence prevention should be used in such a way that the maximum reduction in violence is achieved (Fagan and Catalano, Chapter 20). Rotheram-Borus and colleagues (2012) call for an entirely different approach: disruptive innovations, or the simplification of services so that they will meet the needs of the majority, who may be over-served by traditional programmes. They give the example of mass distribution of cheap over-the-counter spectacles: while a minority will need specialist eye care, the over-the-counter reading glasses are much cheaper, easy to distribute widely, and will meet the needs of most people who need reading glasses.

They call for the following as a research agenda (Rotheram-Borus et al. 2012), offered here as an agenda for taking the field of violence prevention further forward so that population reach can be attained:

i. Identify the common elements across evidence-based interventions, so that we can identify what the 'active ingredients' are in interventions and ensure that those are replicated. In violence prevention, one example is a meta-analysis of studies of parent training programmes that sought to reduce child behaviour problems, and which identified the following as the most effective elements: positive parent-child interactions, emotional communication skills, teaching the use of time out, emphasizing consistency in parenting, and ensuring that parents practiced new skills with their children during training sessions (Kaminski et al. 2008). Identifying these effective elements makes it relatively simple to design an intervention that is likely to be effective across a number of contexts, and helps to build good theory about what works and why.

ii. Experiment with novel delivery formats, such as self-help interventions, brief interventions, using paraprofessionals to deliver services, and using technology and media services. Among the brief interventions that they mention, one with relevance to violence prevention is the Family Check-up, an intervention which focuses on strengths rather than problems to target child behaviour problems, and provides an effective, low-cost alternative to a psychiatric referral (Dishion et al. 2008). Similarly, integrating the use of mobile phone technology into a parent training programme has been shown to improve engagement of low-income parents in parent training to address children's disruptive behaviour disorders, and to improve child outcomes over standard parent training alone (Jones et al. 2013).

Transporting Interventions across Contexts

Both understanding the common elements of effective programmes and novel delivery channels are also likely to assist with transportation of interventions. Violence prevention interventions have often, as the contents of this book attest, been developed and tested in high-income countries, while high rates of violence and the more urgent need for intervention are more likely to be found in LMIC. There is evidence that programmes can effectively be transported from one context to another—for instance, in a systematic review exploring parent training programmes in LMIC to reduce child maltreatment, eight of the 12 studies identified were of programmes transported from one context to another (Knerr et al. 2013). But few of the programmes described in this book have been transported to novel contexts, and few programmes indigenous to LMIC have been evaluated, thus leaving us with a very weak evidence base outside of high-income contexts.

Transporting programmes and taking them to scale both require effective strategies for training and supporting programme staff in the new context, and for adapting programmes to fit the new context and possibly new culture (Bradach 2003; Elliott and Mihalic 2004). More attention to the best way to achieve these will advance prevention science immeasurably. One particular area that must

be explored is the use of paraprofessionals to deliver programmes. Although there is evidence from the United States that paraprofessionals were not as effective as professionals in delivering a home-visiting programme (Olds et al. 2002), in LMIC there simply are too few professionals to implement programmes at scale (Hanson et al. 2010), and ways of capacitating paraprofessionals to deliver programmes effectively must be found.

The Role of Knowledge Translation in Violence Prevention

Ensuring effective programme roll-out (particularly at scale) and transportation require effective knowledge translation (Spoth et al. 2013)—a practice that aims 'to ensure that research findings are implemented appropriately and for the net benefit of patients and the public' (Shea 2011, p.3). Two types of knowledge translation have been identified (Spoth et al. 2013): Type 1, which translates basic research findings into effective programme design; and Type 2, which translates programmes already proven effective into policy and practice, at scale, sustainably, across different populations and settings.

There have been some assessments of what makes for effective Type 1 knowledge translation. For instance, in a systematic review of papers describing knowledge translation projects for enhancing care of abused women and children, Larrivée and colleagues (2012) describe barriers to the uptake of evidence-based practices as related to characteristics of the knowledge (for instance, lack of cultural relevance of evidence-based practices); poor adaptation and dissemination efforts (for instance, practitioners' inability to access training in evidence-based practices); characteristics of practitioners (for instance, resistance to evidence-based practices); organizational characteristics (such as a lack of funding for implementing evidence-based practices); and limitations in interactions between scientists and practitioners (for instance, a lack of a shared language). They also describe facilitators, such as pitching messages in appropriate ways, producing guides to best practice, agencies with strong leadership, and a commitment of both scientists and practitioners to achieving common goals (Larrivée et al. 2012). Whatever the barriers and facilitators, Type 1 knowledge translation involves considerable time and contact between researchers and those implementing the intervention (Wathen et al. 2011) or developing new health policies (Waqa et al. 2013). It should be incorporated explicitly and early into research activities, with attention being paid to collaborative working with a variety of stakeholders, the nature and sources of evidence being used, and the role of the research team in working with the local community (Kitson et al. 2013). In LMIC in particular, attention might have to be paid to power dynamics between researchers and other stakeholders (Huzair et al. 2013), and to capacity-building so that evidence can be understood and used effectively (Kasonde and Campbell 2012).

Type 2 knowledge translation has as yet been the focus of far less research attention, yet it is critical if population impact is to be achieved. Spoth and colleagues (2013) offer a conceptual framework—the Translation Science to Population Impact (TSci Impact) Framework—which both describes how the process might work, and provides a framework for researching effective ways to achieve population impact through knowledge translation. As they view it, the process has four stages: (i) stakeholders (such as policymakers and practitioners) gaining knowledge about the intervention and being persuaded that it has advantages over the status quo; (ii) stakeholders deciding to adopt the intervention; (iii) implementation of the intervention; and (iv) institutionalizing the intervention so that it is sustained. They also outline key research questions at each stage. For instance, how best should knowledge be synthesized and presented to policymakers? What influences practitioners to adopt an intervention? How are evidence-based interventions integrated into existing service systems (for instance, what factors influence whether the intervention is delivered with fidelity)? What influences the long-term availability of a programme within a particular service system?

Both the practice of knowledge translation and researching it are critical to achieving the ultimate goal of preventing violence. As described by Gehring in Chapter 43, the evidence base alone is not sufficient to persuade policymakers to adopt particular policies; and as a field we have been woefully poor at achieving population reach.

Conclusion

While this volume makes it clear that the field of violence prevention has made significant gains, it equally makes it clear that much work remains to be done—more prevalence data, and of better quality, is needed; more needs to be done to understand how risk and protective factors operate with regards to particular forms of violence, in particular groups, and across various contexts; more and better-quality evaluations are needed; and far more attention needs to be paid to knowledge translation, to achieving population reach, and to innovations that can speed up the traditional cycle of prevention research. Violence prevention remains a global health priority, and we look forward to learning what can be built on the existing platform of knowledge.

Acknowledgement

Writing this chapter was supported in part by a grant from the University of Cape Town's Research Committee (URC) to the first author.

References

Aos, S., Lee, S., Drake, E. et al. (2011). *Return on Investment: Evidence-Based Options to Improve Statewide Outcomes*. Olympia: Washington State Institute for Public Policy.

Birckmayer, J. D., and Weiss, C. H. (2000). Theory-based evaluation in practice: What do we learn? *Evaluation Review*, 24, 407–31.

Bradach, J. (2003). Going to scale: The challenge of replicating social programs. *Stanford Social Innovation Review*, Spring, 19–25.

Dishion, T. J., Shaw, D., Connell., Gardner, F., Weaver, C., and Wilson, Melvin. (2008). The family check-up with high-risk indigent families: preventing problem behavior by increasing parents' positive behavior support in early childhood. *Child Development*, 79, 1395–414.

Elliott, D. S., and Mihalic, S. (2004). Issues in disseminating and replicating effective prevention programs. *Prevention Science*, 5, 47–53.

Haegerich, T. M., and Massetti, G. M. (2012). Commentary on subgroup analysis in intervention research: Opportunities for the public health approach to violence prevention. *Prevention Science*, 14, 193–8.

Hanson, K., Cleary, S., Schneider, H., Tantivess, S., and Gilson, L. (2010). Scaling up health policies and services in low- and middle-income settings. *BMC Health Services Research*, 10(Suppl 1), I1–4.

Hutchings, J., and Bywater, T. (2010). *Evidence for the Incredible Years (IY) Programmes in Wales*. http://incredibleyears.com/download/administrators/implementations/wales-IY-evidence-overivew.pdf [Accessed 21 December 2013]

Huzair, F., Borda-Rodriguez, A., Upton, M., and Mugwagwa, J. T. (2013). An interdisciplinary and development lens on knowledge translation. *Science and Public Policy*, 40, 43–50.

Jones, D. J., Forehand, R., Cuellar, J. et al. (2013). Technology-enhanced program for chid disruptive behavior disorders: Development and pilot randomized control trial. *Journal of Clinical Child and Adolescent Psychology*, 43, 88–101.

Kaminski, J. W., Valle, L., Filene, J., and Boyle, C. (2008). A meta-analytic review of components associated with parent training program effectiveness. *Journal of Abnormal Child Psychology*, 36, 567–89.

Kasonde, J. M., and Campbell, S. (2012). Creating a Knowledge Translation Platform: nine lessons from the Zambia Forum for Health Research. *Health Research Policy and Systems*, 10, 31–8.

Kitson, A., Powell, K., Hoon, E., Newbury, J., Wilson, A. and Beilby, J. (2013). Knowledge translation within a population health study: how do you do it? *Implementation Science*, 8, 54–62.

Knerr, W., Gardner, F., and Cluver, L. (2013). Reducing harsh and abusive parenting and increasing positive parenting in low- and middle-income countries: a systematic review. *Prevention Science*, 14, 352–63.

Larrivée, M., Hamelin-Brabant, L., and Lessard, G. (2012). Knowledge translation in the field of violence against women and children: An assessment of the state of knowledge. *Children and Youth Services Review*, 34, 2381–91.

Mrazek, P. J., and Haggerty, R. J. (1994). *Reducing Risks for Mental Disorders: Frontiers for Preventive Intervention Research*. Washington, D.C.: Institute of Medicine.

Olds, D. L., Robinson, J., O'Brien, R. et al. (2002). Home visiting by paraprofessionals and by nurses: A randomized, controlled trial. *Pediatrics*, 110, 486–96.

Petrosino, A., Turpin-Petrosino, C., and Buehler, J. (2003). Scared Straight and other juvenile awareness programs for preventing juvenile delinquency: A systematic review of the randomized experimental evidence. *Annals of the American Academy of Political and Social Science*, 589, 41–62.

Rotheram-Borus, M., Swendeman, D., and Chorpita, B. F. (2012). Disruptive innovations for designing and diffusing evidence-based interventions. *American psychologist*, 67, 463–76.

Rothman, A. J. (2012). Exploring connections between moderators and mediators: Commentary on subgroup analyses in intervention research. *Prevention Science*, 14, 189–92.

Shaw, C., and McKay, H. (1942). *Juvenile Delinquency and Urban Areas*. Chicago: University of Chicago Press.

Shea, B. J. (2011). A decade of knowledge translation research—what has changed? *Journal of Clinical Epidemiology*, 64, 3–5.

Spoth, R., Rohrbach, L. A., Greenberg, M. et al. (2013). Addressing core challenges for the next generation of Type 2 translation research and systems: The Translation Science to Population Impact (TSci Impact) Framework. *Prevention Science*, 14, 319–51.

Waqa, G., Mavoa, H., Snowdon, W. et al. (2013). Knowledge brokering between researchers and policymakers in Fiji to develop policies to reduce obesity: A process evaluation. *Implementation Science*, 8, 74–84.

Wathen, C. N., Sibbald, S. L., Jack, S. M. and MacMillan, H. L. (2011). Talk, trust and time: A longitudinal study evaluating knowledge translationand exchange processes for research on violence against women. *Implementation Science*, 6, 102–16.

Wilkinson, R., and Pickett, K. (2009). *The Spirit Level: Why Greater Equality Makes Societies Stronger*. New York, NY: Bloomsbury Press.

Index